The Handbook of Global Health Communication

Handbooks in Communication and Media

This series aims to provide theoretically ambitious but accessible volumes devoted to the major fields and subfields within communication and media studies. Each volume sets out to ground and orientate the student through a broad range of specially commissioned chapters, while also providing the more experienced scholar and teacher with a convenient and comprehensive overview of the latest trends and critical directions.

The Handbook of Children, Media, and Development, *edited by Sandra L. Calvert and Barbara J. Wilson*

The Handbook of Crisis Communication, *edited by W. Timothy Coombs and Sherry J. Holladay*

The Handbook of Internet Studies, *edited by Mia Consalvo and Charles Ess*

The Handbook of Rhetoric and Public Address, *edited by Shawn J. Parry-Giles and J. Michael Hogan*

The Handbook of Critical Intercultural Communication, *edited by Thomas K. Nakayama and Rona Tamiko Halualani*

The Handbook of Global Communication and Media Ethics, *edited by Robert S. Fortner and P. Mark Fackler*

The Handbook of Communication and Corporate Social Responsibility, *edited by Øyvind Ihlen, Jennifer Bartlett and Steve May*

The Handbook of Gender, Sex, and Media, *edited by Karen Ross*

The Handbook of Global Health Communication, *edited by Rafael Obregon and Silvio Waisbord*

Forthcoming

The Handbook of Global Media Research, *edited by Ingrid Volkmer*

The Handbook of International Advertising Research, *edited by Hong Cheng*

The Handbook of Global Online Journalism, *edited by Eugenia Siapera and Andreas Veglis*

The Handbook of Global Health Communication

Edited by

Rafael Obregon
and
Silvio Waisbord

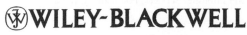

A John Wiley & Sons, Ltd., Publication

This edition first published 2012
© 2012 John Wiley & Sons, Inc

Wiley-Blackwell is an imprint of John Wiley & Sons, formed by the merger of Wiley's global Scientific, Technical and Medical business with Blackwell Publishing.

Registered Office
John Wiley & Sons, Ltd, The Atrium, Southern Gate, Chichester, West Sussex, PO19 8SQ, UK

Editorial Offices
350 Main Street, Malden, MA 02148-5020, USA
9600 Garsington Road, Oxford, OX4 2DQ, UK
The Atrium, Southern Gate, Chichester, West Sussex, PO19 8SQ, UK

For details of our global editorial offices, for customer services, and for information about how to apply for permission to reuse the copyright material in this book please see our website at www.wiley.com/wiley-blackwell.

The right of Rafael Obregon and Silvio Waisbord to be identified as the authors of the editorial material in this work has been asserted in accordance with the UK Copyright, Designs and Patents Act 1988.

Library of Congress Cataloging-in-Publication Data

The handbook of global health communication / edited by Rafael Obregon and Silvio Waisbord.
    p.   ;   cm. – (Handbooks in communication and media)
  Includes bibliographical references and index.
    ISBN 978-1-4443-3862-1 (hardback : alk. paper) – ISBN 978-1-118-24182-0 (ePDFs) –
ISBN 978-1-118-24186-8 (Wiley Online Library) – ISBN 978-1-118-24190-5 (ePub) –
ISBN 978-1-118-24187-5 (Mobi)
I. Obregon, Rafael.   II. Waisbord, Silvio R. (Silvio Ricardo), 1961–   III. Series: Handbooks in communication and media.
  [DNLM: 1. Health Communication.   2. World Health.   WA 590]
    362.1–dc23
                                    2011042670

A catalogue record for this book is available from the British Library.

Set in 10/12.5pt Galliard by SPi Publisher Services, Pondicherry, India

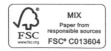

To Laura, Camilo, Andres and Yenis

To Nora and Luis

R. O.

To Sophia, Simone and Julie

S. W.

Contents

Notes on Contributors   x

Acknowledgments   xxi

Introduction   1

Part I   Perspectives on Communication and Global Health   **7**

1 Theoretical Divides and Convergence in Global
   Health Communication   9
   Silvio Waisbord and Rafael Obregon

2 New Perspectives on Global Health Communication: Affirming Spaces
   for Rights, Equity, and Voices   34
   Collins O. Airhihenbuwa and Mohan J. Dutta

3 Rethinking Health Communication in Aid and Development   52
   Elizabeth Fox

4 Toward a Global Theory of Health Behavior and Social Change   70
   Douglas Storey and Maria Elena Figueroa

**Part II   Theoretical Perspectives on and Approaches to Health
          Communication in a Global Context**   **95**

5 The Impact of Health Communication Programs   97
   Jane T. Bertrand, Stella Babalola, and Joanna Skinner

6 Promoting Health through Entertainment-Education Media:
   Theory and Practice   121
   William J. Brown

7 Interpersonal Health Communication: An Ecological Perspective   144
   Rukhsana Ahmed

8 Community Health and Social Mobilization   177
   Catherine Campbell and Kerry Scott

9 Health, News, and Media Information 194
Jesus Arroyave

10 Using Complexity-Informed Communication Strategies to Address
Complex Health Issues: The Case of Puntos de Encuentro, Nicaragua 215
Virginia Lacayo

11 Community Media, Health Communication, and Engagement:
A Theoretical Matrix 233
Linje Manyozo

12 Global E-health Communication 251
L. Suzanne Suggs and Scott C. Ratzan

13 Managing Fear to Promote Healthy Change 274
Merissa Ferrara, Anthony J. Roberto, and Kim Witte

14 Innovations in the Evaluation of Social Change Communication
for HIV and AIDS 288
Ailish Byrne and Robin Vincent

Part III   Case Studies of Applied Theory and Innovation 309

15 Mobile Phones: Opening New Channels for Health Communication
Katherine de Tolly and Peter Benjamin 311

16 Social Marketing and Condom Promotion in Madagascar: A Case Study
in Brand Equity Research 330
*W. Douglas Evans, Kim Longfield, Navendu Shekhar,
Andry Rabemanatsoa, Ietje Reerink, and Jeremy Snider*

17 Participatory Health Communication Research: Four Tools
to Complement the Interview 348
Karen Greiner

18 Egypt's *Mabrouk!* Initiative: A Communication Strategy
for Maternal/Child Health and Family Planning Integration 374
Ron Hess, Dominique Meekers, and J. Douglas Storey

19 Risk Communication and Emerging Infectious Diseases: Lessons
and Implications for Theory–Praxis from Avian Influenza Control 408
Ketan Chitnis

20 Journalism and HIV: Lessons from the Frontline of Behavior
Change Communication in Mozambique 426
Gregory Alonso Pirio

21 jovenHABLAjoven: Lessons Learned about Interpellation,
Peer Communication, and Second-Generation Edutainment
in Sexuality and Gender Projects among Young People 444
Jair Vega Casanova and Carmen R. Mendivil Calderón

22 Changing Gender Norms for HIV and Violence Risk Reduction:
A Comparison of Male-Focused Programs in Brazil and India 469
Julie Pulerwitz, Gary Barker, and Ravi Verma

23   Women's Health and Healing in the Peruvian Amazon: Minga
     Perú's Participatory Communication Approach   488
     Ami Sengupta and Eliana Elias

24   Positive Deviance, Good for Global Health   507
     Arvind Singhal and Lucía Durá

25   Health Promotion from the Grassroots: Piloting a Radio Soap
     Opera for Latinos in the United States   522
     María Beatriz Torres

26   "Children can't wait": Social Mobilization to Secure Children's
     Rights to Social Security   539
     Shereen Usdin and Nicola Christofides

Part IV   Crosscutting Issues   557

27   Capacity Building (and Strengthening) in Health Communication:
     The Missing Link   559
     Rafael Obregon and Silvio Waisbord

28   Institutionalizing Communication in International Health:
     The USAID–Johns Hopkins University Partnership   582
     Jose Rimon II and Suruchi Sood

29   Communication and Public Health in a Glocalized Context:
     Achievements and Challenges   608
     Thomas Tufte

Part V   Conclusions: Rethinking the Field   623

30   Toward Social Justice in Directed Social Change: Rethinking
     the Role of Development Support Communication   625
     Srinivas R. Melkote

31   Conclusions: Why Communication Matters in Global Health   642
     Silvio Waisbord and Rafael Obregon

Index   652

Notes on Contributors

Rukhsana Ahmed, PhD, is Assistant Professor in the Department of Communication, University of Ottawa. Her primary area of research is health communication with an emphasis on interpersonal communication across cultures and within organizations. She is also interested in issues of development, gender, religious diversity, and ethnic media. Her research has been published in *Communication Studies, Intercultural Communication Studies, Women's Health and Urban Life: An International and Interdisciplinary Journal, Journal of Cancer Education, Medical Informatics and the Internet in Medicine,* and in several book chapters. She is currently coediting a book on health communication in media contexts.

Collins O. Airhihenbuwa, PhD, MPH, is Professor and Head of the Department of Biobehavioral Health, the Pennsylvania State University. He is the author of the PEN-3 model used to centralize culture in public health, health promotion, and health communication projects. He has published over 90 articles and book chapters. His books include *Health and Culture: Beyond the Western Paradigm* (1995); the *UNAIDS Communications Framework for HIV/AIDS: A New Direction* (1999); and *Healing Our Differences: The Crisis of Global Health and the Politics of Identity* (2007). He is a fellow of the American Academy of Health Behavior and the Academy of Behavioral Medicine Research.

Jesus Arroyave, PhD, is Director of the School of Communication and Associate Professor at Universidad del Norte in Barranquilla, Colombia. His professional interests focus on health communication and development, and journalism and media studies. He is the author and coauthor of three books and several journal articles and book chapters.

Stella Babalola, PhD, is Associate Professor and teaches Health Communication in the Department of Health, Behavior, and Society at Johns Hopkins University. She is also Senior Research Advisor at the Center for Communications Programs of the same university. Dr. Babalola has a wealth of experience in international health, teaching, communication, and research. She has published extensively. During the last five years,

Dr. Babalola's research has been largely in the areas of HIV risk reduction, childhood immunization, and adolescent reproductive health.

Gary Barker, PhD, is International Director of Instituto Promundo, a Brazilian NGO, with offices in Rio de Janeiro and Washington, DC, that works locally, nationally, and internationally to promote gender equity and to reduce violence against children, women, and youth. He has carried out research on masculinities, violence, gender, health, and conflict in Latin America, sub-Saharan Africa, and Asia and coauthored numerous training materials, including the Program H series.

Peter Benjamin, PhD, MSc, BSC, is the managing director of Cell-Life. His professional interests are in information and communications technology for social change, now focusing on mHealth. He is the author of over 20 chapters and published papers, and has presented at over 50 conferences.

Jane T. Bertrand, PhD, MBA, is the chair of the Department of Global Health Systems and Development at the Tulane School of Public Health and Tropical Medicine. She also holds the Neal A. and Mary Vanselow endowed chair. Her professional interests focus largely on program evaluation and behavior change communication in the areas of HIV prevention and international family planning.

William J. Brown, PhD, is Professor and Research Fellow in the School of Communication and the Arts at Regent University. His academic research interests include health communication, media, and social influence, and the use of entertainment-education for social change. He has published extensively in academic journals and books, including articles in *Health Communication*, the *Journal of Health Communication*, *Communication Research*, the *Journal of Communication*, *Mass Communication & Society*, *International Communication Gazette*, and *The Asian Journal of Communication*.

Ailish Byrne, PhD, is Senior Research Associate with the Communication for Social Change Consortium and a Nairobi-based consultant. Professional interests focus on participatory research and evaluation, action research, and capacity development across sectors, with keen interest in systemic and complexity-informed approaches. She is the coauthor of the *Innovations in the Evaluation of Social Change Communication* (UNAIDS, 2011); the external review report on IDRC's Evaluation Unit, 2005–2010 (2010); Pushing the boundaries: New thinking on how we evaluate, *MAZI* 19, 2009; Evaluating social change and CFSC: New perspectives, *MAZI* 17, 2008; and Working toward evidence-based process: Evaluation that matters, *MAZI* 13, 2007.

Catherine Campbell, PhD, is Professor of Social Psychology at the London School of Economics, and Program Director of the MSc in Health, Community, and Development. Her research focuses on the role of collective action in tackling health inequalities, against the background of her interest in the role of transformative communication in building social capital for health in marginalized communities. She is author of *Letting*

Them Die: Why HIV Prevention Programmes Fail (Indiana UP, 2003), and numerous articles in international health journals.

Ketan Chitnis, PhD, is the Regional HIV/AIDS Specialist with UNICEF Asia Pacific Shared Services Centre, Thailand. His professional and research interests are in health, communication, and empowerment in international development. Currently his work focuses on social protection for children and AIDS, and previously he advised and supported programs to manage behavior and social change interventions across child and maternal health issues. He has published in *The International Communication Gazette*, *Journal of Creative Communications*, *Keio Communication Review*, and *Investigación y Desarrollo*, among others.

Nicola Christofides is senior lecturer in the School of Public Health, University of the Witwatersrand, where she heads up the Masters in Public Health Program. Nicola was responsible for coordinating and developing a new field of study in Social and Behavior Change Communication at the School of Public Health. Prior to this she was a specialist scientist at the Gender and Health Research Unit, Medical Research Council. She has more than 10 years research experience in the area of gender-based violence, HIV/AIDS, reproductive health, and evaluating social and behavior change communication programs and interventions. She has published in a range of different journals.

Katherine de Tolly, MPhil, BA, is mHealth Project Manager and Senior Researcher at Cell-Life. Her professional interests include mHealth (the use of mobile technology in healthcare) and Web communications, with a particular emphasis on government, research, and HIV-related communications. She published her first journal article in 2011 and has presented at five conferences.

Lucía Durá, PhD, is Assistant Professor of Rhetoric and Writing Studies in the Department of English at the University of Texas at El Paso. Her dissertation focused on cultivating a rhetorical disposition for the practice of positive deviance action research, and her research interests focus on rhetoric for social change, methodology, medical rhetoric, technical and professional writing, and organizational communication. Her research collaborations have yielded numerous national conference presentations and publications on positive deviance, social change, methodology, and health education, including a coauthored monograph, *Protecting Children from Exploitation and Trafficking: Using the Positive Deviance Approach* (2009).

Mohan J. Dutta, PhD, is Professor of Communication at Purdue University, where he teaches and conducts research in international health communication, critical cultural theory, poverty in healthcare, health activism in globalization politics, indigenous cosmologies of health, subaltern studies and dialogue, and public policy and social change. Currently, he serves as senior editor of the journal *Health Communication* and sits on the editorial board of seven journals. He is the Associate Dean for Research and Graduate Education in the College of Liberal Arts at Purdue University, a Service Learning Fellow, and a fellow of the Entrepreneurial Leadership Academy at Purdue University where he has been developing a project on communication leadership in social change. He also directs the Center on Poverty and Health Inequities at Purdue University.

Eliana Elias is the cofounder and Executive Director of Minga Perú. Trained in social communication from the University of Lima, Eliana has been recognized as an Ashoka fellow and an AVINA leader and is committed to promoting social justice and human dignity among women in the Peruvian Amazon. She has been designing and implementing communication strategies for social change in the Peruvian Amazon since the early 1990s.

W. Douglas Evans, PhD, is Professor of Prevention and Community Health in the School of Public Health and Health Services at the George Washington University. He has published over 80 peer-reviewed articles and chapters on the effectiveness of health communication and social marketing behavior change interventions. He conducts research on health branding and the development and evaluation of new health technologies. He works both in the United States and in developing countries. In 2008 he published the volume, *Public Health Branding*, and is currently finishing two other books, *Global Social Marketing Research* and the SOPHE-APHA *Guide to Health Communication*.

Merissa Ferrara, PhD, is Assistant Professor at the College of Charleston. Her research interests include health communication and interpersonal communication. Her current line of research investigates social support (or lack thereof) for maintaining a healthy lifestyle. She has published several articles on such topics. She was also a researcher with Johns Hopkins University, working to increase collective efficacy regarding the adoption of certain medications and family planning in hopes to reduce the prevalence of HIV/AIDS in Namibia.

Maria Elena Figueroa, PhD, is Director, Research and Evaluation Division and Director, Global Program on Water and Hygiene, at the Center for Communication Programs at Johns Hopkins University. Dr. Figueroa's research has focused on the understanding of health behavior in developing country settings. She is interested in the use of interdisciplinary research and the use of different theoretical approaches and methodologies for a more comprehensive study of cultural, household, and individual factors that account for health behavior differentials. Dr. Figueroa's current research interests include: developing a better understanding of the social and cultural factors that explain safe water, sanitation and hygiene behaviors, including the role of the household and community traits in such practices.

Elizabeth Fox, PhD, is the Director of the Office of Health, Infectious Diseases, and Nutrition at USAID. Her office is responsible for global leadership in maternal and child health, environmental health, nutrition, health system strengthening, and the prevention and mitigation of infectious diseases, including TB, malaria, and avian and pandemic influenza. Before joining USAID, she was the manager of strategic planning at the International Bureau of Broadcasting, formerly USIA. She lived and worked in Bogota, Colombia, and Buenos Aires, Argentina, between 1968 and 1984, spending 10 years as the social sciences representative for Latin America at the International Development

Research Centre of Canada. She worked in Paris between 1984 and 1989 as a consultant to UNESCO. In 1990 she held the first UNESCO chair in communication at the Universidad Autónoma de Barcelona, She has an honorary doctorate from the Pontificia Universidad Católica of Peru (2007). She is currently adjunct faculty at the School of International Service of American University. She is the author, among other books, of *TV y Comunidad: Cinco Falacias*, Santiago: CENECA, 1986, and *Dias de Baile: El Fracaso de la Reforma de la Televisión en America Latina*, Mexico: Felafacs, 1991.

Karen Greiner, PhD, is postdoctoral scholar at the University of South Florida. Her research focuses on communication interventions designed to promote community-level social change in creative, innovative, and inviting ways. She is the author of "Participatory communication processes as infusions of innovation: The case of 'Scenarios from Africa'" (2009) and "Performance activism and civic engagement through symbolic and playful actions" (2008).

Ron Hess, MPS, currently serves as Director of Private Sector Programs, JHU/CCP. Mr. Hess has worked in communication for over 25 years, beginning as a media producer and entering the field of public health after studying communication theory and research at Cornell University. His work with JHU/CCP has involved alliances with governmental, civil society, and private sector organizations, and has included programs in the Middle East, Asia, the former Soviet Union, and East Africa. He served recently as a Country Director for the USAID-supported Communication for Healthy Living (CHL) project in Egypt.

Virginia Lacayo has more than 18 years of experience in the field of communication for social change. Her professional interests and experience focus on innovative approaches to communication for social change, complexity theory applied to international development and organizational change, and program design and evaluation. These issues have been the topic of her recent publications, presentations, and seminars. She finished her Master's Degree on Communication and Development at Ohio University and is currently working on her doctoral dissertation, focusing on the application of system thinking principles and ideas to communication for social change and social movement building strategies.

Kim Longfield is the Director for Research and Metrics at PSI and has worked for the organization since 2001. She is responsible for a team of more than 40 international researchers and the quality of research implemented in approximately 60 countries. Kim's expertise is in social marketing, qualitative research, and studies among populations at high risk of HIV/AIDS. She earned a PhD in Sociology and International Health and a MPH in International Health/Health Communication and Education, both from Tulane University. She is the author of more than two dozen published journal articles, reports, book chapters, and working papers.

Linje Manyozo, PhD, is lecturer and director of the MSc Programme in Media, Communication, and Development at the London School of Economics and Political Science. His professional interests focus on interrogating citizen voices and participation in development policy formulation and implementation. He is the author of *People's Radio: Communication Change across Africa*.

Dominique Meekers, PhD, is Professor at Tulane University's School of Public Health and Tropical Medicine. He has conducted extensive research on the determinants of health behaviors, and on the effect of social marketing and health communication programs on health behaviors in developing countries. Dr. Meekers served as the principal investigator for the external evaluation of the Health Communication Partnership, of which the Communication for Healthy Living program, Egypt, was a part. His current research agenda focuses on the social and behavioral aspects of global health, with particular emphasis on developing countries.

Srinivas R. Melkote, PhD, is Professor in the Department of Telecommunications at Bowling Green State University. He has worked in the field of communication and media studies for over 30 years. His research interests include the role of communication and media in directed social change, media effects, and health communication. His most recent publications include the widely used text *Communication for Development in the Third World* (coauthored with Leslie Steeves) and *Critical Issues in Communication* (co-edited with Sandhya Rao).

Carmen R. Mendivil Calderón, MA, is professor in the Social Communication and Journalism Program at Universidad Autónoma del Caribe, Colombia. She has worked in the design, implementation, and evaluation of communication strategies for social change on issues related to community media, human rights, ethnic and sexual diversity, gender equality, youth, and sexual and reproductive health. She has worked at regional and international nongovernmental organizations and international cooperation, including agencies and programs of the United Nations. She has published in Colombian communication journals.

Rafael Obregon, PhD, is Associate Professor in the School of Media Arts and Studies and Director of the Communication and Development Studies Program at Ohio University. He has taught and served as director of the Department of Social Communication at Colombia's Universidad del Norte and has taught and conducted research in Africa, Asia, and Latin America. He serves on the editorial boards of several journals, including the *Journal of Health Communication,* and has published articles and book chapters on communication, health, and development. His research interests are communication for development and social change, health communication, capacity strengthening, and monitoring and evaluation. As of September 2011, he joined UNICEF, New York as Chief of Communication for the Development Unit.

Gregory Alonso Pirio, PhD, is President of EC Associates (Empowering Communications) – a firm providing consulting and project implementation services on a variety of international communications, media, and conflict resolution issues. Dr. Pirio has been a global leader in the use of media and communications for constructive social change and a pioneer in the innovate use of ICT-based distance learning for health care professionals. Dr. Pirio is also a Visiting Scholar at the School of Conflict Analysis and Resolution, George Mason University, where he has launched the "Voices of Marginalized Youth Initiative."

Julie Pulerwitz, ScM, ScD, is the Director of the HIV/AIDS and TB Global Program at PATH, managing a diverse portfolio of HIV and TB projects addressing prevention, diagnosis, care, and treatment. She has particular expertise in behavior-change research and programs, as well as gender and male engagement, and stigma. Dr. Pulerwitz has authored over 20 articles in peer-reviewed journals and book chapters. She regularly participates in technical advisory groups, reviews for scientific journals, and guest-lectures at universities.

Andry Rabemanantsoa has a Diploma in Statistics and Information Management and a Diploma in Mathematics and Physics from the Faculty of Science, Antananarivo. He is Senior Research Coordinator at PSI. He has extensive experience with the design, implementation, supervision, and evaluation of large multi-round household studies in a variety of health areas involving different target groups. Prior to joining PSI, Mr. Rabemanantsoa worked as a statistician and information officer for a rural food security program financed by GTZ/Germany.

Scott C. Ratzan, MD, MPA, is Vice President, Global Health, Johnson & Johnson and Editor-In-Chief of the *Journal of Health Communication: International Perspectives*. Dr. Ratzan is co-chair of the United Nations Secretary General's Joint Action Plan on Women's and Children's Health Innovation Working Group. He also serves on the Non-Communicable Disease Network (NCDNet) of the World Health Organisation, officially representing the pharmaceutical industry. His books include *The Mad Cow Crisis: Health and the Public Good*; *Attaining Global Health: Challenges and Opportunities*; and *AIDS: Effective Health Communication for the 90s*.

Ietje Reerink, MPH, MA, currently works as a Senior Technical Advisor for research and communications with PSI Madagascar. She previously held the position of Director, Reproductive Health Department, also for PSI in Madagascar and worked in a similar position for PSI in Myanmar. She has more than 12 years professional experience managing reproductive health programs across the world, and has held positions at the Royal Tropical Institute in Amsterdam and at Family Care International in New York. Her expertise is in strategic planning, applied research for decision making, social franchising, BCC, and monitoring and evaluation.

Jose Rimon II, PhD, is senior officer in the global health policy and advocacy group of the Bill and Melinda Gates Foundation. He covers nutrition, reproductive, maternal, neonatal, and child health. Prior to joining the foundation, he was at Johns Hopkins University as the Director of the Health Communication Partnership, the Senior Deputy Director of the Center for Communication Programs, and a Senior Associate faculty at the Department of Health, Behavior and Society.

Anthony J. Roberto, PhD, is Associate Professor with the Hugh Downs School of Human Communication. His research and teaching interests focus primarily on social influence and health communication. Professor Roberto is lead author of *Influence In Action* (Allyn and Bacon, 2002), and has published over 27 peer-reviewed research articles in a variety of journals, including *Communication Research, Health Communication, Human Communication Research*, the *Journal of Applied Communication Research*, and the *Journal of Health Communication*. He has also authored four book chapters, and five lessons he created have been published in *Communication Teacher*.

Kerry Scott, MA, has worked in community health and community-based monitoring of public health services in collaboration with SATHI, a health advocacy NGO in Maharashtra, India. She has also conducted research in Manicaland, Zimbabwe on community-level facilitators and hinderers of ART access and adherence. She remains involved in the Manicaland Project through work on the links between community mobilization, social capital, and HIV in the region. She is currently in a PhD program at Johns Hopkins' Bloomberg School of Public Health.

Ami Sengupta, PhD, is a communication and development specialist. She has conducted extensive research on women's rights and community-led processes in international development and has published in several peer-reviewed journals. Presently, Ami is an independent consultant based in Bangkok, Thailand. She has over a decade of experience spanning research, training, and consulting with international development agencies.

Navendu Shekhar, MPA, MSc, works at Pathfinder International (PI) as Research and Metrics Advisor. He has 12 years of research experience spanning market research, causal econometric analyses, behavior change research, and large international surveys such as UNICEF's MICS. Prior to PI, he worked at Population Services International where he provided technical assistance and trained teams on research in eight countries of Southern Africa. He has also worked as Senior Project Director at the Indian Market Research Bureau, New Delhi.

Arvind Singhal, PhD, is the Samuel Shirley and Edna Holt Marston Endowed Professor of Communication and Director of the Social Justice Initiative in UTEP's Department of Communication. He is also appointed as the William J. Clinton Distinguished Fellow at the Clinton School of Public Service, Little Rock, Arkansas. Singhal teaches and conducts research in the diffusion of innovations, the positive deviance approach, organizing for social change, and the entertainment-education strategy. He is coauthor or editor of 11 books, including *Inviting Everyone: Healing Healthcare through Positive Deviance* (2010); *Protecting Children from Exploitation and Trafficking: Using the Positive Deviance Approach* (2009); *Entertainment-Education Worldwide: History, Research, and Practice* (2004); and *Combating AIDS: Communication Strategies in Action* (2003).

Joanna Skinner, MHS, MA, is a public health specialist with a focus on health communication for HIV/AIDS prevention among women and youth. She has worked at the United Nations Population Fund, the Johns Hopkins University Center for Communication Programs, and the United Nations Secretariat.

Suruchi Sood, PhD, is currently Assistant Professor in the Department of Medical Science and Community Health at Arcadia University. Prior to this appointment, she was

Assistant Professor, Department of Health Behavior, and Society and Senior Program Evaluation Officer, Center for Communication Programs, both within the Johns Hopkins University, Bloomberg School of Public Health.

Jeremy Snider, MPH, is currently pursuing a PhD in Health Services at the University of Washington in Seattle. Mr. Snider has previously worked for the President's Emergency plan for AIDS Relief and with a USAID-funded Health System Strengthening project. He has also served as a consultant and data analyst for a number of public health studies. His research experience includes using primary data, at the domestic and international level, to examine health resource allocations and evaluate the impact and effectiveness of clinical and public health interventions.

J. Douglas Storey, PhD, is Director for Communication Science at the Johns Hopkins Center for Communication Programs and faculty member in the Department of Health, Behavior, and Society at the Bloomberg School of Public Health. He has 30 years of experience in health and development communication and evaluation research, and has lived and worked in more than 25 countries. He is the author of numerous articles and book chapters on a wide range of topics including health communication theory, communication campaigns, program evaluation, population and reproductive health, maternal/child health and nutrition, emergency preparedness and response, and strategic communication planning.

L. Suzanne Suggs, PhD, MS, CHES, is Assistant Professor of Health Communication and Social Marketing, Institute of Public Communication and Education, Faculty of Communication Sciences at the Università della Svizzera Italiana, Lugano, Switzerland. Dr. Suggs' principal research examines the use of communication technologies and messaging strategies to improve health status and health outcomes, and to facilitate health behavior change. She is an Editorial Review Board member of the *Journal of Health Communication: International Perspectives* and is co-chair of the European Social Marketing Network.

María Beatriz Torres, PhD, is Assistant Professor of Communication at Gustavus Adolphus College. She has worked in different capacities in the field of communication for the last 24 years. She was awarded Mexico's National Council of Science and Technology and Fulbright scholarships. She delivers workshops and presentations on intercultural health communication and effective cross-cultural communication for profit health care and nonprofit organizations. She has produced TV and Radio programs in Mexico, Argentina, and the United States.

Thomas Tufte, MA, PhD, is Professor of Communication at Roskilde University, Denmark. He is co-director of Ørecomm (http://orecomm.net). Since 2000, he has conducted research and undertaken consultancies on health communication, mainly in Africa and related to HIV/AIDS prevention. From 2009–2013, he is the coordinator of a research project: "Media, Empowerment and Democracy in East Africa" (MEDIeA, www.mediea.ruc.dk). He is also a member of the advisory board for the Division of

Social and Behaviour Change Communication, School of Public Health, University of the Witwatersrand, South Africa. He is also a member of Editorial Review Board of the *Journal of Health Communication* (2001–2011).

Shereen Usdin, MBBCh, MPH, is an Executive and founding member of the Soul City Institute for Health and Development Communication. Her professional work includes development communication with a focus on HIV and AIDS, gender, and social justice. She is a co-founder and board member of the Alliance for Children's Entitlement to Social Security. She has received a Shoprite/Checkers Women of the Year award for her contributions to health as well as a Gordon's Institute of Business Science award for social entrepreneurship. She is the author of a book on the politics of global health and another on HIV and AIDS.

Jair Vega Casanov, MSc, is Professor and Researcher at the Social Communication Department at Universidad del Norte, Colombia. His areas of interest are communication and social change, health communication, and communication and politics. He has published in social sciences journals and coauthored *Internationalizing Media Studies* (University of Westminster, Routledge, 2009), and *Trazos de una Otra Comunicación en América Latina* (Ediciones Uninorte, 2011). He has been consultant for the Pan-American Health Organization, PCI, Friederich Ebert Stiftung, Communication for Social Change Consortium, and the Communication Initiative.

Ravi Verma is the Regional Director of the Asia regional office of the International Center for Research on Women (ICRW), based in New Delhi. With a background in social sciences and social demography, he has worked extensively and continues to work on promoting gender equality, working with men and boys in various settings and institutions.

Robin Vincent, BSc, PhD is currently the Senior Advisor for Learning, Evaluation, and Impact at the Panos Institute, London. Robin is a social anthropologist with an interest in understanding complex social change, social movements, and communicative culture. Robin has 14 years experience of working in HIV and health communication for development, and facilitating learning and evaluation in development work and designing communication strategies. Robin has published on complexity and social change in HIV responses, social movements, and learning in development partnerships.

Silvio Waisbord, PhD, is Professor and Associate Director in the School of Media and Public Affairs at George Washington University. He is the editor-in-chief of the *International Journal of Press/Politics*. He has published books and articles about journalism and politics, and the role of media and communication in social change and global health.

Kim Witte, PhD, is an International Health Communication expert with over 75 publications. Dr. Witte has conducted research with approximately 40 different populations worldwide on more than 35 different health-related topics, with a special focus on culturally appropriate risk messages. She has been recognized with the Outstanding Health Communication Scholar Award, the Distinguished Article Award by the National Communication Association (Applied Communication), the Distinguished Book Award by the National Communication Association (Applied Communication), with the Teacher-Scholar Award from Michigan State University, and with nearly a dozen Top Three Papers from national and international conferences. Dr. Witte has received funding from the CDC, the National Institute of Occupational Safety and Health, the American Cancer Society, and elsewhere.

Acknowledgments

We are thankful to the many people who have made this project possible. At Wiley-Blackwell, Elizabeth Swayze believed in this book when it was a rough draft and supported us along the way. Julia Kirk and Allison Kotska superbly shepherded the book throughout the process. Stephen Curtis was a wonderful copy-editor. Hazel Harris made sure the project was completed in due time. The anonymous reviewers who provided feedback on our handbook proposal helped sharpen its focus.

Obviously, this project wouldn't have been possible without the commitment, enthusiasm, and ideas of the contributors. They deserve credit for writing thoughtful chapters that invite us to think rigorously. We are very proud of having assembled a formidable collection of top-notch scholars and practitioners, who made our job intellectually rewarding and helped us turn an idea into a solid book.

It is hard to pin down exactly when we started to develop the idea for the book. We are sure, however, that the support, motivation and many ideas here presented originated in conversations about global health communication and social change with numerous friends and colleagues. We thank Jose Amar, Jesus Arroyave, Gloria Coe, Tito Coleman, James Deane, Warren Feek, Jesus Ferro, Elizabeth Fox, Karen Greiner, Chris Morry, David Mould, Ellyn Ogden, Thad Pennas, Julia Rosenbaum, Bill Smith, Jair Vega and Susan Zimicki.

Finally, we are grateful to our families for their unconditional support and love. To them, we dedicate this book.

Introduction

Over the past decades significant investments have been made in international health and development programs. That effort is illustrated by significant investments that governments and donors have made to address major public health issues. Examples include investments made by the Bill and Melinda Gates Foundation, Rotary International, and the Government of India to eradicate polio; the commitment of the government of Botswana to provide ARVs (antiretrovirals) for people who live with HIV; the USA's PEPFAR program also to provide ARVs to millions of HIV-positive people, especially in Africa; and the international investments to curb emergent pandemics such as avian influenza and SARS. In each of those efforts, communication has played an important role in advocating for healthy policies and environments, mobilizing communities, creating trust between users and providers, promoting healthier behaviors or the adoption of new behaviors, and raising awareness to rapidly and effectively respond to disease outbreaks.

The 66th General Assembly of the United Nations (UN), held in New York in 2011, may be remembered for one reason: the diplomatic efforts of Palestine to be recognized as a full member of the UN, and the subsequent diplomatic efforts for a negotiated solution between Israel and Palestine. Yet, for the international health and development community the main reason to reflect back on that General Assembly is likely to be the high-level meeting on noncommunicable diseases (the second ever to focus on health, after HIV/AIDS), which included a political declaration for the control of noncommunicable diseases (UN Declaration A/66/LI). United Nations Secretary-General Ban Ki-moon stated that "the summit in September in New York is our chance to broker an international commitment that puts noncommunicable diseases high on the development agenda, where they belong."

The human and economic cost of noncommunicable diseases (NCDs) is shocking. An analysis based on the four main NCDs (cardiovascular diseases, diabetes, cancer, and

The Handbook of Global Health Communication, First Edition. Edited by Rafael Obregon and Silvio Waisbord.

chronic respiratory diseases) indicates that "under a 'business as usual' scenario where intervention efforts remain static and rates of NCDs continue to increase as populations grow and age, cumulative economic losses to low- and middle-income countries (LMICs) from the four diseases are estimated to surpass US\$ 7 trillion over the period 2011–2025" (World Health Organisation/World Economic Forum, 2011, p. 3). Reports indicate that nearly 36 million deaths were attributed to NCDs worldwide in 2008. Beyond the obvious alarm that such figures have caused, another important discovery in the past years is that the burden of NCDs has become a global health concern that affects both developed and developing countries.

One of the many events organized to raise awareness about the need for a global response to NCDs was the launch of a special edition of the *Journal of Health Communication* titled "Communicating the Non-Communicable" (Volume 16, Supplement 2, September 14, 2011). This special issue of the journal highlights the role of communication in addressing the main social and behavioral determinants associated with NCDs (unhealthy diet, tobacco and alcohol use, salt intake, and physical inactivity). For each of those determinants communication can also play a pivotal role through strategies and interventions that seek to address individual, community, and social and political factors.

The year 2011 also marked the start of the last five-year period of the Millennium Development Goals (MDGs). At the end of 2015 the international health community will assess to what extent those goals have been achieved. However, three years before the end of MDGs efforts, it is already known that many countries will not have reached the MDGs by 2015. While that outcome should be the focus of many international debates for a few years, what is more important about the MDGs is that they have provided clear goals and targets against which the international development and health community can measure progress. For our purpose, what is most interesting is that six of the eight MDGs focused on, or were related to, health. International and national efforts to address the MDGs have included huge investments in communication. From campaigns aimed at preventing HIV/AIDS and diseases such as malaria and TB to reduction of maternal and child mortality and the empowerment of women and girls, communication is at the core of those efforts.

The international health and development community is at a crossroads. On the one hand, it still faces, and will continue to face, a significant test represented by diseases that are preventable as well as by the quality of health services and systems, particularly in poorer countries. On the other hand, international pressure and advocacy have increased to a point where it is imperative to mobilize globally in order to prevent diseases that affect populations in emerging economies and low- and middle-income countries. The convergence of communicable and noncommunicable diseases somehow closes a circle that, more than ever, demands a collective and coordinated response by international agencies, donors, governments, civil society organizations, communities, and individuals.

This is a particularly important moment in international efforts to address health issues, in which the response of the international health community will require a solid understanding of health communication approaches, lessons learned, and challenges and opportunities at the international and global level. Reflecting upon the role of communication in addressing the health issues we have described above is imperative to understanding the key contributions that communication can make to global efforts to address disease and improve health. The many chapters included in the handbook provide important lessons that should inform research and practice in health communication with an increasingly global perspective.

The Handbook offers a comprehensive view of contemporary theoretical and applied research issues in global health communication, framed from a development and social change perspective. It explores multiple theories and approaches in the study of communication, health, and development, and examines new perspectives such as communication for social change and their application to health issues. Few dispute the centrality of communication in global public health and development efforts, given the extensive research and applications in local and international aid programs. Yet, new questions remain unanswered and new challenges have emerged about the role of communication processes in improving health conditions among communities, and promoting broader social change in international health contexts. This volume provides a comprehensive and up-to-date analysis of these issues through a collection of original contributions that review and analyze the historical, institutional, social, cultural, and political dimensions of global health communication.

In response to the variety and depth of challenges in global health communication and development, the Handbook espouses a broad understanding of communication that transcends conventional divisions between informational and participatory approaches. It offers an integrated view that links communication to the strengthening of health services, the involvement of affected communities in shaping health policies and improving care, and the empowerment of citizens in making decisions about health, and by extension their own, development.

The Handbook features contributions from leading scholars and practitioners in the field who address different communication dimensions and questions in current global health programs primarily in developing regions. The chapters make four key contributions: they propose an understanding of communication as collective actions to redress health inequities and development challenges through a variety of mediated and interpersonal interventions; put forth a vision that synthesizes current perspectives in both research and practice in the field; bring together both research and programmatic perspectives to discuss a common set of theoretical questions; and foster a conversation between academics and practitioners around questions of common interest to inform further research.

The Handbook covers a wide range of communication approaches as well as health issues, and draws insights and experiences from health programs and interventions from around the world. It also addresses key crosscutting issues that are central to institutional and programmatic aspects of global health communication. Such diversity of health topics and communication approaches illustrates the depth of the theoretical perspectives and conceptual debates, and the richness of the field and its many contributions to the study of communication, development, and social change.

This volume attempts to offer a truly global perspective, discuss a broad range of theoretical approaches and case studies drawn from recent health programs, and address a common set of questions that are central for comparative research across health systems, cultures, and politics. It features a cross-cultural selection of cases, and examines long-standing debates and innovative approaches in communication applied to a range of health issues across geographic regions. In structuring it, we have worked towards bringing together chapter contributions around key questions that offer a coherent and integrated set of debates and analyses. Because the Handbook offers a comprehensive survey of the field in terms of conceptual approaches, health and development issues, and communication interventions, we believe that it will be useful for students, scholars and practitioners who are interested in identifying and examining key research questions and arguments.

Organization of the Handbook

In order to address issues and challenges outlined above, the book is divided into four thematic sections:

I. Contemporary Issues and Perspectives in Communication, Global Health, and Development
II. Theoretical Perspectives on and Approaches to Global Health Communication, Development, and Social Change
III. Innovation in Research and Practice in Global Health Communication in Development Contexts
IV. Cross-Cutting Issues for Research and Practice in Global Health Communication and Development.

Part I identifies and discusses key questions and theoretical debates and challenges of global health, communication, and development perspectives. Part II explores the multiplicity of communication theories, processes and approaches that guide research and practice in global health communication and development. Part III focuses on the application of theoretical notions in innovative interventions that put forth new research questions and themes. Finally, Part IV identifies and explores critical dimensions for further research and practice.

Chapters in each section follow a common structure in order to provide a coherent flow and organization. The first section analyzes the state of the art, reviews theoretical debates, identifies and discusses research directions, and analyzes the implications of theoretical developments for research and practice. The second discusses key theoretical concepts, debates, and developments, analyzes how theory informs research and practice, examines the contributions of recent research and practice to refining theoretical concepts, discusses innovative lines of research and programmatic experiences, and identifies questions for future research and debate. The third section provides several innovative case studies; discusses theoretical dimensions of specific projects, and puts forward key recommendations for research and practice. The Handbook concludes with two chapters that draw key lessons from the contributions, and lays out key issues and perspectives for future research and practice in global health communication.

It is our hope that this Handbook will contribute to enriching teaching and learning in many ways and stimulate critical debates and interest among students, scholars, and practitioners to further explore critical global health communication issues and enhance the knowledge base in the field.

Reference

World Health Organisation/World Economic Forum (2011). *From Burden to "Best Buys": Reducing the Economic Impact of Non-Communicable Diseases in Low and Middle-Income Countries.* Geneva, Switzerland: World Health Organisation/World Economic Forum.

Part I

Perspectives on Communication and Global Health

1

Theoretical Divides and Convergence in Global Health Communication

Silvio Waisbord and Rafael Obregon

Introduction

This chapter offers a survey of theories in global health communication. The goals are to analyze the genealogy of key theories and debates, compare concepts and arguments, and their differences, and to discuss the possibility of theoretical convergence.

Global health communication has straddled both academic debates and programmatic interventions. Given this position, theories were not only developed to produce evidence-based generalizations that explain relations among variables and offer predictions about a range of phenomena. They have also been formulated to provide conceptual guidance to health programs aimed at promoting changes and reaching specific outcomes. Such expectations about the empirical implications of theories have not been limited to conceptual frameworks produced in the mold of scientific positivism and empirical research. Theories rooted in the humanities and interpretative frameworks have also maintained close connections with health programs. Scholars in health communication (Fishbein, 2000; Fishbein and Yzer, 2003) and communication for development and social change (Melkote and Steeves, 2001; Morris, 2004; Gumucio-Dagron and Tufte, 2006; Servaes, 2008), the two fields that underpin the theoretical edifice of global health communication, have refined theories to contribute to addressing concrete health challenges. Just like general theories about public health, they are intended not simply to explain phenomena. They were designed to pursue specific programmatic goals based on normative imperatives too – in other words, to pursue social good (Kreps, 1989; Rogers, 1994).

Aside from whether scholars were primarily driven to provide programmatic prescriptions or contribute to academic debates, theoretical paradigms have been increasingly used to provide intellectual justification to global health interventions. The incorporation

The Handbook of Global Health Communication, First Edition. Edited by Rafael Obregon and Silvio Waisbord.

of theory into program design has been far from a linear and predictable process. Instead, given the predominance of biomedical approaches in global health, it has been a bumpy ride. Gradually, as program managers realized the need for social-behavioral approaches and acknowledged the solid conceptual foundations in communication studies, communication scholarship gained a stronger footing.

The main argument presented in this chapter is as follows: the field is still characterized by a theoretical divide between information/media effects and participatory/critical theories that mirrors broad differences in health communication and communication studies at large. Despite efforts to bridge these theoretical traditions, the divide remains grounded on different conceptions of communication and its place in promoting better health worldwide. Finding bridges, let alone reconciling differences, seems unlikely given that theories and models are based on antithetical epistemological and analytical premises and ask different questions about the nature of communication and the conditions required to address challenges in contemporary health that impede cross-pollination across disciplinary and conceptual traditions.

Theories about global health communication have conceptually drawn from theoretical debates in the field of communication at large, and have been empirically informed by hundreds of studies about the role of communication in health programs in diverse international settings. Conceptually, theories and models have been influenced by the evolution of development communication and health communication as two separate branches of communication studies. Therefore, the genealogy of the field is rooted in the convergence of theories originally intended to analyze and explain the role of communication in processes of social, economic, and political development as well as the role of communication in improving health conditions and indicators in the United States. Since then, global health communication has straddled both parallel lines of research in the discipline. Consequently, it has been influenced by theoretical debates and research with different goals.

Empirically, theories have largely been informed by international, rather than global, studies in health communication. This difference is not insignificant. "Global" refers to health and communication issues that affect the world as a whole and, concomitantly, to approaches that analyze them as phenomena with planetary dimensions and implications. Examples of such global framework are theories about the role of communication in addressing health risks and challenges that transcend geographical and cultural borders, whether the spread of infectious diseases or the impact of climate change. Conversely, "international" alludes to the intersection between health and communication in specific local, regional, and national cases throughout the world. Examples are the analysis of the role of communication in immunization campaigns in a given country or strategies to promote care and treatment of people living with HIV/AIDS in a community. Whereas the former put global perspective at the forefront, the latter are focused on specific local dimensions. No question, the vast majority of studies have fallen into this second category. Even as globalization theories and approaches have remarkably influenced contemporary debates in the social sciences, theory-building remains grounded in distinct community and national studies. Moreover, studies are also focused on individual health issues and experiences that reflect the stove piping mindset in global health at large (Brown, Cueto, and Fee, 1996).

The study of health communication in a global context needs to be placed as the prolongation of two scholarly traditions, "development communication" and "health communication," two separate fields of analysis and practice. This section discusses the former; the next section addresses the latter.

Health in Development Communication

Theory-building and conceptual debates in global health communication are linked to the genealogy of "development communication" in the 1950s. Specifically, the study of health communication in international context continued the analytical premises of modernization theory, which was the "dominant paradigm" in the field of development communication in its early decades. Although modernization studies were not primarily concerned with health outcomes, they were based on epistemological premises that are similar to the socio-psychological and communication theories that came to dominate the study of global health communication.

Modernization theory dominated the early generation of development communication studies. One of its basic tenets was that development problems were rooted in cultural obstacles, namely, the persistence of traditional attitudes and knowledge. As long as traditional cultures persisted, modernization theorists argued, development was impossible (McClelland, 1961; Hagen, 1962). Besides its uncritical assumption that development meant the Western model of development, modernization put forth a causal argument inspired by a particular socio-historical interpretation of the West. It was embedded in two key analytical premises. First, it offered a functionalist explanation of society according to which there is a necessary correlation between political, economic, and cultural systems. A "modern" democratic polity and capitalist economy necessitate a "modern" culture characterized by individualism, scientific values, innovation, entrepreneurship, secularism, and so on. Second, modernization argued that "culture" (including psychosocial characteristics as well as knowledge and attitudes) is the independent variable that explains "development." By embracing these premises, modernization offered a cultural-functionalist argument with obvious programmatic implications. Addressing the problems of underdevelopment required cultural change, that is, the transformation of prevalent psychological and cultural traits.

The blend of a view that emphasized the primacy of cultural change in large processes of social transformation with communication theories about powerful media effects set the paradigm that defined the field of development communication. If the mass media have significant impact on psychological and cultural attributes, as several studies have contended, then they could be instrumental in promoting cultural changes in "underdeveloped" countries. Put it differently, seminal writings (Lerner, 1958; Schramm, 1964) in development communication drew from both modernization theories (which were prevalent in international studies) and media studies to argue that exposure to the mass media was vital for cultural change and, subsequently, for "modern development." The "modern" media were viewed as agents of positive change, as they could expose people to "modern" knowledge and attitudes.

Implicit in this line of argument was a conceptual model that basically understood communication as the transmission of information and the study of persuasion. Media technologies were critical because they allowed the mass distribution of information and, as "propaganda" studies suggested, were capable of influencing knowledge and attitudes among large numbers of people. Communication was conceived as a unidirectional process by which those with access to the media can influence the minds of the many who don't. It is about how ideas are disseminated in society, and how people can be persuaded to believe, think, and act in certain ways.

Such an "informational/persuasion" view of communication was present in Everett Rogers' (1962) study about the diffusion of innovations. Rogers suggested that information is a critical yet not sufficient condition for the adoption of new ideas. His well-known model of five stages and his distinction between types of "adopters" stressed the significance of awareness and knowledge of innovations (whether new farming methods or scientific advances) in adopting them. Knowledge does not necessarily lead to effective change, but the latter does require modifications in levels of awareness and knowledge. According to Rogers, development communication was the intentional transference of ideas and information to change belief and behaviors. It is about how sources persuade receivers.

Rogers and Schramm eventually moderated early assumptions about the power of the media. They acknowledged the importance of interpersonal communication in processes of persuasion. Also, they recognized the importance of sociocultural factors in motivating people to change beliefs and behaviors. In response to his critics, Rogers (1976) even admitted that participation should be a key component of communication. For him, communication is a "process in which participants create and share information with one another in order to reach a mutual understanding" (Rogers, 1986, p. 199). Yet the paradigm still espoused the conception of communication as information transmission and persuasion. Even if it was recognized that people participated on more leveled conditions, communication was basically conceived as information sharing. Put it differently, despite the widening of who participated, the basic conception of communication didn't change.

What matters for understanding the intellectual lineage of international/global health communication is that fundamental tenets of modernization theories resonated with the early systematic application of communication theories to health issues as development problems. Just like modernization, those studies subscribed to the view that communication was primarily concerned with information and persuasion – it was a scientific field interested in conditions and strategies that maximize the impact of information transmission on knowledge, attitudes, and behaviors. The role of theory, then, was to identify continuities and develop explanations about how information dissemination and exchange modify awareness, knowledge, and beliefs about health issues and, ultimately, contribute to changing health practices.

The strong push for family planning programs in international aid in the 1960s and 1970s set the stage for a wealth of studies about the impact of communication programs on health indicators. Evidence of this approach was the work of Schramm (1971) and Rogers (1973) who extensively analyzed communication interventions implemented to support population programs worldwide. As a consequence, conclusions and theories about health (as well as development) communication were largely informed by findings about the effect of interventions and media campaigns on beliefs about family size, knowledge of family planning methods, information about health systems, and the like. These studies summarized previous findings and identified key questions that were subsequently addressed by a wealth of studies (Piotrow *et al.*, 1997).

Theories about Health Communication: Behavior Change and Media Effects

At the same time, health communication emerged as distinct scholarly field of inquiry in the United States (Kreps, Bonaguro, and Query, 1988). The combination of pioneering theoretical insights and landmark programmatic experiences (Farquhar and Maccoby, 1975) shaped the flourishing of health communication. Theoretically, the field has been defined by the combination of interdisciplinary approaches (Kreps and Maibach, 2008; Nussbaum, 1989) and concepts grounded in social psychology and the "media effects" research in communication studies. Analytically, it has engaged with a vast range of communication processes and health issues (Parrott, 2004). A detailed analysis of the development of key theories falls outside the scope of this chapter. Several articles have already compared core concepts and arguments as well as the applicability of theoretical constructs across health issues and settings (Brashers and Babrow, 1996; Noar and Zimmerman, 2004).

What matters for understanding theory in global health communication is how theoretical concepts and methodological approaches developed by health communication, primarily in US academia, exerted a notable influence. First, because groundbreaking studies were rooted in social psychological theories, communication has been typically understood as a human process of information transmission and reception. This also explains why the focus has been on individuals rather than on broad social, political, and economic forces. The impact of the latter on health communication has been eclipsed by the paramount interest in barriers and motivations at the individual level. Questions about individual cognition and psychological and social attributes in exposure to and the processing of health information have been dominant. Second, individualistic premises underlay the research on the impact of health information on behaviors. Collective behaviors were basically conceived as the aggregation of individual practices rather than as distinct phenomena explained by specific dynamics and causes. Third, the tradition of empirical research and applied knowledge in health communication also influenced the research agenda of global health communication. Theory was meant to provide solid conceptual footing and evidence to guide interventions to affect health behaviors. Finally, the ascendancy of the media effects tradition also left a clear mark on studies about health communication worldwide.

The field of health communication was born out of scholarly interest in issues located at the intersection of information, individual decision making, and health behaviors. Because it was located at the crossroads of various disciplines, "communication" has been used interchangeably with other terms such as education, promotion, marketing, and information. Such loose usage certainly helped to define a broad field of interdisciplinary inquiry which included communication, psychology, education, and public health (Glanz, Marcus Lewis, and Rimer, 1990). Also, it allowed scholars to reach out to academic communities, journals, and professionals across disciplines. It put in place, however, the conditions for persistent conceptual confusion. Communication is not identical with information (Berry, 2004), promotion and other adjacent concepts. Certainly, such confusion isn't unique to global health communication. One could reasonably argue that it mirrors the perennial conceptual cacophony in the study of communication at large (Craig, 1993, 1999) which also resulted from the convergence of dissimilar disciplinary and theoretical traditions.

As the field of health communication progressively embraced behaviorist theories and goals, communication became associated with information dissemination, materials, interventions (campaigns), target audiences, and messages. Questions have been focused on the factors that contribute to the promotion of healthy behaviors. Put it differently, as behavior change issues became dominant in the literature, communication was synonymous with information and its role in health behaviors. Such an understanding of communication is one among several possible competing definitions.

Health communication was born with the unmistakable imprint of social psychology. Just as the study of human communication partially developed as a branch of psychology in previous decades, the study of health communication carried over basic premises and questions from psychological studies. Between the mid 1960s and mid 1970s, socio-psychological theories laid the conceptual bedrock. They asked questions and put forth propositions that remain central to theoretical inquiry and practical interventions. During those formative years, key writings were published about social learning and modeling (Bandura, 1963, 1969, 1971) health beliefs (Rosenstock, 1966), media effects (McGuire, 1969), persuasion (Tichenor, Donohue, and Olien, 1970), and individual rationality (Fishbein and Ajzen, 1975).[1]

During the 1970s, studies similarly informed by sociopsychological theories built on previous work. They refined original arguments about the role of cognition, individual attributes, and personal attitudes on health behaviors (Becker and Maiman, 1974). These theoretical perspectives left a powerful imprint as they articulated basic principles and propositions that informed countless studies since then.

The rise of social marketing (Kotler, 1972; Kotler and Zaltman, 1971) also contributed to the consolidation of health communication in the United States. Social marketing was neither a "theory" *stricto sensu* not solely preoccupied with health issues. Rather, it encompassed a set of approaches that proposed the utilization of commercial marketing techniques to promote social behaviors, including health practices and outcomes. It aimed to promote social goods by drawing upon theories of consumer behavior that conceptualized the processes of needs creation and consumer decision-making (Novelli, 1990). At the core of social marketing was the exchange model according to which individuals, groups, and organizations receive perceived benefits in exchange for purchased products.

With social-psychological theories, social marketing shared the interest in understanding individual behaviors as well as the factors that influence decision making. Whereas scholarly theories were primarily concerned with explaining health behaviors and drawing propositions for further testing, social marketing applied to health issues was mainly interested in affecting behaviors (Andreasen, 1994). In doing so, it proposed that it was necessary to produce nuanced understandings about the factors that influence behavior change. Systematic, research-based information about consumers was deemed indispensable for effective interventions. Marketing research techniques are valuable for finding out thoughts and attitudes about a given issue that help prevent possible failures and position a product. For its advocates, one of the main strengths of social marketing is that it allows products and concepts to be positioned in traditional belief systems. Social marketing's emphasis on research and the segmentation of "target" publics implicitly put less emphasis on information as the main driver of behavior change. Social marketing's well-known "4 P model" outlined several factors that may affect health decision making: product, price, place, and promotion. Promotion, social marketing's term to refer to communication and information, was theorized as one factor affecting practices.[2]

The field of health communication matured during the 1980s and early 1990s. It became consolidated in academic units, conferences, and journals as well as in terms of public and private funding (Ratzan, 1996; Rogers, 1994). Studies developed more nuanced theoretical models to fill gaps in previous research (Janz and Becker, 1984; Rosenstock, Strecher, and Becker, 1988). The number of studies applied to a range of health issues proliferated. Questions about the role of information in modifying individual knowledge, beliefs, and health behaviors sprang to the forefront.

Dominant approaches continued to theorize communication in terms of information dissemination intended to change individuals' perception of threats and benefits, and readiness to act. The cybernetic model underlay the study of communication in terms of information disseminators, interpreters, and input/output flows (Donohew and Ray, 1990). Theories that defined central questions in the research agenda in subsequent decades, most notably the Theory of Reasoned Action (Fishbein, 1980) and the Theory of Planned Behavior (Ajzen,1985), proposed that individual attitudes and subjective norms determine behavioral intentions. Likewise, models such as the Precede–Proceed, outlined a multistage development of health behaviors. Concepts such as self-efficacy (Rosenstock, Strecher, and Becker, 1988) were proposed to better understand multiple factors that affect individual decisions to perform specific health behaviors. Scholars (Freimuth, 1990) made calls to close the extensively documented gap between information and practices. Interest in the range of interpersonal and mediated communication on health behaviors remained central in the study of social norms (Lapinski and Rimal, 2006).

The interest in behavioral and cognitive issues dovetailed with the tradition of "media effects" in communication studies. Going back to the beginnings of the field, the literature on "media effects" has remained central, particularly in the United States. The blend of social-psychological approaches with long-standing interest in media effects steered the field in a definite direction: the study of the impact of information dissemination through mediated and interpersonal channels on individual behaviors. Given the dominant interest in media effects, key arguments and findings in the health communication literature have been adjacent to the extensive literature on media effects. Just as the behaviorist bent meant that health communication offered extensive and sophisticated theories about behavior change, the focus on media effects similarly made its conclusions directly relevant within the tradition of media effects in communication studies.

Interest in media effects has driven research on key components of information processes and media effects: audiences, channels, and messages (Flay, DiTecco, and Schlegel, 1980; Maibach and Parrott, 1995). Underlying this line of inquiry has been the intention to understand how to maximize the impact of communication interventions on health knowledge, attitudes, and behaviors. Scholars refined ways to theorize audience segmentation (Slater, 1996), and understand the psychosocial characteristics of specific audiences (Keller and Lehmann, 2008). Studies have analyzed the social, cultural, and psychological characteristics of various audiences differentiated by age (Greene *et al.*, 1996) , education (Salmon *et al.*, 1996), race (Kreuter *et al.*, 2003; Pratt *et al.*, 2003), gender, and other variables (Dearing, 2004). Questions about impact have also informed research about channels. Studies have assessed the merits of different channels to maximize reach, reception, comprehension, and other factors. From the use of various channels in a multi-media world (Randolph and Viswanath, 2004) to the strengths of tailored print materials (Kreuter and Wray, 2003; Skinner *et al.*, 1999), they have produced a rich literature. The issue of effectiveness has also driven research on message design. Studies have assessed the quality of messages to promote health behaviors by keeping and holding attention from various audiences (Donohew, Lorch, and Palmgreen), and using different appeals (Witte and Allen, 2000).

This body of literature has offered nuanced approaches to the study of media effects. It has addressed immediate and long-term, intentional and unintentional, positive and negative effects of communication interventions (Cho and Salmon, 2007; Salmon and Atkin, 2003). Also, media effects issues have been the subject of numerous meta-analyses of information campaigns across health issues (Snyder, 2007; Noar, 2006). This wealth of data has contributed to refining theoretical concepts and informed conclusions about the need for integrated approaches to health communication interventions

Global Health Communication Theories

Rogers's theory of diffusion of innovations applied to health (Bertrand, 2004) and dominant theoretical approaches in health communication set the course for global research. Those paradigms laid the fundamental epistemological and analytical premises and raised the theoretical questions that defined the field. Consequently, much of global health communication has been focused on behavioral change and media impact. It has been primarily driven to produce applied knowledge to help inform aid programs and local interventions. It has largely subscribed to the individualistic premises of social-psychological theories focused on behavior decisions and obstacles at the personal level. It has embraced the concept of communication as information dissemination through interpersonal and mediated channels.

From these perspectives, two set of interests have animated research on international health communication. On the one hand, scholars have been concerned with how communication interventions support programs to address health challenges that disproportionately affect the global South. Much of the literature has focused on the linkages between communication and three health issues: family planning/reproductive health, child health (including nutrition and immunization), and HIV/AIDS. When population growth and nutrition issues dominated international health and aid in the 1960s and 1970s (Robinson and Ross, 2007), the agenda of international health communication was focused on those issues, too. The experiences of communication programs in support of child health (Hornik *et al.*, 2002) and family planning (Piotrow *et al.*, 1997) behaviors provided plenty of cases for theory building. The HIV/AIDS crisis from the 1980s onwards shifted considerable attention to questions about how communication affects sexual behavior. Ongoing research has particularly paid attention to how communication relates to stigma, social norms, and gender roles as key behavioral determinants.

Given the close proximity between theory and practice, it is not surprising that much research has dealt with issues that have received significant levels of funding from aid agencies during the past decades. Certainly, other priorities in international health and aid have been examined, such as specific infectious diseases (malaria and tuberculosis most notably). The bulk of the attention, however, has remained closely aligned with the main priorities of major aid donors.

On the other hand, global health communication has offered opportunities to conduct research on the same questions that drove interest in the field of health communication, and test the applicability of theories originally formulated mainly in the United States. International cases bring up a wealth of evidence to determine the explanatory power of propositions regarding behavioral and media-impact issues. Underlying this approach is the assumption that scientific theories should be able to generalize and predict results regardless of social and cultural settings. Theories make universal claims that need to be probed across settings. Variations help us to refine the explanatory and predictability power of theories. This premise has animated decades-long research and theory in global health communication.

International experiences thus have offered countless cases to determine the strength of theoretical hypotheses with respect to the interaction between information processes and health behaviors. Like the field of health communication at large, much of the literature has been interested in assessing the mechanisms that contribute to activating or moderating intervention/campaign effects at the individual and social levels.

Whereas conclusions generally agree that "ideational" factors play an important role in health behaviors, studies have analyzed the impact of different communication (information) issues and strategies on social-psychological behavioral determinants. It is impossible to summarize the state of the findings across communication programs and health issues within the scope of this chapter. The impressive body of evidence does not lend itself to parsimonious and categorical conclusions. Studies have confirmed the circuitous process of interpersonal and mediated influence on health behaviors, and the multiple ways in which we should study the linkages between interventions and effects (Piotrow and Kincaid, 2001). Recent studies have documented the small to moderate effects of programmatic interventions in changing various behavioral determinants at the individual and social levels (e.g., knowledge, attitudes, perceptions, social norms) and promoting healthy behaviors.

Besides the intention to contribute to program design and thus to the improvement of health conditions, this body of literature is characterized by an interest in assessing the explanatory power of central propositions in health communication. Studies have shown the strengths of key theories and approaches to explain the contributions of communication programs to modifying behavioral determinants in health behavior. There is no shortage of examples of research conducted around the world on various health issues similarly interested in testing key theories in health communication. An illustrative sample includes studies on the theory of reasoned action (Kwadwo, 2001; Pick, 2007), social marketing (Agha, Karlyn, and Meekers, 2006), the health belief model, the extended parallel process model (Witte, 1998), self/collective efficacy (Smith, Ferrara, and Witte, 2007; Storey *et al* 2007), risk perception (Agha, 2003), social cognition (Smith, Downs, and Witte, 2007), and social networks and interpersonal communication (Sood, Shefner-Rogers, and Sengupta, 2006 ; Valente, Paredes, and Poppe, 2006).

How have behavioral and information processing theories helped to understand what works at the programmatic level? It is difficult to offer a summary of findings that captures the wealth of experiences documented in dozens of studies. Whereas studies have helped to refine theoretical understanding of information questions, we still lack a parsimonious explanation about the link between information processes and health behaviors. The data show that information campaigns and other interventions positively affect knowledge, attitudes, risk perception, and other components of the ideational processes (Bond and Valente, 1999; Boulay and Valente, 1999). Evidence, however, is more ambiguous about whether changes in information and attitudes are mirrored in transformations in health behaviors. Also, because most studies have analyzed the impact of single interventions around a specific health issue, we still lack comparative analyses to know whether information interventions have a similar impact across health programs and behavioral determinants. Even meta-studies of campaign effects, which offer a comprehensive overview across interventions, are focused on single health programs.

The Dominant Paradigm and its Critics

The widespread application of behavioral and "media effects" theories in global health communication has been the subject of several criticisms. Informed by a range of interpretative/cultural and participatory theories, scholars have targeted the conceptual and epistemological assumptions of those theories, and have tried to reorient the field around different sets of questions and theoretical premises. The focus and tenor of the critiques reflect similar arguments in both the fields of health communication (Zoller and Kline, 2008) and development communication (Morris, 2004; Servaes, 1996). The critique can be summarized as follows: the tradition of media effects on health behaviors is premised on narrow understandings of both communication and health. It carries specific theoretical and epistemological premises that are problematic for studying the rich and complex relation between communication and health in a global context.

One set of criticisms has questioned the prevalent definition of communication in behavioral and media effects studies. From participatory and ritualistic perspectives, the notion of communication *qua* information dissemination is conceptually incorrect for it focuses exclusively on the transmission of information from, put in the parlance of traditional cybernetic studies, "senders" (health programs, campaign organizers) to "receivers" (individuals). Absent is a conception of communication that stresses the exchange of ideas and participation in public life and the development of critical consciousness. The focus on "health/communication" campaigns, which has attracted considerable analytical and theoretical attention, denotes a misguided conceptualization of communication that fails to rigorously distinguish communication from information. Put simply, campaign communication is not communication, but rather, it is an instance of massive distribution of information by certain (typically powerful) actors, who carefully assess how target audiences may react to key messages. Health communication, instead, should bring to the fore questions of how people talk and make sense of issues related to health, disease, and well-being. It is about how citizens participate in public spaces through debating health issues, identifying challenges and solutions, and determining courses of action. Several studies have shown how communication skills are central to the process by which people identify, understand, discuss, and act upon health challenges (Campbell and Jovchelovitch, 2000; Campbell and MacPhail, 2002). This should be the analytical focus of communication research: how societies problematize health and disease, and establish priorities for action.

Another set of writings has questioned the individualistic premises of the behaviorist/media effects paradigm. This critique has centered on the dominant epistemology in much health communication research. Scholars have questioned the applicability of individual-centered models in non-Western societies (Airhihenbuwa, Makinwa, and Obregon, 2000; Buhler and Kohler, 2002). In societies where communal values are dominant, they argue, it is mistaken to theorize about health communication based on the premise that the individual is the core social actor. Such approaches may apply in Western societies characterized by strong individualism, but they are inappropriate where the concept of personhood is subsumed under a broad set of group identities.

This line of criticism should not be interpreted as simply stating that "culture matters," and calling on us to consider cultural diversity as a central dimension of global health communication. In fact, the question of how culture underpins health communication in international settings has been present in much of the research on innovations and behavior change (Rogers and Shoemaker, 1971). The critique pushes the field in a different direction: It is not just about considering the weight of community issues such as norms and attitudes as they influence individual behaviors, but rather, the need to rethink the epistemology of global health communication, basically shifting the analytical focus from individuals to communities. Community and cultural context should not be considered another set of behavioral determinants that affect individual decisions and practices; instead, they should be foregrounded in the analysis.

This criticism is linked to a questioning of the rationalistic, modernistic premises of health behaviorism and communication (Dutta and de Souza, 2008). Much of global health communication follows the model of individual rational decision making underpinning health communication and behavioral research. For example, the "knowledge–behavior gap," an issue that has been extensively discussed in the literature, is premised on the notion that knowledge should lead to behavior change. If individuals were aware and properly informed about health risks, they would act "rationally" to maximize individual benefits and therefore practice healthy behaviors. Such an assumption needs to be questioned on the grounds that "individual rationality" needs to be contextualized.

What rationality means in one context, either defined in terms of the articulation of means and ends in utilitarianism philosophy or incentives and benefits in behavioral economics, is different across cultural contexts. Rationality is culturally defined according to social expectations, norms, and attitudes. This makes it necessary to understand how communities and individuals experience, think, and make decisions about health in order to better comprehend communicative processes.

Scholars have also raised questions about the behavioral focus of global health communication research. Communication studies, they argue, should be primarily concerned with participation and power, issues largely absent in much of the literature (Lupton, 1994). Behavioral and campaign theories are not primarily concerned with issues surrounding power, such as the influence of political-economic forces on health, gender inequity, the impact of health and other (e.g. labor, environmental) policies on the well-being of individuals and communities, the struggles of underrepresented and subaltern groups to improve health conditions, and so on (Melkote, Muppidi, and Goswami, 2000). Questions such as how power shapes health communication or how communication about health can transform power are notoriously absent. Such questions are absent given that dominant theories are primarily concerned with different set of questions. Socio-psychological theories and health campaign/communication theories are primarily interested in questions about information processing, behavior modeling, and media effects and therefore offer propositions to explain such phenomena.

What is troubling if health communication research focuses on those issues at the expense of power and participation? The silence on macro-power structures and emphasis on individual behaviors implicitly assumes that health is, above all, a matter of individual responsibility. Health communication focuses on the power of individuals who weigh different information and other considerations in making decisions about health. What is missing in this approach is the analysis of how power and policies structurally affect health conditions before individuals are confronted with information or options (Airhihenbuwa, Makinwa, and Obregon, 2000; Erni, 2004). Therefore, it is necessary to consider power asymmetry at different levels to properly assess the role of personal, interpersonal, and social forces in health communication.

Communication needs to consider how citizens participate to change conditions that affect health, and how they mobilize to advocate for policies to improve access to better health (Diop, 2000; Ford, Odallo, and Chorlton, 2003; Waisbord, Michaelides, and Rasmuson, 2007). Growing interest in community participation in health policy and health advocacy (Usdin *et al.*, 2000) shows the importance of questions about power, policy, gender, and politics for health communication research and practice. Likewise, participatory experiences designed to address a range of health issues, such as HIV/ AIDS (Gao and Wang, 2007) and tuberculosis (Waisbord, 2010), attest to the strengths of community–based approaches to promote health goals in various countries.

Linked to this argument is another criticism: standard health communication theories uncritically accept the model of power embedded in the biomedical model of health. Biomedical notions largely dominate global health programs. Implicit in the biomedical model is a definite conceptualization of power with respect to knowledge and authority that has great implications for theorizing health communication. Whereas medical experts are granted full power, citizens are cast as passive actors. Standard discourse is reflective of such premises. Whereas experts are assigned central, unchallenged authoritative roles in determining appropriate behaviors, people are cast as "patients" who are expected to "adhere/comply" with prescribed actions. Issues of "lay" knowledge and contestation over knowledge/power, to put it in Foucault's terms, are typically absent. In light of these relatively unexplored ideological assumptions, critical perspectives favor the examination of assumptions about health knowledge and expertise, and propose multilayered analyses of communication in the construction of power relations in health (Waisbord, 2008).

Critical approaches also question standard methodologies used in global health communication research (Zoller and Kline, 2008). They find the dominant position of positivist and experimental research troubling. It overshadows interpretive and qualitative analyses which, in their minds, are better suited to analyzing the social construction and representation of health and illness. Drawing from anthropology and critical social studies, they underscore the need for discourse analysis, ethnography, and other qualitative, in-depth methods to grasp how societies define certain understandings of health, how health inequalities are formed and maintained, how public debate informs health decisions, and so on. These problems, which are viewed as central to the overall intellectual enterprise in health communication, need be approached with methodologies that capture the relationship between critical dimensions of communication, such as sense-making processes (Dutta-Bergman, 2004), cultural difference, and dialogue (Lambert and Wood, 2005), and the socioeconomic and political conditions of health systems around the world.

This range of criticisms reflects theoretical divides in the field of communication. Theories start from different epistemological premises, are interested in different dimensions of the intersection between health and communication, and are driven by different questions. Not surprisingly, then, they have produced quite different explanations, propositions, and predictions.

Whereas such theoretical eclecticism reflects the diversity and inclusiveness of the field, it also exposes significant divides. One could argue that these two theoretical traditions, one focused on information processing and behavioral change and the other concerned with power, participation, and public debate, have existed in parallel. One could perfectly well conduct research within one tradition without having to reach out or recognize alternative theories. Doubtlessly, the task of finding common ground between these two streams of research is not easy. Both paradigms are rooted in quite different theoretical and intellectual traditions.

Towards Theoretical Convergence?

Difficulties notwithstanding, it is important to recognize several attempts to incorporate analytical insights and issues that had been hitherto separated in two theoretical streams in global health communication. Although such efforts have not put to rest long-standing divisions, they herald a phase of theoretical efforts to condense conceptual insights and findings from different traditions. These efforts suggest the rise of scholarship receptive to cross-theoretical pollination that recognizes the strengths of theoretical models grounded in different epistemologies and academic traditions.

Efforts towards theoretical convergence are animated by the perception that although original theories still provide basic foundations, they are insufficient to assess the complexity of social determinants of health, and inform strategic thinking about actions to promote changes at both individual, social, and policy levels (Freimuth and Crouse Quinn, 2004). Key scholars working in the tradition of behavior change and media effects have made persuasive arguments about the need to produce more nuanced, multi-leveled analysis of behavioral determinants, and rethink the meaning of communication interventions to address health challenges. Behavior change theorists have acknowledged the need to conceptualize interventions as part of broad actions for social change in countries with enormous power and social inequalities as well as persistent disparities in access to healthcare. By the same token, single interventions ("campaigns") need to be included as part of comprehensive, collective, and multi-actor strategies to change a range of conditions that negatively affect health. It is not simply about "the power of the media" or one single campaign, but rather, the combined power of broad-based actions.

Approaches grounded in social psychological theories have stressed the need to adopt multiple levels of analysis to address the influence of social and policy factors in health behaviors (Fishbein and Yzer, 2003). Examples are the transtheoretical/stages of change model (Prochaska, Norcross, and DiClemente,1994), and the ecological model (Abroms and Maibach, 2008) which propose ways to address a range of individual, social, and policy factors that affect health behaviors.

Recent studies in global health communication have reached similar conclusions. They make calls for integrated behavioral theories and multivariable analysis to understand communication issues around health practices, and guide interventions (Murray-Johnson *et al.*, 2005; Odutolu 2005; Vijayakumar, 2008) Particularly applied to HIV/AIDS prevention and family planning/reproductive health issues, they subscribe to basic principles of the ecological model on account of its offering an integrated perspective to analyze a range of behavioral determinants. At the individual level, it emphasizes the importance of knowledge and attitudes about transmission, prevention, and care, risk perception about certain practices, self efficacy to successfully implement new behaviors, and perceived norms informing behavioral choices. At the level of social networks, the model stresses the role of partners, family members, and peers in relation to power, trust, influence and gender and other social norms underlying prevention and care practices. At the level of the community, it indicates the need to consider issues related to social capital, participation, empowerment, access to information and resources, and collective attitudes and efficacy to practice and change behaviors. At the societal level, the model emphasizes the need to assess the influence of large social and political structures, the policy and media environment, cultural and religious norms, and economic factors influencing practices related to HIV prevention and care.

Another important point of convergence is the call to theorize the role of community mobilization in processes of behavior change. None other than Albert Bandura (1998), author of seminal writings underpinning behavioral theories in health communication, has stressed the importance of linking health promotion/communication to collective actions for social change and policy to transform environmental/social factors affecting health. Likewise, several studies in global health communication (Rogers and Storey, 1987) have examined the positive impact of collective mobilization. Interest in community mobilization and health communication resonates with a rich literature on community-based health services, and the role of social mobilization in health/development.

Perhaps no area of study in global health communication suggests growing interest in theoretical integration as clearly as research on "education-entertainment" (E-E). E-E has not only become the focus of much attention in the field in the past decades, given its application in family planning, HIV/AIDS and other health programs around the world. Equally important, its intellectual trajectory has made E-E a leading case in assessing the possibilities of blending different theoretical approaches. It has attracted attention from studies informed by different conceptual and epistemological premises (Brown, in Chapter 6 of this volume, provides a detailed account of the evolution and conceptual premises of E-E).

Both the history and key findings of E-E have been extensively analyzed elsewhere. It is generally understood as the application of entertainment strategies to disseminate information in order to promote healthy behaviors and, more broadly, social good. For the purpose of this chapter, it is important to highlight that E-E is a theoretical hybrid embedded in analytical premises from a range of frameworks and models. Miguel Sabido's original ideas drew from Bandura's (1977) social learning theory, specifically, the notion that individuals learn behavior by observing role models in the media. Imitation and influence are the expected outcomes of interventions. Pioneering E-E *telenovelas*, for example, were based on Bandura's model of cognitive subprocesses: attention, retention, production and motivational processes that help understand why individuals imitate socially desirable behavior. This process depends on the existence of role models in the messages: good models, bad models, and those who transition from bad to good. Besides social learning, entertainment-education strategies are based on the idea that expected changes result from self-efficacy, the belief of individuals that they can complete specific tasks (Bandura, 1994; Maibach and Murphy, 1995). Evaluation analyses have concluded that interventions based on E-E principles have had several positive consequences: they prompt conversations about health (including many hard-to-talk-about issues), increase sensitivity about specific issues, and reinforce messages and social norms (Farr *et al.*, 2005; Piotrow *et al.*, 1992; Singhal and Rogers, 1999). Evidence about impact on behavior change, however, is more ambiguous as studies haven't always found significant increase in demand for health services (Yoder, Hornik, and Chirwa, 1996; Westoff and Rodriguez, 1995).

The rich trajectory of E-E illustrates a dynamic process of theoretical borrowing and increased openness to insights from various frameworks. In their landmark book, Singhal and Rogers (1999, p. xii) defined E-E as "the process of purposely designing and implementing a media message to both entertain and educate, in order to increase audience knowledge about an educational issue, create favorable attitudes, and change overt behavior." Later (Singhal and Rogers, 2002), they expanded their original understanding beyond individual-centered knowledge and behaviors to include community and social change and actions.

Recent studies show the possibility of theoretical convergence around E-E. Scholars have praised not only the impact of E-E on collective agency and social change, but also the participatory nature of the design of E-E programs. Research has shown that E-E programs have positive effects, including the activation of social networks and collective efficacy, issues which are critical for promoting wide changes (Papa *et al.*, 2000; Sood, 2002).

Simultaneously, studies informed by critical and participatory theories have assessed the potential of E-E to facilitate opportunities for the expression and empowerment of the disempowered actors. Positions are clearly divided: whereas some scholars recognize that E-E can adequately provide opportunities for participation (Tufte, 2005), others conclude that the epistemological premises and conditions of global health programs hamper the participatory ambitions of E-E. The former position argues that E-E programs offer opportunities for marginalized populations to think critically, gain a better understanding of their circumstances, and become empowered in the process. The experience of Soul City, originally in South Africa and later in other countries in the region, and of the NGO Puntos de Encuentro (Meeting Points) in Nicaragua, powerfully demonstrates the potential of E-E to approach communication within a wide agenda for spearheading social change (Tufte, 2000). Not only it is premised on core emancipatory ideals that put people at the center of social change, it also tackles obstacles at multiple levels. Along similar lines, Jacobson and Storey (2004) have argued that, if they are designed on the basis of participatory premises, E-E experiences can effectively advance ideals of democratic communication.

Dutta (2006) has eloquently expressed reservations about such arguments. For him, E-E is inevitably hamstrung by individualistic and universalistic premises, as well as the overall limitations of health programs supported by international donors. Despite the rhetoric of participation, E-E programs are top-down vehicles for predetermined ideas and agendas that reflect Western interests in the global South. They leave untouched the modernizing ambitions of traditional global health communication. Subaltern groups are not fully involved in the identification of problems and the selection of the strategies best suited to addressing problems of exclusion and disempowerment.

How do we interpret the fact that critical scholars draw opposite conclusions? Scholars like Tufte, Jacobson, Storey, and others who positively assess the potential of E-E to bridge theoretical divides and promote participatory ideals, draw conclusions from single experiences. These experiences show that, indeed, E-E designed with participatory ideals in mind can advance objectives linked to better health and equality. One is left wondering, however, whether E-E necessarily achieves such objectives. Entertainment programs can simply include health/social messages aimed at changing specific health knowledge and attitudes, without being part of collective actions to facilitate critical consciousness, question power inequalities, or modify structural factors. Put it differently, we lack sufficient evidence to conclude inductively from a few cases that E-E interventions necessarily bridge theoretical divides and advance participatory goals. At best, they show the potential of E-E to support different goals and illustrate various theoretical arguments.

Nor does it seem that Dutta's sharp critique applies *in toto* to E-E. The diversity of experiences doesn't lend itself to drawing categorical, normative generalizations. It is a mistake not to differentiate between entertainment programming with social messages broadcast by major, profit-driven media corporations and those aired by rural community-owned radio stations. They are part of very different media structures with different linkages to audiences/communities. E-E is not simply a way to advance commercial goals and deepen the entertainment, profit-driven characteristics of media industries.

Nor is it obvious that, just because E-E programs are funded by major aid donors, they act as the tools of the economic-political forces that perpetuate global health inequalities, or promote a monolithic set of values (e.g., a population control agenda). The reality of health aid programs, including communication experiences, is more messy and unpredictable than Dutta acknowledges. Nothing in the theoretical premises of E-E necessarily tilts the overall experience (from design to broadcast to evaluation) in favor of certain principles. The Soul City experience, for example, foregrounds the participatory ideal in ways that may not be typical across E-E interventions, which mainly aim to modify ideational factors to affect health behaviors. Moreover, if "active audience" theories have it right, just because certain texts are designed to promote certain values (e.g. reproductive health choices, safe sex, family planning), we should not conclude *a priori* that publics wholeheartedly embrace those ideals or adopt them in health practices. In fact, evaluation research echoes arguments about the inherent openness of media texts and the problem of inferring "effects" from the conditions underlying media production or the motivations of media producers. The fact that E-E programs have resulted in contested meanings and conversations, and that participatory evaluation yielded a wealth of complex consequences not predicted during the design phase, should make us cautious about drawing generalizable conclusions. Without comparative analysis across several experiences, we lack sufficient evidence to draw positive or negative conclusions about the impact of E-E.

This debate illustrates the fact that E-E remains a fertile ground not only to explore further the possibilities of combining theoretical traditions, but also to assess how theoretical convergence may be feasible. It encapsulates the theoretical tensions and methodological differences in the field.

Conclusions

Beyond E-E, the field needs to examine a diversity of experiences to assess how theoretical convergence is possible and why it is desirable.

It is important not to lose sight of the fact that, despite growing interest in exploring the possibilities of theoretical convergence, this goal is rarely at the forefront of program design. Frequently, donor-funded programs are mainly driven by short-term and pragmatic considerations. "Theory-testing" is hardly a main priority. This is particularly problematic if future theory-building efforts in global health communication remain largely dependent on aid funding. The question is, then, how scholarly objectives, specifically the continuous need for theory refining and experimentation, can be pursued in the context of aid programs subjected to bureaucratic imperatives and the complex politics of donors and local actors (governments, non-government organizations, the private sector) (Waisbord, 2008). Programs aren't necessarily embedded in critical, participatory principles because stakeholders aren't aware of those premises or narrow theoretical scholarship undergirds conceptual guidelines and design. Rather, too often partners in both the North and the global South are primarily interested in goals, such as program visibility and political gain (Tomaselli, 1997), which are better served by run-of-the-mill, informational interventions rather than innovative programs aimed at testing theoretical breakthroughs and promoting participatory ideals.

Future directions to continue exploring theoretical convergence include conducting comparative research across communities/countries and health issues. The bulk of the literature features single cases at the community or national levels focused on specific health challenges. This division reflects broad compartmentalization of health programs in separated, silo-like structures according to "disease" and "country." Consequently, we have a significant amount of findings by "disease" (HIV/AIDS and family planning/reproductive health surely rank atop), but little comparative research to argue convincingly that theoretical propositions apply across experiences/communities and health issues. This is unfortunate, given that comparative studies may help to test the applicability of theories across programs, and thus produce solid evidence to support broad claims.

One possible path to further cross-theoretical research is to identify common questions that are both theoretically and practically relevant. If research questions remain bounded within the conceptual confines of any given theory, it is unlikely that scholars would try to find theoretical bridges. Theory-specific questions continue to provide much of the intellectual impetus for theory-building in the field (e.g., What works in persuasion? Do communication interventions prompt social networks to talk about health? What leads people to participate in order to redress health conditions? How does health advocacy affect health behaviors?). Therefore, it is not surprising that, like ships passing the night, scholars embedded in different theoretical traditions only occasionally communicate with each other.

From a perspective that believes that global health communication should be linked to broad thinking about social change, we believe that it is important to ask questions that cut across a wide swath of research in the field. To mention some examples: When does collective action make a difference in health conditions? How does communication contribute to promoting and maintaining community participation in health? How do consciousness-raising activities lead people to overcome feelings of disempowerment around health matters? What do we know about effective programmatic sequences to promote changes at individual, social, and policy levels?

Although we believe in the merits of probing the prospects of theoretical convergence, we are mindful about inherent limitations given deep theoretical cleavages in the field Just like the adjacent fields of health communication (Babrow and Mattson, 2003) and communication for global/development and social change (Waisbord, 2000), the prospects for theoretical synthesis are caught in underlying tensions that do not seem easy to resolve. Nor we can expect that theoretical ambitions will be mainly interested in resolving those tensions or addressing the vast range of issues that fall in the agenda of global health communication research.

As long as communication is defined in antithetical terms (information/participation), it seems implausible that different traditions would easily converge on key principles. As long as researchers assume that different health determinants (individual/social/system) should be the focus of theoretical development and practice, it is hard to envision a common set of questions that might bring cross-theoretical collaboration. As long as some scholars remain primarily concerned with questions about information and persuasion, and others prioritize issues of power, resistance, and participation, theoretical cross-pollination seems improbable. As long as there is no consensus on the purpose of academic enterprise in global health communication, whether to support changes in health behaviors, promote health changes through participatory strategies, or question the modernizing goals of health and development programs, the search of common questions and theoretical frameworks is elusive. Put it differently, the persistence of different theoretical questions and research interests, grounded in the multidisciplinary genealogy of the field, undercuts the possibilities for bringing traditions closer together. Despite occasional and valuable ventures across the theoretical divide, conceptual fragmentation and parallel scholarship may still define the field in the future.

Notes

1   It is also important to point out that several studies examining interpersonal communication in medical settings were published around that time. This line of inquiry, however, did not become as influential as socio-psychological approaches in international health communication which has remained focused on mass campaigns and interventions.
2   Since then, global health programs have used social marketing to promote condom use, breast-feeding, and immunization. For Chapman Walsh *et al.* (1993, p. 108), "The first nationwide contraceptive program social marketing program, the Nirodh condom project in India, began in 1967 with funding from the Ford Foundation." The substantial increase in condom sales was attributed to the distribution and promotion of condoms at a subsidized price. The success of the Indian experience informed subsequent social marketing interventions such as the distribution of infant-weaning formula in public health clinics. The application of social marketing wasn't free of criticisms. Analysts questioned the motivations of commercial sponsors to promote health products and the effectiveness of programs. The well-known controversy around the marketing of powdered milk in the global South encapsulated skeptics' doubts about social marketing. They questioned the validity of promoting commercial products at the expense of other healthy practices (e.g. breastfeeding) and the unintended negative consequences in resource-poor settings (e.g. price prompted people to dilute powdered milk; lack of access to safe water to mix formula caused diarrheal diseases).

References

Abroms, L. C. and Maibach, E. W. (2008). The effectiveness of mass communication to change public behavior. *Annual Review of Public Health, 29*, 219–234.

Agha, S, Karlyn, A. and Meekers, D. (2006). The promotion of condom use in non-regular sexual partnerships in urban Mozambique. *Health Policy and Planning, 16*(2), 144–151.

Agha, S. (2003). The impact of a mass media campaign on personal risk perception, perceived self-efficacy and on other behavioral predictors. *AIDS Care, 15*(6), 749–762.

Airhihenbuwa, C. O., Makinwa, B. and Obregon, R. (2000). Toward a new communications framework for HIV/AIDS. *Journal of Health Communication 5*(1), 101–111.

Ajzen, I. (1985). From intentions to actions: A theory of planned behavior. In J. Kuhl and J. Beckmann (Eds.), *Action-Control: From Cognition to Behavior* (pp. 11–39). Heidelberg: Springer.

Andreasen, A. R. (1994). Social marketing: Its definition and domain. *Journal of Public Policy and Marketing, 13*(1), 108–114.

Armitrage, C. J. and Conner, M. (2001). Efficacy of the theory of planned behavior: A meta-analytic review. *British Journal of Social Psychology, 40,* 471–499.

Babrow, A. and Mattson, M. (2003). Theorizing about health communication. In T. Thompson, A. Dorsey, K. Miller and R. Parrott (Eds.), *Handbook of Health Communication* (pp. 35–61). Mahwah, NJ: Lawrence Erlbaum Associates.

Bandura, A. (1963). The role of imitation in personality, *The Journal of Nursery Education, 18*(3), 207–215.

Bandura, A. (1969). Social-learning theory of identificatory processes. In D. A. Goslin (Ed.), *Handbook of Socialization Theory and Research* (pp. 213–262). Chicago: Rand McNally.

Bandura, A. (1971). Analysis of modeling processes. In A. Bandura (Ed.), *Psychological Modeling: Conflicting Theories.* Chicago: Aldine-Atherton.

Bandura, A. (1977). Self-efficacy: Toward a unifying theory of behavioral change. *Psychological Review, 84,* 191–215.

Bandura, A. (1998). Health promotion from the perspective of social cognitive theory. *Psychology and Health, 13*(4), 623–649.

Becker, M. H. and Maiman, L. (1974). The health belief model: Origins and correlates in psychological theory. *Health Education Monographs, 2,* 324–508.

Berry, D. (2004). *Risk, Communication and Health Psychology.* Maidenhead: Open University Press.

Bertrand J. T. (2004). Diffusion of innovations and HIV/AIDS. *Journal of Health Communication, 9*(S1), 113–121.

Bond, K. and Valente, T. W. (1999). Social network influences on reproductive health behaviors in urban northern Thailand. *Social Science and Medicine, 49*(12), 1599–1614.

Boulay, M. and Valente, T. W. (1999). The relationship of social affiliation and interpersonal discussion to family planning knowledge, attitudes and practices. *International Family Planning Perspectives, 25*(3), 112–119.

Brashers, D. and Babrow, A. (1996). Theorizing communication and health, *Communication Studies, 47*(3), 243–251.

Brown, T., Cueto, M., and Fee, E. (2006). The World Health Organisation and the transition from "international" to "global." *American Journal of Public Health, 96*(1), 62–72.

Buhler, C. and Kohler, H. P. (2002). Talking about AIDS: The influence of communication networks on individual risk perceptions of HIV/AIDS infection and favored protective behaviors in South Nyanza District, Kenya. Typescript.

Campbell, C. and Jovchelovitch, S. (2000). Health, community, and development: Towards a social psychology of participation. *Journal of Community and Applied Social Psychology, 10,* 255–270.

Campbell, C. and MacPhail, C. (2002). Peer education, gender and the development of critical consciousness: Participatory HIV prevention by South African youth. *Social Science and Medicine, 55*(2), 331–345.

Chapman Walsh, D., Russ, R. E., Moeykens, B. A., and Moloney, T. W. (1993). Social marketing for public health. *Health Affairs, 12*(2), 104–119.

Cho, H., and Salmon, C. T. (2007). Unintended effects of health communication campaigns. *Journal of Communication, 57,* 293–317.

Craig, R. T. (1993). Why are there so many communication theories? *Journal of Communication, 43*(3), 26–33.

Craig, R. T. (1999). Communication theory as a field. *Communication Theory, 9*(2), 119–161.

Dearing, J. W. (2004). Improving the state of health programming by using diffusion theory. *Journal of Health Communication, 9,* 21–36.

Diop, W. (2000). From government policy to community-based communication strategies in Africa: Lessons from Senegal and Uganda. *Journal of Health Communication,* 5(1 S1), 113–117.

Donohew, L. and Ray, E. B. (1990). *Communications and Health: Systems and Applications.* Hillsdale, NJ: Lawrence Erlbaum Associates.

Donohew, L., Palmgreen, P., and Lorch, E. P. (1994). Attention, need for sensation, and health communication campaigns. *American Behavioral Scientist,* 38, 310–322.

Dutta, M. (2006). Theoretical Approaches to entertainment education campaigns: A subaltern critique. *Health Communication,* 20(3), 221–231.

Dutta, M. and de Souza, R. (2008). The past, present, and future of health development campaigns: Reflexivity and the critical-cultural approach. *Health Communication,* 23(4), 326–339.

Dutta-Bergman, M. (2004). The unheard voices of Santalis: Communicating about health from the margins of India. *Communication Theory,* 14(3), 237–263.

Erni, J. N. (2004) Global AIDS, IT and critical humanism: Reframing international health communication. In M. Semati (Ed.), *New Frontiers in International Communication Theory* (pp., 71–88). Lanham, MD: Rowman and Littlefield.

Farquar, J. W. and Maccoby, N. (1975). Communication for health: Unsettling heart disease. *Journalism of Communication,* 25(3), 114–126.

Farr, A. C., Witte, K., Jarato, K., and Menard, T. (2005). The effectiveness of media use in health education: Evaluation of an HIV/AIDS radio campaign in Ethiopia. *Journal of Health Communication,* 10(3), 225–235.

Fishbein, M. (1980). A theory of reasoned action: some applications and implications. In H. E. Howe, Jr. and M. M. Page (Eds.), *Nebraska Symposium on Motivation, 1979* (pp. 65–116). Lincoln, NB: University of Nebraska Press.

Fishbein, M. (2000). The role of theory. *AIDS Care,* 12(3), 273–278.

Fishbein, M. and Ajzen, I. (1975). *Belief, Attitude, Intention, and Behavior: An Introduction to Theory and Research.* Reading, MA: Addison-Wesley.

Fishbein, M. and Yzer, M. C. (2003). Using theory to design effective health behavior interventions. *Communication Theory,* 13(2), 164–183.

Flay, D. R., Ditecco, D., and Schlegel, R. P. (1980). Mass media in health promotion: An analysis using extended information-processing model. *Health Education Quarterly,* 7(2), 127–147.

Ford N., Odallo, D., and Chorlton, R. (2003). Communication from a human rights perspective: Responding to the HIV/AIDS Pandemic in Eastern and Southern Africa. A working paper for use in HIV and AIDS Programmes. *Journal of Health Communication,* 8(6), 599–612.

Freimuth, V. S. (1990) The chronically uninformed: Closing the knowledge gap in health. In E. B. Ray and L. Donohew (Eds.), *Communication and Health: Systems and Applications* (pp. 171–186). Hillsdale, NJ: Lawrence Erlbaum Associates.

Freimuth, V. and Crouse Quinn, S. (2004). The contributions of health communication to eliminating health disparities, *American Journal of Public Health.* 94(12), 2053–2055.

Gao, M. Y. and Wang, S. (2007). Participatory communication and HIV/AIDS prevention in a Chinese marginalized (MSM) population. *AIDS Care,* 19(6), 799–810.

Glanz, K., Marcus Lewis, F., and Rimer, B. K. (Eds.) (1990). *Health Behavior and Health Education: Theory, Research, and Practice.* San Francisco: Jossey-Bass.

Greene, K., Rubin, D., Hale, J. L., and Walters, L. H. (1996). The utility of understanding adolescent egocentrism in designing health messages. *Health Communication,* 8, 131–152.

Gumucio-Dagron, A. and Tufte, T. (Eds.) (2005). *Communication for Social Change Anthology: Historical and Contemporary Readings.* South Orange, NJ: Communication for Social Change Consortium.

Hagen, E. F. (1962) *On the Theory of Social Change.* Chicago: Dorsey.

Hornik, R. C., McDivitt, J., Zimicki, S. *et al.* (2002). Communication in support of child survival: Evidence and explanation from eight countries. In R. C. Hornik (Ed.), *Public Health Communication: Evidence for Behavior Change* (pp.219–248). Mahwah, NJ: Lawrence Erlbaum Associates.

Jacobson, T. L. and Storey, J. D. (2004). Development communication and participation: Applying Habermas to a case study of population programs in Nepal. *Communication Theory, 14*(2), 99–121.

Janz, N. K. and Becker, M. H. (1984). The health belief model: A decade later. *Health Education and Behavior, 11*(1), 1–47.

Keller, P. A. and Lehmann, D. R. (2008). Designing effective health communications: A meta-analysis. *Journal of Public Policy and Marketing, 27*(2), 117–130.

Kotler, P. (1972). A generic concept of marketing. *Journal of Marketing, 36*(2), 46–54.

Kotler, P. and Zaltman, G. (1971). Social marketing: An approach to planned social change. *Journal of Marketing, 35*(3), 3–12.

Kreps, G. L. (1989). Setting the agenda for health communication research and development: Scholarship that can make a difference. *Health Communication, 1*(1), 11–15.

Kreps, G. L., Bonaguro, E. W., and Query, J. L. Jr. (1998). The history and development of the field of health communication. In L. D. Jackson and B. K. Duffy (Eds.) *Health Communication Research: Guide to Developments and Directions* (pp. 1–15). Westport, CT: Greenwood Press

Kreps, G. L. and Maibach, E. W. (2008). Transdisiciplinary science: The nexus between communication and public health. *Journal of Communication, 58*, 732–748.

Kreuter, M. W., Lukwago, S. N. Bucholtz, D. C. *et al.* (2003). Achieving cultural appropriateness in health promotion programs: Targeted and tailored approaches. *Health Education and Behavior.* 30(2), 133–146.

Kreuter, M. W. and Wray, R. J. (2003). Tailored and targeted health communication: Strategies for enhancing information relevance. *American Journal of Health Behavior, 27*(Supplement 3), 227–232.

Kwadwo, B. (2001). Determinants of condom use intentions of university students in Ghana: An application of the theory of reasoned action. *Social Science and Medicine, 52*(7), 1057–1069.

Lambert, H. and Wood, K. (2005). Comparative analysis of communication about sex, health and sexual health in India and South Africa: Implications for HIV prevention. *Culture, Health and Sexuality, 7*(6), 527–541.

Lapinski, M. K. and Rimal, R. N. (2005). An explication of social norms. *Communication Theory, 15*(2), 127–147.

Lerner, D. (1958). *The Passing of Traditional Society: Modernizing the Middle East.* Glencoe, IL: The Free Press.

Lupton, D. (1994). Toward the development of critical health communication praxis, *Health Communication, 6*(1), 55–67.

Maibach, E. and Parrott, R. (Eds.) (1995). *Designing Health Messages: Approaches from Communication Theory and Public Health Practice.* Thousand Oaks, CA: Sage.

McClelland, D. C. (1961). *The Achieving Society.* Princeton, NJ: Van Nostrand.

McGuire, W. J. (1969). The nature of attitudes and attitude change. In G. Lindzey and E. Aronson (Eds.), *Handbook of Social Psychology*, 2nd edn., vol. 3 (pp. 136–314). Reading, MA: Addison-Wesley.

Melkote, S. R., Muppidi, S. R., and Goswami, D. (2000). Social and economic factors in an integrated behavioural and societal approach to communications in HIV/AIDS. *Journal of Health Communication, 5*, 17–27.

Melkote, S. and Steeves, L. (Eds.) (2001). *Communication for Development in the World: Theory and Practice for Empowerment*, 2nd edn. New Delhi, India: Sage.

Morris, N. (2004). A comparative analysis of the diffusion and participatory models in development communication. *Communication Theory, 13*, 225–248.

Murray-Johnson, L., Witte, K. Boulay, M. *et al.* (2005). Using health education theories to explain behavior change: A cross-country analysis, *International Quarterly of Community Health Education, 25*(2), 185–207.

Noar, S. M. (2006) A 10-year retrospective of research in health mass media campaigns: Where do we go from here? *Journal of Health Communication, 11*(1), 21–42.

Noar, S. M. and Zimmerman, R. S. (2004). Health behavior theory and cumulative knowledge regarding health behaviors: Are we moving in the right direction? *Health Education Research, 20*(3), 275–290.

Novelli, W. D. (1990). Applying social marketing to health promotion and disease prevention. In K. Glanz, F. Marcus Lewis and B. K. Rimer (Eds.), *Health Behavior and Health Education* (pp. 342–369). San Francisco: Jossey-Bass Publishers.

Nussbaum, J. (1989). Directions for research within health communication. *Health Communication, 1*(1), 35–40.

Odutolu, O. (2005). Convergence of behavior change models for AIDS risk reduction in sub-Saharan Africa. *International Journal of Health Planning and Management 20*(3), 239–252.

Papa M. J., Singhal, A., Law, S. *et al.* (2000). Entertainment-education and social change: An analysis of parasocial interaction, social learning, collective efficacy, and paradoxical communication. *Journal of Communication, 50*(4), 31–55.

Parrott, R. (2004). Emphasizing "communication" in health communication. *Journal of Communication, 54*, 751–787.

Pick, S. (2007). Extension of theory of reasoned action: Principles for health promotion programs with marginalized populations in Latin America. In I. Ajzen, D. Albarracin, and R. Hornik (Eds.), *Prediction and Change of Health Behavior: Applying the Reasoned Action Approach* (pp. 223–241). Mahwah: Lawrence Erlbaum Associates

Piotrow, P. and Kincaid, D.L. (2001). Strategic communication for international health programs. In R. Rice and C. Atkin (Eds.), *Public Communication Campaigns*, 3rd edn. (pp. 249–266). Thousand Oaks, CA: Sage.

Piotrow, P., Kincaid D. L., Hindin M. J. *et al.* (1992). Changing men's attitudes and behavior: The Zimbabwe male motivation project. *Studies in Family Planning, 23*(6), 365–375.

Piotrow, P. T., Kincaid, D. L., Rimon, J. G. I., and Rinehart, W. (1997). *Health Communication: Lessons from Family Planning and Reproductive Health*. Westport, CT: Praeger Publishers.

Pratt, C. A., Ha, L., Levine S. R., and Pratt, C.B. (2003). Stroke knowledge and barriers to stroke prevention among African Americans: Implications for health communication. *Journal of Health Communication, 8*(4), 369–381.

Prochaska, J. O., Norcross, J., and DiClemente, C. C. (1994). *Changing for Good: The Revolutionary Program That Explains the Six Stages of Change and Teaches You How to Free Yourself from Bad Habits*. New York, NY: William Morrow and Co., Inc.

Randolph, W., and Viswanath, K. (2004). Lessons learned from public health mass media campaigns: Marketing health in a crowded media world. *Annual Review of Public Health, 25*, 419–37.

Ratzan, S. (1996). The status and scope of health communication. *Journal of Health communication, 1*(1), 25–42.

Robinson, W. C. and Ross, J. A. (Eds.) (2007). *The Global Family Planning Revolution: Three Decades of Population Policies*. Washington, DC: The World Bank.

Rogers, E. M. (1962). *Diffusion of Innovations*. New York: Free Press

Rogers, E. M. (1973). *Communication Strategies for Family Planning*. New York: Free Press.

Rogers, E. M. (1976) (Ed.). *Communication and Development: Critical Perspectives*. Beverley Hills, CA: Sage.

Rogers, E. M. (1986). *Communication Technology: The New Media in Society*. New York: Free Press.

Rogers, E. M. (1994). The field of health communication today. *American Behavioral Scientist*, *38*(2), 208–214.

Rogers, E. M. and Shoemaker, P. (1971). *Communication of Innovations: A Cross-cultural Approach*. New York: Free Press.

Rogers, E. M. and Storey, J. D. (1987). Communication campaigns. In C. R. Berger and S. H. Chafee (Eds.), *Handbook of Communication Science* (pp. 817–846). Thousand Oaks, CA: Sage.

Rosenstock, I. M. (1966). Why people use health services. *Milbank Memorial Fund Quarterly 44*, 94–124.

Rosenstock, I. M. (1974). Historical origins of the health belief model. *Health Education Monographs*, *2*(4), 328–335

Salmon, C. and Atkin, C. (2003). Using media campaigns for health promotion. In T. L. Thompson, A. M. Dorsey, K. I. Miller, and R. Parrott (Eds.), *Handbook of health communication* (pp. 449–472). Mahwah, NJ: Lawrence Erlbaum Associates.

Salmon, C., Wooten, K., Gentry, E., Cole, G., and Kroger, F. (1996). AIDS knowledge gaps in the first decade of the epidemic and implications for future public information efforts. *Journal of Health Communication*, *1*, 141–155.

Schramm, W. (1964). *Mass Media and National Development*. Stanford, CA: Stanford University Press.

Schramm, W. (1971). *The Process and Effects of Mass Communication* (rev. edn.). Urbana, IL: University of Illinois Press.

Servaes, J. (1996). Communication for development in a global perspective. The role of governmental and non-governmental agencies. *Communications*, *21*(4), 407–418.

Servaes, J. (Ed.) (2008). *Communication for Development and Social Change*. London: Sage.

Singhal, A. and Rogers, E. M. (1999). *Entertainment Education: A Communication Strategy for Social Change*. Mahwah, NJ: Lawrence Erlbaum Associates.

Singhal, A., Rogers, E. M., and Sood, M. (1999). The gods are drinking milk! Word-of-mouth diffusion of a major news event in India. *Asian Journal of Communication*, *9*(1), 86–107.

Slater, M. D. (1996). Theory and method in health audience segmentation. *Journal of Health Communication*, *1*(3), 267–284.

Smith, R. A., Downs, E., Witte, K. (2007). Drama theory and entertainment education: exploring the effects of a radio drama on behavioral intentions to limit HIV transmission in Ethiopia. *Communication Monographs*, *74*(2), 133–153.

Smith, R. A., Ferrara, M., and Witte, K. (2007). Social sides of health risks: Stigma and collective efficacy. *Health Communication*, *21*(1), 55–64.

Snyder, L. B. (2007). Health communication campaigns and their impact on behavior, *Journal of Nutrition Education and Behavior*, *39*(2), S32–S40.

Sood, S. (2002). Audience involvement and entertainment-education. *Communication Theory*, *12*(2), 153–172.

Sood, S., Shefner-Rogers C. L., and Sengupta, M. (2006). The impact of a mass media campaign on HIV/AIDS knowledge and behavior change in North India: Results from a longitudinal study. *Asian Journal of Communication*, *16*(3), 231–250.

Storey, D., Boulay, M., Karki, Y. *et al.* (1999). Impact of the integrated Radio Communication Project in Nepal, 1994–1997, *Journal of Health Communication*, *4*(4), 271–294.

Tichenor, P. J., Donohue, G. A. and Olien, C. N. (1970). Mass media flow and differential growth in knowledge. *Public Opinion Quarterly, 34*, 159–170.

Tomaselli, K. (1997). Action research, participatory communication: Why governments don't listen. *African Communication Review, 11*(1),1–9.

Tufte, T. (2001). Entertainment-education and participation, *Journal of International Communication, 7*(2), 25–51.

Tufte, T. (2005). Entertainment-education in development communication: Between marketing behaviors and empowering people. In O. Hemer and T. Tufte, (Eds.), *Media and Glocal Change: Rethinking Communication for Development* (pp. 159–176). Buenos Aires: CLACSO.

Usdin, S., Christofides, N., Malepe, L., and Maker, A. (2000). The value of advocacy in promoting social change: Implementing the new domestic violence act in South Africa. *Reproductive Health Matters, 8*(16), 55–65.

Valente, T. W. (1996). Social network thresholds in the diffusion of innovation. *Social Networks, 18*(1), 69–89.

Valente, T. W., Paredes, P. and Poppe, P. R. (2006). Matching the message to the process: The relative ordering of knowledge, attitudes, and practices in behavior change research. *Human Communication Research, 24*(3), 366–385.

Valente, T. W. and Saba, W. P. (2001). Campaign exposure and interpersonal communication as factors in contraceptive use in Bolivia. *Journal of Health Communication, 6*(4), 303–322.

Vijaykumar, S. (2008). Communicating safe motherhood: Strategic messaging in a globalized world. *Marriage and Family Review, 44*(2 and 3), 173–199.

Waisbord, S. (2000). *Family Tree of Theories, Models and Approaches in Development Communication.* prepared for the Rockefeller Foundation. Retrieved from http://www.communicationforsocialchange.org/pdf/familytree.pdf

Waisbord, S. (2008). The institutional challenges of participatory communication in international aid. *Social Identities, 14*(4), 505–522.

Waisbord, S. (2010). Participatory communication for tuberculosis control in prisons in Bolivia, Ecuador, and Paraguay. *Pan American Journal of Public Health, 27*(3), 168–174.

Waisbord, S., Michaelides, T. and Rasmusson, M. (2007). Communication and social capital in the control of avian influenza: Lessons from behaviour change experiences in the Mekong region, *Global Public Health, 3*(2), 197–213.

Westoff, C. F. and Rodriguez, G. (1995). The mass media and family planning in Kenya. *International Family Planning Perspectives, 21*(1), 26–31.

Witte, K. (1998). A theoretically based evaluation of HIV/AIDS prevention campaigns along the Trans-Africa Highway in Kenya. *Journal of Health Communication 3*(4), 345–363.

Witte, K., and Allen, M. (2000). A meta-analysis of fear appeals: Implications for effective public health campaigns. *Health Education and Behavior, 2*(5), 591–615.

Yoder, P., Hornik, R., and Chirwa, B. (1996). Evaluating the program effects of a radio drama about AIDS in Zambia. *Studies in Family Planning, 27*, 188–203.

Zoller, H. M. and Kline, K. N. (2008). Theoretical contributions of interpretive and critical research in health communication. In C. Beck (Ed.) *Communication Yearbook Vol. 32* (pp. 89–134). Mahwah, NJ: Lawrence Erlbaum Associates.

2

New Perspectives on Global Health Communication
Affirming Spaces for Rights, Equity, and Voices

Collins O. Airhihenbuwa and Mohan J. Dutta

Introduction and Background

Communication represents the undeniable nexus in the production, acquisition, and distribution of knowledge across the globe (Airhihenbuwa, Makinwa, and Obregon, 2000; Dutta and Pal, 2010; Pal and Dutta, 2008a, 2008b). Ultimately, it is through communication that knowledge gets represented globally, and the values attached to it are circulated in the realms of developing policies and interventions targeting global health problems (Dutta, 2008). Health comprises the expression and representation of the totality of the human condition in a society, even though health is typically expressed by the absence or presence of illness and death (Airhihenbuwa, 2007; Thompson, 2003). Since the process of representing knowledge is in itself a production of knowledge, the assumed product location of communication has moved from that of a message to be disseminated among audiences to one of engaging the very processes of producing knowledge about specific subjectivities and political configurations in the global landscape (Dutta, 2010). Increasingly, health (ranging from the physical to the economic, social, mental, and spiritual) has become a defining factor in how we judge the life and indeed the vitality of a community and the agency of the people who live in it (Airhihenbuwa, 2007). Health has also emerged globally as the rationale for the development of global interventions, bringing forth economic, political, social, and cultural interventions that are seemingly deployed to address issues of health (Brown, Cueto, and Fee, 2006; Dutta and Basnyat, 2008a, 2008b, 2008c; Garrett *et al.*, 2009; Koplan *et al.*, 2009). The agency of the people is, in turn, judged by how well they adhere to health information to which they have been exposed or are supposed to have been exposed (Dutta, 2008; Lupton, 1994). All these occur with little attention to how health information and public health agendas are aligned or misaligned with the identity of the

The Handbook of Global Health Communication, First Edition. Edited by Rafael Obregon and Silvio Waisbord.
© 2012 John Wiley & Sons, Inc. Published 2012 by John Wiley & Sons, Inc.

people to whom the information is directed (Airhihenbuwa, 1995, 2007; Airhihenbuwa and Obregon, 2000; Dutta-Bergman, 2004a, 2004b). Also, limited attention is paid to interrogating the marginalizing communicative practices through which public health agendas create and sustain oppressions and economic exploitations across the globe (Dutta, 2008; Zoller and Dutta, 2008a, 2008b). It is not surprising, therefore, that health communication has gained unprecedented attention in how we define and represent identities, cultures, and the role that systems, structures, and language play in identity in general and in the cultural anchors of these identities in particular (Airhihenbuwa, 1995, 2007). The evolution of health communication has also brought a shifting, yet richer, terrain in which matters of culture, identity, politics, and meaning assume a central location in the definition and deployment of public health (Zoller and Dutta, 2008a, 2008b). Especially worth noting in the domain of global productions of knowledge about health are the interpenetrations of power and control in determining both the scope of health communication and, simultaneously, the policies and interventions that are then deployed in order to address global health challenges (Dutta, 2006, 2007, 2008, 2010; Prasad, 2009). These challenges present questions such as: What are the communicative practices and processes through which public health agendas are determined, problems framed, and correponding solutions articulated? How do these communicative productions of knowledge about public health policies and practices engage with increasing global inequalities and the marginalization of the poor against the backdrop of global neoliberal governance? And what, specifically, are the possibilities for social change and structural transformation, having regard to the material and symbolic markers of inequalities constituted in the neoliberal economic order?

A critical aspect of this necessary and emerging new terrain of health communication has been tocentralize the identity of those in whom knowledge has been produced – even though their voices have never been acknowledged – so as to create entry points that celebrate their own agency in the production of health and communication knowledge (Airhihenbuwa *et al.*, 2009; Dutta, 2008; Dutta-Bergman, 2004a, 2004b). Noting the inequalities in the material and symbolic terrains of health communication theory and praxis, a growing body of scholarship in health communication foregrounds the capacity of local communities to actively participate in determining health choices that are meaningful to the communities locally (Dutta-Bergman, 2004a, 2004b; Yehya and Dutta, 2009). The emphasis, therefore, is on the capacity of community members to actively participate in defining the scope of health problems that are relevant to them and determining corresponding and equally relevant solutions. To arrive at this culture-centered voicing of articulations that have historically been rendered silent has meant realigning the epistemic landscape that defines and shapes health communication globally (Dutta, 2008; Airhihenbuwa, 2007). Culture-centered projects of health communication point toward a fundamental restructuring of health communication theory and practice, with the focus placed on the participatory and self-determinatory capacity of local communities to serve as active agents in the determination of their health choices, and on individual and collective rights to health care, health policies, and specific health communication programs (Dutta, 2008).

The critical thoughts noted in this chapter represent an epistemic redirection that at once renegotiates the boundaries and essence of health communication while rendering them always promising and seamless. There is no doubt that the recognition of identity and language as critical to our understanding of communication and health has ushered in a renewed and galvanizing interest in health communication, particularly with a focus on culture (Airhihenbuwa, 2007; Dutta, 2008). The question of how culture defines, and is defined by, health and communication also means a welcome opportunity to examine the question of where cultural identity is best located on the health communication landscape. A location where health and communication intersect with culture and identity offers great promise not only of showcasing how matters of culture are important in health communication, but also of unpacking the often loaded representations of identity and culture into operative codes. These codes are then used to develop solutions that are culturally sensitive and culturally appropriate, while asking health and communication and other health professionals to become culturally competent and engaged with structures in the contexts of human rights, capacities, and access to basic health resources (Dutta, 2008; Gruskin, Mills, and Tarantola, 2007). As argued by Airhihenbuwa (2007), competency, for example, assumes a threshold above which professionals can claim to have mastered the skills necessary to address a particular area of knowledge deficit. Thus, cultural competency has limited utility in health communication since it focuses on individual-level (professional, client, or community member) analysis such as how a professional needs to communicate with a client or a community. In this chapter, we present strategies that offer a multilevel strategy to address the centrality of culture in health communication programs, the articulations of health care policies, frames of human rights in health care, and the politics of structural transformation (Airhihenbuwa 1995, 2007; Dutta, 2006, 2007, 2008, 2009, in press). Such an approach necessarily requires an examination of health meanings in the context of systems, structures, languages, and communities for a robust analysis of how and where health, communication, culture, and identity converge, and the processes through which academic–community partnerships create avenues for disrupting the inequities that are perpetuated through neoliberal health care policies and practices (Airhihenbuwa, 2007; Dutta, 2008).

A cultural approach examines structures and systems to offer meanings to cultural sensitivity, and to situate meanings within articulations of power, control, and resistance. Thus, sensitivity is not discounted, but rather presented in its distinctive role within a culture-centered analysis, as an entry point to interrogating the structures that constitute health (see Dutta, 2007). As noted by Airhihenbuwa (1995, 2007), culture is at the core of language and communication about health and other values that are central to our world. Thus, to understand culture is to understand the structure, systems, and language with which experiences are shared and values are transmitted. To engage health communication scholarship at the birth of an era of increased globalization and increased representation of minorities in US culture means that interdependency becomes the reality of the future. In an interdependent world, the student and scholar of the future will be the one who may not know a language but understands the process by which a culturally anchored communication of health is produced (Airhihenbuwa, 2007; Dutta, 2008, 2009, in press). It is the educators and teachers who have profound appreciation for how group identity is not only about the ability to translate health messages into another language, but also about understanding the role that language plays in the structures and systems that nurture particular forms of producing, transmitting, and acquiring knowledge. This emphasis on the contexts of health and behavior, rather than on the individual decisions of individual actors, was the conclusion that was reached in 1999 in a UNAIDS project in which Airhihenbuwa and colleagues developed and published a new framework on health communication processes and strategies for Africa, Asia, Latin America, and the Caribbean (Airhihenbuwa *et al.*, 1999; Airhihenbuwa, Makinwa, and Obregon, 2000). In this chapter, we bring together a review of emerging scholarship to help frame and shape future thinking in health communication. As a collective, these scholars have brought to us fresh insights into the processes and strategies for health communication in the new millennium. Through their collective voices, the reader should have a deeper appreciation of how health, communication, identity, and culture cohabit to frame our contexts and how we relate in these contexts.

Theoretical Entrypoints to Global Health Communication

The emerging theoretical approaches to global health communication constitute a communicative lens for understanding the public health landscape of the globe. These approaches simultaneously depart from existing health communication approaches by going beyond the message-based framework embodied in health interventions to look at the communicative processes through which specific interpretations of health are circulated in health policies and programs (Airhihenbuwa, Makinwa, and Obregon, 2000; Basu and Dutta, 2009; Dutta, 2008). The communicative lens foregrounds the interpretive processes through which specific sets of meanings of health are privileged while others are backgrounded or erased. It is within this dynamic relationship between the material and symbolic realms of representation that health policies are introduced, disseminated, circulated, and reified. It is through communicative processes that specific forms of governance and public health policies are diffused within the broader populations of funders, program planners, policy makers, etc. Therefore, health communication is constituted in the processes of interpretation, collaboration, and transformative politics that are directed toward challenging and changing the unhealthy structures within which experiences of health at the margins are situated.

Structures of inequity

Increasingly, health communication scholars have drawn attention to the unequal structures within which experiences of health are situated (Dutta, 2007, 2008, 2009; Dutta-Bergman, 2004a, 2004b). The emphasis on these unequal structures calls attention to the political and economic foundations of the inequalities perpetuated through unhealthy policies across the globe, drawing out the linkages between economics and health (Coburn, 2000, 2004). Health outcomes are constituted amidst the neoliberal logics of contemporary governance that place increasing emphasis on the privatization of resources, minimization of state intervention and regulation, and the minimization of barriers to foreign trade and investment. Neoliberal governance perpetuates the hegemony of transnational capitalism by emphasizing the privatization of the lifeworld of citizens across the globe, turning them into consumers of commodities manufactured by transnational companies (TNCs). The commoditization of health has been shaped by the increasing emphasis on the technologies of health that can be purchased by consumers in the global South, thus creating markets for TNCs. Worth noting are the linkages between global foundations such as the Bill and Melinda Gates Foundation and TNCs such as GlaxoSmithKline. Also relevant are the tremendous stores of power in the hands of global TNCs as they take over the center of policy making on health issues, thus serving as the conduits for the neoliberalization of global health.

Public health scholars studying the health effects of neoliberal governance point out that neoliberalism has been accompanied by increasing gaps between the rich and the poor, the increasing marginalization of the poor, and the increasing lack of access to basic health care infrastructures among the poorer sectors of global economies (Millen and Holtz, 2000; Millen, Irwin, and Kim, 2000). Specifically, the global diffusion of neoliberalism through the structural adjustment programs (SAPs) pushed by international financial institutions (IFIs) has resulted in increasing unemployment, poverty, and deprivation in the agricultural sectors in the global South. A communicative lens on these structural constraints attached to neoliberalism examines the ways in which the rhetoric of neoliberalism is perpetuated globally, while at the same time erasing the narratives of structural violence that are tied to the oppressions created by neoliberal governance (Farmer, 1992, 1999, 2003). Attention is drawn to exploring the ironies written into neoliberal discourses of empowerment, democracy, and participation, which foreground the local community as an entry point for the commodities manufactured by TNCs (Dutta and Basnyat, 2008a, 2008b). Empowered communities are defined in terms of their capacity to participate in the market economy and to purchase commodities. In the domain of health, the language of empowerment shifts responsibility for health infrastructures into the hands of local communities, thus drawing attention away from the role of the state in creating health infrastructures and capacities. Communities become the focus of interventions that promote individual behaviors and lifestyle changes without attending to the structural elements of neoliberalism that create and sustain the unhealthy conditions. In response to this erasure of structures from neoliberal frameworks of health promotion, critical health communication theorists increasingly draw attention to the need for theorizing the role of structures in understanding marginalizing processes in health care (Airhihenbuwa, 2007; Dutta, 2008, 2010; Ford and Airhihenbuwa, 2010).

Human rights and the politics of identity

Health scholars studying human rights articulate health as a right, and note that individuals and collectives ought to have specific rights in the context of their health (Gruskin, Mills, and Tarantola, 2007; Mann et al., 1999). Whereas the health-as-a-human-right frame on the one hand draws attention to explicit forms of violence such as torture, state-sponsored murder, state-sponsored interrogation techniques, rape, etc. that threaten health (Hargreaves and Cunningham, 2004; Miles, 2004), on the other hand, the frame also attends to the fundamental absence of basic human rights in the domain of access to health resources (Gruskin, Mills, and Tarantola, 2007; Mann *et al.*, 1999). Mann and colleagues (1999) articulate the relationship of health and human rights in terms of the effects on health of the promotion, delivery, and absence of human rights, as well as the effects on human rights of public health policies and health promotion programs.

The debate around human rights in the context of health and communication at the global level has centered on the tension between individual rights and group rights (An-Na' im and Hammond, 2002; Ignatieff, 2001). The WHO definition of health notes the right of every human being to the highest attainable level of health, laying out the role of governments in terms of creating structures and processes that promote the human right to health. The ensuing responsibility of the state for the health of its citizens also means that it is obliged to provide health coverage to individuals as of right regardless of the cost of services or the nature of services needed. Beyond the responsibility of states, the debate on the binarism, individual versus group, has been most salient in cultures (Africa, Asia, Latin American, Caribbean and their diasporas in Western countries) where identity operates at the group level. When questions arise about the failure of the health care system to care for US ethnic minorities, a typical universalist response is that individuals should do more to help themselves. It has been documented that a history of institutional racism and structural discrimination accounts for much of the persistent health inequity between different groups in the United States and whites (Ford and Airhihenbuwa, 2010). Moreover, the right of the individual is only as attainable as the rights of the group with which the individual identifies. For example, certain gendered issues that are of interest to civil societies invite the question of where individual rights end and group rights begin. Issues of gender roles and the position of women in society are common sites of contestation over rights. Beyond the popular ones that focus on African female genitalia or the status of women in marriage, there are several other sites of contestation over individual versus group rights globally. Examples include the right to refuse to allow one's child to be immunized against childhood diseases, the right to refuse blood transfusion, the right of women to wear the Muslim face veil in France, and the right of individual Catholics to use condoms when the church is against it.

A cultural interrogation of human rights discourses situates human rights in a pivotal position between the symbolic representations that constitute health for individuals and groups, drawing attention to the ways in which human rights claims are made by activist and advocacy groups in the context of harmonizing local and global structures. The popular expression "to think globally and act locally" is advanced readily, even though the local considers the global to be a structural and systemic erasure of its space and voice. Whereas, on the one hand, human rights frames resist the political and economic agendas of transnational hegemony, those very same frames often get utilized to carry out further agendas of human rights violations through economic policies of liberalization and privatization. A cultural approach offers strategies to unpack the tension in the individual versus group rights debate by engaging with the dynamic and constitutive relationships between the local and global sites of enunciation in processes of social change and structural transformation.

Erasure of cultures

Whereas structures are typically missing from the dominant discourses of health communication and health promotion, also absent are the multiple cultural entry points to meanings of health (Airhihenbuwa, 1995, 2007; Dutta, 2008). Based on Enlightenment logic, specific locally situated interpretations of health are circulated as universals, based on West-centric articulations and understandings of health situated amidst the centers of power. The universal effectiveness of Enlightenment logic lies in the erasure of the culturally situated roots of Enlightenment concepts and in the artic- ulation of these concepts as value-free science. Who gets to define the scope and mean- ing of health is intrinsically tied to the positions of power in global discursive spaces, with the logic of the sender and receiver of health interventions being shaped by the political and economic agendas of dominant power structures. Hegemonic configura- tions of health rooted in Western ontologies are diffused as the markers of develop- ment, thus driving an entire industry of top-down health interventions based on assumptions of the universalizing of theory from the West directed toward spaces in the Third World. Cultural interpretations and meanings are erased from the discursive spaces of health interventions that operate in the realms of legitimacy through appeal to the language of rational science.

As noted by Airhihenbuwa (1995, 2007), most theories of health communication and health promotion operate on the basis of fundamental West-centric assumptions about human values and human behavior. For example, conventional theories of health promo- tion such as the health belief model and the theory of reasoned action are essentially individualistic in their conceptualization, focusing on the individual and his or her behav- ior (Airhihenbuwa and Obregon, 2000; Dutta-Bergman, 2005). The decision making is situated at the individual level, thus completely ignoring the cultural variability across various spaces of the globe in how health decisions are made. The unit of analysis is the individual, and health decisions are conceptualized as individual-level decisions situated outside the contexts of the collective. Although individualism here is very much a cultur- ally situated value and lies at the heart of the conceptualization of the dominant theories of health communication, it remains hidden from the discursive spaces of health commu- nication theorizing. In effect then, the hegemony of West-centric health communication theorizing is carried out through the erasure of culturally anchored individual value bases, which makes them seem to be universals, the markers of human progress and rationality.

In instances when culture is indeed taken into account, it is conceptualized as a vari- able that operates as a barrier to the effective dissemination of the intervention in the target population (see Airhihenbuwa 2007; Dutta, 2008; Dutta and Basu, in press). Cultural categories are treated as static entities on the basis of value-based ontological schemes imposed by Western experts who study the relevant cultural characteristics in order to generate health messages that target the barriers to the adoption of the health behavior in the population. Culture here is conceptualized as antithetical to the ration- ality of Enlightenment thinking, as something that needs to be overcome through messages disseminated by campaign planners. The effectiveness of an intervention depends upon its ability to address the culture. The goal of the intervention then is to address the culturally situated barriers that prevent the widespread adoption of the behavior. Worth noting once again is the expert position of the sender of the message situated in the West who gets to observe the behavior, script it, develop categorical schemes, and then target the population with the intervention. The voice that is privileged is still the voice of the West-centered expert working in the Western academy or at an international institution in the West. Missing from the discursive spaces are voices and interpretive frameworks of cultural members of the global South, who get framed as passive objects of interventions. Postcolonial criticisms of the global arena of knowledge production in health communication raise questions about the absence of scholars and theories emanating from the global South from the mainstream platforms of health communication (books, journals, conferences, etc.). What are the implications of these absences? What are the implications of the geospatial biases in the representation of certain sectors of the globe as producers of knowledge whereas other sectors are rendered invisible? What are the political implications of such power differentials in knowledge production, especially as knowledge defines the terrains of policy and praxis? Increasingly, cultural theories of health communication seek to address this erasure of culture from the spaces of knowledge production in health arenas by foregrounding methodologies for listening to the voices of cultural communities. Also, the increasing presence of scholars from the Third World/South in academic spaces in the West has created openings for postcolonial interventions that have started critically engaging with the values embedded in health interventions.

Cultural identities

Culture offers a critical gateway through which human interactions occur and is the context within which such relationships are framed and defined (Airhihenbuwa, 2007). The location of culture in health communication has assumed centrality in communication discourses in the past decades. The reasons for this centrality can be traced to the call for alternatives to the individual-centered logic of conventional models and theories that have dominated the health and communication intellectual landscape on the one hand, and the increased echo of the voices of the subaltern in framing a new approach on the other. The PEN-3 (Airhihenbuwa, 1995, 2007) cultural model and the culture-centered approach to health communication intervention are two examples of alternative turned central approaches to knowledge production that not only critique the limits of conventional models but offer more robust frameworks for understanding the importance and critical nature of culture in health communication.

Cultural identity, therefore, becomes a primary anchor on which behaviors and ideas are shared as forms of communication either interpersonally or through media. This broader approach to addressing the context of health communication was the subject of the UNAIDS/Penn State communication framework for HIV and AIDS published in 1997 (Airhihenbuwa, Makinwa, and Obregon, 2000). In this framework, culture was identified as one of the five main domains of contexts that defined behaviors and communication related to prevention and care for HIV and AIDS. Although government and policy, social economic status, gender, and spirituality were identified along with culture as the five critical domains, it was clear that culture was the cross-cutting domain that defined each of the other domains both in terms of their meaning and their relevance to communication. For example, government policy around HIV disclosure in South Africa requires that no-one living with HIV and AIDS should be identified without their consent. But some elders in communities in South Africa wondered how this policy intersected or conflicted with the cultural expectation that requires or obligates them to call a family meeting once it is determined that a member of the family is sick and needs help (Airhihenbuwa *et al.*, 2009). Both policy and culture provide frameworks for the protection of members of society. Policy tends to focus on individuals, while culture focuses on the collective. The individual does not usually reject the protection of the culture unless such protection requires him or her to sacrifice their privacy. Socioeconomic status is another domain of importance in terms of individual resources to support treatment and care at the individual level and sustain the provision of affordable drugs at the policy level. However, the bimodal distribution of HIV and AIDS in South Africa (the very poor and the very rich have the highest risk) suggests that the message of prevention should target not only the poor but also the rich who have resources to travel and visit multiple risk environments (Shisana *et al.*, 2005). This bimodal distribution tends to typify the two visible classes observed in poorly resourced countries – the haves and the have-nots. However, while the rich are considered to have agency, the poor are considered to be voiceless, and yet the work of Dutta and Basu revealed that the poor and vulnerable such as sex workers have agencies. These agencies must be given space to have a voice so that effective communication strategies can emerge. Gender – and specifically the role of women – is another domain in the framework. The agency of womanhood and motherhood has such deep cultural meanings that the important contributions of motherhood have been ignored in HIV and AIDS literature (Iwelunmor, Zungu, and Airhihenbuwa, 2010). When women are framed as vulnerable and in need of help from civil society, their multiple roles as daughters, sisters, aunts, wives and mothers are fused into a single wasteland of powerlessness. Yet one of the most powerful and critical agencies of women is motherhood. A cultural model offers an opportunity to capture the power and strength inscribed in such an agency in ways that are ignored in the conventional individual-based social psychological models. Spirituality is the final domain of interest in the framework and arguably the one that is not discernable without an understanding of the culture that defines it. Spirituality is as much a cultural value as it is a cultural practice. The US Native American spiritual worldview centralizes the earth as its core, compared to Christianity that centralizes the individual, particularly the child.

Values in health

As noted in the previous section, the dominance of specific configurations of health promotion is tied to the dominance of specific sets of values as the markers of progress. Although typically taken for granted in the spheres of articulation of health, it is worth noting that particular frameworks of health that are circulated in certain interventions are situated within specific constellations of values (Dutta, 2008). These values then determine the evaluative framework that is attached to interventions, the ways in which the objectives are established, strategies are determined, tactics are employed, and programs are implemented. For example, the values of conquering germs underlying Western biomedicine frame much of the public health agenda of contemporary global institutions as opposed to values of harmony, balance, and synergy. The war metaphor predominates in much of the public discursive space around health. Simultaneously, the political economy of the contemporary public health industry is driven by the global security frame, constituting health as an issue of global security and defining public health agendas as germ warfare. The privileging of a specific set of values then determines the entire landscape of health communication and health intervention, the ways in which human beings are conceptualized, the articulation of their relationship with their environment, and the specific solutions that are proposed for the challenges facing communities across the globe.

A global awareness of health communication draws attention to the contested terrains of values, thus creating openings for the explicit articulations of values underlying specific solutions being proposed and the creation of opportunities for engagement in dialectical-dialogical conversations about these values. The culturally situated nature of health communication is highlighted in the discursive space, thus creating frames for understanding the cultural foundations of multiple health communication principles that are otherwise circulated as scientific universals. Health communication knowledge is no longer treated as sacred and beyond interrogation, but rather becomes a dynamic and contested terrain for the articulation of multiple values from multiple worldviews. The goal here is to create entry points for diverse forms of knowledge about health, particularly attending to those values that have historically been erased by hegemonic Western discourses of health. Subaltern rationalities find their entry points into the landscape of values, thus creating opportunities for shaping alternative value frames for the articulation of health. Other ways of theorizing, measuring, and practicing health are foregrounded within the discursive space as legitimate ways of knowing, engaged in dialogue with mainstream platforms of health.

Methodological Issues

As opposed to dominant approaches to health communication that take an intervention-based approach to solving health problems based on top-down assessments of problems and corresponding solutions, emerging approaches to health communication highlight the relevance of community-based strategies for participating in processes of structural transformation. Because these emerging approaches emphasize the intersections of the community and structural transformations, the methodologies of critical health communication theorists emphasize solidarity and reflexivity. It is in friendships with local communities that challenge the dominant assumptions of expertise that spaces are created for transformations in unhealthy global structures. Furthermore, given the multiple engagements of critical approaches to health communication with a variety of stakeholders, the emphasis of such approaches is on using multiple modes of knowing to participate in the co-creation of knowledge.

Multimodal approaches

Cocreation of knowledge in dialogue with the subaltern sectors of the globe is dependent upon the ability of health communication scholars to deconstruct mainstream knowledge configurations, precisely through engagement with methodologies that are quintessential to the development of arguments in the mainstream. This calls for critical health communication scholarship to be engaged in the very languages of articulation that are accessible to the mainstream platforms. Methodological access to such language creates the space for rendering impure the mainstream theories of health, raising fundamental questions about the claims of effectiveness and effects that often go unchallenged in the community of expert campaign planners in spite of evidence to the contrary. Therefore, critical engagements in health communication raise questions about the measures of effects and effectiveness, and furthermore situate these questions of effects against the backdrop of a wide variety of outcome measures. Questions are also raised about the sustainability of interventions in bringing about long-term changes in communities through intervention-based approaches to public health. The adoption of multiple methods fosters the journey between the local and the global. The rich in-depth articulations of the local are complemented by the quantitative articulations in global spaces that harness the potential for structural transformation through the processes of listening to the local narratives of local communities. The harmonious relationship among multiple methods creates entry points for social change by capitalizing on the strengths of multiple methods to put forward arguments on global stages that render impure the traditional categories of conceptualization and measurement.

Reflexivity

The complicity of academic structures in the perpetuation of structural and communicative marginalization by neoliberalism calls for the continual interrogation of the oppressive elements of dominance and control that are embedded in the academic processes of knowledge production. Therefore, reflexivity fundamentally turns the historically outward-driven lens inward, raising the questions "Who gets to produce knowledge?" "With what agendas?" and "What are the implications of the violence enacted in the privileging of certain knowledge claims over others?" The taken-for-granted notions of the inherent altruism in academic knowledge production of interventions are interrogated, attending to questions of power and control. Attention is drawn to the privilege written into the position of the scholar, and the ways in which this privilege is complicit in the creation of global inequalities.

The deconstruction of altruistic interventions draws emphasis to the political economy of the interventions industry, demonstrating the ways in which the very expertise of the scholar amidst West-centric structures is tied to the erasure of subaltern voices from global discursive spaces. This erasure is quintessential to the deployment of expert-driven interventions that perpetuate the violence of the dominant structures by continuing to reify the marginalization of the subaltern sectors. Therefore, critical engagements with health communication in the globalization landscape continually interrogate the ways in which the position of the scholar is tied to the perpetuation of global inequities, raising questions about voice, access, and the politics of scholarship in the production of inequities.

Reflexivity is built on the quest to continually undo one's privilege as a scholar based on deep awareness of the impossibilities of listening to the "other" that are written into expertise-driven models of scholarship. The traditional tendencies to impose knowledge on subaltern communities based on the distanced and objective nature of the knowledge in question are brought under scrutiny, with a focus on fostering openings for listening that are attentive to local community needs. The quest for reflexivity is founded on the principles of humility and self-reflection, encouraging the scholar to continually consider the ways in which her/his politics of scholarship can coparticipate in undoing the erasures that have historically marginalized spaces of knowledge production in mainstream structures.

Solidarity

Because the cultural approach to health communication continually seeks to nurture spaces for the articulation of alternative rationalities from those spaces that have historically been placed at the margins of mainstream discursive spaces, one of the core methodological tools of a cultural approach is solidarity. Solidarity refers to the networks of friendship and mutual support that are created among partners, and, in this context, is descriptive of the relationship of partnership that is created between academic and community partners with the goal of disrupting inequitable knowledge structures and creating alternative entry points for subaltern rationalities. Solidarity reflects the principle of working together and, therefore, methodologically defines the scope of health communication projects in terms of their ability to work together with local communities in building the capacities of the latter. Once the specific structures are identified, health communication programs are then directed toward transforming these structures, and the scholar stands as a co-participant with the community in identifying resources and developing strategies for challenging these structures.

Entrypoints for Praxis

Culturally based health promotion

An important premise of health promotion is the pivotal role of social and physical environments in promoting health. At its core is the role of culture in shaping the values and meanings embodied in those social and physical environments (Airhihenbuwa and Obregon, 2000). There is much written today about the built environment. In Amsterdam, bicycling is a part of the culture and thus having bicycle paths is very important, perhaps more important than having automobile routes. In France, having wider sidewalks for pedestrians is a critical aspect of city design. In the United States the centrality of the automobile in the industrial growth of the country has also meant that catering for it assumes dominance over provision for other systems of individual transport, such as the bicycle, that may be more health-promoting. In each of these countries, the cultural production of movement has become a central aspect of how daily living is organized, how new structures for public health improvements are advanced, and indeed how communication is structured. The national epidemic of obesity in the United States, for example, requires a careful examination of how systemic behaviors have been cultured in ways that define and differentiate population health and wellness. Obesity has differential levels of severity in these three countries, and their social and physical structures have much to do with behaviors that have led to obesity, from food production and consumption to energy expenditure as a part of transportation, and even how we co-construct and communicate about health and disease. The critical role of culture in health promotion is a premise on which the PEN-3 (Airhihenbuwa, 2007) model was based. The PEN-3 model was developed to engage communities at multiple levels of their lives. In PEN-3, one always begins with the positive aspects of the community and its culture and people. This critical departure from individual-based psychological models posits that there are positive elements in every community and these positive cultural values are the elements on which sustainable health communication interventions are based. In PEN-3, researchers that fail to identify the positive aspects of the culture may eventually contribute to the problem that brought them to the community in the first place.

Culture-centered health communication

The cultural centering in the PEN-3 model is further built upon in the culture-centered approach, which puts forward the argument that the praxis of health communication ultimately ought to emerge from within local communities, through the participation of local community members in projects that are directed toward addressing problems that are most relevant to their community (Basu and Dutta, 2008a, 2008b, 2009; Dutta-Bergman, 2004a, 2004b). Therefore, the praxis of health communication is centered in the local culture, with local communities defining the scope of the problem and the specific range of solutions to be applied in the health communication intervention. Culture here is not simply a static set of values, beliefs, and practices, but rather a dynamic and communicatively constituted field that is continually negotiated by cultural members (Airhihenbuwa, 1995, 2007; Dutta and Basnyat, 2008c). In this sense, culture is both constitutive and transformative, at once creating the broader framework for communicative practices and at the same time being actively constituted through communicative practices. Culture becomes meaningful in the shifting local context, rendered visible in the interpretive frames of local communities.

The intervention, rather than being a tool of the expert targeted toward the community, becomes a tool in the hands of the community directed toward specific structures in order to address the health needs that are most salient to the community. The role of the academic partner then is one of working with the community to identify and create resources that fulfill local needs. The emphasis, therefore, is continually on the capacity of the community to define the scope of its problems and to create strategies and tactics to address these problems. Local agency is conceptualized as perhaps the most important tool in the creation of knowledge, and the rationality of local voices is privileged in the definition of health problems and solutions over universally circulated biomedical and public health interpretations.

The so-called scientific foundations of traditional health interventions are questioned in terms of their legitimacy (for instance, referring to the actually fairly small and short-term effect sizes of traditional campaigns). Instead, it is argued that valuable resources should be placed in the hands of the local communities so that they can work together in addressing the health issues that fall within the definitional realms of local communities. The deconstructive element of the culture-centered approach, therefore, continually questions the legitimacy of the so-called science of traditional health interventions, pointing out that the science is situated within specific political and economic configurations and draws upon certain cultural markers. For example, the interrogation of the actual effect sizes and sustainability of traditional health interventions draws attention to the unscientific basis of the "science of interventions," the legitimacy of which is often based on the political and economic powers of the interventions industry rather than on the foundations of scientific evidence. Such deconstructions create openings for disrupting the unchallenged hegemony of the techno-scientific apparatus in public health, and for listening to the voices of local communities as legitimate producers of knowledge. Even more, the culture-centered deconstructions draw attention to the postcolonial nature of health interventions, the racist and imperial underpinnings of many health discourses, and the violence enacted in the erasure of local communities. Deconstruction of the participatory rhetoric of traditionally top-down health interventions demonstrates the ways in which the languages of participation and democracy have been co-opted within neoliberal health discourse to serve the political-economic and geostrategic agendas of neo-imperial powers. Participation is turned into a tool for accessing the new subaltern and for turning her into a market for the commodities of neoliberalism.

Building on the space that is opened up through the deconstructive move, culture-centered projects engage in co-creating participatory spaces in solidarity with local communities in order to listen to their voices in the articulation of health problems and the formulation of corresponding solutions. The local community becomes the focal point of knowledge production, with the aim of shifting participatory decision-making capacities into the hands of community members. Simultaneously, the scholar shifts his or her role to one of listening and primarily works with the community in creating community capacities and working to address structures. Structures here refers to the organizations, institutions, and processes that constrain or enable the capacity of the community to seek out health resources. Therefore, health communication scholars work with the community in negotiating and transforming these structures so that health solutions conceived by the community become achievable. In this domain, the culture of the community is defined as a dynamic and shifting space where local voices are articulated. Therefore, the academic–community partnership focuses on foregrounding these voices so that they may create entry points for transforming structures. Agency is defined in terms of the capacity of the community to participate in creating interpretive frames that are meaningful to community members and in engaging with these frames to bring about changes in structures. The emphasis on agency in the culture-centered approach hinges on the notion that listening to the voices of local community members is the first step toward addressing inequities in health. The communicative erasure of local communities is resisted, and it is through this very resistance that avenues are created for addressing structural violence and global inequalities in health care.

Health activism

The emphasis of the culture-centered approach on engaging with structures is further built upon in projects of health activism that emphasize processes of social change directed at transforming unequal structures across the globe (Zoller, 2005). Health care activism takes a resistive stance to the traditional structures of health, noting the inequities perpetuated by neoliberal structures and therefore seeking to create conditions for better health by fundamentally challenging these inequities. The health as a human right frame creates spaces for structurally directed activist politics of social change (Gruskin, Mills, and Tarantola, 2007). Health is approached within the broader social, cultural, economic, and political context, and the emphasis of projects of health activism is on transforming the sociopolitical contexts of health. Explicit emphasis is placed on negotiating the terrains of power and control that shape the landscape of health communication, with an emphasis on creating resources and structures for ensuring the fundamental rights of communities and individuals to the basic capacities of health (Gruskin, Mills, and Tarantola, 2007; Mann and Tarantola, 1998). Therefore, for Zoller (2005), health activism is some form of explicit challenge to the status quo and the ways in which the status quo has fostered a lack of access to health care. Existing relationships of power are challenged, with an emphasis on bringing about changes in the ways in which these relationships foster inequities and are detrimental to the health of communities. For example, the Sonagachi HIV/AIDs Intervention Project (SHIP) articulated its health activism through the participation of sex workers in challenging the unequal structures of health and terrains of power surrounding sex work (Basu and Dutta, 2009).

Projects of health communication that take on an activist stance emphasize communicative processes of organizing in order to build collectives and create collective resources that are then directed toward challenging unequal structures. Emphasis is placed on communicative processes of mobilizing and organizing in order to pull together resources and build collective capacities in seeking changes in unequal structures. Activist projects begin with the questioning of the individual lifestyle approach to health, advocating instead a structurally based approach that examines the deeper structural factors underlying lack of access to health and seek to change these structural factors. Once specific structural determinants of health have been identified, health activist projects work toward bringing about changes in these determinants through rhetorical strategies that are structurally based. Zoller (2005) defines the processes of activist organizing in terms of issue identification, articulation of an interpretive frame for understanding the causation of health and illness, the construction of solutions, followed by public appeals.

Conclusion

In this chapter we have drawn upon the emerging scholarship in health communication to situate the discussion of the theorizing, methodology, and application of health communication against the backdrop of globalization processes. Our discussion of health communication processes challenges health communication scholars to consider the ways in which culture is central to public health interventions thereby shaping health care structures, health inequalities, and the depleting access to basic health resources among the poorest of the poor. Placing emphasis on global structures and structures of epistemic violence at local community levels, we call for health communication scholarship that attends to the intersections of macro and micro social structures and the political economy of these structures to eliminate the exploitation of the poorest sectors of the globe. The theorization of health communication on this terrain calls for the creation of culturally anchored spaces co-constructed with local communities. This should foreground the capacity of communities to create health solutions and simultaneously foster health capacities with the goal of challenging unhealthy political economic structures surrounding health.

References

Airhihenbuwa, C. O. (1995). *Health and Culture: Beyond the Western Paradigm*. Thousand Oaks, CA: Sage.

Airhihenbuwa, C. O. (2007). *Healing Our Differences – The Crisis of Global Health and the Politics of Identity*. Lanham, MD: Rowman and Littlefield.

Airhihenbuwa, C. O., Belete, F., Ndiaye, K., and Niang, C. I. (2009).Communications strategies for HIV/AIDS in Africa: Lessons learned in Ethiopia and Senegal. In R. G. Marlink and S. J. Teitelmann (Eds.), *From the Ground Up: A Guide to Comprehensive HIV/AIDS Care in Resource-Limited Settings*. Elizabeth Glaser Pediatric AIDS Foundation. Retrieved from http://ftguonline.org/ftgu-232/index.php/ftgu/article/download/2038/4073

Airhihenbuwa, C. O., Makinwa, B., Firth, M., and Obregon, R. (1999). *Communication Framework for HIV/AIDS: A New Direction*. A UNAIDS /PennState Project. Geneva: UNAIDS.

Airhihenbuwa, C. O., Makinwa, B., and Obregon, R. (2000). Toward a new communication framework for HIV/AIDS. *Journal of Health Communication, 5* (Supplement), 101–111.

Airhihenbuwa, C. O. and Obregon, R. (2000). A critical assessment of theories/models used in health communication for AIDS. *Journal of Health Communication, 5* (Supplement), 5–15.

Airhihenbuwa, C. O., Okoror, T. A., Shefer T. *et al.* (2009). Stigma, culture, and HIV and AIDS in the Western Cape, South Africa: An application of the PEN-3 cultural model for community based research. *Journal of Black Psychology, 35*(4), 407–432.

An-Na' im, A. A. and Hammond, J. (2002). Cultural transformation and human rights in African societies. In A. A. An-Na'im (Ed.), *Cultural Transformation and Human Rights in Africa* (pp. 13–37). Zed Books, London.

Basu, A. and Dutta, M. (2008a). Participatory change in a campaign led by sex workers: Connecting resistance to action-oriented agency. *Qualitative Health Research, 18,* 106–119.

Basu, A. and Dutta, M. (2008b). The relationship between health information seeking and community participation: The roles of motivation and ability. *Health Communication, 23,* 70–79.

Basu, A. and Dutta, M. (2009). Sex workers and HIV/AIDS: Analyzing participatory culture-centered health communication strategies. *Human Communication Research, 35,* 86–114.

Brown T. M., Cueto, M., and Fee, E. (2006). The World Health Organisation and the transition from international to global public health. *American Journal of Public Health, 96*, 62–72.

Coburn, D. (2000). Income inequality, social cohesion and the health status of populations: The role of neoliberalism. *Social Science and Medicine, 51*, 135–146.

Coburn, D. (2004). Beyond the income inequality hypothesis: Class, neo-liberalism, and health inequalities. *Social Science and Medicine, 58*, 41–46.

Dutta, M. J. (2006). Theoretical approaches to entertainment education campaigns: A subaltern critique. *Health Communication, 20*(3), 221–231.

Dutta, M. (2007). Communicating about culture and health: Theorizing culture-centered and cultural sensitivity approaches. *Communication Theory, 17*(3), 304–328.

Dutta, M. (2008). *Communicating Health: A Culture-Centered Approach.* London: Polity Press.

Dutta, M. (2009). Theorizing resistance: Applying Gayatri Chakravorty Spivak in public relations. In Ø. Ihlen, B. van Ruler, and M. Fredrikson, *Social Theory on Public Relations* (pp. 68–79). Abingdon: Routledge.

Dutta, M. (2010). The critical cultural turn in *Health Communication*: Reflexivity, solidarity, and praxis. *Health Communication, 25*, 534–539.

Dutta, M. (in press). Cultural theories of health communication. In S. Littlejohn and K. Foss (Eds.), *Encyclopedia of Communication Theory.* Thousand Oaks, CA: Sage.

Dutta, M. and Basnyat, I. (2008a). Interrogating the Radio Communication Project in Nepal: The participatory framing of colonization. In H. Zoller and M. Dutta, M. (Eds.), *Emerging Perspectives in Health Communication: Interpretive, Critical and Cultural Approaches* (pp. 247–265). Mahwah, NJ: Lawrence Erlbaum Associates.

Dutta, M. and Basnyat, I. (2008b). The Radio Communication Project in Nepal: A critical analysis. *Health Education and Behavior, 35*, 459–460.

Dutta, M. and Basnyat, I. (2008c). A critical response to participatory hegemony. *Health Education and Behavior 35*, 462–463.

Dutta, M. and Basu, A. (in press). Cultural theories of health communication. In T. Thompson, J. Nussbaum, and R. Parrott (Eds.), *Handbook of Health Communication.* Abingdon: Routledge.

Dutta, M., and Pal, M. (2010). Dialogue theory in marginalized settings: A Subaltern Studies approach. *Communication Theory, 20*, 363–386.

Dutta-Bergman, M. (2004a). The unheard voices of Santalis: Communicating about health from the margins of India. *Communication Theory, 14*, 237–263.

Dutta-Bergman, M. (2004b). Poverty, structural barriers and health: A Santali narrative of health communication. *Qualitative Health Research, 14*, 1–16.

Farmer, P. (1992). *AIDS and Accusation: Haiti and the Geography of Blame.* Berkeley, CA: University of California Press.

Farmer, P. (1999). *Infections and Inequalities: The Modern Plagues.* Berkeley, CA: University of California Press.

Farmer, P. (2003). *Pathologies of Power: Health, Human Rights and the New War on the Poor.* Berkeley, CA: University of California Press.

Ford, C. and Airhihenbuwa, C. O. (2010).The public health critical race methodology: Praxis for antiracism research. *Social Science and Medicine, 71*, 1390–1398.

Garrett, L., Mushtaque, R., Chowdhury, R., and Pablos-Mendez, A. (2009). All for universal health coverage. *The Lancet 372*, 1294–1299.

Gruskin, S., Mills, E., and Tarantola, D. (2007). Health and human rights 1: History, principles, and practices of health and human rights. *The Lancet, 370*, 449–455.

Hargreaves, S. and Cunningham, A. (2004). The politics of terror. *The Lancet, 363*, 1999–2000.

Ignatieff, M. (2001). Human rights and politics. In M. Ignatieff with A. Guttman (Ed.), *Human Rights as Politics and Idolatry* (pp. 3–52). Princeton, NJ: Princeton University Press.

Iwelunmor J., Zungu M., and Airhihenbuwa C. O. (2010). Rethinking HIV/AID disclosure among women within the context of motherhood in South Africa. *American Journal of Public Health, 100*(8), 1393–1399.

Koplan, J. P., Bond, T. C., Merson, M. H. *et al.* (2009). Towards a common definition of global health. *The Lancet, 373*(9679), 1993–1995.

Lupton, D. (1994). Toward the development of a critical health communication praxis. *Health Communication, 6*(1), 55–67.

Mann, J. M., Gruskin, S., Grodin, M. A., and Annas G. J. (1999). *Health and Human Rights. A Reader.* New York: Routledge.

Mann, J. M. and Tarantola, D. (1998). Responding to HIV/AIDS: A historical perspective. *Health and Human Rights, 5*, 5–8.

Miles, S. H. (2004). Abu Ghraib: Its legacy for military medicine. *The Lancet, 364*, 725–729.

Millen, J. and Holtz, T. (2000). Dying for growth, Part I: Transnational corporations and the health of the poor. In J. Y. Kim, J. V. Millen, A. Irwin, and J. Gershman (Eds.), *Dying for Growth: Global Inequality and the Health of the Poor* (pp. 177–223). Monroe, ME: Common Courage Press.

Millen, J., Irwin, A., and Kim, J. (2000). Introduction: What is growing? Who is dying? In J. Y. Kim, J. V. Millen, A. Irwin, and J. Gershman (Eds.), *Dying for Growth: Global Inequality and the Health of the Poor* (pp. 3–10). Monroe, ME: Common Courage Press.

Pal, M. and Dutta, M. (2008a). Public relations in a global context: The relevance of critical modernism as a theoretical lens. *Journal of Public Relations Research, 20*, 159–179.

Pal, M. and Dutta, M. (2008b). Theorizing resistance in a global context: Processes, strategies and tactics in communication scholarship. *Communication Yearbook, 32*, 41–87.

Prasad, A. (2009). Capitalizing disease: Biopolitics of drug trials in India. *Theory, Culture, and Society, 26*, 1–29.

Shisana, O., Rehle, T., Simbayi, L. C., *et al.* (2005). *South African National HIV Prevalence, HIV Incidence, Behaviour and Communication Survey.* Cape Town: HSRC Press.

Thompson, T. L. (2003). Introduction. In T. L. Thompson, A. M. Dorsey, K. I. Miller, and R. Parrott (Eds.), *Handbook of Health Communication* (pp. 1–5). Mahwah, NJ: Lawrence Erlbaum Associates.

Yehya, N. and Dutta, M. (2010). Health, religion, and meaning: A culture-centered study of Druze women. *Qualitative Health Research, 20*, 845–858.

Zoller, H. (2005). Health activism: Communication theory and action for social change. *Communication Theory, 15*, 341–364.

Zoller, H. and Dutta, M. (2008a). Introduction: Communication and health policy. In H. Zoller and M. Dutta (Eds.), *Emerging Perspectives in Health Communication: Interpretive, Critical and Cultural Approaches* (pp. 358–364). Mahwah, NJ: Lawrence Erlbaum Associates.

Zoller, H. and Dutta, M. (2008b). Afterword: Emerging agendas in health communication and the challenge of multiple perspectives. In H. Zoller and M. Dutta (Eds.), *Emerging Perspectives in Health Communication: Interpretive, Critical and Cultural Approaches* (pp. 449–463). Mahwah, NJ: Lawrence Erlbaum Associates.

3

Rethinking Health Communication in Aid and Development

Elizabeth Fox

This chapter proposes some questions that have to be sorted out in order to rethink health communication in aid and development. First, around which health issues should the rethinking be done? Rethinking health communication around the best-funded health areas is problematic because high levels of attention and pressure to produce results are not necessarily conducive to experimentation. The second question, how to gauge rethinking, looks at issues of indicators and measurement. The third, how to value rethinking, examines the status (or lack thereof) of health communication. The second part of the chapter examines some of the conditions needed to rethink health communication and two of the specific health areas, polio and malaria, with enough resources to do so. The chapter concludes with a section on building the capacity in developing countries to rethink health communication and a call to stop changing the name of health communication every time we come up with something new. A final reflection asks readers to recognize the limits of the field and the unintended consequences of bad programming and where the demand for health communication has gone.

Where to Rethink

A number of things have to be sorted out in order to rethink health communications in aid and development. The first of these is: around which health issues should the rethinking be done? Rethinking health communication around those issues that currently receive the most funding is problematic. High levels of attention and pressure to produce results quickly are not conducive to experimentation. In order to rethink you need to fail and then be forced to come up with something new. Or you need to have the type of learning environment that allows for and demands experimentation, critical outside peer review,

The Handbook of Global Health Communication, First Edition. Edited by Rafael Obregon and Silvio Waisbord.
© 2012 John Wiley & Sons, Inc. Published 2012 by John Wiley & Sons, Inc.

and analysis of results. Neither of these conditions is present today in most of the larger health communication areas in aid and development.

As can be expected, the majority of activities relating to health communication fall in those areas that receive the most funding. Currently, in terms of US Government funding, these are HIV/AIDS, followed by maternal and child health, reproductive health, malaria, and TB and other infectious diseases.

The health areas receiving the greatest amounts of funding also receive the most attention from donors. The organizations, including governments, carrying out these programs are under enormous pressure to show results and show them often within a year or so. As might be expected, this high level of pressure does not allow time for much rethinking of health communication. Actually, it sometimes leads to just the opposite: not rethinking, but reaching automatically for the current thinking, the existing models, and the usual ways of doing things.

Being in the international spotlight, up against international goals such as the Millennium Development Goals (MDGs), and having to respond to broad public support and demands for results does not leave much room for innovation and risk taking.

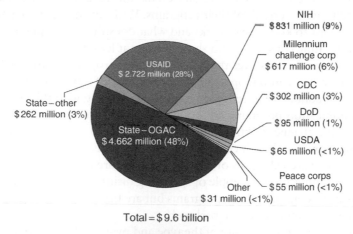

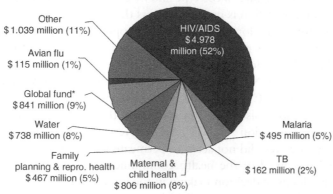

Figure 3.1 US government funding in global health in 2008.

Program managers and their funders tend to rely on what could be seen as the tried and true model of health communication. Why not? This model has been used successfully over the last 40 or so years – for example, to introduce Oral Rehydration Therapy (ORT), support vaccination campaigns, and raise awareness about contraceptives.

The tried and true model is not necessarily wrong. But it has been around for a while without being subject to much review. Although critiqued and built upon incrementally, it has seldom been subject to the level and type of rigorous academic review and analysis that leads to radical rethinking. To date, the application of theories such as the health belief model, stages of changes, theory of planned behavior or social cognitive theory, used in social marketing, community mobilization, and other planning frameworks and coupled with pretesting, implementation, and evaluation has been the hallmark of the majority of the health communication programs in aid and development. This is largely the case for programs in HIV/AIDS and malaria.

There is a reason for this lack of review. The donor community rarely sets the bar very high on measuring actual changes in behaviors as a result of health communication programs. And, the people carrying out communication programs resist using the more complex and often costly monitoring and evaluation measures that could show actual changes in behavior as a result of their programs. Without this data on actual changes in behavior, it is hard to know what works and what doesn't. The requirement to fund big programs under time constraints and show funders at least process indicators such as the number of people reached leaves the people running programs neither the time nor the data needed to venture into more experimental waters of health communication.

Although not conducive to rethinking, nothing is wrong with this situation as long as health communication programs are doing what they are supposed to do – bringing about sustainable changes in knowledge and behaviors to achieve public health impact. In many cases, however, health communication programs are not delivering results, and in some cases they are failing. In others they actually are causing harm, for example, by stigmatizing certain groups of people or spreading disinformation. Often, the failures are not linked back to communication programs but are blamed on the "ignorance" or inaction of the target communities themselves.[1]

HIV/AIDS seems to be a failure of the type and magnitude needed for a call for some rethinking of how communication is used to address the epidemic. The current ratio of two new people on treatment for every five new people contracting the disease can hardly be called a success. This rethinking, however, is fairly recent and not yet mainstreamed (Global HIV Prevention Working Group, 2008).

Over the past ten years, the UN Communication Roundtable, the UNAIDS Framework, the Communication for Social Change (CFSC) debates, and similar arguments made in a handful of public health journals called and suggested the need for serious rethinking about how health communication for HIV/AID prevention was designed and carried out. That rethinking, however, did not seem to permeate the larger public health debate and remained largely confined to the health communication community, with limited influence in the upper levels of decision making in the international/global public health community. An editorial in the prestigious British medical journal, *The Lancet,* published ahead of the International AIDS Conference in Vienna, Austria expressed the hope that this conference could provide such a forum for discussion.[2]

The statement that failure and/or a learning environment that allows for, and demands, experimentation and critical outside peer review and analysis of results are necessary conditions for rethinking health communication requires a caveat. It mainly applies to the large health communication programs funded by foreign donors and governments, and not to the smaller health communication activities that generally do not receive large amounts of international aid. While these small community-, faith-, or political-based activities often demonstrate innovations and creativity that are not seen in some of the larger-scale projects, sadly they too often implement watered-down versions of their richer cousins.

Failure, on the other hand, large-scale failure, on the scale of the failure in HIV/AIDs prevention, the inability to reduce significantly the number of women who die every year in childbirth, or the startlingly high rates of malnutrition and poor nutrition worldwide in the face of both scarcity and abundance, is another story. The failures in HIV/AIDS prevention are beginning to force some serious rethinking in health communication programs. The old models simply are not working: behaviors and social norms are not changing, even in the face of the mounting toll of the epidemic. Likewise, nutrition advocates are beginning to suspect that well-crafted jingles and solid social marketing campaigns for fortified products are not going to achieve the normative shifts in infant and young child feeding practices that need to occur to produce lasting change in the nutritional status of populations. Maternal health programs, faced with continued high ratios of maternal mortality, even with increased access of women to hospitals and pre-natal care, are beginning to focus far greater attention on how to change crucial inter-personal communication practices of the health provider and within the family.

The flip side of the question of where to rethink health communication is that rethink-ing actually is occurring, but in different health programs, not in those that are the major focus of aid and development. We need to look to these programs for new ideas. The attention to health communication in the United States for lifestyle issues such as smoking cessation, substance abuse, teenage drinking, obesity, and chronic diseases prevention, often generates new ways to reach people using different theories, platforms, and techniques.

Some of the reasons why these domestic programs are able to rethink health commu-nication while heath development programs cannot have to do with how long and at what level they are funded. Domestic programs in the United States often have enough funding and time for researchers to experiment and track results over longer periods. Competition among companies to carry out these programs is high, and companies need to show a high level of innovation to stay in business. Another reason is that funding usually is provided for independent outside evaluations of what is working and what is not, which are then fed into new program designs. The dispersal of funds is sometimes more decentralized, including at community level, allowing more room for experimenta-tion and innovation on a smaller scale. Finally, the dynamics of the power relations between health communicators and targeted communities can be different in the devel-oped and developing world.

In the former, local interest groups often demand a higher level of accountability to show results for the use of public funds. In the latter, targeted communities usually have no voice in how funds are spent.

Part of the answer of where to rethink health communication for aid and development may be found in those health areas that traditionally have been the focus of the more developed countries and societies. There may be ways to rethink health communication using the advances in marketing from the private sector or from domestic programs that have had the luxury of longer-term research programs and more rigorous peer review.

In order to be useful, however, the benefits of this rethinking must be reaped in the contexts and cultures where development occurs. This is a challenge given the pressures for health communication to carry out large-scale programs and achieve measurable results within set timeframes. This leads to another of the questions that needs to be sorted out in order to rethink health communication – how to measure the results or the impact of rethinking

How to Gauge Rethinking? Problem of Indicators and Measurement

The truism that what is easiest to measure is usually not worth measuring has been the case for much of the monitoring and evaluation of health communication programs over the years. It is easy to measure process indicators such as the number of pamphlets printed, radio spots aired, or meeting held. It is relatively easy to measure reach and determine if radio programs are aired at the right time to reach the intended audiences or if village health workers meet with the intended audiences to encourage the use of bed nets. It is much harder to measure the actual impact of the health communication programs. Assuming that rethinking should be based on data on impact and effectiveness of programs and on the accumulation of evidence of what works and why, this lack of data constitutes a barrier to innovation.

The problem of measurement also has to do with the length of health communication programs in developing countries. Many programs have a three- to five-year time span, not long enough for rigorous testing. Shifts in priorities in development aid often work against the ability to carry out longitudinal studies on program effectiveness.

Why is it so hard to get good data on what works and why? Partly it is a function of costs. Research on big enough samples and with enough time and controls to be representative of populations is costly and time-consuming. Few donors are willing to make the levels of investment necessary to "prove" what works in health communication, the way you might carry out a vaccine trial or test a new delivery mode for commodities. On top of that, the research methodologies are complicated and messy because people are complicated and messy. It is hard to control information flow, hard to separate control groups and sample groups, and hard not to contaminate one group with another. Adding in ethical considerations makes it even trickier. How can a program advise one group of a life-saving intervention and not the other in order to test a health communication campaign? How can information be withheld? The short answer is that it can't.[3]

Another barrier to getting sufficient data, data robust enough to rethink health communication, is that the data should begin to build toward a body of evidence. Even if research designs are not perfect and some of the studies cannot be replicated, there should be a way to accumulate the evidence of what works and what doesn't by using standard enough indicators across health communication interventions by health areas. This, however, is seldom the case. Although efforts are underway to develop standardized indicators, for example, in the case of health communication for programs advocating the correct use of bed nets in malaria programs, health communication programs, for the most part, lack common indicators.

A lack of common indicators and of data that can be accumulated over time and across different settings makes it hard to form a clear picture of the conditions and circumstances under which successes and failures occur. Without this picture, rethinking is fairly baseless. The magic of health communication, when it works, is lost because it cannot be replicated. The many changing factors that make programs effective are impossible to tease out because of the lack of data. Although the same standards of scientific research that build new and effective vaccines cannot be applied in the field studies of health communication, more can be done to accumulate evidence and demand a minimum level of measurement or evaluation of impact. This evidence and measurement of impact are the building blocks of any rethinking.

The dearth of data and of robust research around health communication is both the cause and effect of another factor that limits rethinking of the field – its lack of status.

How to Value Rethinking, the Status of Health Communication or the Lack of It

Health programs, by definition, are largely run by health professionals. The doctors, nurses, pharmacists, epidemiologists, and public health professionals who design and manage health programs in aid and development were trained in disciplines that address how to prevent or cure disease. Their tools are for the most part proven, effective public health interventions: vaccines, micronutrients, antibiotics, contraceptives, condoms, bed nets, HIV/AIDS and TB drugs, and clean water.

Significant parts of the public health community have a certain amount of impatience with health communication. As a field or profession, health communicators point out that, just because the solution exists, people will not necessarily use it. "Why not?" health professionals ask. "It's obvious that X or Y works; make it available and they will come or they will use it. Why bother with health communication at all?"

Sometimes, the public health profession is right, they do come. More often, however, they don't, and the reasons they don't are not clear. That is when the health communication people are called in. Health communicators, however, cannot come to the table with a tried and true set of interventions that are proven to work. Their first reactions tend to be more questions than solutions. Their data and numbers are softer and less convincing than those of their medical colleagues. All this contributes to lowering the prestige both of the professional and the profession.

The health professional attempting to get a straight answer from a health communicator may sometimes doubt if the health communication field is doing any thinking at all. Sometimes they are right. Some health communication programs have become jargony and formulaic, others repetitive, still others little more than crude copies of earlier campaigns. Since programs are not routinely measured and evaluated, health communicators often get away with it.

It becomes a vicious circle. Because health communication is often held in low esteem and not given sufficient funding for rigorous evaluation, the field does not progress. Since it does not progress, it is held in low esteem. When decisions are made between funding more vaccines and more bed nets versus more radio spots or more community meetings, funders will tend to go for the proven interventions, further eroding the ability of health communicators to carry out and evaluate effective, innovative programs.

The relative lack of stature of health communication is so pervasive that it is not even recognized as a field. International aid organizations increasingly interested in building health systems, for example, usually do not include health communication as a component of a health system that needs to be built. In some cases health communication is made an essential part of all the components of a health system – finance, governance, commodities, information systems, human resources, and services. Making health communication a part of everything, however, effectively makes it no one's responsibility. By becoming all-pervasive, health communication becomes impossible to hold accountable, measure, and therefore to rethink and improve.

What Are the Conditions Needed to Rethink Health Communication?

Rethinking a field or discipline can occur with the appearance of various conditions: a scientific breakthrough, the entrance of new partners, a significant setback or failure of existing thinking or ways of doing things, or a "visionary movement" that introduces new questions, challenges, or innovations. Rethinking usually requires a forum or community of knowledge of some nature as well as champions of new ways of doing things. Some of these conditions are present in the field of health communication. Others are lacking.

Health communication has been around for a while. While no magic bullet has appeared to change the field, it has experienced some breakthroughs, its share of failures, various and sundry movements to change it and bring in new theories and techniques, as well as a few strong champions of rethinking and forums where rethinking has occurred.

Almost 50 years ago, in 1962, the UNESCO General Conference commissioned Wilbur Schramm, the Director of the Institute for Communication Research at Stanford University, to examine the role of the mass media in promoting economic and social progress. Schramm's study, "Mass Media and National Development" drew a direct line between mass media and health: "To improve the health and vigor and extend the life span of the population requires not only the provision of medical and pharmaceutical services, but also the teaching of new health habits, which in turn require in many cases the adoption of new attitudes" (Schramm, 1962, p.31). The fifty years since Schramm wrote these words have witnessed the ebb and flow of health communication in aid and development across donors and developing countries. The field grew from Schramm s original vision of "teaching new health habits" to encompass sophisticated advances in commercial marketing and advertising. Health communication integrated new concepts and theories of individual, group, and community behaviors and social networks.

Health communication was applied along with policy changes and advocacy to achieve widespread shifts in behaviors around issues as diverse as seatbelt use, alcohol and drug abuse, smoking cessation, and teen pregnancy. Health communication applied in developing countries successfully introduced Oral Rehydration Therapy (ORT), supported mass vaccination campaigns against smallpox and polio, and increased knowledge and sometimes the practice of family planning. Along the way, some of the limits of health communication became apparent.

These limits are obvious, though they were not necessarily so at the time. The overly optimistic vision of teaching new health habits ran up against scarcities of health supplies and services. Programs also bumped up against the limits of increasing knowledge without changing environments to support new behaviors and strengthening the power and ability of individuals and groups to perform them. Health programs began to realize the stigma produced by health messages that essentially blamed the victim for not doing the right things for themselves and their health even when it was not under their control to do so. (The current debate about obesity programs is fast discovering some of these same limitations.) Essentially, it became apparent that "communication experts" are not necessarily experts in changing behavior.

Measurement and evaluation tools grew sharper. Public opinion research, for example, became more sophisticated in its ability to identify and track individual and group behaviors and to segment audiences to deliver more targeted messages and incentives to high-risk individuals and groups. Smaller, more cost-effective "hyper-targeted" interventions replaced some mass campaigns. The field learned more about normative, generational, and longer-term behavior shifts and how to reach individuals and groups to influence behaviors well before they are at risk.

Some of the greatest advances in health communication occurred in the media themselves, the main delivery vehicles for health communication and behavior change messages. Technological advances – first radio and television, satellites, video cameras, cell phones, computers, and the Internet – increased access and distribution channels in many regions, transforming prior concepts of scale and financial sustainability and opening the door to new partnerships with public and private media alike. Media markets grew, increasing the globalization of actors and the diversity of sources and shifting the financial equations for earnings and reach. At the same time, small media and community-based outlets showed their effectiveness in reaching individuals and groups with health communication messages.

As the health communications field for aid and development grew, it developed its own vocabulary, models, concepts, and a host of actors who could carry out programs around the world. Health communication became a successful "industry." The health communication industry, however, was not always that successful in terms of achieving real and lasting shifts in behavior around key public health issues. Yet, for many years, scientific breakthroughs, new partners, setbacks or failures, or a movement introducing new questions, challenges, or innovations were either not present or not strong enough to cause real change in the field.

Innovations, when they occurred, became additive rather than game-changing. New technologies were introduced and applied on top of existing programs or existing programs were retrofitted into the new technologies. The hope of radical change in health communication programs as a result of television, satellites, Internet, and maybe even cell phones fell short when measured against the lack of evidence of commensurate shifts in health behaviors. Witness the sobering statistics on the failure to stem the tide of HIV/AIDS infections.

Aid programs funded experts meetings on health communication. UN Agencies set up task forces and forums on health communication. Donors commissioned studies and literature reviews. Somehow, a critical mass of evidence of success and failure through the gradual accumulation of data did not reach a tipping point to produce rethinking. Over the years, new actors and movements such as critical communication, participatory communication, communication for social change sprang onto the scene, but somehow were unable to significantly alter the practice of health communication in aid and development.

Health communication did not develop the necessary critical mass to become a field or discipline with a way to systematically assess success and failure, carry out peer-reviewed research, or accumulate evidence. Health communication in aid and development remained a practice, a good practice, in some cases a community of practices, with different theories, schools, and tools. It did not grow into a field that collectively examined itself critically on the basis of 50 years of accumulated evidence of success and failure.

Rethinking Health Communication around Specific Health Areas: Who Has Time? Who Has Money?

Despite the statement above on the general lack of critical thinking, critical rethinking is taking place in some health areas. The editors of this book and some of the contributors provide in-depth analysis of how this has occurred across the field. There is one specific health area, however, where health communication is beginning to be rethought, polio eradication. With polio, partly as a result of the threat of failure and partly as a result of significant funding being available, a group of thinkers and practitioners has begun to rethink health communication.

What they have done in the case of polio is to rethink health communication in a more integrated manner, specifically within public health intervention. They have not rethought health communication in the abstract as a field or as a set of concepts or theories.

This may be the only way to tease out new approaches to health communication – within the context of specific health problems and barriers. Or at least it may be the only way that the field and the practitioners working in it will have the resources and support to analyze what works and what doesn't and submit health communication programs and results to a process of rigorous peer review.

Health communication for polio eradication is being rethought not because health communication was succeeding, but because polio eradication had reached a crisis and communication programs were "failing." Vaccination efforts had been halted in northern Nigeria, leading in only two years to the spread of polio virus to 21 polio-free countries and adding hundreds of millions of dollars to the eradication effort. The setbacks or failures of the polio eradication program were related to communication, the toxic combination of misinformation and misdirected communication efforts.

A 2010 review of communication for polio eradication explained some of the factors behind this failure in Nigeria:

> 2003 was a watershed year, however, for the polio eradication initiative, when a large, well organized misinformation campaign in several states in northern Nigeria resulted in a boycott of polio immunization campaigns. ... Unfounded rumors that the vaccine caused HIV/ AIDS and sterility, as well as the absence of effective communication strategies, led to widespread rejection of immunization in parts of west and central Africa and to a lesser degree India. Communication efforts have been key in addressing the controversy and subsequent mistrust that remains and sporadically re-emerges (Waisbord *et al.*, 2010, p. 11).

Before 2003, the polio communication effort had for the most part been run fairly independently of the other parts of the eradication program. When polio eradication entered into crisis, however, the communication specialists and the public health specialists who ran the program began to rethink this independence and how communication goals were being set, data gathered and analyzed, and programs run. Up till then, the goals of the polio communication program had been mainly awareness and information goals. After the "crisis" they became more integrated into the goals of the overall initiative in terms of reaching the unvaccinated and improving compliance with vaccination.

This shift resulted in a stronger link between the communication programs and the epidemiological analysis and an increased use of indicators that brought the social data together with the epidemiological data on the characteristics and spread of the disease. This forced the communication specialists to get inside the heads of the polio eradicators and their audiences. It forced them to rethink and to challenge standard explanations for why people failed to turn up to be vaccinated or hid their children when vaccinators knocked on the door. Concepts such as "resistance," "fear," or misinformation were pulled apart and analyzed with real data and in greater detail from the different target audiences. Other possible explanations for nonvaccination were proposed, examined, and held up to criticism. More generalized explanations evolved into more localized, more culturally specific, and, sometimes, counterintuitive explanations. People running health communication programs developed impact indicators for communication program that could be tracked over time with trend analysis and linked to measurable health outcomes (Taylor and Shimp, 2010).

One could ask if what happened in polio communication was rethinking or simply carrying out evidence-based health communication programs the way they should be done in the first place. In other words, we don't have to wait for failure to rethink. When health communication is provided with appropriate resources and a living, working link to the other health aspects of the program, it will be more effective and result in a rethinking of some of the old ways of doing business.

A similar process of rethinking health communication should, and in some places is, taking place today within the global effort to eliminate malaria as a major public health threat in Africa. This effort involves major new funding from the US Congress, private donors and foundations, the private commercial sector, and countries across Africa. The goal is to make the use of four effective antimalaria interventions the social norm in malaria endemic countries. These are: correct bed net use, indoor residual spraying, treatment with antimalarials for pregnant women, and prompt and appropriate treatment for children under five with malaria.

Partly because the funds are there to carry out significant communication programs, and partly because the four interventions are so closely tied with behaviors, health communication is playing an important role in the malaria effort.

Using a net, seeking care, or allowing sprayers into your house are behaviors that can be measured and tracked using data that can link back to communication programs. The different populations that are at risk from malaria are known and can be identified and described. The current malaria elimination effort has not failed. It is a success, measurable in dropping rates of child deaths from malaria. To date, the success of the malaria elimination effort, however, has not led to a rethinking of health communication. While health communication is a component of the effort, it has not yet been adequately challenged to do things differently or to critically question its assumptions about what works.

This challenge, however, will come. Keeping malaria transmission low in future, after the tremendous push of the elimination program recedes, will present challenges not yet addressed by health communicators. Some of these – for example, how to keep preventive efforts going when risk is low and visible signs of the disease are infrequent – are important questions that have yet to be fully understood.

Meanwhile, the health communication efforts in the malaria program are generally following the methodologies, concepts, models, and theories that have been carried out over the last 30 or so years. This does not mean that health communications programs for malaria elimination are not good. They are. But they, to date, have not been forced to critically examine their assumptions about what they are doing and how they are reaching people. And, perhaps more importantly, the other health professionals working in the malaria program have not yet come to the point where they cannot move forward without first working more closely with their health communication colleagues. Free bed net distributions, teams with insecticides to spray houses, and the availability of effective drugs are working well to reduce transmission, along with fairly modest investments in communication programs.

Health communication for malaria will probably not have to be rethought until national malaria programs face the challenges of how to maintain preventive behaviors without the visible risk of disease and the massive donor investments occurring today in drugs and commodities. By that time, with luck, the investments in infrastructure, housing, and sanitation that eliminated malaria in developed countries may have occurred, making individual and community health communication programs less necessary. It is more likely, however, that they will not have occurred, and malaria will continue to be a threat.

The fact that health communication for malaria does not have to be rethought in the near future, however, does not mean that it should not be rethought now. Programs could be far more evidenced-based, with indicators much more closely linked to health indicators; trend data could be more systematically collected within and across countries to track what is working and what is not to redirect programs. New concepts and indicators for social norms and cultural shifts around malaria treatment and prevention could be developed and explored.

If all this sounds familiar to health communicators, it is the type of questioning that is slowly and finally taking place today around health communication and HIV/AIDS. The enormous and public failure on the part of the HIV/AIDS prevention program to reduce risky behaviors has led to a great deal of rethinking about the limits of cognitive communication approaches within complex social contexts and human sexuality. Fear, spirituality, violence and gender, social networks – all have come into play in rethinking health communication around HIV/AIDS. The conditions are right, programs are failing, funds are available, and nothing else is working.

Building the Capacity to Rethink Health Communication

Even with the necessary conditions of failures, funds, and frustration, rethinking is not possible if nobody is around to do it. That is where capacity building comes in. Historically, health communication for aid and development has been carried out through a heavy dose of technical assistance from academics and practitioners from developed countries. Given the short time frames and high performance demands on foreign assistance funds, capacity building in health communication often gets ignored or downplayed. It is easier to send in a team to put together a health communication strategy, develop indicators, and management structures than to support the riskier and more time-consuming task of building local capacity. As a result, public sector health communication departments in ministries of health and other government departments have been underfunded and understaffed and, consequently, have underperformed.

Nor do most universities in developing countries have robust academic communication programs, let alone health communication programs. Over the last two decades or so, the lack of leadership from developing country universities as sources of rethinking health communication has been profound, especially in Africa. The reasons are many: political strife, lack of resources, and government crackdowns on intellectual life in universities across the developing world, to name a few. While universities in some countries have escaped this pattern, for example, Brazil, Mexico, or lately South Africa, NGOs largely have filled the vacuum in critical thinking around health communication left by the universities. Yet, with few exceptions, these NGOs are more oriented toward social action than towards critical rethinking of social issues and development approaches. And most NGOs lack students and professors and anything more than basic applied research capabilities.

Funding has not been available in most developing countries to support the programs and students or to build a critical mass of professors and researchers in health communication. In the past, the shortage of employment opportunities in health communication for professionals from developing countries, especially at higher levels of research, design, planning, and evaluation, completed the vicious cycle. While this is beginning to change, with increased employment opportunities opening up in the communication field, funding and capacity for health communication training and research in developing countries continues to lag.

As a result of the lack of funding and capacity, health communication programs in the public sector carry out scant formative research to develop messages and materials and even less evaluative or impact research to gauge the outcome of communication programs. Failures are not identified, and lessons learned are not collected, analyzed, or used. The planning function for health communication within ministries, since most of the activities are donor planned and funded, is often hastily organized, limited in scope, and reduced to meeting the immediate demands of programs.

When programs are designed not on the basis of research and evidence but on the basis of other factors such as funding available or convenience, the field of health communication loses the ability to rethink what it is doing. When a program does not result in the desired behavior change or shift in attitudes, without data, planners can't know which parts did or didn't work, what was the most efficacious mix of media and channels, or which messages were most appropriate.

The lack of capacity in countries, coupled with the lack of funding for and attention to health communication programs, especially in the public sector, severely limits the ability to rethink the field. Successes cannot be verified, evidence cannot be accumulated, and failures cannot be examined. Meanwhile, gaps between knowledge and behavior, misinformation and misconceptions, and low levels of adoption of basic health behaviors by large sectors of the population continue to bedevil public health programs throughout the developing world. Even countries with sophisticated media markets and significant investments in health communication face these challenges.

While the need for rethinking is clear, the national capacity to do so is generally weak. The motivation of funders to build this capacity is limited by pressing demands to show results. That said, the health communication community of practice in developing countries is working with national academic resources and those of developed countries to slowly forge the types of programs and partnerships that will enable rethinking to occur. Examples of this include the ongoing work in health communications of the Consortium of Universities in Lima, Peru, the health communications programs at the University of the Witwatersrand in South Africa, and more.

Rethinking the Name

Over the years, health communication has had many labels: Health Education, Health Literacy, Information, Education, Communication (IEC), Behavior Change Communication (BCC), Social Marketing, Communication for Social Change, Social and Behavior Change Communication. Every time a group or school of thought wants to rethink the field and take it in a new direction, it gives the field a new name. This is a problem. It's a problem because it creates a situation where, instead of evolving and maturing as a discipline, health communication looks as if it is many different disciplines.

If biology or psychology changed their name with each new discovery or theory the slow accumulation, sharing, and testing of knowledge that a field needs to evolve could not occur. The field would become fragmented. Philosophy has many different schools; so too comparative literature, but they are still philosophy or literature. The passion with which new labels for health communication are developed and launched, often accompanied by the demonization of the previous label, makes it hard to build a field on the basis of the accumulation of evidence. It also confuses the user.

Health communication as both a discipline and a practice is a part of wider public health programs and efforts. The field interacts with doctors and nurses, epidemiologists, sanitation engineers, pharmacists, and many other disciplines. The debates, evolution, and new labels in the field of health communication are of less interest to these professions than is the ability of health communication to contribute to public health results. Just as a social scientist does not have to understand the latest debates and discoveries in electrical engineering in order to use a new hand-held computer, health professionals do not have to get inside the theories and evolving schools of health communication to make health communication an integral part of public health programs. Rethinking health communication means making it more accessible, less full of jargon, and easier for other health professionals to interact with and use.

Rethinking the Limits and the Stigma of Health Communication

Health communication programs in aid and development, no matter how good they are, don't always work. The right information and messages developed by, with, or for the appropriate populations, in the appropriate language and tone, and addressing the correct barriers or incentives can still fail. Failure often is the result of environmental, contextual, or biological factors that are beyond the control of the individual, group, or even the community. Health communication programs against obesity in developed countries come to mind. Healthy food choices are not available, labeling is not clear, sports and exercise are unavailable, etc. Meanwhile health messages continue to advocate weight loss, creating or adding to the social stigma already surrounding the obese.

Something similar may be happening with health communication for aid and development. Easy funding available for mass media campaigns around HIV/AIDS, family planning, or even child nutrition may actually stigmatize the infected, the noncompliant, or the malnourished.

Part of rethinking could be thinking more modestly, in a more measured way, and with more awareness of the environmental and contextual determinants and constraints facing the individual and the group. This rethinking is already occurring in well-thought-out and carefully researched and planned health communication programs. Yet, we still keep forgetting the limitations of our field and fall back into campaign mode, often ignoring the context within which the individual or group functions.

Rethinking Demand for Health Communication – Where Has It Gone?

Health communication in aid and development in all its many forms has been around for 50 years or so. Investments in health communication, however, probably have gone down in the last 10 years relative to other investments in health such as commodities and as part

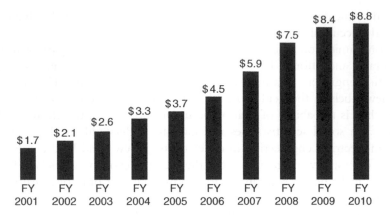

Figure 3.2   Funding for US global health programs FY2001–FY 2010 (in billions).

of overall health budgets. While health as part of foreign assistance has grown exponentially over the last 10 years, health communication budgets have not kept pace. By the end of 2009, for example, the Global Fund had disbursed US$10 billion: US$ 5.7 for HIV/AIDS programs, US$ 1.5 billion for Tuberculosis programs; and US$ 2.8 billion for malaria programs.[4] Cumulative expenditure on health communication for the three diseases was around 1 percent for the TB programs, 5 percent for Malaria programs, and 7 percent, for HIV/AIDS. The percentage of funds spent on health communication in US global health programs follows a similar distribution. Approximately 5 percent of the funds for the President's Malaria Initiative, for example, were designated for health communication in 2010.

This is the result of the increase in effective, proven treatments for AIDS, TB, and malaria and the rising costs of commodities and drugs as a part of overall health budgets. It also is the result of complacency on the part of health programs. Once certain health behaviors such as the use of oral rehydration therapy (ORT) achieved the targeted level of use, health communication programs directed at this behavior tended to drop off. Data shows that the use of ORT then experienced a parallel drop-off. When public health programs took their eye off the ball and did not continue to support communication programs around early successes in breastfeeding or ORT, these behaviors showed real slippage in country after country.

It also is the result of the failure to accumulate evidence about impact and effectiveness, including the cost-effectiveness, of health communication. Other social health interventions such as community distribution of antibiotics or training in neonatal survival techniques have been subjected to these standards of evidence and have shown impact and effectiveness. Health communication, as noted above and for many reasons including costs, methodological considerations, and even ethical considerations, with few exceptions, has not. As a result, when planners ask how much we can expect from our investments in health communication, the answers are not readily available. Health communication programs increasingly are being held to the same standards of evidence of impact as other investments and interventions. Rethinking health communication requires rethinking how to respond to the question of impact and effectiveness in a way that can be used by planners and implementers of health programs in aid and development.

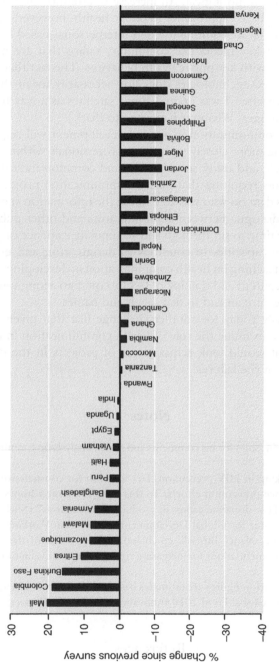

Figure 3.3 Increases and decreases in ORT coverage since 2000 in countries conducting Demographic and Health Surveys (DHS).
Source: DHS.

Finally, and paradoxically, a possible reason for the drop-off in demand for health communication is the advent of innovations in communication and information technology. Now, that doesn't sound logical. An increase of attention and funding to IT, cell phones, and other web-based approaches to public health, however, may have siphoned funding away from nonflashy community- and interpersonal-based health communication programs and low-key media like community radios that are necessary to reach mothers and caretakers with key public health behaviors. The fact that health communication programs use new technologies does not necessarily mean that they are more effective. (I remember when I was excited about satellites as a way to reach the world with development messages. Whatever happened to that?)

Rethinking health communication in aid and development will require many things. It will require working more closely with other professionals within health areas, conducting better research, and using sounder data and common indicators. Some of this could start with donors requiring that health communication programs provide more accountability such as data on who was able to use the information successfully and why. It will require more dialogue between communicators and other public health professionals. It will require time to sift through and accumulate evidence of past successes and failures and build the capacities in countries to design, run, and evaluate programs. Improving university teaching on health communication in developing countries through advances in teaching content and training of faculty could go a long way towards advancing the field. It will require an end to new labels and names.

Perhaps we are ready today for another challenge like that given Wilbur Schramm almost 50 years ago to examine the role of health communication in promoting health and development that would look across scores of projects in the developing world, including a hard look at the failures.

Notes

1   I am grateful to Martin Alilio for his comments and added analysis on monitoring and evaluation and on failures.
2   "[Professionals working in HIV prevention] lack a forum for constructive fact-to-face debate to discuss and advance prevention efforts. To this end, *The Lancet* hopes AIDS 2010 can fill this void and unite these disparate camps in productive discussions" (Shelton, 2010, p. 2).
3   The report of the Center for Global Development's Evaluation Working Group (William D. Savedoff, Ruth Levine, Nancy Birdsall, co-chairs) explores some of these barriers in greater detail and offers recommendations for increasing rigorous impact evaluation (Center for Global Development, 2006).
4   The health communication figures are estimates based on the grants information on the Global Fund website and the Global Fund 2010 Innovation and Impact Report.

References

Center for Global Development (2006). When will we ever learn? Improving lives through impact evaluation. Report of the Evaluation Working Group. Retrieved from http://www.3ieimpact.org/doc/WillWeEverLearn.pdf

Global HIV Prevention Working Group (2008). Behavior change and HIV preventions: [Re] Considerations for the 21ˢᵗ century. Retrieved from http://www.globalhivprevention.org/pdfs/PWG_behavior%20report_FINAL.pdf

Schramm, W. (1964). *Mass Media and National Development: The Role of Information in the Developing Countries*. Stanford, CA: Stanford University Press.

Shelton, P. (2010). AIDS 2010. *The Lancet, 376*(9734), 2–3.

Taylor, S. and Shimp, L. (2010). Using data to guide action in polio health communications: experience from the polio eradication initiative (PEI). *Journal of Health Communications, 15*(51), 48–65.

Waisbord, S., Shimp, L., Ogden, E., and Morry, C. (2010). Communication for polio eradication: Improving the quality of communication programming through real-time monitoring and evaluation. *Journal of Health Communications, 15*(51), 9–24.

4

Toward a Global Theory of Health Behavior and Social Change

Douglas Storey and Maria Elena Figueroa

Introduction

Our goal in this chapter is to describe an evolution of theories of health behavior and social change and describe some practical models and case studies that reflect this evolution. We argue here, as elsewhere (Kincaid, Delate, Storey, and Figueroa, in press), that for many years our field has been moving away from the idea of communication as a one-time one-way communicative "act" toward a view of communication as an iterative social process (precisely a multilevel dialogue) that unfolds over time. The practice of health communication has changed as global health concerns have changed, as our understanding of the complexity of health determinants has improved, and as new opportunities and approaches to health communication have emerged. As communication technologies have become more diverse, accessible and affordable – closing gaps between continents and within communities alike – it makes sense to aspire to a global theory of health communication.

The Nature of Theory

Theories are analytical tools for understanding, explaining, and making predictions about topics of conceptual or practical interest. *Scientific* theories rely on formalized rules for gathering and evaluating evidence and on standards for quantifying and logically linking constructs, while everyday theories, in practice, tend to rely on commonsense observation and reasoning for sense-making and consensus building.

Theories generate hypotheses that can be tested (Hempel, 1952; Popper, 1963). In the traditional scientific sense this means designing an experiment in order to test a

The Handbook of Global Health Communication, First Edition. Edited by Rafael Obregon and Silvio Waisbord.
© 2012 John Wiley & Sons, Inc. Published 2012 by John Wiley & Sons, Inc.

hypothesis and refine theory. In a programmatic context, hypothesis testing means (1) designing a program with a change model in mind; (2) implementing the program; (3) verifying that change occurred according to the rationale that informed the program; then (4) deriving lessons and applying them to a new program. Testing hypotheses and refining theories, whether in a scientific or programmatic sense, proceeds haphazardly unless guided by systematic measurement, so any dream of a global theory carries with it some empirical obligations. As Obregon and Waisbord note elsewhere in Chapter 1 of this volume, there are few examples of global comparative research. Yet, there is an abundance of research at the national level that might be considered a form of "replication with variation" (to borrow a concept from Charles Darwin) (Dennett, 1995). Drawing on our personal experience with applied health communication programs and program research over the past 30 years in at least 30 countries, across world regions, our goal in this chapter is to provide a theoretical synthesis for global health communication.

In the sections that follow, we describe the evolution of theories in health behavior and social change and the concurrent evolution of methods and measurements. We then provide four short case studies that illustrate aspects of the evolution and conclude with some suggestions for the next stages of global theorizing.

An Evolution of Thinking

How do theories progress? A recent article by Neuman and Guggenheim (2011) analyzed citation patterns for over 20,000 communication journal articles dating back to 1933 and found evidence of six clusters of media effects theories that are roughly chronological but overlapping. Considering over 70 years of theoretical scholarship, they concluded that the history of theory is not a series of successive repudiations of earlier models. Rather, it more closely resembles the biological evolution of a simple organism into a more complex one. From a "starting point of a simple model of persuasion and transmission", theories have progressed toward a complex amalgam of constructs combining aspects of active audience processing, social context, technical attributes of channels, societal/political/institutional context, and interpretation of meaning (Neuman and Guggenheim, 2011, pp. 188–189). The result is a multilevel, richly cross-referenced body of theory, not a paradigm victory of participation over dissemination or of critical theory over modernization.

Although studies of communication sometimes use different vocabulary rooted in different traditions, the overall body of literature demonstrates clearly and consistently that communication can strengthen many aspects of human agency, whether in the domain of individuals acting to manage their own and their family's health, or in the domain of communities engaging with and challenging health systems to improve access to and quality of services, or in the domain of national governments setting health priorities and committing politically (or not) to redress health imbalances and other inequities. Today, most health communication interventions that attempt to create change – whether at the individual level or at higher levels of society – use some combination of informational, participatory, and structural change approaches in a complementary way. Therefore, an emerging global theory of health communication must account for all levels of social engagement from individual action to structural change and for interactions among them.

Our own experience as scholar-practitioners reinforces this view. Early applications of theory in health communication emphasized individual-level theories of learning, persuasion, and decision making as they related to health behavior and, especially, behavior change. Programs used psychosocial theories such as Reasoned Action/Planned Behavior (Fishbein and Ajzen, 1975; Ajzen and Fishbein, 1997) and Social Cognitive Theory (Bandura, 1986, 1995) to guide strategic planning, then evaluated the programs guided by the same frameworks (e.g., did communication affect efficacy beliefs and did efficacy beliefs in turn affect behavior?). The systematic application and testing of theories in this way over time, in varied settings and for many health issues demonstrated that it *was* possible to measure communication processes and outcomes reliably, spurring the field away from the notion of communication impact as an unobservable "black box" process (Friedenberg and Silverman, 2006, pp. 85–88) and toward more sophisticated models of change.

It is true that the early modern history of communication theory, including its application to health issues, overemphasized individual-level behavior change. This was soundly criticized, particularly by Latin American scholars (Beltrán, 1974; Diaz Bordenave, 1976), who noted a lack of attention to structural factors in social change and to power inequities that can stifle change. In response, more structurally oriented theories of change arose (Rogers, 1976) that acknowledged additional higher-order determinants of health, such as network structures and access to resources, *as well as* individual-level psychosocial factors. For example, by the third edition of *Diffusion of Innovations*, Rogers (1983) had moved beyond an information dissemination model of communication toward the convergence model (Kincaid, 1979, 2009; Rogers and Kincaid, 1981). Convergence describes a process of change grounded in socially situated dialogue, not the result of simple exposure to new information. Thus, behavioral choices take into account the appropriateness of a new practice within the social milieu; the social, economic, and, presumably, cultural costs of a change in practices; the relative advantage – economic, social, material – of a new practice over an existing one; the complexity of the practice, including access to the resources and social support one needs to actualize change; and whether it is possible to see what happened to others who have tried to change. This version of diffusion also implicitly acknowledged the importance of power – the capacity to exercise control over others – as a function of network structures and of the relationships between communicators that sometimes distort and sometimes strengthen communication and the process of change. Although commonly measured at the individual level, most of the factors listed above are inherently social and structural, not strictly individual, because they require consideration of one's neighbors, of what is acceptable and possible in one's community and society, of control over resources and access to social support and, in the case of some new practices, the extent to which one can or must collaborate with others to achieve (or resist) change.

Demand for Accountability

At the same time that a shift was happening toward more social and structural views of communication, more and more opportunities for applied research in diverse settings were being funded under a series of global procurements for health communication technical assistance by, among others, the United States Agency for International Development (USAID). These agreements included The Mass Media and Health Practices (MMHP) project (1978–1985) and its successors, the Healthcom project (1985–1994), the Population Communication Services project (1982–2004), the Health Communication Partnership project (2003–2009) and the C-Change project (2009 to date). USAID's virtually unbroken 35-year investment in health communication helped drive theory development through demands for objective evidence of the nature and magnitude of communication effects on health behavior and health outcomes as a condition for funding.

Particularly in the area of population and reproductive health, a rapid expansion of funding for family planning programs in the 1980s (Piotrow *et al.*, 1997; Blanc and Tsui, 2005) focused attention on the role of communication in global fertility change (reduction in the average number of children borne in a woman's lifetime) and on subsequent declines in population growth rates that threatened economic development. Along with a series of multiyear, multicountry global contracts for health communication between the late 1970s and the present came demands to conclusively link communication inputs to outcomes and impact and to develop *predictive* models of change at the level of individual behavior (e.g., contraceptive use), as well as at the level of societal health outcomes (e.g., contraceptive prevalence (CPR)) that would guide future planning and investment. Especially after the year 2000, the requirements for sophisticated research and evaluation approaches intensified.

Admittedly, most of the funding available through these initiatives went toward the development and implementation of programs at the national level; little funding was made available for comparative research across the many countries where these projects operated. What synthesis did occur was usually the result of global project staff and researchers working in multiple countries and on multiple health issues who carried lessons learned from one project to another and from country to country. Some visionary program directors, like Phyllis Piotrow (Piotrow *et al.*, 1997) of the PCS project, helped foster this synthesis by insisting that all communication initiatives allocate at least 10 percent of their budget to research. Later, under the HCP project, core funding was dedicated to secondary analysis of data, resulting in the publication of over 120 peer-reviewed, project-related articles over a six year period.

One example of the synthesis this generated was the concept of *ideation*, derived from Cleland and Wilson's iconoclastic (1987) work on global fertility transition. Ideation was defined as a set of knowledge, attitudinal, social support, and social interaction variables (all of which could be influenced by communication) that together predicted the use of contraception and CPR across a variety of national settings, resulting in a reliable model of global fertility change (Kincaid, 2000) based on psychosocial and cultural factors, rather than just on levels of education or economic development. A five-country study in Nepal, The Philippines, Tanzania, Honduras, and Egypt (Kincaid *et al.*, 2007a) confirmed that ideation had a significant effect on the use of contraception, increasing the odds of family planning use by 20 to 30 percent, even after controlling for a wide variety of other socioeconomic factors. Since that study, the ideation model has been used and tested in programs addressing numerous health issues, including safe water handling, handwashing and hygiene, HIV/AIDS stigma reduction, democracy and governance, and avian influenza prevention, among others, lending further support to the generalizability of this concept.

The Role of Community

Yet, even as research confirmed the predictive value of psychosocial theories, it became clear that there were missing theoretical elements, notably community-level processes and how they contribute to health outcomes. In our view, this omission generally was not an intentional result of an individual level paradigm bias. Rather, it was the result of a lack of appropriate tools and methods for *measuring* community phenomena. Most of the early evidence of community processes and effects on health outcomes was anecdotal or qualitative in nature; there were few quantitative measures available that were not merely the sum of individual-level changes. Aggregated individual data at the community-level – the percent using a contraceptive method, for example – are useful for analyzing population trends (e.g., contraceptive prevalence rate), but do not capture collective phenomena (e.g., resource equity or social cohesion). And while qualitative assessments of community processes by themselves can be richly informative, they cannot generate population-based estimates of disease prevalence or program impact, hampering the ability to predict program results with any precision or to generalize research findings to the larger population.

Two models that helped bridge this gap were the Integrated Model of Communication for Social Change (Figueroa *et al.*, 2002) and the more recent Communication for Participatory Development Model (Kincaid and Figueroa, 2009). Kincaid and Figueroa (2009) identified eight issues that any comprehensive theoretical model needed to address and be able to measure, focusing in particular on community level processes. Models should: (1) reflect human development in local communities, as well as change at the national (structural/political) level; (2) emphasize dialogue as a symmetrical, two-way process of communication; (3) reconcile the demand for social change at the community level with the need for change at the individual level; (4) feature local ownership of the change process in order to minimize reliance on external stimuli and resources; (5) recognize the importance of self-determination as well as the catalytic and facilitative role of external change agents; (6) acknowledge the inevitability of local conflict and suggests ways to manage or resolve it; (7) allow for self-assessment during the change process to sustain collective action; and (8) acknowledge the importance of access to mass media as well as to local media, such as community radio, posters/billboards, traveling theater groups, and – increasingly – mobile technologies that allow individuals and groups to produce and exchange their own content, rather than rely primarily on external sources of content.

Ecological Models of Behavior

Models like this challenged practitioners and theorists alike to think holistically, leading toward a social-ecological perspective on health communication. In the biological sciences, *ecology* refers to the complex interrelationships among organisms and the environment in which they live, in essence a biophysical "dialogue." By extension, *social* ecology is "the study of the influence of the social context on behavior, including institutional and cultural variables" (Sallis and Owen, 2002, p. 462). Social ecological approaches take into account the interconnected influences of family, peers, community and society on behavior (Sallis and Owen, 2002; Jamison *et al.*, 2006; Powell *et al.*, 2006). From

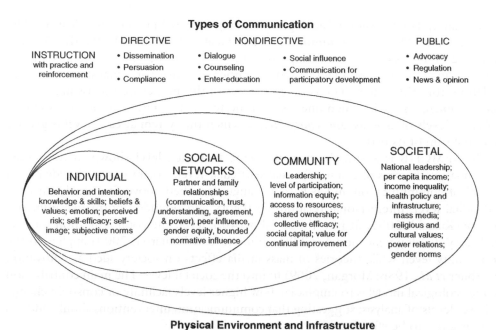

Figure 4.1 Social ecology model of communication and health behavior.
Source: Kincaid, D. L., Figueroa, M. E., Storey, J. D. and Underwood, C.R. (2007b). A social ecology model of communication, behavior change, and behavior maintenance. Working paper. Center for Communication Programs, Johns Hopkins Bloomberg School of Public Health.

this perspective, health communication programs must be seen as a form of dialogue, too. If conceptualized as a *dialogue* with the audience, then a communication program can be reconceptualized as a self-correcting feedback process, defined dynamically as a diminishing series of under-and-over corrections *converging* on a goal (Kincaid, *et al.*, in press). Effective communication begins with the audience and continues over time as a process of mutual adjustment and convergence (Piotrow, *et al.*, 1997). Properly conducted, formative research and pretesting of activities and materials is a "conversation" between members of the audience and those who design and conduct the program. It gives the audience or stakeholders a chance to speak first – to provide valuable information about their own situation, beliefs and values, current and past behavior, hopes and dreams for a better life. Monitoring research tells us who and how many are listening or otherwise participating. Impact evaluation measures how many have been affected, in what ways, and why, enabling improvements in the next "conversation." From start to finish, this process is designed to reduce the gap between the initial state of the audience or community and its desired state, as specified by the audience or community itself and the objectives of the program (Kincaid *et al.*, in press).

Ecological thinking is not new. As early as 1946, the World Health Organisation drew attention to the fact that many of the barriers to change at one level can be found in conditions at higher levels of the social system (WHO, 1946). Unfortunately, none of these early ecological models explicitly mention communication. Figure 4.1

depicts an updated version of ecological thinking that includes communication. The Social Ecology Model of Communication and Health Behavior (SEMCHB) (Kincaid et al., 2007b) describes the complexity, interrelatedness, and wholeness of the components of a complex adaptive system, rather than just particular components in isolation from the system. The two key features of this model are the assumptions of *embeddedness*, a state in which one system is nested in a hierarchy of other systems at different levels of analysis, and *emergence*, in which the system at each level is greater than the sum of its parts.

The SEMCHB is a *metatheory* in the sense that each level shown in the model encompasses theories of change for that particular level. For example, the ideational model of communication and behavior change described above fits largely into the individual level; interpersonal relationship theory and bounded normative influence theory (Kincaid, 2004) fit into the social network level; the communication for participatory development model (CFPD) (Kincaid and Figueroa, 2009) applies to the community level; while theories of mass media effects on society such as cultivation (Gerbner et al., 1986; Morgan, 2009) fit into the societal level. The main contribution of the ecological model is to emphasize how higher levels facilitate or constrain change at lower levels of analysis; suggesting that communication interventions should address all four levels to be effective.

The model also implies that if individual change is facilitated and supported by social changes at higher levels it is more likely to be self-sustaining. Individuals who go against prevailing norms, who attempt to change without support and complementary change from other family members, or who defy local community leaders or power brokers will find it difficult to maintain new behavior even if highly motivated to change. An anecdotal example of societal-level constraints on community leaders is the case of a traditional chief in KwaZulu Natal, South Africa, with whom we worked, who reached the conclusion in 2007 that the AIDS epidemic was so severe in his village that everyone should be tested for HIV infection. However, political pressures and lack of attention to HIV/AIDS issues that arose during national and provincial elections that year sidetracked his plan. What would this traditional chief have done if the leaders of his party and national leaders had publicly encouraged local leaders to advocate HIV testing in their communities?

While SEMCHB portrays health within an ecological context, it is not an operational model because it provides little specific guidance for the design and implementation of programs. Ideal strategies do not just implore people to change or decry inequities that suppress change. They must identify specific desired outcomes of a communication program, specify the direct and indirect determinants of those outcomes, and detail how communication will influence those determinants. When we speak of direct and indirect determinants, we refer to individual health actions and the social psychological drivers of behavior, as well as to community engagement and participation and the effectiveness of and access to health care delivery systems, all supported by enlightened health policy. All of these determinants, of course, can be influenced by communication.

Health Competence

Closer to an operational or predictive model of health communication is the Pathways™ to Health Competence model (Storey *et al.*, 2006). The concept of health competence reflects the continuing evolution of multilevel ecological theories of behavior. In early 2002, the Office of Population and Reproductive Health of the United States Agency for International Development (USAID) issued a Request for Applications for a global health communication project (USAID, 2002). USAID was at the time undergoing structural change through which divisions responsible for population and reproductive health, child survival, maternal and child health, HIV/AIDS, and infectious disease would be organized into a single Global Bureau for Health. This procurement, which became the Health Communication Partnership (HCP) project, was intended to serve the health communication needs of the entire Bureau in an efficient manner, cutting across health domains to "employ communication effectively to improve health, stabilize population, and advance a health-competent society" (USAID, 2002, p. 6). A health-competent society is one in which individuals, communities, and institutions have the knowledge, attitudes, skills, and resources needed to improve and maintain health (Storey *et al.*, 2006).

Conceptually, the Pathways™ model emerged from an extensive review of theories and evidence regarding levels or domains of communication activity and impact. For example, at the individual and interpersonal level, competence factors related to decision-making and behavior are derived from such theories as reasoned action/planned behavior (Ajzen and Fishbein, 1997), social learning (Bandura, 1986), diffusion (Rogers, 2003), and risk management (Witte and Allen, 2000) models, as well as theories of emotion (Zajonc, 1984), social comparison and influence (Festinger, 1954; Suls, 1977), subjective norms (Fishbein and Ajzen, 1975; Ajzen and Fishbein, 1997), self-efficacy and collective efficacy (Bandura, 1986, 1997), self-image (Triandis, 1972), subjective risk (Becker, 1974), and personal advocacy (Piotrow *et al.*, 1997).

At the community level, other frameworks such as health literacy (e.g., Kickbusch and Nutbeam, 1998; Nutbeam, 2000) and social capital (Putnam, 1993, 2001; Kawachi, Kennedy, and Lochner, 1997) inform health competence. Both concepts have cognitive dimensions (e.g., trust and reciprocity) and structural dimensions (e.g., patterns and levels of participation in groups). For example, in terms of health, social capital facilitates social mobilization for health improvement, structurally enhances access to and the flow of information and increases the likelihood of social, emotional and material support for behavioral decision-making.

Also at the community level, the previously mentioned *Integrated Model of Communication for Social Change* (Figueroa *et al.*, 2002) informs health competence through its focus on the process of community dialogue leading to collective action, which is itself based on theories of development communication (Beltran, 1974; Diaz Bordenave, 1994), theories of group dynamics, conflict resolution, and network/convergence (Kincaid, 1979), as well as less often considered perspectives on such topics as

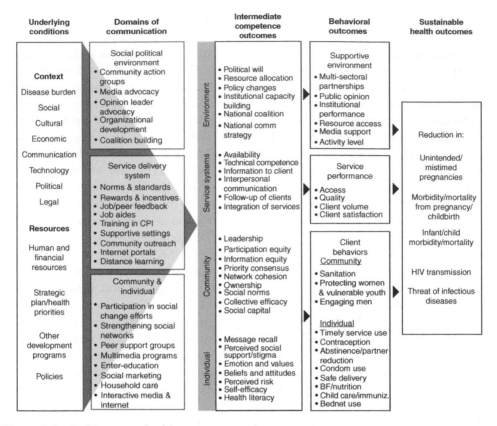

Figure 4.2 Pathways to a health-competent society.
Source: Center for Communication Programs, Johns Hopkins Bloomberg School of Public Health.

leadership (e.g., Senge, 1994; Stodgill, 1974; Lord and Brown, 2004; Tirmizi, 2002; Chemers, 2000) and equity (Gumucio-Dagròn, 2001; White, 1994; Moser, 1993).

Because health competence is determined by the combination of many interrelated factors, it is not an either/or condition; rather it lies along a continuum from low to high. A health-competent society is one in which competence is strong at multiple levels. People who are health-competent act appropriately and consistently to improve and/or maintain health across whatever health areas become personally relevant (e.g., infection prevention, healthy lifestyles, maternal and child health, reproductive health) or at the levels where they exercise responsibility (e.g., the household, the community, the delivery of services, the formulation and implementation of policy).

According to this perspective, *health-competent environments* enact policies that create opportunities for communities and individuals to flourish, allow decision making through debate and dialogue among the media, community and civil society, and provide universal access to health information. *Health-competent service delivery systems* provide access to quality services and products; have adequate capacity in their workforce (leadership, management, training, professionalism); and have governance structures through which stakeholders can access and be involved in the design and operation of health systems. *Health-competent communities* are involved in setting health agendas, have structures and systems that allow members to participate in planning, setting priorities and ensuring that the means of communication are available to all. At the *individual* level, people participate in local governance, express appropriate demand for care-seeking/providing behaviors, make health-enhancing lifestyle choices across a range of health issues (e.g., reproductive health, diet, substance use, and child care), and adhere to treatment protocols, because they understand and realize the benefits of such actions.

Communication influences health competence and health-competent behavior in a variety of ways and can be used instrumentally in social and behavior change programs to help individuals, communities, service delivery systems and whole societies progress toward sustainable health outcomes. While the model has an implicit left-to-right orientation, suggesting causal order and progression toward (pathways to) improved health, consistent with common models of social and behavior change, it should not be interpreted as endorsement of a strictly linear communication and change process. In fact, all levels and stages of change interact to reinforce each other.

Evolution of Methods and Measurement

No discussion of theory is complete without consideration of the research methods and measurement approaches upon which the theory is based. As theories in health communication have evolved so the research methods and the measures to monitor the process of health communication and its effects have developed over time. In fact, many of the advances in ecological theory would not have been possible without the simultaneous evolution of methods and measures in response to donor demands for reliable evidence of impact and causal attribution. From reliance on simple associations between program exposure and outcomes used in the late 1980s to the measurement of the direct and indirect effects of communication in the 1990s, to sophisticated multivariate and multilevel analyses in the 2000s, applied health communication research has been informed by – and has informed – the development of theories. At our Center, if not elsewhere, four principles have consistently guided applied research during this extended period: (1) formative research should be interdisciplinary (including the use of local theories and local knowledge) in order to explore the multilevel factors that affect health practices; (2) program monitoring and outcome monitoring should aim to learn from the communication process as it unfolds by systematically tracking the implementation process and intermediate outcomes, respectively; (3) impact evaluation should be future-oriented and theory-based (Chen, 1990) in order to understand the program's transformation processes (i.e., *how* the communication worked) and determine how to improve the program, and (4) program implementation and program research and evaluation should be fully integrated across the entire program cycle and should involve local expertise from the start in order to tap local wisdom and build local capacity.

The Contribution of Methods and Measurement
to Theory

It is beyond the scope of this chapter to thoroughly describe the many ways in which
these four principles of health communication research have contributed to bring health
communication theory and practice to where it is today.

Briefly, *formative research* helps bring the "voices" of people into the design of the
program. While most programs in the late 1980s and early 1990s focused on the individual as the main audience, much of the formative research attempted to identify social
and structural influences on individual motivations and choices, including the influence
of secondary audiences such as husbands, mothers-in-law, health providers, community
leaders, and others who exert positive or negative social pressure. As early as 1996,
formative research for the *Puentes* project in rural Peru (see more below) used a triangulation approach to identify higher-level factors that had resulted in lack of, and untimely
use of, health services.

Formative research methods and approaches evolved as health issues grew in complexity and as dissatisfaction with the quality of information derived from traditional methods such as focus groups and in-depth interviews increased. Participatory research
methods expanded dramatically in the mid 1990s, introducing new ways to gain deeper
insight into prevailing mental models and sense-making related to wellness, disease, and
health decision making. Recently, projective techniques such as photo-elicitation were
used in Mozambique to help stakeholders articulate culture-based values and beliefs
related to gender and sexual norms by projecting their thoughts onto photographs of
couples and events. Other methods being used in Mozambique include the "photovoice" technique, which uses photography taken by youth and music to reflect attitudes
toward health. Content analysis of newer forms of communication such as text messages
and Twitter feeds, as well as analysis of the networks formed using social media, offer
additional opportunities to bring people's reality and voices into the development of
media content and to understand how that content is used.

Monitoring research is used to track whether or not a program is being implemented
as planned, is reaching the intended end users, and is generating the expected reactions
to communication activities and materials. Depending on the program timeframe and
resources, monitoring can also contribute to the development of audience-centered
communication content. For example, (Singhal and Durá, 2010) used a system of "cultural scorecards" to assess initial success at achieving desired health outcomes. The growing access to interactive and social media such as text messaging and Facebook creates
opportunities for qualitative and participatory program monitoring that allow people to
openly and in "real time" express their reactions to the content of a program. These
same phone- and Internet-based technologies allow health communication programs to
analyze mass response from audiences that has always been there but was hard to access.
New data capture methods like these contribute to our theoretical understanding of
social communication in ways we could not have imagined just a few years ago.

Program evaluation also has become increasingly theory-driven, as opposed to
method-driven. Theory-driven evaluation is designed to both measure the effect of a

program on desired outcomes while simultaneously explaining how and why change occurred in order to improve future program efforts. Quantitative methods have become increasingly rigorous and sophisticated, requiring considerable training to be used correctly and effectively. Methods have evolved from simplistic treatment-control experimental designs that can manipulate only one variable at a time, to complex, dynamic, multivariate approaches (often paired with qualitative methods) that are appropriate for evaluating large-scale, population-based, multimedia programs over time, and which also permit modeling of sophisticated social and behavioral theories. Examples of some of these newer methods include the measurement of communication dose response (Kiragu *et al.*, 1996), the measurement of indirect exposure and effects (Boulay *et al.*, 2002), the role of ideation (Kincaid *et al.*, 2007a), the use of time-series analyses (Kincaid *et al.*, 2002), propensity score matching (Babalola and Vondrasek, 2005; Kincaid and Do, 2006) and Multivariate Casual Attribution (MCA) analyses (Babalola and Kincaid, 2009) and multilevel analysis (Babalola, 2008).

Despite the vast body of evaluation literature, however, health communication scholars continue to struggle to keep up with theory, particularly ecological theory. The quantification of social and structural factors, although steadily improving, is still based largely on the aggregation of individual data to the group or cluster level, thereby still falling short of operationalizing collective aspects of theory. Qualitative methods fare somewhat better at describing higher conceptual levels, but themselves fall short on generalizability and on the generation of population-based estimates of effects. These methodological limitations will continue to challenge us as we attempt to develop a global theory of health communication, but the effort to address those challenges and develop the appropriate methodologies to match our theories will be worthwhile.

Applications of Multilevel Ecological Models

Ecological models like Pathways™ to health competence can help theorists and practitioners identify and interpret needs and opportunities for health communication within and across levels of society. They also provide a framework for global comparative research, but to date only limited comparative research has been done using this model (Storey, Kaggwa, and Harbour, 2006). Little work has examined the impact of political/environmental level factors on health outcomes because this would require cross-national comparisons. Such research opportunities are limited by the existing funding structures for health communication that are oriented primarily toward national, subnational or even community-based programs. For example, although the health competence model was designed for use in the global Health Communication Partnership program (http://hcpartnership.org/) that eventually operated in 21 countries, the resources for research were usually insufficient for tests of the health competence model across all competence levels within each country, let alone at all levels in multiple countries. So while there are few *global* research projects, there may be growing opportunity for *international* synthesis across a growing body of programs that use a multilevel ecological approach.

Aman Tirta: Public–private partnerships and policy change for safer water

Unsafe drinking water is a major cause of diarrhea, which is the second leading killer of children under five in Indonesia. Boiling water in Indonesia is a universal practice. However, stored drinking water at home is often found contaminated with E.coli, a bacterial indicator of fecal contamination.

Initially, *Aman Tirta* began as a solely private venture. In partnership with CARE International Indonesia, two commercial companies – PT Tanshia Consumer Products and Ultra Salur – developed a public–private partnership (PPP) approach to create the first fully sustainable (non-subsidized, self-financing) commercial model to promote a specific safe water systems product: *Air RahMat*. This low-cost water disinfection technology was introduced in Indonesia in 2005 to provide households with an alternative technology to prepare their drinking water. When used correctly in conjunction with proper storage, *Air RahMat* is 15 times cheaper than boiling water and studies have shown that it reduces the risk of diarrhea up to 85 percent. Commercial manufacturing and distribution of *Air RahMat* plus community participation and media promotion activities that engage communities (including locally produced sociodramas, puppet shows, and youth group activities) created demand for the product and for safe water practices.

Advocacy communication with the Ministry of Health (MOH) created an enabling environment for household water treatment and safe storage by introducing several methods of water treatment (filtration, chlorination, and others) to Indonesian households, who have consistently used boiling but not fully benefitted from safe water. By introducing and actively promoting a Community-Based Total Sanitation policy beginning in 2008, the MOH focused public attention on a hygiene behavior cluster that included five practices: no open defecation, hand washing with soap, household water treatment and safe storage, solid waste management, and waste water management. This new policy also endorsed several treatment technologies, including *Air RahMat,* that were totally unknown to Indonesian households when the program started. At the same time the Ministry of Health decided to scale up the program and set a goal of implementation in 330 districts or 20,000 villages by 2014, ensuring the sustainability of household water treatment, safe water storage and other hygiene practices.

Puentes: Bridging services and community

The *Puentes* (Bridges) project in Peru (1997–2004), was a USAID-funded initiative implemented by a partnership of the Johns Hopkins Center for Communication Programs, Save the Children and the Peru Ministry of Health (MOH). In rural Peru, the relationship between clients and providers was a major barrier to utilization of reproductive health services: cultural power relationships and educational and socio-economic gaps between clients and providers lead to poor communication. Traditionally, efforts to improve the utilization of health services focus on the supply side by strengthening providers' clinical skills (training); improving management systems, logistics and finances; formalizing and enforcing standards for service delivery, and so on. But the supply side approach may not address community concerns and perspectives, i.e., the demand side.

To correct this imbalance, *Puentes* "listened" to community members and providers then tried to develop shared responsibility between health providers and community members and increase communities' sense of ownership in achieving quality public health services. *Puentes* established a local project team for planning, implementing and monitoring the project. Led by Save the Children, the team was trained in community mobilization principles, facilitation skills, participatory techniques, and interpersonal communication skills. Communities were identified where there was interest in participating in the project, where the need to improve relations had been identified, and where women could be involved in the development of the project. Together, communities and health personnel conducted a self-diagnosis using participatory videos. Using the video as stimulus, the community and health service groups met over two days to develop a definition of "quality" and a joint action plan that focused on such improvements as affordable medicines in stock, shorter waiting times, 24-hour access to care, understandable information, confidentiality and privacy, more equitable balance of power between communities and service providers, more mutual respect, and more female service providers.

What changed as a result? Health officials and community members reported increased use of health services, the formation of joint committees to coordinate, monitor, and document activities, regular meetings between communities and service providers to review progress toward the quality goals, expanded hours of service, and better drug stocks. In terms of health impact, a comparison between villages in project and non-project areas showed significant increases in family planning use and lower incidence of acute respiratory infection (seasonally adjusted) in project areas only. Finally, the methodology was adopted by the Ministry of Health's national quality improvement project, although not without some initial problems as higher power structures shut down some of the joint efforts by communities and providers.

One lesson illustrated by *Puentes* is that structural change at the community (no less at the national and even global) level is often needed as a precondition to improvements in health. Efforts to promote reform in such things as media policy and donor agency priorities, while important, should not take precedence over efforts to change conditions at the national and community levels where investments in health communication and communication capacity building can have direct and immediate impact on health outcomes. Global theories of health behavior and social change should, therefore, acknowledge global structural issues while focusing attention on practical national- and community-level efforts where change can be most readily achieved. Furthermore, by focusing on activities by and with national and local institutions and groups, local capacity to design, implement, and evaluate health and development programs is enhanced, leading to more sustainable change.

Communication for Healthy Living: Health as an entry point to civil society

"Healthy Families, Healthy Communities" was the focal point for this community-based component of the USAID-funded Communication for Healthy Living project in Egypt (2003–2011). For a full description of this program, see Hess, Meekers, and Storey,

Chapter 18 in this volume. One key strategy was to create capable community development associations (CDAs). CDAs already exist throughout Egypt with the purpose of providing community services and providing local leaders with mechanisms for using available resources, but their capacity varies widely. Some, with greater experience and capacity, were identified as "veteran" CDAs, while those with less experience and capacity were identified as "novice" CDAs. Veteran CDAs received some initial training and seed funds to learn how to transfer their experience to novice CDAs and support them to initiate community activities.

CDAs take on the role of mobilizing their community and promoting behavior change in four health areas: family planning and reproductive health; maternal and child health; infectious disease prevention (including avian influenza, H1N1, and hepatitis; and healthy lifestyles (including hygiene, safe water, and chronic disease prevention). Specific priorities and activities were determined by the communities themselves. Over time, 49 CDAs implemented community activities in five governorates of rural Upper Egypt, reaching a population of about 1.7 million people.

Interventions are implemented primarily *for and by* women, who work as change agents at the village level. Using the Arab Women Speak Out (AWSO) women's empowerment curriculum (Underwood and Jabre, 2008), CDAs train female volunteers, who then become locally recognized role models in their families and communities. Approximately 24,000 women received AWSO training and from these, 1400 volunteers became formal outreach workers in their communities, thus bridging the gap between knowledge and action. Together with the CDA, these women develop activities tailored to the local community, based on CHL's Family Health Package, consisting of integrated family planning, reproductive health, and maternal and child health topics, as well as information on water and hygiene, nutrition, female genital cutting, tobacco, safe injection practices and HIV/AIDS.

By the end of the program, three out of four pregnant women in focal villages were receiving at least five prenatal check-ups, compared with only one in three before the program. Ninety-nine percent of births to women in the intervention villages met the WHO standards for average birth weight, compared to only 86 percent in the rest of Upper Egypt. Over 80 percent of women in the intervention villages were using family planning in the postpartum period, compared with 48 percent before the program started. The percent of children classified as malnourished in intervention villages declined from 30–40 percent at the beginning of the program to 2–5 percent at program's end.

Not only women were involved. *Dawar* meetings, a term referring to traditional weekly gatherings of male heads of households usually from a single extended family, were used as an opportunity to engage men in program activities. The main objectives of this component were to increase dialogue around family health issues among men, to increase access among men to health information, to mobilize their support of women's participate in program activities, and to mobilize community dialogue on health priorities and solutions to the village's health and environmental problems.

Community participation helped overcome barriers to public discussion of health issues and built confidence in community ability to mobilize for community improvements in schools facilities, road repair, health unit functioning and waste management.

After three years of CDA activity at the village level, the program was scaled up when several veteran CDAs began offering community training to villages at the district level. Many communities developed their own successful spin-off health programs based on the Family Health Package, generating demand in neighboring communities for assistance from the "veteran" communities. Guide manuals and materials developed for the initial intervention villages in five governorates were rolled out at the national level in 2009 and have now been adopted by nine governorates. The successful "modeling" of effective community response has encouraged new villages to adopt the approach. Village councils have come to acknowledge the role of CDAs in health advocacy and health improvement.

In terms of financial sustainability, within one year the average annual cost of implementing community-based activities in the intervention villages declined from $15,000 to $5,000 because participating villages themselves mobilized cash and in-kind resources, thereby increasing the sustainability of the program. CDAs used skills they learned during the training and mentoring process related to resource mobilization, financial management, fund raising and proposal development increased the financial stability of these organizations. Veteran CDAs that had mentored new CDAs frequently formed ongoing working relationships to submit proposals to government agencies and donors for funding support. Most CDAs developed multiple sources of funding beyond the original funding support from USAID.

Tsha-Tsha and *Scrutinize*: Mass media for cultural change

Beginning in 2003, the South African Broadcasting Corporation (SABC) began airing a television drama series, *Tsha Tsha*, produced by the Centre for AIDS Development, Research and Evaluation (CADRE) and Curious Pictures, with technical assistance from Johns Hopkins Health and Education in South Africa (JHHESA), a locally registered and run NGO. *Tsha Tsha* was part of a five-year USAID-funded effort to develop, implement, and evaluate high-profile HIV prevention, care and support, and treatment campaigns that would promote and reinforce positive behaviors and attitudes and shift social norms and cultural values.

The primary audience for *Tsha Tsha* was youth and young adults aged from 16 to 35. Although it was focused on HIV/AIDS, it covered a wide spectrum of related issues including care and compassion for people living with AIDS, stigma reduction, voluntary counseling and testing, risk reduction behaviors including condom use, secondary abstinence, faithfulness, and partner reduction. Avoiding a didactic tone, the series focused on the choices young people make as they transition to adulthood and how those choices are tied up with culturally driven questions of identity and social influences. Compelling and highly popular characters modeled self-reflection and how to become active agents choosing the shape of their own lives.

The *Tsha Tsha* scripts were informed by extensive formative research, both qualitative and quantitative, as well as by extensive pretesting. An independent national survey at the end of the first year of broadcasting used a battery of items to measure psychosocial variables associated with behavioral choices, including detailed questions about program recall, character identification, empathy, cultural norms and values, and social influences. Exposure to 17 other HIV/AIDS programs, both media-based and community-based, was also measured. The use of propensity score matching techniques (Babalola and Kincaid, 2009; Kincaid and Do, 2006) to adjust for exposure bias and other control variables found a 14 percentage point increase in getting an HIV/AIDS test and a 13 percentage point increase in condom use resulting from exposure to *Tsha Tsha*, even after controlling for exposure to other HIV/AIDS programs.

On the heels of the *Tsha Tsha* success, a subsequent initiative, *Scrutinize*, was developed in 2009 to increase awareness of risk behaviors among young people (18–32 years of age) related to HIV infection including: the risk of having two or more partners at the same time; the linkage between alcohol, sex, and HIV; and the exchange of sex for money or material goods. *Scrutinize* is a joint effort by JHHESA, Levi Strauss's *Red for Life* campaign, USAID, PEPFAR, and other partners. It was comprised of eight animated advertisements (animerts) broadcast on national channels and in the waiting rooms of 307 clinics nationwide. YouTube versions of the final seven animerts used in the campaign are available on-line at the JHHESA website, http://www.scrutinize.org.za, and the Matchboxology website, http://www.matchboxology.com/. *Scrutinize* also included promotional items such as bar coasters, stickers, umbrellas, hats, HIV risk cards, Levi *Scrutinize* T-shirts, and posters that showed how to use condoms correctly and one that illustrated sexual networks, many of which linked the *Scrutinize* theme to football (soccer). Unplanned publicity occurred when one of South Africa's most popular DJs, Cleo, showed dancers in one of his music videos wearing the Levi T-shirts. Coverage of the campaign also appeared in newspapers (Kincaid *et al.*, in press).

A national impact evaluation of the *Scrutinize* campaign (Kincaid *et al.*, in press) found that correct recall of the animert on the risks associated with having multiple concurrent sexual partners (MSP) had a *positive* direct impact on knowledge of MSP risks and a direct *negative* impact on MSP behavior. Using propensity score matching techniques again, analysis of survey data indicated a 3.2 percentage point decrease in MSP behavior attributable to exposure to the MSP spot. Because the survey was population-based, it was possible to extrapolate to the number of people reached and affected by the campaign. Of the 10.8 million South Africans aged 16–32 who reported being sexually active in the year preceding the survey, 32.4 percent or 3.5 million people correctly recalled the MSP animert (32.4 percent). Based on the PSM estimate, 3.2 percent of this group or 111,886 people avoided multiple sexual partnerships as a result of exposure to the spot.

Together, *Scrutinize*, *Tsha Tsha* and other high profile mass media offerings are beginning to shift social norms in South Africa.

Developing a Global Model

As the foregoing project sketches suggest, research and practice continue to evolve as they integrate individual, social, and structural factors into ecological frameworks like the Pathways™ to Health Competence. Programs like *Puentes* in Peru and *Aman Tirta* in Indonesia can mobilize communication resources to strengthen political and service delivery systems (including in some cases the private sector) in order to create an enabling

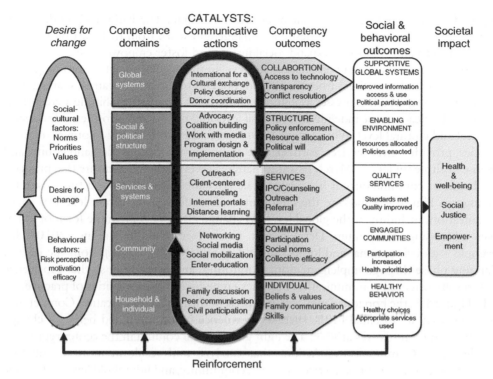

Figure 4.3 Global model of health communication and competence.
Source: Center for Communication Programs, Johns Hopkins Bloomberg School of Public Health.

environment. Communities can come together and work collectively for the common good of their members, to advocate for their needs, and to build mutually supportive partnerships with service providers. Local leaders and civil society organizations can use communication, as in *Puentes* and Egypt's CHL program, to advocate for policy change and program support, build coalitions, conduct and support outreach, monitor public health conditions and needs, network with like-minded groups, and design, implement, and evaluate health communication activities. Families, as in Egypt's CHL program, can be involved to set health priorities consistent with their family life-stage and work together to seek and use the services they need. And projects like *Tsha Tsha* and *Scrutinize* can use mass media to catalyze public dialogue and interpersonal communication in order to shift behavioral norms and generate cultural change.

However, while the Pathways™ model is a useful and dynamic guide to theory and practice across countries and programs, it is becoming clear that the missing level of analysis at this stage of evolution is the global one. Figure 4.3 is our attempt to introduce this global level into existing ecological thinking. At the far left of the model, we place the engine that drives all social development efforts: the desire for change. Societies, communities, service delivery systems, families and individuals tend to have an inherent desire to improve their lives, but often face resistance or obstacles that leave them complacent about the status quo, discouraged about opportunities for improvement, or actively opposed to social, political, economic or behavioral change. The Pathways™ model needs to account for the initial level of desire for change and work from that starting point to increase health and wellbeing, expand social justice and foster empowerment.

Fresh desire for change can originate at any level in the system, sometimes coming from the top down and sometimes from the bottom up. Desire for change can be sparked with communication, which expresses aspirations and creates *demand* by shifting perceptions of risk and efficacy at the individual behavioral level and norms and priorities at the socio-political and cultural level. When people *want* change they will allocate resources, enforce policies, provide better services, participate in community processes, demand equity, and choose healthier practices. Merely desiring change, however, does not ensure that progress will begin or continue once it has started. The arrows circulating around the Desire for Change in Figure 4.3 indicate the importance of reinforcement across levels of social organization, including at the global level. As change efforts begin–in the form of initiatives addressing Millennium Development Goals (see United Nations, 2010), for example – global, national and local stakeholders must *learn by doing*, from the earliest planning phase through implementation, monitoring, and evaluation, so that experience with results-oriented communication becomes embedded in communities of practice.

In Figure 4.3, the horizontal grey arrows represent the five communication Competence Domains that are essential to the success of evidence-based social and behavior change communication initiatives at scale. The light grey vertical column in the center represents five levels of Communicative Actions that catalyze and result in more Competent Outcomes at global, national, service delivery, community, and household levels. Dynamic arrows encircle the Communicative Actions column, suggesting how actions at the various levels can reinforce each other. Strategic communication programs work hard to optimize such reinforcement across levels so that competence is enhanced system-wide.

Global competence is characterized by transparency in international relations and committed efforts to avoid and resolve conflicts between nations as well as among national populations, national governments, and transnational organizations. Examples include a committed effort to join forces when health is threatened, such as the global efforts to prevent avian and pandemic influenza or to provide timely support for emergency relief efforts after an earthquake or tsunami. Public and private entities can collaborate to avoid overexploitation of natural and human resources worldwide, prevent human trafficking, and ensure optimal access to and use of communication and other technologies in the public interest. These competencies result from broad-based participation in international fora for cultural exchange and policy discourse, and through websites and the use of innovative technologies such as GPS resources and satellite imaging that can track and monitor disease. Donor agencies, the private sector, and philanthropic foundations can coordinate their efforts to minimize redundancy and avoid reinventing the wheel, support and promote proven methods and program approaches, and direct resources to programs, issues, and geographic areas where need is greatest, based on evidence. When these and other factors are in place, the result is Supportive Global Systems.

Political Competence is characterized by such things as appropriate formulation and enforcement of health policies, sufficient allocation of resources to systems development and functioning, and the political will to address health challenges in the first place. It is primarily at this level that national structures and institutions must deal with international and transnational forces that influence priorities and access to and investments in health programs, communication technologies and other development resources. Changes in health competence at the political structural level can shift development priorities for the greater good, respond to or influence public opinion, increase media coverage of and support for specific health issues or programs, improve access to resources, strengthen partnerships, and raise national levels of collaboration and participation in health improvement. Communication advocacy directed toward the media or opinion leaders (e.g., legislators) can build support for health policy changes or increased budgets, or strengthen political will to address controversial or difficult issues. Advocacy by community or activist groups can serve to publicize concerns or draw municipal attention to health problems. Communication within and among organizations can enhance coordination and build or mobilize coalitions around health improvement efforts or result in consensus around a national communication strategy. When these and other factors are in place, the result is an Enabling Environment.

Service Competence is characterized by such things as systematic client-oriented outreach, coordinated referral systems, and the correct use of technical skills including interpersonal communication and counseling (IPC). Within the *Service Delivery* domain, a great deal of communication occurs among providers and between clients and providers. Health service systems need to communicate norms and standards of practice, and provide rewards, incentives, and training to personnel. Information and job aids that health workers need for their work must be provided, and workers must be trained to use them effectively, perhaps through distance learning or interactive media such as mobile phones that are now being used to link health practitioners to high-quality professional resources and personnel at a distance. Health workers themselves must communicate effectively with clients, sometimes in facility-based venues, sometimes through outreach. These kinds of communication extend the availability of quality services, improve the technical skills of personnel, and improve the effectiveness of information delivered to and interactions with clients. Communication at this level can also improve coordination or integration among services, including referral and follow-up systems, resulting in increased and more effective use of quality services by clients. When these and other factors are in place, the result is the availability and delivery of Quality Services anywhere they are needed.

Community Competence is characterized by such things as participation in health improvement efforts by members of the community, the expression of positive social norms around health behaviors, and a collective belief in the community's ability to tackle health challenges. At the community level, many types of communication play a role. Interpersonal communication related to health among community members within social networks, peer groups, and the family can be encouraged or facilitated. Sometimes interpersonal contact with change agents or outreach workers provides links between the community and service domains. Mass and interactive media can provide information on demand, connect people with each other, stimulate reflection and dialogue, arouse emotions, model behaviors, and motivate action, including service utilization or advocacy for better services. Various communication strategies from social marketing to entertainment education to web-based messaging and, now, social media can play a role. Health competence outcomes of such communication can include more equitable access to information within a community, increased opportunity to participate in local health-improvement efforts, more community dialogue (if not consensus) around health priorities or other social issues, expanded or strengthened networking and collective efficacy, and increased commitment to health improvement by community leaders – all outcomes related to social capital. When these and other factors are in place, the result is Engaged Communities.

Individual Competence is characterized by such things as a belief in the value of good health as something worth pursuing, the practice of open and honest family communication about health and how to achieve it, and self-confidence in one's ability to achieve desired health outcomes. Many familiar individual-level outcomes also result from health competence communication at this level: recall of relevant health information, knowledge of health determinants and practices (health literacy), shifts in or reinforcement of health beliefs and attitudes, change in perceived risk or improved emotional coping with perceived threats to health, increased perceptions of social support for difficult health practices, reduced stigma attitudes, and increased self-efficacy. Improvements in these health-competence outcomes increase the likelihood of positive health behaviors related to hygiene, reproductive health, safe pregnancy and delivery, child feeding and immunization, and prevention of infectious diseases. When these and other factors are in place, the result is more Healthy Behavior, including appropriate and timely Service Utilization.

While it is unlikely that any one program could – or would even try to – address all of the elements described in the Global Model of Health Communication and Competence, most programs that produce measureable change in health status work holistically to at least some extent, addressing multiple levels of competence and employing multiple modes of communication. Research must inform decisions about what to address and how, helping planners choosing the combination of levels, paths, and strategies that are most likely to result in program objectives, given available program resources.

Advances in communication technology, especially newer mobile technologies and social media, and the democratization of their use – while not perfect – have dramatically improved prospects for effective health communication globally. In addition, the emergence of health issues like pandemic influenza and grand-scale environmental disasters with global impact, as well as more frequent international calls for a global response to issues such as HIV/AIDS, malaria, nutrition, and perinatal mortality, increase the need for a global theory of health behavior and social change. In this chapter we have described an evolution of theory and research that can help us conceptualize a new generation of ecological approaches to health communication and behavior. A global theory is possible if we continue to seek the elusive opportunities for cross-national comparative research, be systematic in our use of theories and research methods at the national and sub-national levels and honor the empirical obligations of our discipline. Evolution proceeds through replication with variation.

References

Ajzen, I. and Fishbein, M. (1997). *Understanding Attitudes and Predicting Social Behavior*. New York: Prentice-Hall.

Babalola, S. (2008). Correlates of the uptake of childhood immunization in northern Nigeria: A multilevel analysis. *Maternal and Child Health Journal, 13*(4), 550–558.

Babalola, S. and Kincaid, D. (2009). New methods for estimating the impact of health communication programs. *Communication Methods and Measures, 3*(1), 61–83.

Babalola, S. and Vondrasek, C. (2005). Communication, ideation, and contraceptive use in Burkina Faso: An application of the propensity score matching method. *Family Planning and Reproductive Health Care, 31*(3), 207–212.

Bandura, A. (1986). *Social Foundations of Thought and Action.* Englewood Cliffs, NJ: Prentice-Hall.

Bandura, A. (1995). *Self-efficacy in Changing Societies.* New York: Cambridge University Press.

Becker, M. H. (1974). The health belief model and personal health behavior, *Health Education Monographs 2,* 324–473.

Beltrán, S. L. R. (1974). Rural development and social communication: Relationships and strategies. In *Proceedings of the Corner-CIAT International Symposium on Communication Strategies on Rural Development, Cali, Colombia, 17–22 March* (pp. 11–27). Ithaca, NY: Cornell University.

Blanc, A. K. and Tsui, A. O. (2005). The dilemma of past success: Insiders' views on the future of the International Family Planning Movement. *Studies in Family Planning, 36*(4), 263–276.

Chemers, M. M. (2000). Leadership research and theory: A functional integration. *Group Dynamics: Theory Research and Practice, 4,* 27–43.

Chen, H. T. (1990). *Theory-driven evaluations.* Newbury Park, CA: Sage.

Cleland, J. and Wilson, C. (1987). Demand theories of fertility transition: An iconoclastic view. *Population Studies, 41,* 5–30.

Dennett, D. (1995). *Darwin's Dangerous Idea.* New York: Simon and Schuster.

Díaz Bordenave, J. (1976). Communication of agricultural innovations in Latin America: The need for new models. *Communication Research, 3*(2), 135–154.

Díaz Bordenave, J. (1994). Participative communication as a part of building the participative society. In S. A. White, N. K. Sadanandan, and J. Ascroft (Eds.), *Participatory Communication: Working for Change and Development* (pp. 35–48). New Delhi: Sage Publications.

Festinger, L. (1954). A theory of social comparison processes. *Human Relations, 7,* 117–140.

Figueroa, M. E., Kincaid, D. L., Rani, M. and Lewis, G. (2002). Communication for social change: A framework for measuring the process and its outcomes. *Communication for Social Change Working Paper Series.* Retrieved from http://www.communicationforsocialchange.org/pdf/socialchange.pdf

Fishbein, M. and Ajzen, I. (1975). *Belief, Attitude, Intention and Behavior: An Introduction to Theory and Research.* Reading, MA: Addison-Wesley.

Friedenberg, J. and Silverman, G. (2006). Mind as a black box: The behaviorist approach. In J. Friedenberg and G. Silverman (Eds.), *Cognitive Science: An Introduction to the Study of Mind* (pp 85–88). Newbury Park, CA: Sage Publications.

Gerbner, G., Gross, L., Morgan, M., and Signorielli, N. (1986). Living with television: The dynamics of the cultivation process. In J. Bryant and D. Zillman (Eds.), *Perspectives on Media Effects* (pp. 17–40). Hilldale, NJ: Lawrence Erlbaum Associates.

Gumucio-Dagrón, A., (2001). *Making Waves: Stories of Participatory Communication for Social Change.* New York: The Rockefeller Foundation.

Hempel, C. G. (1952). *Fundamentals of Concept Formation in Empirical Science.* Chicago, IL: The University of Chicago Press.

Jamison, D. T., Breman, J. T., Measham, A. R. *et al.* (Eds.) (2006). *Disease Control Priorities in Developing Countries.* Washington, DC: The World Bank and Oxford University Press.

Kawachi, I., Kennedy, B. P., and Lochner, K. (1997). Long live community: Social capital as public health. *The American Prospect, 35,* 56–59.

Kickbusch, I. and Nutbeam, D. (1998). *Health Promotion Glossary.* World Health Organisation. Geneva.

Kincaid, D. L. (1979). *The Convergence Model of Communication.* Honolulu: East-Est Communication Institute, Paper 18.

Kincaid, D. L. (2000). Social networks, ideation, and contraceptive behavior in Bangladesh: Longitudinal analysis. *Social Science and Medicine, 50,* 215–231.

Kincaid, D. L. (2004). From innovation to social norm: Bounded normative influence. *Journal of Health Communication, 9* (Supplement 1), 3757.

Kincaid, D. L. (2009). Convergence theory. In S. W. Littlejohn and K. A. Foss (Eds.), *Encyclopedia of Communication Theory.* Thousand Oaks, CA: Sage.

Kincaid, D. L., Delate, R., Storey, J. D. and Figueroa, M. E. (in press). Closing the gap in practice and theory: Evaluation of the Scrutinize HIV campaign in South Africa. In R. Rice and C. Atkins (Eds.), *Public Communication Campaigns,* 4th Edition. Thousand Oaks, CA: Sage.

Kincaid, D. L., and Do, M. P. (2006). Multivariate causal attribution and cost-effectiveness of a national mass media campaign in the Philippines. *Journal of Health Communication, 11* (Supplement 2), 1–21.

Kincaid, D. L., and Figueroa, M. E. (2009). Communication for participatory development: Dialogue, collective action, and change. In L. Frey and K. Cissna (Eds.), *Handbook of Applied Communication* (506–530). Mahwah, N.J.: Lawrence Erlbaum Associates.

Kincaid, D. L., Figueroa, M. E., Storey, J. D., and Underwood, C. R. (2007a). Communication, ideation and contraceptive use: The relationships observed in five countries. *Proceedings of the World Congress on Communication for Development.* Washington, DC: World Bank.

Kincaid, D. L., Figueroa, M. E., Storey, J.D., and Underwood, C.R. (2007b). A social ecology model of communication, behavior change, and behavior maintenance. Working paper. Center for Communication Programs, Johns Hopkins Bloomberg School of Public Health.

Kincaid, D. L., Merritt, A. P., Nickerson, L. *et al.* (2002). Impact of a mass media vasectomy promotion campaign in Brazil. In R. C. Hornik (Ed.), *Public Health Communication: Evidence for Behavior Change* (179–196). Mahwah, NJ: Lawrence Erlbaum Associates.

Kiragu, K., Krenn, S. C., Kusemiju, B. *et al.* (1996). Promoting family planning through the mass media in Nigeria: Campaigns using public service announcements and a national logo. IEC Field Report (5). Baltimore: Johns Hopkins Centre for Communication Programs.

Lord, R. G. and Brown, D. J. (2004). *Leadership Processes and Follower Self-Identity.* Mahwah, NJ: Lawrence Erlbaum Associates.

Morgan, M. (2009). Cultivation analysis and media effects. R. L. Nabi and M. B. Oliver (Eds.), *The Sage Handbook of Media Processes and Effects* (pp. 69–82). Thousand Oaks, CA: Sage.

Moser, C. O. (1993). *Gender Planning and Development: Theory, Practice and Training.* London and New York: Routledge.

Neuman, W. R. and Guggenheim, L. (2011). The evolution of media effects theory: A six-stage model of cumulative research. *Communication Theory, 21,* 169–196.

Nutbeam, D. (2000). Health literacy as a public health goal: A challenge for contemporary health education and communication strategies into the 21st century. *Health Promotion International, 15,* 259–267.

Piotrow, P. T., Kincaid, D. L, Rimon, J. G., Rinehart, W. E. (1997). *Health Communication: Lessons from Family Planning and Reproductive Health.* Westport, CN: Praeger.

Popper, K. (1963). *Conjectures and Refutations,* Routledge and Kegan Paul, London.

Powell K. E., Mercy J. A., Crosby A. E. *et al.* (1999). Public health models of violence and violence prevention. In L. R. Kurtz (Ed.), *Encyclopedia of Violence, Peace, and Conflict.* (vol. 3) (pp. 175–187). San Diego (CA): Academic Press.

Putnam, R. D. (1993). The prospective community: Social capital and public life. *The American Prospect, 13:* 1–8.

Putnam, R. D., (2001). Social capital: Measurement and consequences. ISUMA. *Canadian Journal of Policy Research*. Retrieved from http://www.oecd.org/dataoecd/25/6/1825848.pdf

Ratzan, S. C. (2001). Health literacy: Communication for the public good. *Health Promotion International*, *16*(2), 207–214.

Rogers, E. M. (1976). Communication and development: The passing of the dominant paradigm. In E. M. Rogers (Ed.). *Communication and development: Critical perspectives* (pp. 121–148). Beverly Hills, CA: Sage.

Rogers, E. M. (1983). *Diffusion of innovations*, 3rd edn. New York: Free Press.

Rogers, E. M. (2003). *Diffusion of innovations*, 5th edn. New York: Free Press.

Rogers, E. M. and Kincaid, D. L. (1981). *Communication Networks: A New Paradigm for Research*. New York: Free Press.

Sallis, J. F. and Owen, N. (2002). Ecological models of health behavior. In: Glanz, K., Rimer, B.K., Lewis, F.M. (Eds.) *Health Behavior and Health Education: Theory, Research, and Practice*, 3rd edn.). San Francisco: Jossey-Bass, pp. 462–484.

Senge, P. M. (1994). *The Fifth Discipline: The Art and Practice of the Learning Organization*. Currency Doubleday, New York.

Singhal, A. and Durá, L. (2010). Tarjetas de valoracion cultural: un llamado para desarrollar sentidos participativos de monitereo y evaluacion [Cultural scorecards: A call for participatory means of monitoring and assessment]. *Folios, 23*(January–June), 161–180.

Snyder, L. (2007). Health communication campaigns and their impact on behavior. *Journal of Nutrition Education and Behavior*, *39*, S32–S40.

Snyder, L., Johnson, B., Huedo-Medina, T. *et al.* (2009). Effectiveness of media interventions to Prevent HIV, 1986–2006: A meta-analysis. Paper presented at the Annual meeting of the American Public Health Association, Philadelphia, November 8–11.

Stodgill, R. M. (1974). *Handbook of Leadership: A Survey of the Literature*. New York: Free Press.

Storey, J. D., Kaggwa, E. and Harbour, C. (2006). Health competence research brief: Pathways to health competence for sustainable health improvement – Examples from South Africa and Egypt. Technical Report. Baltimore, MD: Johns Hopkins Center for Communication Programs.

Suls, J. M. (1997). Social comparison theory and research. In J. M. Suls and R. L. Miller (Eds.), John Wiley: New York.

Tirmizi, S. A. (2002). The 6-L framework: A model for leadership research and development [Electronic version]. *Leadership and Organization Development Journal*, *23*, 269–279.

Triandis, H. (1974). *The analysis of subjective culture*. New York: Wiley.

UNAIDS (1999). Communications framework for HIV/AIDS: A new direction. New York: UNAIDS. Retrieved from http://www.unaids.org/en/media/unaids/contentassets/dataimport/publications/irc-pub01/jc335-commframew_en.pdf.

United Nations (2010). Millenium development goals report 2010. Retrieved from http://www.un.org/millenniumgoals/reports.shtml.

USAID (United States Agency for International Development) (2002). Request for application (RFA) No. USAID M/OP-02-470. Washington, DC: Office of Population and Reproductive Health. Washington, DC.

Wakefield, M. A., Loken, B., and Hornik, R. C. (2010). Use of mass media campaigns to change health behavior. *The Lancet, 376*, 1261–1271, DOI:10.1016/S0140-6736(10)60809-4.

Westoff, C. and Bankole, A. (1997). *Mass Media and Reproductive Behavior in Africa*, Demographic and Health Surveys Analytical Reports, No. 2. Calverton, MD: Macro International.

White, S. A. (1994). The concept of participation: Transforming rhetoric to reality. In S. A. White, K. S. Nair, and J. R. Ascroft (Eds.), *Participatory Communication: Working for Change and Development*. New Delhi: Sage Publications.

Witte, K. and Allen, M. (2000). A meta-analysis of fear appeals: implications for effective public health campaigns. *Health Education and Behavior 27*, 591–615.

World Health Organisation. (1946). WHO definition of health. Preamble to the Constitution of the World Health Organisation as adopted by the International Health Conference. New York: WHO.

Zajonc, R. B. (1984). On the primacy of affect. *American Psychologist, 39*(2), 117–123.

Part II

Theoretical Perspectives
on and Approaches to Health
Communication in a Global Context

5

The Impact of Health Communication Programs

Jane T. Bertrand, Stella Babalola, and Joanna Skinner

Background

This book explores the many different types of health communication programs, the vast majority of which are designed to bring about some type of change. Whether one labels the interventions as information-education-communication (IEC), behavior change communication (BCC), or social and behavior change communication (SBCC), these programs seek to achieve specific results. This chapter focuses on impact: broadly speaking, the extent to which such programs achieve their objectives. Whereas non-evaluators might use the word in the loose sense of observing a change in the desired direction, evaluators seek greater rigor in establishing causality (i.e., that the observed change can be attributed to the communication program), as well as the magnitude of the change. In this chapter, we define "impact," describe the methods used to demonstrate change and causality, and present the results on the effectiveness of health communication for three illustrative health issues. We then discuss the most commonly used study designs for evaluating BCC programs, given that randomized control trials (RCTs) are rarely an option for communication programs, especially those with a mass media component. The chapter ends with a discussion of methodological challenges and future directions for research.

The evaluation of health communication programs can address any of four types: mass media, community-level activities (that often go under the umbrella term "community mobilization"), interpersonal communication/counseling (IPC/C), and electronic media. As described in several chapters of this book, most programs recognize the social ecological framework, whereby the actions of an individual are affected by the concentric circles of influence around them: spouse/partner, family, community, and society (Sallis and Owen, 2002). Increasingly, the design of programs takes into account these other

The Handbook of Global Health Communication, First Edition. Edited by Rafael Obregon and Silvio Waisbord.
© 2012 John Wiley & Sons, Inc. Published 2012 by John Wiley & Sons, Inc.

levels of influence and may explicitly target secondary audiences in addition to the primary audience. Although some researchers have attempted to capture these other levels of effect in their evaluations (e.g., Sweat and Dennison, 1995), in the vast majority of cases evaluation measures change in the knowledge, attitudes, risk perceptions, and behaviors of the individual.

One type of intervention closely related to health communication programs is advocacy. In general, we think of communication programs as directed toward the primary beneficiary (be it for family planning, HIV prevention, smoking cessation) as well as secondary audiences (e.g., spouses/partners, families, friends). By contrast, advocacy is a form of persuasive communication directed to changing the attitudes and actions of policy makers and decision makers that relate to structural factors, such as funding for a program, favorable regulations, or changes in legislation. Most of the work to assess the impact of advocacy has taken the form of policy analysis, case studies, and other qualitative assessments. Although advocacy is crucial to the change process, it is beyond the scope of this chapter.

Evaluators measure impact based on the stated objectives of a given health communication program. Well-designed programs often have an explicit conceptual framework that shows the pathways that lead from the program intervention to the desired change – often a behavior (e.g., use of seatbelts, condoms, contraception, bed nets). However, staged theories of behavior change indicate that individuals often go through different changes in knowledge, attitude, risk perception, self-efficacy, and other psychosocial factors (also called ideational factors) before acting on a specific behavior. Thus, many programs include such changes in their stated objectives (e.g., to increase awareness, knowledge of how to perform a specific task, risk perception, and so forth), even if behavior change is the primary objective. The conceptual framework will usually show the long-term outcome in terms of health status (e.g., morbidity, mortality, fertility), indicating the "big picture" goal for this type of program, even if it is not measured as part of the evaluation (see Figure 4.2, Pathways to a health-competent society, in the preceding chapter). For example, smoking cessation programs are designed to contribute to reductions in rates of lung cancer and other chronic ailments related to smoking, which may appear as the final desired result on the conceptual framework (or logic model) for the program. Yet the evaluation does not attempt to make this link, nor does it need to, given the strong epidemiological evidence linking smoking to lung cancer and other diseases.

Some Definitions

"Impact" is what programs seek to achieve. Yet the term has different meanings for different people. In the anecdotal sense, it can be an unmeasured aspiration that a program has some positive benefit. Even the smallest NGO can discuss the desired "impact" of its project, whether or not there are plans to evaluate it. However, if we consider the meaning of impact where some type of evaluation occurs, it generally has one of three meanings:

1   Ultimate change in health status that a program or intervention seeks to achieve, whether or not (and usually not) the evaluation design attempts to determine causal

attribution. For example, reducing incidence is the ultimate goal of almost any HIV prevention intervention, and many see their own intervention as contributing to this "impact," even if they don't attempt to measure incidence in their evaluation (or evaluate at all);

2   A change in the output or outcome indicator, consistent with the objectives of the program, assessed by quantitative methods that allow one to establish cause and effect; and

3   A definable benefit, as assessed by qualitative methods (e.g., most significant change method).

"Effectiveness" is an alternative term used in evaluation research, but again it may carry a slightly different meaning for different persons. Effectiveness, as defined by Shadish, Cook, and Campbell (2002) refers to "how well an intervention works when it is implemented under conditions of actual implementation" (p. 507). In this sense it overlaps with the second definition of impact above (i.e., measurable cause-and-effect). However, others may use it more casually to describe a measurable change consistent with the objectives of the intervention ("if the desired change occurred, my program was effective").

"Efficacy" refers to the expected change when an intervention is administered under tightly controlled circumstances, such as in a clinical trial for a new drug. It measures whether the product can effect change under ideal, controlled conditions, which is often referred to as theoretical effectiveness. To illustrate, consider the efficacy versus effectiveness of condom use. The efficacy of condom use may be 98 percent (when used properly and consistently), yet the effectiveness of condom use is generally far lower, given the tendency of men and women to forget to use it, prefer not to use it in the heat of the moment, use it incorrectly if intoxicated, or do some other thing that detracts from its potential benefit.

The evaluation of communication programs focuses on effectiveness (change under real world conditions), not efficacy. Because of the high methodological bar required to establish "impact" in the sense of causal attribution and the difficulty of applying true experimental designs to the evaluation of full-scale comprehensive communication programs, evaluators often prefer the term "effectiveness." By contrast, policy makers and program managers often prefer "impact," because it communicates a sense of success that everyone can grasp.

Evidence of Impact from Health Communication Programs

The question central to this chapter is "do health communication programs work?" That is, "do health communication programs produce measurable change, consistent with their objectives?" A national politician campaigning for office has little doubt of the "effects" of communication; similarly, even well-known brands of soft drinks or fast foods continue to spend millions on marketing campaigns because of their demonstrated effects on sales.

This question continues to be asked of health communication campaigns, and even more so when they involve multi-million dollar budgets, in part because most campaigns don't have a quick, routine, inexpensive means of measuring impact (such as sales). Because the answer to this question is complex, it is often misinterpreted as "maybe not – if it takes that much to explain." The answer is complex because:

- Campaigns generally have multiple objectives, and the results generally vary by objective (e.g., increasing knowledge versus changing behavior);
- Campaigns are not standard in media intensity or duration, resulting in differing levels of effects; and
- Campaigns on certain topics have shown greater effects than on other topics.

Let us begin with the conclusion and work backward from there. Health communication campaigns have shown measurable effects over a series of outcomes (i.e., knowledge, attitudes, risk-perception, self-efficacy, behavior) on numerous health topics in both industrial and developing countries. That being said, not every campaign achieves its desired behavioral outcomes; some are more effective than others.

Some health communication topics have been more extensively evaluated than others. In the industrialized world (primarily the United States), youth substance abuse and nutritional interventions (fruit and vegetable consumption, dietary fat intake) are the most widely evaluated topics. In the developing world, family planning and HIV prevention head the list (see Snyder, 2007a). Reasons include the urgency of the topic as a public health issue, the level of funding invested in interventions, including communication programs, on this topic (more costly programs require greater levels of accountability), and the need to demonstrate effectiveness to skeptics (e.g., in the case of international family planning).

Rather than addressing the simple question "are campaigns effective?" it is more useful to determine the magnitude of campaign effects, according to Dr. Leslie Snyder, one of the leading scholars assessing campaign impact using meta-analyses of multiple campaigns. She argues that determining the effect size of a given campaign allows one to determine how it has done in comparison to other campaigns on the same or other topics. In addition, it allows the researcher to identify variables related to effect size, such as reach (Snyder, 2001).

The level of effectiveness of health campaigns that include some form of the media depends in part on the specific behavior being presented (Snyder, 2007a), as shown in Figure 5.1. It establishes a benchmark against which to compare the effects of specific campaigns and helps to establish realistic goals for new campaigns (Snyder, 2007a). (An effect size of $r=0.05$ roughly translates into 5 percent more people performing the behavior after the campaign than before it.) Seat belt campaigns ($r=0.15$), dental care campaigns ($r=0.13$) and adult alcohol reduction ($r=0.11$) have had the greatest levels of success. Topics with moderate effect sizes include family planning ($r=0.06$), youth smoking prevention ($r=0.06$), and heart disease prevention (such as diet and physical activity behaviors ($r=0.05$)), sexual risk-taking ($r=0.04$), mammography screening ($r=0.04$), adult smoking cessation ($r=0.04$), youth alcohol prevention and cessation ($r=0.04$ to 0.07), and tobacco prevention campaigns ($r=0.04$). Programs with the least success to date include youth drug and marijuana campaigns ($r=0.01$ to 0.02). Campaigns

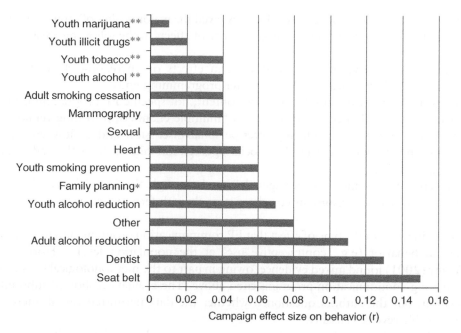

Figure 5.1 Average campaign effect size (r) on behavior across different health topics. *Source*: Snyder (2007b).

that have an enforcement (coercion) component, such as seat belt use and alcohol checks for minors, generally show a stronger effect (r=0.17) than those relying entirely on persuasion (not using messages about the legal enforcement of a behavior)(r=0.05) (Snyder and Hamilton, 2002).

In this chapter we present results on the impact of communication programs for three health topics: international family planning, HIV prevention, and smoking cessation.

International family planning programs

In the 1970s and 1980s, many developing countries became increasingly committed to decreasing rapid population growth; consequently, they developed strong family planning (FP) programs, often with a national-level media campaign to promote contraceptive use. The United States Agency for International Development (USAID) was a major funder of international family planning and supported much of this communication work through the Johns Hopkins Bloomberg School of Public Health/Center for Communication Programs (CCP). USAID wanted to determine the effectiveness of such campaigns, in part to address skeptics that questioned the value of the investment in family planning.

Hornik and McAnany (2001) conducted a very thorough and systematic analysis of the effects of media on fertility change (not just family planning use), as part of a review for the National Academy of Sciences. They reviewed the major studies of campaign effects published from 1970–1999. They found evidence of effects in the following areas:

- Campaigns do have measurable short-term effects on increasing clinic demand, though the effect appears to dissipate after programming ends;
- Access to media (exposure to ordinary content, not specific FP programming) may have societal-level effects; they observed "multiple channels, providing reinforcing messages, over time, producing inter-personal discussion and a slow change in values, and working at a level of social aggregation higher than the individual" (pp. 234–235);
- Self-reported attention to messages delivered through the IEC efforts of general pro-family planning programs correlates strongly with fertility behaviors.

However, in terms of the type of effect that FP communication programs aim to achieve – change in behavior (e.g., contraceptive use) at the population level – Hornik and McAnany (2001) found mixed evidence, owing in part to the methodological limitations in evaluating communication programs cited above. The evaluation showed substantial association, but the authors questioned whether the data permitted causal inference, citing possible reverse causality.

Snyder and colleagues have conducted several meta-analyses of the available evaluations of international family planning programs, which have quantified the effect size and yielded more positive results on the impact of FP communications program. Snyder *et al.* (2003) performed a meta-analysis of 39 family planning campaigns carried out with technical assistance from CCP between 1986 and 2001. On average, the greatest campaign effect for men and women was on knowledge of modern family planning methods ($r=0.15$). There were also positive effects for partner communication about family planning ($r=0.10$), approval of family planning ($r=0.09$), behavioral intentions ($r=0.07$), and use of modern methods of family planning ($r=0.07$).

International HIV prevention programs

Over the last two decades, the spread of HIV/AIDS has become one of the foremost public health problems, particularly in sub-Saharan Africa where its impact is having devastating effects. Funding and subsequent programming for HIV treatment and prevention have grown dramatically under the US President's Emergency Plan for AIDS Relief (PEPFAR), and communication interventions have been a primary strategy used in fighting the epidemic. The high levels of funding have supported both communication programs and evaluations of their effectiveness.

Snyder *et al.* (2009) performed a meta-analysis of media interventions to prevent HIV conducted from 1986 to 2006 in both developed and developing countries.[1] The authors examined three key outcomes: condom use, practical knowledge, and number of sex partners. On average, the greatest effects of media interventions were found to be on condom use ($r=0.36$) and also for practical knowledge ($r=0.31$). Effect sizes were stratified by development status using the Human Development Index (HDI), which revealed even higher levels of effect for interventions implemented in low HDI countries (r=0.46), compared to mid HDI countries (r=0.25) and high HDI countries (r=0.12). The research also underscored the importance of matching outcome evaluation with the goals of the program: the analysis showed that those interventions in low HDI countries that had a stated goal of condom promotion had a stronger effect than those without. On the other hand, those with a goal focused on abstinence showed lower effect sizes on condom use. Condom distribution was also found to be a mediating program factor that increases the effect size on condom use in low HDI countries, signaling the benefit of addressing supply and demand issues simultaneously.

By contrast, HIV campaigns have not had measurable impact on reducing the number of sexual partners (r=0.01) (Snyder *et al.*, 2009). Programs with this explicit objective are relatively new. Although Uganda had used the concept of "zero grazing" since 1987 and programs worldwide had included the phrase "be faithful" in many of their campaigns, the epidemiological importance of multiple concurrent partners to the spread of the epidemic only surfaced in the past five years. Programs in sub-Saharan Africa are now taking more explicit aim at this behavior (e.g., the *Scrutinize* campaign in South Africa). But the lack of measurable impact on this behavior from campaigns in previous years is not surprising, given the major focus on condom use and abstinence.

The review included those interventions that used mass media, such as TV and radio, those that use mass media plus interpersonal activities, such as peer outreach and counseling, and those that used interpersonal activities combined with small media such as posters and handouts. Of these, mass media combined with interpersonal activities showed the greatest effect in low HDI countries (r=0.51).

Results are also available on the effectiveness of peer education programs utilizing interpersonal communication channels in developing countries. Medley *et al.* (2009) conducted a meta-analysis that showed positive effects for HIV knowledge, equipment sharing among injection drug users, and condom use. The majority of evaluations reviewed measured HIV knowledge and showed moderate effect sizes (OR: 2.28, 95% confidence interval [CI]: 1.88, 2.75). Condom use was also a common outcome measured and showed similarly positive effects among a range of target populations, including injection drug users, commercial sex workers, transport workers, heterosexual adults, and miners, with a statistically significant impact when combined (OR: 1.92; 95% CI: 1.59, 2.33). The analysis did not find any effect on sexually transmitted infections (STIs). Although the results of the meta-analysis are illuminating, the authors point out the need for operations research to gain a fuller understanding of *how* peer education programs differ in implementation, *which* ones show the greatest effect and *why*, so that it is possible to identify and replicate best practices.

Smoking cessation

Smoking cessation has been the focus of many campaigns, primarily in the developed world, with mixed results as to impact. Snyder (2007b) found an effect size of r=0.04, putting adult smoking cessation at the lower end of campaign effectiveness. Much of the available evidence comes from studies conducted in northern America and Europe.

More than two decades ago, Flay (1987) reviewed findings from the evaluation of 40 domestic and international mass media campaigns that were designed to influence cigarette smoking. The 40 campaigns reflected the three methods of media use for smoking cessation: (1) provide information on the negative consequences of smoking and motivate smokers to quit; (2) promote smoking-cessation-related actions (e.g., quit for a day, call a help line, request information or self-help materials, visit a clinic); and (3) provide smoking cessation self-help media clinics. Of the campaigns that Flay reviewed, nine were informational/motivational in nature, 11 were designed to promote specific smoking cessation actions and 20 provided media self-help clinics for smoking cessation. In general, the 40 campaigns reached a large segment of the intended population. Nonetheless, not all were successful in influencing smoking prevalence, even in the short term. For example, of the nine informational/motivational campaigns, only five were associated with significant decreases in smoking prevalence. The 11 campaigns that promoted specific steps to permanent quitting showed promise with evidence of associated decreases in smoking prevalence. Evidence on the effectiveness of the 20 media self-help clinics indicate that for smokers who already display knowledge, attitudes and intention that are consistent with smoking cessation, the media can provide effective self-help clinics to enable them to stop smoking.

More recently, Bala, Strzeszynski, and Cahill (2009) reviewed 11 studies that assessed the effectiveness of mass media interventions for adults in Australia, South Africa, England, and the USA. The studies showed mixed results regarding the effectiveness of the media for smoking prevalence, cigarette consumption, quit attempts, and quit rates. The review also revealed mixed results for the effectiveness of smoking cessation media campaigns on intermediate variables, including knowledge about negative consequences of smoking, attitudes toward smoking, social pressure to quit and smoking-related norms. Overall, eight of the 11 programs showed some positive effects on smoking behavior.

A rigorous evaluation of England's Health Education Authority's anti-smoking advertisement campaign found that, after 18 months, exposure to the media-only component of the campaign increased the odds of *not* smoking by 53 percent while exposure to both the media campaign and community anti-smoking activities increased the odds by 67 percent compared to non-exposure (McVey and Stapleton, 2000), a statistically significant difference.

The published literature contains many studies on the effectiveness of smoking cessation communication programs *among youth*. These studies tend to show somewhat more positive effects than for the population as a whole (largely adults). Farrelly, Niederdeppe, and Yarsevich (2003) reviewed studies on mass media campaigns for youth and found that most campaigns showed significant positive effects. Farrelly and colleagues found evidence of effectiveness in both experimental studies targeting a narrow, clearly defined geographic area and in statewide, broad-coverage interventions. In one experimental study, researchers found that a four-year advertising campaign led to considerable reductions in smoking prevalence; the positive effects persisted two years after the intervention ended (Flynn *et al.*, 1992). In another experimental study in Norway, adolescents in one county that received a set of three smoking cessation media interventions were compared with their counterparts in a control county (Halfstad *et al.*, 1997). The study found that nonsmokers at baseline were less likely to smoke at follow-up in the intervention county compared to the control county. The study also found that adolescent girls (but not adolescent boys) who smoked at baseline were more likely to have stopped smoking at follow-up in the intervention county compared to the control country. The positive results persisted one year after the end of the interventions. This study is significant in that it is one of the few that found positive effects for a stand-alone (as opposed to being combined with community-based or school-based activities) smoking cessation media intervention.

A number of statewide campaigns were found to be effective for youth smoking behaviors, including the Massachusetts anti-tobacco media campaign (Commonwealth of Massachusetts, 2002; Siegel and Biener, 2000), the Truth campaign in Florida (Bauer *et al.*, 2000) and to some extent the Question It campaign in Mississippi (Fisher, 2001). However, other studies on the effects of statewide interventions for youth did not demonstrate positive results, partly because of the difficulty of isolating the effects of a specific full-coverage media intervention in a context of larger, more comprehensive approaches to tobacco control.

One consistent finding does emerge from studies on the literature on communication programs and their effect on smoking behavior: media programs that are implemented as part of a comprehensive approach to tobacco control are more effective than stand-alone media programs (Flay, 1987; Murray, Prokhorov, and Harty, 1994; Farrelly, Niederdeppe, and Yarsevich, 2003; Bala, Strzeszynski, and Cahill, 2009). Other factors that appear to enhance the effectiveness of communication programs for smoking cessation include intensive and high frequency programming, extended reach, long duration and sociodemographic characteristics of program recipients (Flay, 1987; McVey and Stapleton, 2000; Farrelly, Niederdeppe, and Yarsevich, 2003; Bala, Strzeszynski, and Cahill 2009).

Cost-effectiveness

Media are often more cost-effective at reaching people than interpersonal channels, because they can reach very large numbers after the initial investment required to produce the message, whereas interpersonal channels incur ongoing salary and other costs in reaching relatively small numbers at a given event or setting. To calculate cost-effectiveness, it is necessary to first establish effectiveness, then determine the costs of the program, to arrive at an estimate of cost per unit of change. Given the methodological challenges of evaluating the effectiveness of communication programs, evaluating their cost-effectiveness further raises the bar. Nonetheless, a number of researchers have estimated the cost per unit of change for different types of communication programs.

These cost-effectiveness studies fall into two main categories: (1) comparing the cost effectiveness of a communication program to other types of interventions designed to achieve the same objectives, and (2) establishing the cost per unit of change as a programmatic indicator of interest to donor agencies and program directors. In terms of examples of the first type, Cohen, Wu, and Farley (2004) evaluated the cost-effectiveness of different types of HIV/AIDS interventions in developed and developing countries using modeling techniques. Of the 26 interventions evaluated, including biomedical, structural, and individual behavior change programs, mass media programs were found to be one of the most cost-effective approaches. Another study that examined different types of interventions in developing countries found that mass media, peer education, and treatment of STIs for sex workers were the most cost-effective options available (Hogan *et al.*, 2005). By comparison, school-based education activities had a high cost per disability adjusted life year (DALY) averted (Hogan *et al.*, 2005; Cohen, Wu, and Farley, 2004).

Some of these studies comparing interventions have also been carried out in the context of specific country epidemics. For example, in Peru, one study found that mass media was among the four most cost-effective interventions, along with peer education, treatment of STIs and voluntary counseling and testing (Aldridge *et al.*, 2009). In the Dominican Republic, a comparison between a communication intervention and an intervention that added a structural component through policy regulation found that both approaches were cost effective per DALY, but that cost-effectiveness increased when the policy approach was added (Sweat *et al.*, 2006). In India, Sood and Nambiar (2006) compared the cost of three television-based components of a single mass media campaign. They found that the most expensive component – the TV drama series – was also the most cost-effective, based on per-user increased condom use; the authors argued that *cost-effectiveness* – not the total cost of the component – should be a primary consideration in decision making regarding programming.

Several studies of the second type (establishing the cost per unit of change for programmatic purposes) have been conducted in relation to international family planning programs. Robinson and Lewis (2003) estimated the cost of giving a client sufficient knowledge and motivation to lead them to seek out and adopt a contraceptive method in the Egypt program to be approximately US$3.00. Kincaid and Do (2006) used a series of multivariate techniques to support the conclusion that the observed 6.4 percentage point increase in modern contraceptive use following a communication program in the Philippines could be attributed to the national mass media campaign and to its effects on attitudes toward contraceptives. This net increase represented 348,695 new adopters in the population of married women at a cost of US$1.57 per new adopter.

Long-term effects

Surpassing the challenges of measuring short-term effects of health communication programs are the difficulties and complexities of measuring and understanding long-term effects. A larger public health impact, such as a decline in disease incidence or prevalence, is often the ultimate long-term goal of health communication programs, but this level of impact is rarely measured. In some cases, this is because the evidence linking the behavior to the disease outcome is so well established, as is the case with smoking and lung cancer, that it can safely be assumed that reductions in smoking will lead to long-term reductions in lung cancer incidence (Wakefield, Loken, and Hornik, 2010). In other cases, the feasibility of measuring disease incidence over time among the vast target audience of typical communication programs, compared to smaller cohorts of randomized control trials for example, is a significant barrier.

More frequent, albeit still rare, are measures of long-term impact in terms of sustaining changes in knowledge, attitudes, or behaviors over time. A recent summary of mass media campaigns to change health behavior noted that the behavioral impact tends to decrease when the intervention ends. This is particularly true for changes in behavior that require ongoing action, such as physical activity or tobacco prevention, rather than campaigns that target one-off actions such as immunization (Wakefield, Loken, and Hornik, 2010). In part, this is due to the continual influence of competing factors, such as tobacco advertising or the abundant availability of junk food.

In the case of smoking cessation, a systematic review of school-based programs found very few studies that measured the long-term impact, a reflection of the difficulties in allocating scarce resources for long-term follow-up. Nevertheless, of those interventions that did conduct follow-up, little evidence of long-term effectiveness was found (Wiehe *et al.*, 2005). However, results from another review of school-based tobacco prevention programs that focused on social influences did find significant long-term effects ranging from 2–15 years, although the great variability in the rigor of evaluations included in the study is a limitation. The authors hypothesize that long-term effects are more likely to be found for those programs that demonstrated strong short-term effects (Skara and Sussman, 2003).

HIV prevention programs that measure long-term impact are also limited, again a reflection of the lack of resources allocated to this type of follow-up. A systematic review of mass media programs for promoting HIV testing in developed countries found no long-term effects despite short-term changes in behavior, possibly due to the short campaign durations (Vidanapathirana *et al.*, 2005). However, another study comparing the effectiveness of fear-inducing campaigns compared to HIV counseling and testing on perceived risk, knowledge, and condom use found that, although fear campaigns are not an effective intervention, both short-term and long-term effects were found for counseling and testing. For these interventions, the authors found that initial increases in condom use grew over time, leading them to hypothesize that a longer timeframe gives participants greater opportunity to reflect on their behavior and for the environment to reinforce the behavior being promoted (Earl and Albarracin, 2007).

These studies suggest we can be cautiously optimistic about the effects of health communication programs on sustaining long-term behavior change. However, the challenges identified in measuring long-term effectiveness highlight the need for greater investment in long-term programs that meet the realities of the ongoing competing messages and external environmental factors encountered when trying to change ongoing behaviors.

Commonly Used Study Designs for Evaluating BCC programs

How does a researcher conduct a study to measure the impact of a communication program? Communication evaluation uses the same methods available in other realms of public health evaluation to measure impact. For some purposes it is adequate simply to demonstrate that the desired change occurred; however, in many situations the challenge for the researcher is to demonstrate that the intervention *caused* the desired change (and to measure the magnitude of the change). To answer this question of cause and effect, the researcher must select from among a number of different study designs. The strength of the causal inference (that is, the claim that the campaign caused the observed change in behavior) depends directly on the rigor of the study design used. The three main categories of study design include:

- experimental study designs (of which randomized control trials [RCTs] are one type);
- quasi-experimental designs (possibly the most widely used in program evaluation at present); and
- nonexperimental designs (fraught with biases but nonetheless used extensively on the grounds that they are better than nothing).

In the next section we outline the most widely used study designs for evaluating the impact of communication programs and determining causality, starting with the least rigorous and moving to the most rigorous.

Most evaluation manuals and introductory epidemiology textbooks present the full range of study designs for demonstrating cause and effect, with a description of the advantages and disadvantages of each. These bibliographic references range from the classic texts (Campbell and Stanley, 1963; Cook and Campbell, 1979) to user-friendly versions for field personnel (e.g., Fisher and Foreit, 2002). The section below is by no means an exhaustive list of study designs but rather those most commonly used in the evaluation of communication programs.

Nonexperimental designs

Cross-sectional designs with no pretest

1 Cross-sectional designs with no pretest (also known as a correlational or passive observational designs) yield data that can be used to assess if certain attributes tend to co-occur, but lack the desired elements for plausible causal attribution such as pretests and control groups. For example, a researcher might be interested in the degree to which people who are exposed to a communication program on family planning tend to use contraceptive methods. To answer the research question, the research might conduct a household survey among the intended audience and ask questions regarding campaign exposure and condom use.

2 *"Before/after" or pretest–posttest design with no control group.* This design is widely used because it answers a very pressing question: did the desired change occur? It involves comparing the percent performing the behavior before and after the campaign. If the difference is statistically significant, one can claim to have demonstrated change.[2]

Nonexperimental designs are fairly easy to implement; the major limitation to this type of design is that it does not control for potential confounding factors. For example, in the scenario described above, the data may show a strong correlation between campaign exposure and condom use. The data, however, cannot demonstrate a cause and effect relationship because the study has not controlled for alternative explanations of the observed correlation, including selection bias, the influence of a third variable, and reverse causation.

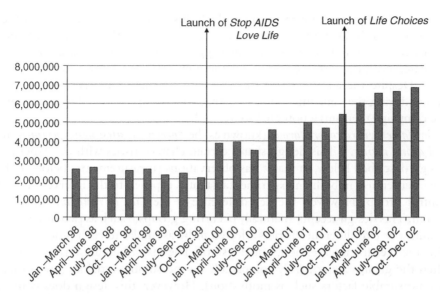

Figure 5.2 Condom sales in the Ghana social marketing program: A time series analysis. *Source*: Tweedie *et al.* 2002.

Quasi-experimental designs

A common feature of quasi-experimental designs is the use of control groups and/or pretest outcome measures to infer what would have happened in the absence of the intervention. Also common to quasi-experimental designs is the absence of random assignment of individuals or groups to treatment or control conditions. In quasi-experimental design, the researcher must identify all alternative explanations of the expected relationship prior to the study and devise plans to address them through design, logic, measurement or analysis (Shadish, Cook, and Campbell, 2002). The caveat is that it is not always easy or feasible to enumerate and address all the potential alternative explanations. Four quasi-experimental designs used in the evaluation of health communication programs are listed below (1–4):

1   *(Interrupted) time series analysis.* This method tracks the desired result of a given intervention both before and after the intervention, but in contrast to the simple before/after design, it does so over a number of points prior to, and a number of points after, the intervention. Time series lends itself to evaluations where the desired result is measured through routinely collected service statistics (e.g., number of clinic visits, number of condoms sold) or some other statistic that is available at regular intervals over time. For example, some communication campaigns are designed to increase service utilization at a network of facilities or to increase the volume of sales for a specific product. For such cases, time series is an excellent method that involves little additional expense for the evaluation. The graph in Figure 5.2 illustrates the volume of condom sales before and after a condom social

marketing campaign in Ghana in the early 2000s. The fact that the slope of the line changed sharply after the launch of the campaign and the intercept of the line increased significantly at the same time suggests that the communication campaign increased both the absolute number of condoms and the rate of increase in condom sales. Despite the advantages of this method, "history" (that is, some event that occurs during the same interval of time that affects the outcome but is unrelated to the campaign) remains a potential source of bias.

2 *Before/after with a control group* (known as the *"pretest–posttest nonexperimental control group design."*) This design shares certain characteristics with the experimental design described below, in that it has observations (measurements) before and after the intervention in both an experimental (that is exposed to the intervention) and a control group. However, the key difference is the *lack of randomization* in this design. This design accepts "naturally occurring groups," such as two different communities or two different districts selected to be as similar to each other as possible. One receives the intervention, one does not. The major limitation is selection bias: often the groups are not truly comparable on measurable variables (and worse yet, nonmeasurable factors such as motivation). However, this design does control for testing and history, making it much stronger than the simple before/after design with no control group.

3 *Pretest–posttest separate sample design* (also known as the *"one-group pretest–posttest design,"* according to Shadish, Cook, and Campbell (2002)). This design is very similar to the nonexperimental design of pretest–posttest with no control group, mentioned above, except that the two different samples are randomly selected for the before and after measurement. By randomly selecting members of the study population, the evaluators can control for selection bias (theoretically, the random selection will yield two highly similar groups on key compositional variables) and for testing effect (since few if any of the respondents on round 1 will be in round 2). It does have the major limitation that it does not control for history.

4 *Post-test only with advanced statistical controls.* Increasingly, evaluators are turning to a quasi-experimental one-group posttest-only design that applies statistical controls to reduce the potential bias of confounding variables, allowing one to make claims of plausible attribution. This approach comprises a group of techniques that Babalola and Kincaid (2009) referred to as Multivariate Causal Analysis (MCA). Included in this class of methods is propensity score matching (PSM) (Rosenbaum and Rubin, 1983, 1984). The technique is used to create a control group (not exposed to the campaign) that is statistically equivalent to the treatment group (exposed to the campaign) on all measureable sociodemographic and other relevant factors. It yields the "net effect" of the program, after removing the effects of pre-intervention differences between those likely to see or hear a campaign versus those not exposed to it (selection bias). PSM relies on two key assumptions: the common support assumption (that is, there is an overlap between the characteristics of program participants and nonparticipants) and the conditional independence assumption (CIA). CIA posits that if all the variables that jointly affect treatment and outcome have been observed, then the potential outcome of nontreatment is independent of treatment participation. This assumption requires that we have

information on all the variables that can potentially influence both the treatment and the outcome.

To use this technique, one must first predict the propensity (probability) of treatment or exposure from a vector of measured variables that are related to both treatment and outcome. The resulting probability measure is then used to match individuals who are exposed to the intervention with their statistically equivalent counterparts who are not exposed (Deheijia and Wahba, 2002). PSM helps to overcome an important dimensionality problem since respondents are matched, not on a vector of variables, but on a single summary variable. PSM is applicable to situations where the treatment variable is a categorical variable that has only two mutually exclusive categories and to multiple treatment programs (Babalola and Vondrasek, 2005; Lechner, 2002).

One limitation of PSM is that it can only control for the effects of measured confounding variables. There are other techniques available to researchers to quantify and adjust for unmeasured confounding variables. These methods include sensitivity analysis after PSM to simulate the effects of a potential unmeasured confounder on the PSM estimates. For example, Babalola and Kincaid (2009) estimated that the unmeasured confounder that would completely negate the observed effects of exposure to communication programs on condom use in Tanzania would be one that increases the odds of exposure almost seventeenfold; they concluded that such a variable was difficult to envisage. Other methods that can be used to assess and correct for the potential effects of unmeasured confounders include bivariate probit analysis (estimates a model with two covarying endogenous variables; e.g., exposure and immunization uptake) and multivariate probit analysis (estimates a model with three or more covarying endogenous variables; e.g., exposure, attitudes, and condom use) (Hutchinson and Wheeler, 2006; Monfardini and Radice, 2008; Babalola and Kincaid, 2009).

Experimental design

Pretest–posttest experimental control group design. This design yields the most rigorous results, because it controls for all the major threats to validity (testing, selection, history, and others). Randomized control trials (RCTs) are one type of experimental design. A unique aspect is that the researcher must randomly allocate subjects to the experimental or control group before exposing the experimental group to the intervention. It is virtually impossible to meet this condition in the case of large-scale communication programs, except where the researcher can control the "stimulus" (to ensure that one group gets exposed to the communication and the other does not). Evaluators cannot use this design to evaluate communication programs that have a radio or TV component, because all persons in the catchment area are potentially exposed to the program; they have no means of randomly allocating certain people to a "non-exposure" group. The only case in which the evaluator can use this design is where one can control the placement of (exposure to) the intervention. For example, if a mass media campaign only used written pamphlets, one could distribute these to randomly selected households and withhold them from randomly selected controls. (However, mass media programs generally employ mutually reinforcing channels, making this a poor approach to the campaign.) With regard to community mobilization, theoretically one could randomize communities (not individuals) to receive a given set of activities and withhold them from communities randomly selected as the controls; however, we were unable to find any examples of such communication programs in the published literature. Of the three types of communication programs, this design lends itself best to the evaluation of interpersonal communication/counseling, especially in a clinical setting where one can randomly assign clients to receive (or not) a given intervention.

Methodological Challenges in Determining Causality in Health Communication Programs

Determining causality – the chain of events that leads to an observed effect – has been of utmost importance to scientists and philosophers since the eighteenth century (see, e.g., Hume 1978 [1739]). Almost 50 years ago, Bradford Hill (1965) created a list of the conditions necessary but not sufficient for inferring causation, among which were the following:

1   Empirical association or correlation between the posited cause and effect. The stronger the association between two variables, the more likely it is that one causes the other. It is important to note, however, that, whereas there can be no causation without correlation, the presence of correlation does not necessarily imply causation;
2   Theoretical coherence: the linkage must be consistent with what we already know about the issue;
3   Plausibility: it must make theoretical or intuitive sense;
4   Graduated relationships: larger doses of the cause produce greater effects;
5   Consistency: the relationship has been observed in different settings over time;
6   Specificity: there are no alternative explanations for the effect: the association is not due to other causes;
7   Temporal precedence and spatial contiguity: the cause must precede the effect in time and space. In other words, X must cause Y, and *not* vice versa;
8   Responsiveness to experiment: changing the cause (X) leads to a change in the effect (Y).

Of the different study designs for measuring program effectiveness outlined, the RCT is the only one that definitely demonstrates conditions 6–8 above, which is the reason the RCT is often been touted as the golden standard for program impact evaluation (Rossi, Lipsey, and Freeman, 2004; Shadish, Cook, and Campbell 2002; St. Pierre, 2004). Nonetheless, RCTs have serious limitations that make them difficult or even impossible to apply in reality (Habicht, Victora, and Vaughn, 1999; Norman, 2003; Victora, Habicht, and Bryce, 2004; Grossman and MacKenzie, 2005; Sanson-Fisher *et al.*, 2007; West *et al.*, 2008). For example, in evaluating a national-level communication campaign, it is not possible to randomly assign subjects or even communities to a treatment and a control area. Sanson-Fisher and his colleagues (2007) have eloquently discussed the limitations of RCTs for evaluating population-based health interventions even when it is possible to perform some form of randomization. These limitations include lack of sufficient population groups for efficient randomization (especially in community or cluster randomized studies), potential for contamination (when the intervention inadvertently reaches the control group), premature evaluation (when, for practical reasons, the study does not allow enough time for the intervention to have effects before conducting the follow-up), and threats to external validity (because the study groups and/or individuals are not representative of the larger population or the intervention is not typical of what would have been obtained in real life). Other shortcomings of RCTs include relative costs, ethical concerns, differential attrition, and limited applicability across types of interventions.

As a result, evaluators have instead used alternative methods more suited to the nature of communication programs, such as quasi-experimental designs that use cross-sectional data. However, such designs cannot entirely eliminate or control for the bias due to selectivity and endogeneity inherent in cross-sectional data. Nonetheless, it is vexing to researchers in this field that results produced using *the most appropriate study designs for large-scale communication programs*, as well as increasingly sophisticated analytic techniques borrowed from econometrics, still do not carry the weight of RCTs in some scientific circles.

More often than not, health communication programs are evaluated with cross-sectional data collected at one or more points in time. There are significant problems inherent in cross-sectional data, including selection bias. Estimating program effect requires knowing not only what happened in the presence of the program but also what would have happened had the program not occurred (the counterfactual). With cross-sectional data, we cannot infer the counterfactual from the behavior of people who are not exposed to the program. In the absence of randomization, exposure to a health communication intervention is subject to volitional control. It is possible, and actually likely, that the persons exposed to the intervention are different from those not exposed along key variables that are also associated with the outcome of interest. This situation creates a selection bias. If all the relevant variables along which the treatment and control groups differ are measured, it is possible to correct for selection bias using appropriate regression methods, including propensity score matching, discussed earlier. The situation gets complicated when, as it is often the case, some of the key variables associated with exposure and outcome are not measured, resulting in an endogeneity problem.

Another challenge in evaluating the impact of health communication interventions is the issue of reliability and validity of self-reported data. Most of the behaviors that a health communication program seeks to promote cannot be observed by the researcher, making it imperative to rely on responses provided by respondents. The extent to which such self-reported data can be trusted has been repeatedly questioned (Krieger *et al.*, 2005; Del Boca and Noll, 2000; Weinhardt *et al.*, 1998; Brody, 1995). Self-reports are subject to memory lapse and intentional misrepresentation, resulting in measurement error. Some researchers have argued that study participants tend to understate stigmatized behaviors while overstating normative behaviors (Brody, 1995). The type of question asked, the context in which the question is asked and the person asking the question are all factors that can affect the accuracy of self-report data. Data for evaluating health communication interventions are collected using one or more of the following modes: self-administered questionnaire, interviewer-administered face-to-face questionnaire, telephone interview, postal questionnaire, diaries for self-monitoring, audiotape-administered interview, computer-assisted interview and audio computer-assisted self-interview (ACASI). Whereas computer-assisted interviews and ACASIs are becoming more popular in developing countries, their use is still relatively limited due to technology availability and cost of procuring the devices.

Some have asked the question: Are there health or social issues that are more difficult than others to measure using standard evaluation approaches and methodologies? Whereas the study designs are similar across health topics, one important variant is the behavioral outcome used to measure "success" in a given program. Specifically, is there a single robust behavioral outcome that is used consistently to evaluate this program? Is this measure strongly correlated to the mortality, morbidity, or fertility outcome of interest? And how credible is self-report on this behavioral measure/outcome? Family planning and HIV prevention offer a useful contrast. For example, in family planning evaluation, this "single robust measure" is current contraceptive use among married women of reproductive age. This behavioral outcome correlates strongly with fertility rates (except in the few countries with high levels of induced abortion). And the FP research from over three decades demonstrates that women tend to report accurately on their contraceptive use, if interviewed in private by a respectful, nonjudgmental interviewer. By contrast, measuring HIV prevention behaviors is more challenging. First, there are multiple behaviors that prevent HIV. Even if one limits oneself to the most common – condom use – there is no "single robust measure" that is used consistently across evaluations. Common measures include "condom use at last sex," "condom use at last sex with a casual partner," "consistent condom use," and "consistent condom use with a casual partner," to name a few. In terms of relating this measure to HIV transmission, there is no standard conversion, since the likelihood of HIV transmission will depend in part on HIV prevalence in the community under study. Moreover, self-report on condom use is not highly reliable. A final challenge of evaluating HIV prevention relates to measuring HIV transmission (although generally health communication programs stop at evaluating behavior change). Ideally, one would like to measure HIV incidence (i.e., the rate of recent infection), whereas most studies employing biomarkers can only measure HIV prevalence. However, HIV programs continue to be among the most widely evaluated, because they represent such a large financial investment and the stakes are so high.

Conclusion

In this chapter, we have addressed the question "Do health communication programs work? Do they produce measurable change, consistent with their objectives?" This review of the evidence points to several conclusions:

1   Health communication campaigns have shown measurable effects over a series of outcomes (i.e., knowledge, attitudes, risk-perception, self-efficacy, behavior) on numerous health topics in both developed and developing countries.
2   Consistent with staged behavior change theoretical perspectives, health communication tends to have greater effects on knowledge and attitudes than on behaviors.

3   The strength of these communication effects varies by topic, as shown in Figure 5.1. Data presented herein showed higher effect sizes for HIV prevention than for family planning campaigns in developing countries.

4   The effects of the campaign may vary by the characteristics of the socioeconomic status of the population, as Snyder (2009) demonstrated for HIV: the effect sizes were higher for the HIV campaigns implemented in less developed compared to developed countries.

5   Campaigns that have an enforcement (coercion) component, such as seat belt use and alcohol consumption among minors, generally show a stronger effect than those relying entirely on persuasion (not using messages about the legal enforcement of a behavior) (Snyder, 2002).

6   The two topics that have received the most extensive and continuous funding (both for the communication programs and their evaluation) in developing countries – family planning and HIV prevention – show strong positive effects on behavior, as well as on several ideational factors, including knowledge, approval of FP, and social norms for condom use.

7   Having high levels of funding does not mean a campaign will necessarily be effective, as shown by the results for substance abuse campaigns among youth in the United States. This highlights the importance of well-designed campaigns based on knowledge of what program works for a specific target audience and health topic.

Factors that tend to reduce the effectiveness of communication campaigns include the following:

Complexity of the required change. It is widely recognized that persuading an audience to change brands of toothpaste is far easier than persuading it to adopt a new behavior in place of one that is strongly rooted in cultural norms or personal identity. Also, a change that requires a one-time action may be easier to effect than one that requires consistent practice over time. Nowhere has this lesson been more apparent than in efforts to promote safer sex for HIV prevention. Where the behavior requires personal sacrifice, continued input, constant vigilance (e.g., use a condom every time), learning a complicated skill, or related challenges, change is more difficult to achieve.

Insufficient intensity or low quality of the campaign. There are no hard and fast rules regarding the number of channels to use, the length of a campaign, the frequency of messages, and related factors. Nor is there an objective measure of quality of programming. Most often, these decisions are dictated by the available funding for the activity. Program evaluations that measure exposure to (or recognition of) campaign messages indicate that the extent to which the campaign reached the intended population influences the outcome. Low-budget or poorly designed campaigns may be ineffective if the intensity or quality of the program is not sufficient to draw the attention of the intended audience. While measuring quality is difficult, more attention needs to be paid to this in order to build our understanding of what works, under what circumstances, and why.

Premature evaluation of the campaign. Premature evaluation can result in negative results for programs which, given enough time, would have shown to be effective. There are no clear guidelines regarding the time necessary for behavior change to take place. Nonetheless, some behaviors are easier to change than others; changes in some behaviors can be observed within a relatively short time whereas others may take longer. For example, a significant increase in condom use may take a shorter time than significant reductions in number of sex partners or age at sexual debut. The timing of impact evaluation should take into consideration the length of time necessary to see significant changes.

A lack of evaluation data (or limited data) on the effectiveness of communication programs on a given health topic should not be interpreted as "no effect." For example, in developing countries we know little about the effects of communication programs on partner reduction, prevention for HIV positives, immunization, cancer prevention, and smoking cessation. Some health communication programs targeting these health topics are ongoing in developing countries. Rigorous evaluations are needed of these types of programs to strengthen our knowledge base of the effectiveness of communication programs in these arenas.

Communication programs are evolving over time, and thus we should not judge the potential of future communication programs by the programs of the past. For example, in recent years, health communication approaches for HIV transmission reduction have shifted toward the greater use of multiple strategies, particularly those integrating mass media, community mobilization and interpersonal approaches, with promising results (Noar *et al.*, 2009). The most recent meta-analysis of HIV programs from developing countries (Snyder *et al.*, 2009) indicated that those that incorporated both mass media and interpersonal components, compared to mass media alone, were more effective. Thus, as more programs evolve toward more comprehensive models, we have reason to believe that future campaigns may have greater effects on average than those evaluated to date (Bertrand *et al.*, 2006).

The field of health communication program evaluation is moving towards the use of more sophisticated analytic methods that help to control for the key threats to internal validity, including selectivity and endogeneity biases. As additional and more rigorous evaluations are conducted, we will learn more about what specific strategies work better than others or how different populations respond to similar interventions. Through such evaluations, we will have the opportunity to improve and refine health communication programs to maximize their effectiveness for HIV prevention.

Although this article has focused entirely on measuring the impact of communication programs, we encourage researchers (and the funding agencies that support them) to go beyond evaluating the narrow question of "did the program have an impact?" to understanding why and how the program has worked (or not). To this end, the evaluation should be theory-driven, using an appropriate causal framework to guide data collection and analysis. A comprehensive review of literature and rigorous qualitative formative research should help to determine the appropriate pathways of influence to specify in the causal framework. Health communication program evaluation should also include process evaluation, conducted post-launch of the program to document reach and audience reaction. Qualitative evaluation methods may provide useful insights from the intended audience of the reach and perceived effectiveness of the program activities. For example, the Most Significant Change method can be used to document what the intended population perceives as the most relevant impact of the program. Whereas program planners and donors tend to focus on the question "Was the communication program effective?", we should continue to invest in these other types of research and evaluation that allow us to increase the effectiveness of health communication programming.

Notes

1 Snyder's meta-analyses include many of the studies cited in three synthesis papers on the effects of communication programs on HIV-related behaviors: Bertrand *et al.*, 2006; Bertrand and Anghang, 2006; and Noar *et al.*, 2009. Thus, we present her findings that incorporate key results from these other three synthesis articles.
2 Some authors classify this design as quasi-experimental (Shadish, Cook, and Campbell, 2002), whereas Fisher and Foreit (2002) consider it nonexperimental.

References

Aldridge, R. W., Iglesias, D., Caceres, C. F., and Miranda, J. J. (2009). Determining a cost effective intervention response to HIV/AIDS in Peru. *BMC Public Health, 9*, 352.

Babalola, S. and Kincaid, D. L. (2009). New methods for estimating the impact of health communication programs. *Communication Methods and Measures, 3*(1), 61–83.

Babalola, S. and Vondrasek, C. (2005). Communication, ideation and contraceptive use in Burkina Faso: an application of the propensity score matching method. *Family Planning and Reproductive Health Care, 31*(3): 207–212.

Bala, M., Strzeszynski L., and Cahill K. (2008). Mass media interventions for smoking cessation in adults. *Cochrane Database of Systematic Reviews*, Issue 1. Art. No.: CD004704. DOI: 10.1002/14651858.CD004704.pub2.

Bauer, U. E., Johnson T. M., Hopkins R.S., and Brooks R. C. (2000). Changes in youth cigarette use and intentions following implementation of a tobacco control program: findings from the Florida Youth Tobacco Survey, 1998–2000. *Journal of American Medical Association, 284*, 723–728.

Bertrand, J. T. and Anhang, R. (2006). The effectiveness of mass media in changing HIV/AIDS-related behavior among young people in developing countries. *World Health Organisation Technical Report Series, 938*, 205–241.

Bertrand, J. T., O'Reilly, K., Denison, J. *et al.*, (2006). Systematic review of the effectiveness of mass communication programs to change HIV/AIDS-related behaviors in developing countries. *Health Education Research, 21*(4), 567–597.

Brody, S. (1995). Patients misrepresenting their risk factors for AIDS. *International Journal of STD and AIDS, 6*, 392–398.

Campbell, D. T. and Stanley, J. C. (1963). *Experimental and Quasi-Experiment Designs for Research*. Boston: Houghton Mifflin Co.

Cohen, D. A., Wu, S. Y., and Farley, T. A. (2004). Comparing the cost-effectiveness of HIV prevention interventions. *Journal of Acquired Immune Deficiency Syndromes (1999), 37*(3), 1404–1414.

Commonwealth of Massachusetts (2002). *Preventing Tobacco Use among Massachusetts Youth: Programs and Results*. Boston: Commonwealth of Massachusetts Department of Education.

Cook, T. D. and Campbell, D. T. (1979). *Quasi-Experimentation: Design and Analysis for Field Settings*. Chicago, IL: Rand McNally.

Dehejia, R. H. and Wahba, S. (2002). Propensity score matching methods for nonexperimental causal studies. *Review of Economics and Statistics, 84*(1), 151–161.

Del Boca, F. K. and Noll, J. A. (2000). Truth or consequences: the validity of self-report data in health services research on addictions. *Addiction, 95*(Supplement 3), 347–360.

Earl, A. and Albarracin, D. (2007). Nature, decay, and spiraling of the effects of fear-inducing arguments and HIV counseling and testing: A meta-analysis of the short and long-term outcomes of HIV-prevention interventions. *Health Psychology, 26,* 496–506.

Farrelly, M. C., Niederdeppem, J., and Yarsevich, J. (2003). Youth tobacco prevention mass media campaigns: past, present, and future directions. *Tobacco Control, 12,* i35–i47.

Fisher, A. A. and Foreit, J. R. (2002). *Designing HIV/AIDS Intervention Studies: an Operations Research Handbook.* New York: The Population Council.

Fisher, L. (2001). Mississippi: The unsung hero of tobacco control, USA. *Cancer Causes and Control, 12*(10), 965–967.

Flay, B. R. (1987). Mass media and smoking cessation: A critical review. *American Journal of Public Health, 77,* 153–160.

Flynn, B. S., Worden, J. K., Secker-Walker, R. H. *et al.* (1992). Prevention of cigarette smoking through mass media intervention and school programs. *American Journal of Public Health, 82,* 827–834.

Grossman, J. and Mackenzie, F. J. (2005). The randomized controlled trial: Gold standard or merely standard? *Perspectives in Biology and Medicine, 48*(4), 516–534.

Habicht, J. P, Victora, C. G. and Vaughn, J. P. (1999). Evaluation designs for adequacy, plausibility and probability of public health program performance and impact. *International Journal of Epidemiology, 28*(1), 10–18.

Halfstad A., Aaro, L. E., Engeland, A. *et al.* (1997). Provocative appeals in anti-smoking mass media campaigns targeting adolescents – the accumulated effect of multiple exposures. *Health Education Research, 12,* 227–236.

Hill, A. B. (1965). The environment and disease: Association or causation? *Proceedings of the Royal Society of Medicine, 58,* 295–300.

Hogan, D. R., Baltussen, R., Hayashi, C. *et al.* (2005). Cost effectiveness analysis of strategies to combat HIV/AIDS in developing countries. *BMJ (Clinical Research Ed.), 331*(7530), 1431–1437.

Hornik, R. and McAnany, E. (2001). Mass media and fertility change. In J. Casterline (Ed.), *Diffusion Processes and Fertility Transition: Selected Perspectives* (pp. 208–239). Washington, DC: National Academy Press.

Hume, D. (1978 [1739]). *A Treatise of Human Nature,* edited by L. A. Selby-Bigge and P. H. Nidditch, Oxford: Clarendon Press.

Hutchinson, P. and Wheeler, J. (2006). Advanced methods for evaluating the impact of family planning communication programs: Evidence from Tanzania and Nepal. *Studies in Family Planning, 37*(3), 169–186.

Kincaid, D. and Do, M. P. (2006). Multivariate causal attribution and cost-effectiveness of a national mass media campaign in the Philippines. *Journal of Health Communication, 11* (Supplement 2), 69–90.

Krieger, N., Smith, K., Naishadham, D. *et al.* (2005). Experiences of discrimination: Validity and reliability of a self-report measure for population health research on racism and health. *Social Science and Medicine, 61*(7), 1576–1596.

Lechner, M. (2002). Program heterogeneity and propensity score matching: An application to the evaluation of active labor market policies. *The Review of Economics and Statistics, 84*(1), 151–161.

McVey, D. and Stapleton, J. 2000. Can anti-smoking television advertising affect smoking behavior? Controlled trial of the Health Education Authority for England's anti-smoking TV campaign. *Tobacco Control, 9,* 273–282.

Medley, A., Kennedy, C., O'Reilly, K., and Sweat, M. (2009). Effectiveness of peer education interventions for HIV prevention in developing countries: A systematic review and meta-analysis. *AIDS Education and Prevention, 21*(3), 181–206.

Monfardini, C. and Radice, R. (2008). Testing exogeneity in the bivariate probit model: A Monte Carlo study. *Oxford Bulletin of Economics and Statistics*, *70*(2), 271–282.

Murray, D. M., Prokhorov, A. V., and Harty, K. C. (1994). Effects of a statewide antismoking campaign on mass media messages and smoking beliefs. *Preventive Medicine*, *23*, 54–60.

Noar, S. M., Palmgreen, P., Chabot, M. *et al.* (2009). A 10-year systematic review of HIV/AIDS mass communication campaigns: Have we made progress? *Journal of Health Communication*, *14*(1), 15–42.

Norman G. (2003). RCT=results confounded and trivial: The perils of grand educational experiments. *Medical Education*, *37*, 582–584.

Robinson, W. C. and Lewis, G. L. (2003). Cost-effectiveness analysis of behavior change interventions: A proposed new approach and an application to Egypt. *Journal of Biosocial Science*, *35*(4), 499–512.

Rosenbaum, P. R. and Rubin, D. B. (1983). The central role of the propensity score in observational studies for causal effects. *Biometrika*, *70*(1), 41–55.

Rosenbaum, P. R. and Rubin, D. B. (1984). Reducing bias in observational studies using subclassification on the propensity score. *Journal of the American Statistical Association*, *79*, 516–524.

Rossi, P. H., Lipsey, M. W., and Freeman, H. E.(2004). *Evaluation: A Systematic Approach* (7th edn.). Thousand Oaks, CA: Sage Publications.

Sallis, J. F. and Owen, N. (2002). Ecological models of health behavior. In K. Glanz, B. K. Rimer, and F. M. Lewis (Eds.), *Health Behavior and Health Education: Theory, Research, and Practice*, 3rd edn. (pp. 462–484). San Francisco: John Wiley and Sons.

Sanson-Fisher, R. W., Bonevski, B., Green, L.W., and D'Este, C. (2007). Limitations of the randomized controlled trial in evaluating population-based health interventions. *American Journal of Preventive Medicine*, *33*,155–161.

Shadish, W., Cook, T. D. and Campbell, D. T. (2002). *Experimental and Quasi-Experimental Designs for Generalized Causal Inference*. Boston: Houghton Mifflin Harcourt.

Siegel, M. and Biener, L. (2000). The impact of an antismoking media campaign on progression to established smoking: results of a longitudinal youth study. *American Journal of Public Health 90*, 380–386.

Skara S. and Sussman S. (2003). A review of 25 long-term adolescent tobacco and other drug use prevention program evaluations. *Preventive Medicine*, *37*(5), 451–474.

Snyder, L. (2001). How effective are mediated health campaigns? In R. Rice and C. Atkin (Eds.), *Public Information Campaigns*, 3rd edn (pp.181–190). Thousand Oaks, CA: Sage.

Snyder, L. (2007a). Health communication campaigns and their impact on behavior. *Journal of Nutrition Education and Behavior*, *39*(2), S32–S40.

Snyder, L. (2007b). Meta-analyses of mediated health campaigns. In R. W. Preiss, B. M. Gayle, N. Burrell *et al.* (Eds.), *Mass Media Effects Research: Advances through Meta-analysis* (pp. 327–345). Mahwah, NJ: Lawrence Erlbaum Associates.

Snyder, L., Badiane, L., Kalnova, S. and Diop-Sidibe, N. (2003). Meta-analysis of family planning campaigns advised by the Center for Communication Programs at Johns Hopkins University compared to campaigns conducted and advised by other organizations. Unpublished draft paper for the Johns Hopkins Bloomberg School of Public Health and Agency for International Development.

Snyder, L. and Hamilton, M. (2002). Meta-analysis of US health campaign effects. In R. Hornik (Ed.), *Public Health Communication: Evidence for Behavior Change* (pp. 357–383). Mahwah, NJ: Lawrence Erlbaum Associates.

Snyder, L., Johnson, B., Huedo-Medina, T. *et al.* (2009). Effectiveness of media interventions to prevent HIV, 1986–2006: A meta-analysis. Presentation at the American Public Health Association Meeting, November 2009, Philadelphia, PA.

Sood, S. and Nambiar, D. (2006). Comparative cost-effectiveness of the components of a behavior change communication campaign on HIV/AIDS in north India. *Journal of Health Communication, 11* (Supplement 2), 143–162.

St. Pierre, R. G. (2004). Using randomized experiments. In J. S. Wholey, H. P. Hatry, and K. E. Newcomer (Eds.), *Handbook of Practical Program Evaluation,* 2nd edn. (pp. 150–175). San Francisco, CA: Jossey-Bass.

Sweat, M. and Dennison, J. A. (1995). Reducing HIV incidence in developing countries with structural and environmental interventions. *AIDS, 9* (Supplement A), S251–257.

Sweat, M., Kerrigan, D., Moreno, L. *et al.* (2006). Cost-effectiveness of environmental-structural communication interventions for HIV prevention in the female sex industry in the Dominican Republic. *Journal of Health Communication, 11* (Supplement 2), 123–142.

Tweedie, I., Boulay, M., Fiagbey, E., Banful, A., and Lokko, K. (2002). *Ghana's Stop AIDS Love Life Program Phase 1: Evaluation Report February 2000–June 2001.* Accra: Ghana Social Marketing Foundation; Baltimore: Johns Hopkins Bloomberg School of Public Health, Center for Communication Programs.

Victora, C. G., Habicht, J. P., and Bryce, J. (2004). Evidence-based public health: Moving beyond randomized trials. *American Journal of Public Health, 94,* 400–405.

Vidanapathirana J, Abramson, M. J., Forbes, A., and Fairley, C. (2005). Mass media interventions for promoting HIV testing. *Cochrane Database of Systematic Reviews* 2005, Issue 3. Art. No.: CD004775. DOI: 10.1002/14651858.CD004775.pub2.

Wakefield, M. A., Loken, B., and Hornik, R. C. (2010). Use of mass media campaigns to change health behavior. *The Lancet, 376,* 1261–1271.

Weinhardt, L. S., Forsyth, A. D., Carey, M. P. *et al.* (1998). Reliability and validity of self-report measures of HIV-related sexual behavior: Progress since 1990 and recommendations for research and practice. *Archives of Sexual Behavior, 27,* 155–180.

West, S. G., Duan, N., Pequegnat, W. *et al.* (2008). Alternatives to the randomized controlled trial. *American Journal of Public Health, 98*(8), 1359–1366.

Wiehe, S. E., Garrison, M. M., Christakis, D. A. *et al.* (2005). A systematic review of school-based smoking prevention trials with long-term follow-up. *Journal of Adolescent Health, 36,* 162–169.

6

Promoting Health through Entertainment-Education Media
Theory and Practice

William J. Brown

The promotion of public health through entertainment media has become a growing communication practice during the past several decades. Commonly known as the *entertainment-education communication strategy*, media professionals and health communication scholars and practitioners now collaborate throughout the world to purposefully use the powerful influence of entertainment to promote specific health beliefs and behavior (Singhal and Rogers, 2004). A comprehensive discussion of how entertainment-education health initiatives have diffused internationally would fill several books (see Singhal *et al.*, 2006); therefore, this chapter will focus on widespread applications of specific theoretical perspectives that have been used to promote health globally.

The intentional use of entertainment to address public health, which predates the emergence of broadcast media, is as old as the tradition of storytelling. Unfortunately, little research has been done to assess systemic health promotion through entertainment in both oral and text-centric cultures. The influence of entertainment on health through novels, for example, has been underinvestigated. Not until after World War II did health communication professionals, government agencies, nonprofit organizations, and academic scholars begin to collaborate to systematically plan entertainment-education programs for development and social change, primarily through electronic media. This chapter will begin by discussing the family planning radio dramas in Jamaica during the late 1950s and 1960s and will end by discussing a hearing safety campaign in the Netherlands in 2009–2010 through an online webisode drama series. In between these two periods a number of other health interventions will be discussed, including entertainment programs designed to promote HIV prevention and sexual responsibility, oral rehydration therapy, alcohol abuse prevention and designated drivers, breast cancer awareness, environmental safety, and better treatment of children with disabilities.

The Handbook of Global Health Communication, First Edition. Edited by Rafael Obregon and Silvio Waisbord.

Family Planning Serial Dramas

Inspired while in Britain by the BBC's radio drama, *The Archers,* the longest-running entertainment-education radio program in history, Elaine Perkins produced a remarkable body of creative work in Jamaica to promote public health. Her entertainment-education radio programs advocated numerous health beliefs and behavior over several decades, beginning in 1958. Perkins' early *radionovelas* promoted mosquito eradication, rural development, rural-to-urban migration acculturation, and tourism for the government of Jamaica. During the 1980s, Perkins created one of her most famous radio dramas, *Naseberry Street,* to promote family planning and encourage sexual responsibility. *Naseberry Street* was a fictitious street in a poor neighborhood of Kingston. One of the main characters of the series was a health educator and nurse who provided family planning information to people in the community. The program reached an audience of about one million people daily, which at that time was 40 percent of the total Jamaican population (Hazzard and Cambridge, 1988). It was especially popular with women of lower socioeconomic status, those in greatest need of family planning information. A study of the program's effects indicated that listeners were more likely to adopt family planning practices, to be more sexually responsible, and to delay sexual relations until marriage than those who did not follow the program (Population Reports, 1986).

Perkins' *radionovelas* achieved a wide variety of educational goals (Hazzard and Cambridge, 1988; Cambridge, 1992; Stone, 1986). Although she did not formalize a theory for producing effective entertainment-education *radionovelas,* Perkins understood the importance of *perceived realism, perceived similarity,* and *cultural proximity,* three important theoretical constructs applied to entertainment-education productions. When audiences perceive that characters in fictional dramas are real people with similar life experiences, they are more likely to learn from those characters (Buenting and Brown, 2009; Hoffner and Buchanan, 2005). Scholars have studied perceived realism and perceived similarity in a variety of communication contexts, finding that in mediated contexts both variables influence how audiences respond to mediated messages (Busselle, Ryabovolova, and Wilson, 2004; Green, 2004). Perkins demonstrated through her *radionovelas* that creating fictional characters that audience members believed were authentic (perceived as "real people") led audiences to identify more strongly with those characters, thus facilitating more engagement and learning from them (Busselle and Bilandzic, 2008).

To create perceived realism and perceived similarity, Perkins' *radionovelas* featured nonprofessional actors who had been personally involved with the health issues her dramas addressed. She believed that audience members would form a stronger emotional connection to common people than to professional actors. Perkins also recognized that her stories were more powerful when they emanated from the culture, explaining: "Jamaica has an oral culture, and the history of the community has always been stored and transmitted through storytelling" (Perkins, 2000). Greater cultural proximity increases audience receptivity to media productions (Burch, 2002; Trepte, 2008). Narratives with greater *cultural proximity* are more likely to create audience involvement and be sources of social change than those which are more culturally dissimilar (Buenting, 2007; Singhal and Udornpim, 1997).

Perceived similarity tends to cultivate credibility and trust, enabling audience members to connect their own personal experiences with the experiences of media personalities (Krugman, 1965), which can then lead to emotional and psychological involvement with them (Rubin, Perse, and Powell, 1985; Rubin and McHugh, 1987). Audiences prefer media programs that are cultural proximate to them because they are more relevant (Straubhaar, 1991). Cultural proximity is complex, may lie below the surface (that which is easily visible), and includes sharing a common language, history, stories, social norms, beliefs, values, and rituals. While examining cultural proximity in soap operas, La Pastina and Straubhaar (2005) wondered why southern Italians liked a Brazilian *telenovela* more than northern Italians and why Brazilians preferred a Mexican *telenovela* to Brazilian *telenovelas* of higher quality. They concluded that soap opera viewers often relate to the characters of these serials beyond the surface-level variables of language and geographical region. Southern Italians related to the Brazilian *telenovela* because the narrative included issues regarding Italian immigration to Brazil, which had personally affected the lives of many Italian viewers. Brazilian women in their study liked a Mexican *telenovela* because it featured romantic themes to which they could relate as compared to their Brazilian counterparts which at that time focused on the struggles of modern life.

Perkins touched audiences at these deeper levels of perceived similarity, inspiring other Latin American countries to produce similar entertainment-education programs. In Costa Rica, educators created *Dialogo* (Dialogue), a radio talk show intended to provide information on family planning and sexual responsibility. Broadcast for ten minutes weekdays at 7:00 a.m. on five national and regional radio stations from 1970 to the mid 1980s, the host of the program, an Episcopalian minister named Padre Carlos, answered questions about sex, pregnancy, and planning for children. Hearing a Christian minister openly discuss sex gave *Dialogo* a large audience estimated to be 40 percent of the population. Research indicated that the program effectively increased knowledge of and positive attitudes toward family planning among Costa Ricans (Risopatron and Spain, 1980). Like *Naseberry Street* in Jamaica, *Dialogo* created the space for public dialogue about topics traditionally considered taboo.

Indonesia created an entertainment-education radio soap called *Butir Butir Pasir di Laut* (*Grains of Sand in the Sea*) to promote family planning during the late 1970s and 1980s. Beginning in 1977, a total of 3500 episodes of the program were aired over a 12-year period, providing relevant information about family planning practices (Singhal and Rogers, 1989). Although data were not collected to document the number of radio listeners who adopted family planning practices as a result of the program, the program's longevity likely had a cumulative effect in encouraging Indonesians to seek out family planning information.

The popularity of *Dialogo* (Dialogue) in Costa Rica and of *Butir Butir Pasir di Laut* (*Grains of Sand in the Sea*) in Indonesia shows how entertainment-education programs can have an agenda-setting effect by initiating dialogue about important health beliefs and practices, even ones previously considered to be taboo. Although initially derived from the study of how news media create public dialogue about certain topics (McCombs, 2005; Rogers and Dearing, 1993), agenda-setting research shows that many forms of media, including entertainment programs, not only influence what people talk about but also influence how people think about certain topics (McCombs and Shaw, 1993). Since both professional entertainers and fictional characters can invigorate public discussion of publicly debated issues, agenda-setting provides an important theoretical perspective to consider when designing and evaluating entertainment-education programs intended to promote health.

While radio dramas were captivating audiences and inspiring public discussion during the 1960s and 1970s, *Simplemente Maria* (*Simply Mary*), a 1969 Peruvian *telenovela*, was motivating audiences to adopt educational goals and prosocial practices throughout Latin America during the 1970s (Singhal, Obregon, and Rogers, 1994). After observing *Simplemente Maria*'s phenomenal period of success, Miguel Sabido, Vice-President of Research for *Televisa*, Mexico's National Television Network, reasoned that the entertainment-education strategy used so successfully in radio dramas could be even more powerful if applied to television drama (Singhal, Rogers, and Brown, 1993a). Through Sabido's leadership, Mexico began broadcasting the first of 180 episodes of *Accompáñame* (*Come Along with Me*), a 30-minute television serial, in late 1977. The *telenovela* attracted a loyal audience, achieving an average audience rating of 29 percent (Church and Geller, 1989).

The setting for *Accompáñame* was a lower-class neighborhood in Mexico City where three sisters lived. While creating the series, Sabido applied Jung's (1981) theory of archetypes, Bandura's (1977) social learning theory, Bentley's (1967) dramatic theory, MacLean's triune brain theory (1973), and Rovigatti's circular model of communication (Televisa's Institute of Communication Research, 1981). Bandura (1977, 1986) observed that individuals learn not only by formal education, but also by observing the behavior of others both in real life and in fictional stories and by modeling behavior that leads to positive consequences. Three types of role modeling identified by Bandura (1977) have been applied in entertainment-education productions: (1) *prestige modeling* illustrated by characters who demonstrate culturally admired behaviors, (2) *similarity modeling* illustrated by characters who appeal to different audience segments by demonstrating benefits of prosocial behavior, and (3) *transitional modeling* illustrated by characters who change from antisocial behavior to prosocial behavior (Singhal and Rogers, 1999).

In *Accompáñame*, Sabido created one sister in a family as a negative role model who suffers through an unwanted pregnancy and the resulting stress that follows. A second sister, representing the positive role model, enjoys a happy marriage and discusses with her husband how to plan their children and use contraception methods to prevent unwanted pregnancies. A third sister, whom Sabido created as a transitional role model, initially rejects the family planning practices being promoted, but then changes over time and decides to adopt family planning, resulting in a transformation from an unhappy marriage to a peaceful and contented marriage.

Drawing on the work of Carl Jung, Sabido's fictional characters also represented the archetypes of married couples who lived in family harmony and married couples who lived in conflict. *Accompáñame* provided valuable information resources for couples who wanted to learn about family planning methods and motivated couples to go to family planning counseling centers and seek out family planning advice (Nariman, 1993). Mexico's national family planning program also received an average of 500 calls a month during the period of the broadcasts and gained 2500 volunteers to help promote family planning, both dramatic increases; and more than 562,000 individuals adopted family planning methods provided by government health clinics, a 33 percent increase in one year (Sabido, 1981). Televisa's positive experience with *Accompáñame* encouraged leaders at the network to produce a second telenovela to promote family planning in 1981 and 1982 called *Por Amor* (For Love), followed by many additional entertainment-education television series that addressed important health issues (Singhal, Rogers, and Brown, 1993b).

Aware of Sabido's methodology, Johns Hopkins University's Population Communication Services (JHU/PCS) and David Poindexter, founder of the nonprofit organization Population Communication International (PCI) in New York, helped to diffuse the entertainment-education communication strategy to several other countries to promote family planning. These efforts further promoted the application of Savido's theoretical framework. Nigeria was one of the first countries in Africa to use entertainment television to promote family planning. In collaboration with JHU/PCS, the Nigerian National Television Authority (NTA) broadcast *In a Lighter Mood* in 1986–1987 to promote family planning. The program hosts discussed various methods of contraception and the benefits of adequately spacing the birth of children and promoted smaller family sizes. *In a Lighter Mood* also advertised the services of family planning clinics in three cities where viewers could get family planning information. In a survey of visitors to clinics in Enugu and Ibadan, nearly 50 percent said they had watched episodes of the program; among those who watched, 79 percent of the Enugu respondents and 99 percent of the Ibadan respondents recalled the family planning messages in the program (Piotrow *et al.*, 1990). Inspired by the successful use of entertainment for health education in other countries and encouraged by David Poindexter, the government of Kenya produced its first entertainment-education radio soap opera, *Ushikwapo Shikimana* (*When Given Advice, Take It*), in 1987. The dramatic program reached an estimated seven million people, about 40 percent of the population of Kenya in 1987 (Singhal and Rogers, 1989). By 1989, the series was reaching 60 percent of the population, a projected 75 percent of which reported that they understood the family planning messages (Mazrui and Kitsao, 1988).

The setting for the radio series was the home of Mzee Gogo and his four wives, children, and grandchildren. Producers of the series applied the elements of perceived realism and perceived similarity that Perkins' *radionovelas* emphasized and the role modeling of fictional characters that Sabido's *telenovelas* employed. A total of 219 episodes were broadcast, reaching 40–50 percent of the population of Kenya. A mailed survey study sponsored by the Kaiser Family Foundation found that 84 percent of the survey respondents had listened to the program and 72 percent of them felt that the program helped listeners to adopt family planning (Advocates for Youth., 1998).

A summative study of *Ushikwapo Shikimana* indicated that many women said the radio program motivated their husbands to permit them to seek family planning services (Ligaga, 2005; Population Communication International, 2005). An analysis comparing the 1984 and 1989 Kenyan Demographic Health Surveys revealed that the decline in desired family size from 6.3 children to 4.8 children and the 58 percent increase in contraceptive usage was due in substantial part to mass media family planning messages such as those contained in television and radio serials (Advocates for Youth, 1998).

One of the most interesting experiments with an entertainment-education family planning campaign was Egypt's television mini-series called *Ana Zananna* (*I'm Persistent*), also the name of the lead character of the series. Similar in genre to the Taster's Choice commercial mini-series in the United States, *Ana Zananna* was a series of 14 one-minute dramas that incorporated humor and positive and negative role models. Broadcast nationwide in 1988, each episode aired an average of 100 times and reached 90 percent of Egyptian households (Singhal and Rogers, 1989). Research indicated that 98 percent of Egyptian television viewers understood *Ana Zananna's* family planning messages and 74 percent could recall the specific phrases used by the lead role model for family planning, Ana Zananna (Singhal and Rogers, 1989). The respondents were also able to correctly identify the positive and negative role models in the mini-drama series, which they found to be both entertaining and educational.

In summary, family planning soap operas broadcast on radio and television around the world have achieved commercial success and promoted favorable attitudes towards family planning and the adoption of family planning practices. These programs applied theories about perceived realism and perceived similarity, cultural proximity, social learning, and role modeling through character archetypes. Experiences with entertainment-education dramas to promote family planning inspired new entertainment-education projects in the 1990s that took on a variety of other health education needs and applied new theoretical perspectives, which are discussed next.

Reducing Sexually Transmitted Infections

One of the most pressing world health needs of the twenty-first century is reducing the spread of sexually transmitted infections, particularly HIV/AIDS, which is the leading cause of death in many nations. By the beginning of 2009, more than 60 million people had been infected with HIV, more than 25 million people had died of AIDS-related illnesses worldwide, and more than 33 million people were living with HIV (World Health Organisation, 2010). Children have been especially devastated by the AIDS epidemic. In sub-Saharan Africa alone, there are now more than 14 million children who have been orphaned because of AIDS (World Health Organisation, 2010).

Policy planners and health educators have focused their use of the entertainment-education communication strategy on slowing the rate of HIV transmission and, more generally, promoting sexual responsibility (Singhal, 2005). One of the greatest challenges in reducing sexually transmitted diseases is getting people to talk about it (Brown, 1991). Dramatic serials provide a solution to this problem, particularly in regions of the world where radio listening and television viewing is communal.

Tanzania was one of the first countries that implemented an entertainment-education campaign intervention for HIV-prevention. With private and government funding for research and production, Tanzania launched a five-year radio project in 1993, leading to the broadcast of a highly popular radio soap opera, *Twende na Wakati* (*Let's Go with the Times*). The series overall promoted sexual responsibility and addressed a number of issues, including family planning and empowerment of women, and developed a powerful storyline that addressed HIV and AIDS.

Through the extensive use of formative research, including dozens of focus groups, the creators of *Twende na Wakati* created a likable character, a truck driver named

Mkwaju, who transported goods up and down the trans-African highway which runs north to south through the center of Tanzania. The well-travelled truck route is notorious for its brothels at major truck stops, which became primary centers for HIV transmission throughout East Africa. In the radio serial, Mkwaju is a sexual adventurer who has many sexual encounters with girlfriends along his truck routes, unbeknownst to his wife, Tunu. As he drifts away from his wife and children, Mkwaju begins to get sick repeatedly. Although he does not understand what is happening to him, the radio audience eventually discerns that he has all the symptoms of being infected with HIV.

The drama is heightened when the *Twende na Wakati* listeners begin to speculate which girlfriend transmitted HIV to him, and whether or not his wife Tunu would also become sick. Bentley's (1967) dramatic theory postulates that the greater the dramatic tension in a story the greater emotional and psychological involvement audience members will develop with the characters of the story. Eventually Mkwaju develops AIDS and despite his irresponsibility, his wife cares for him until he dies. But the dramatic story does not end with his death. *Twende na Wakati* continues the HIV/AIDS theme with Mkwaju's son, Kibuyu, who at first seems to be following in the irresponsible lifestyle of his father. However, Kibuyu becomes a transition role model who changes his behavior before he acquires the same disease that killed his father.

The program writers created Mkwaju and Kibuyu as empathetic characters so the audience would develop parasocial relationships with them, eventually leading to identification. Parasocial interaction and identification are two closely related forms of involvement with both fictional and real media personas that increase the cognitive and behavioral effects of personas on audiences (Brown, 2010; Brown and deMatviuk, 2010). Parasocial interaction takes place when audience members form psychological and emotional bonds with media personas, forming pseudo-relationships called *parasocial relationships* (Horton and Wohl, 1956). Parasocial interaction includes both the affective and cognitive forms of involvement of audience members with mediated personalities. Over decades of research, parasocial relationships have been observed between television viewers and newscasters, talk show hosts, soap opera stars, situation comedy characters, celebrities, professional athletes, and religious leaders (Bae, Brown, and Kang, 2010; Brown, 2009, 2010; Brown and Basil, 1995; Brown, Basil, and Bocarnea, 2003a; 2003b; Cohen, 2004; Cole and Leets, 1999; Levy, 1979; Rubin and Perse, 1987). Radio listeners developed strong parasocial relationships with the characters of *Twende na Wakati* (Vaughan *et al.*, 2000).

Identification with media personas is a stronger effect that often follows parasocial interaction (Bae, Brown, and Kang, 2010; Fraser and Brown, 2002; Brown and de Matviuk, 2010). Conceptualized by Kelman (1961) as a process of social influence, identification occurs when audience members adopt the attitudes, beliefs, values and behavior of media personas with whom they have established a self-defining relationship. Identification has resulted in the adopting of HIV-prevention behaviors (Basil, 1996; Brown and Basil, 1995), the adoption of wildlife conservation values (Brown, 2010), the adoption of drug abuse prevention attitudes and beliefs (Brown and de Matviuk, 2010), and giving assent to organ donation (Bae, Brown and Kang, 2010). Health and media professionals have utilized the identification process by creating characters in media productions that audiences identify with and look to as role models, as in the MARCH model developed by the CDC to combat HIV/AIDS (Galavotti, Pappas-DeLuca, and Lansky, 2001).

The producers of *Twende na Wakati* collaborated with social scientists to set up a randomized controlled study for HIV prevention by blocking the broadcast of the radio series in one city of Tanzania, Dodoma, which became the control group. This enabled researchers to make direct comparisons of the health beliefs and practices between those who listened to the radio series and those who did not. A study by Vaughan *et al.* (2000) found that *Twende na Wakati* had a measurable effect on reducing HIV in Tanzania, including: (1) increasing perceptions of personal risk of contracting HIV/AIDS, (2) increasing self-efficacy with respect to preventing HIV and AIDS, (3) increasing interpersonal communication about HIV and AIDS, (4) increasing identification with the role models of the program, (5) decreasing the number of sexual partners by both men and women, and (6) increasing condom use. The series also promoted the adoption of family planning (Rogers *et al.*, 1999). An amazing 82 percent of the listeners of *Twende na Wakati* adopted at least one method of HIV-prevention and 23 percent adopted one or more family planning methods, and Tanzania experienced a 153 percent increase in condom distribution during the time the program aired (Vaughan *et al.*, 2000).

Neighboring Kenya, keen observers of the effects of Tanzania's *Twende na Wakati*, launched a new health initiative in 1998 with the sponsorship of Populations Communications International (PCI), which also helped to fund *Twende na Wakati,* and First Voice International (FVI). Kenya resurrected the radio drama it had first broadcast in the late 1980s. The new radio series, *Ushikwapo Shikamana* (*If Assisted, Assist Yourself*), focused on HIV and AIDS but also addressed other health-related issues, including teen sexuality and gender discrimination. Four episodes of *Ushikwapo Shikamana* were aired each week over a 26-week period each season during a five-year period, which ended in June 2004. Recurring themes in the series included how HIV is transmitted, having compassion for people living with AIDS, and caring for children orphaned by AIDS.

In addition to the radio series, the program sponsors and creative team produced comic strips that were published three times a week in Kenya's leading Kiswahili newspaper, *Taifa Leo*. These weekly comic strips were eventually compiled into one comic book and printed in December 2001. The comic book was distributed through a variety of outlets, including bookstores, church groups, and literacy programs.

Feedback from listening groups indicated *Ushikwapo Shikamana* increased awareness of the causes of HIV and AIDS and helped girls protect themselves from HIV and sexual abuse (Poindexter, 2004). Primary and secondary school children also created soap opera drama clubs based on the series (Populations Communications International, 2005). In April of 2005, Kenya began rebroadcasting *Ushikwapo Shikimana* by satellite.

Based on the early success of *Twende na Wakati* in promoting HIV prevention practices, Tanzania launched a new radio soap opera called *Mkwaju* (*Walking Stick*). Like its predecessor, *Mkwaju* featured the life of a truck driver and his battles with sexual responsibility and HIV. The program also achieved national popularity and through audience involvement with *Mkwaju,* three-fourths of its regular listeners changed their sexual practices to reduce their HIV risk (Sawyer, 2002).

In South Africa, the Soul City Institute for Health and Development Communication has become a pioneer in producing entertainment-education media throughout Africa.

The first 13 episodes of its first television series focused on children's health and HIV/ AIDS prevention. Soul City's second television series, broadcast in 1996, focused on HIV/AIDS, TB, and smoking prevention, followed by a third series in 1997, which also concentrated on HIV/AIDS prevention messages as well as other health-related themes. All three series achieved high audience ratings, became some of the most popular prime-time television programs on South African television, and reached an estimated 20 million people (Japhet and Goldstein, 1997).

In 2001 and 2003, the fifth and sixth *Soul City* television series were produced and broadcast in South Africa. Like the first four series, the programs consistently achieved high audience ratings and won numerous awards for excellence in television drama. Extensive summative research indicates the programs increased knowledge and adoption of HIV/AIDS prevention practices (Usdin *et al.*, 2004). Soul City has conducted evaluation studies of each television series to document the influence of the programs on viewers. In addition to promoting sexual responsibility, Soul City programs have advocated family planning, HIV/AIDS prevention, drug and alcohol abuse prevention, and other prosocial beliefs and practices in South Africa and in many nations in Southern Africa.

One example of Soul City's extensive regional impact is its *OneLove* campaign, launched in January of 2009 in South Africa to stimulate public discussion about the practice and negative consequences of having multiple sexual partners. The three-year campaign, which has diffused to Lesotho, Swaziland, Zambia, Zimbabwe, Tanzania, Malawi, Namibia, and Mozambique, is already having an impact by directly addressing entrenched cultural practices that exacerbate the spread of HIV (Rassool, 2009).

Another important program used to combat sexually transmitted infections in southern Africa is *Sesame Street*. The South African version of the children's television series, *Takalani* (*Be Happy*), was launched in July of 2000 with funding from USAID and Sanlam. Through a collaboration of the South African Broadcasting Corporation, the Department of Education, and the Sesame Street Workshop, the producers of the series decided to address how children were responding to the HIV crisis. By 2005, the number of children living with HIV in South Africa had surpassed two million, with an HIV prevalence rate among children age 2–9 of 5.6 percent (Human Sciences Research Council, 2005). In order to help children understand other children living with HIV, the producers of *Takalani* created an HIV-positive muppet. Formative research with young children was conducted to help the creative producers understand how children would relate to the HIV/AIDS messages in the program (Clacherty and Kushlick, 2004).

Oral Rehydration Therapy

Dysentery is one of the leading causes of death among young children in the world today. Inability to access potable water has contributed to alarming rates of dysentery deaths in much of the underdeveloped world. Diarrhea-related diseases such as cholera, dysentery, typhoid fever, and rotavirus claim the lives of nearly two million children and account for a high percentage of infant mortalities worldwide (London, 2005). One simple but effective technique to save a child's life when dysentery strikes is through oral rehydration therapy (ORT), a sodium and glucose solution developed by medical researchers in Bangladesh and India during the 1970s. By mixing salt, sugar, and water, common ingredients in every household, an oral rehydration solution can save a dehydrated child's life.

Egypt, a country with a high infant death rate, successfully implemented a $50 million ORT campaign using entertainment to teach parents how to administer ORT. By using well-known film and television stars to promote ORT, the public service announcement campaign attracted a great deal of attention. Celebrity-driven health campaigns also work through the degree of involvement that audience members form with celebrities. Results of the campaign were phenomenal. Awareness of ORT reached 98 percent of the population in five years and usage of ORT reached 82 percent (Abdulla, 2004). Infant mortality rates were cut almost in half during the campaign and by 1991, at the end of the campaign, nearly all mothers (more than 99 percent) knew about ORT and more than 96 percent used ORT. Infant mortality rates were reduced by 70 percent by the end of the campaign, saving the lives of more than 100,000 children in the first two years of the entertaining public service television ads (White, 1991). Other nations also have made ORT a commonly known life saving technique through entertainment-education media.

John Riber, an American filmmaker based in Tanzania, has produced numerous entertainment-education films in India, Bangladesh, Sri Lanka, Zimbabwe, and Uganda, each a big commercial success. Riber's films have promoted a number of health education and social change goals. His award-winning film *Consequences* promoted family planning, his films *It's Not Easy* and *More Time* promoted HIV/AIDS prevention, and *Neria*, another award-winning film, promoted the status of women. One of Riber's most successful films was *Sonamoni* (*Golden Pearl*), which featured oral rehydration therapy. The film tells the story of Gafur and his wife Rohima, who are persecuted by a village ruffian and cut off from safe drinking water. Forced to use polluted river water for their family, their baby soon gets dysentery and dehydration threatens the child's life. Fortunately Gafur learns about ORT, saves his child, and exposes to the community that the villain's cattle had been contaminating their village's drinking water. This popular film was seen by 20 million Bangladeshis, teaching millions of parents about ORT (Riber, 1992). Riber's films provide realistic characters with whom audiences identify, giving his films great popular appeal and creating strong audience involvement (Buenting, 2007).

Alcohol Abuse Prevention

Another important health issue addressed by entertainment programming is alcohol abuse and responsible drinking. One of the early communication campaigns designed to promote responsible drinking and driving through entertainment programming was orchestrated during the 1980s by the Harvard School of Public Health. Stung by the tragic death of a popular Boston news reporter, husband, and father to young children, who was killed by a drunk driver, Jay Winsten, associate dean of the School, asked Hollywood television producers to help them launch the National Designated Driver Campaign (NDDC) to advance the social norm that drivers should abstain from alcohol and that groups of friends planning to drink should choose a designated driver (Winsten, 1994).

The responsible drinking and driving campaign was launched on network television on a 1989 episode of *My Two Dads*, a popular US television series. In the episode, two dads get drunk and then drive home together in their inebriated condition. Their irresponsible drinking and driving angers their daughter, who tells them they should have decided who would be the "designated driver" before they began drinking. Similar prosocial messages encouraging the designated driver concept were included in 76 other US television programs as part of a two-month campaign between Thanksgiving and New Years (the heavy drinking season in the United States) of 1989, causing an increase in viewer awareness of the designated driver concept (Dejong and Winsten, 1990). Through the partnership of Hollywood leaders, the national campaign, valued at over $100 million dollars in advertising space, placed designated driver messages in more than 160 entertainment programs (Winsten and DeJong, 2001).

The campaign drew from social learning theory and was predicated on capitalizing on the cognitive and affective involvement of television viewers with celebrities and with the television characters they played. Many famous actors and actresses were involved in promoting the no drinking and driving concept. An assessment of the campaign indicated the adoption of the designated driver practice was successfully diffused, especially among males (Dejong and Winsten, 1990). Now the idea and practice of choosing a designated driver is quite common. Not only has it helped those who don't like to drink alcohol to go out with a group and not feel pressured to drink, but it has saved lives by reducing the number of drunk drivers on the road.

Portrayals of alcohol consumption on entertainment television programs in the United States are common (Wallack *et al.*, 1990). Researchers have examined how entertainment contributes to viewers' perceptions of various social norms such as drinking alcohol. For example, one episode of the television program, *Party of Five*, portrayed a detailed drinking and driving incident in which Bailey, one of the main characters, gets in a drunk driving accident, injuring his girlfriend. The episode made the abstract problem of drinking and driving very real, particularly to college students targeted by the episode (Kean and Albada, 2003).

The popular America television situation comedy *Growing Pains* included a powerful episode on drunk driving (Winsten and DeJong, 2001). In the episode, the oldest daughter of the family, Carol Seaver (played by Tracey Gold), had a boyfriend named Sandy who had dropped her off from a date the night before. Owing to his overconsumption of alcohol during the evening, he gets in a serious car accident and is hospitalized. When Carol visits Sandy in the hospital during the next day, he is conscious and appears to be on the road to recovery. Carol tells him he narrowly escaped death and now has a second chance on life, and makes him promise never to drink and drive again. Later that evening, Carol's brother Mike receives a shocking call from the hospital informing his family that Sandy has died from internal hemorrhaging. When Mike breaks the terrible news, Carol cries out in anguish, asking her family through her tears, "What happened to his second chance?" The episode was so powerful that *NBC Nightly News* ran a story about it, indicating the producers had intended to send a powerful message about drinking and driving.

Hollywood writer, producer and director Peter Engel also took on the issue of alcohol abuse, as well as other relevant practices that teenagers struggle with from day to day in his popular television series, *Saved by the Bell*. Engel purposefully sought to blend a highly rated entertainment program for teenagers that featured stories involving everyday moral dilemmas that teens encountered. By showing the struggles of his characters in making the right moral decisions, the program promoted responsibility among its teenage viewers who followed the lives of the program's characters into adulthood. *Saved by the Bell* and its many spin-offs became some of the most highly rated television programs among teenagers in television history. Engel and producers of similar programs demonstrated that popular entertainment could effectively help teenagers to discuss important moral issues such as drinking and driving (Calvert *et al.*, 2002). Engel sought to create engaging characters that his audience could strongly identify with to encourage teenagers to adopt the prosocial values and behavior they modeled.

The designated driver campaign, *Growing Pains,* and *Saved by the Bell* are but a few examples among many in which entertainment television has been used to reduce the abuse of alcohol and reduce drunk driving accidents and fatalities. Although not all dramatic stories dealing with alcoholism or drunk driving necessarily communicate abuse prevention messages, those that do can be very effective. Television writers and producers wishing to address alcohol abuse and other health issues now have support from the Hollywood, Health and Society (HH&S) project the University of Southern California's Norman Lear Center, which provides expert consultation, education, and resources for entertainment professionals who develop scripts with health storylines and health information (Beck, 2004). In partnership with the CDC, HH&S also gives the Sentinel for Health Awards to honor Hollywood writers and producers who address health and social issues. Creators of CBS's *The Young and the Restless,* for example, received a Sentinel Award for an episode on alcoholism (Norman Lear Center, 2010).

Television programs overseas have also dealt with alcohol abuse. For example, India's first long-running television soap opera, *Hum Log,* aired several episodes with an alcohol abuse subplot (Singhal and Rogers, 1988). In the epilogues, film star Askok Kumar warned viewers about the disastrous effects of alcohol abuse. In one of Tanzania's first television soap operas, *Maisha,* the negative effects of alcohol abuse also were prominently featured (Brown, Kiruswa, and Fraser, 2003). South Africa's radio and television series *Soul City* also has addressed responsible alcohol use through positive and negative role models.

Increasing Breast Cancer Awareness

Another important health issue that has been embedded into entertainment storylines is breast cancer. Breast cancer is one of the most critical health issues facing women in the United States. One of the first times that breast cancer was featured in an entertainment program was in an early 1970s episode of *All in the Family*. Edith, Archie Bunker's wife in the series, gets breast cancer and has to have a mastectomy. In a scene between Edith and Irene, one of her good friends, she breaks down in tears because of the fear that Archie may not love her in the same way after she has a breast removed. In a dramatic twist, Irene reveals that she had had a mastectomy and that her husband loved her in exactly the same way. Edith tries not to look at Irene's bust to see if she can determine which breast is real, but despite proclaiming to Irene that she is not looking, Edith can't help herself, to the roaring laughter of the live audience.

The magic of Norman Lear's *All in the Family* was its combination of humor, real life, and important issues that people did not openly discuss. Through the use of humor on a national television program, taboo communication was broken about breast cancer as well as many other sensitive subjects. The characters exposed commonly held prejudicial attitudes, beliefs, and stereotypes in a way to create self-reflection among audience members; although the satirical content also reinforced racial stereotypes among some viewers (Vidmar and Rokeach, 1974).

A decade after Norman Lear's use of entertainment-education to address breast cancer, one of the most popular situation comedies in the United States, *Thirtysomething*, featured an episode in which one of the main characters gets breast cancer. Viewers who followed the breast cancer storyline were both cognitively and emotionally influenced, creating a greater awareness of the issues surrounding breast cancer (Sharf and Freimuth, 1993). The telephone hotline provided to viewers to call after the episode lit up with a dramatic increase of telephone calls, mostly from women requesting more information on breast cancer.

Popular daytime television soap operas such as *One Life to Live* and *The Young and the Restless* also have dealt with the issue of breast cancer. In 2002, producers of *The Young and the Restless* launched a storyline in which Ashley, one of the program's major characters, is diagnosed with breast cancer. The audience walks through this challenge with Ashley for several weeks as she goes through her treatments to a successful conclusion. During the storyline, accurate information was provided to viewers on breast cancer screening, diagnosis, and treatment options. In order to facilitate behavioral responses to the storyline, public service announcements on breast cancer were broadcast by the Cancer Information Service providing a toll-free 800 number for viewers who wanted further information (Beck, 2004).

In these television dramas, audience involvement with the on-screen characters helped to facilitate learning more about breast cancer screening, prognosis, and various options for treatment. The added dimension of having a person available to talk to through a toll-free phone number increased the overall effectiveness of these programs.

Environmental Health

A growing health issue of the 21st century concerns environmental safety. The increased toxicity of our environment through the accumulation of waste and toxic compounds has contributed to the increase of cancer and other harmful diseases, costing some developed nations billions of dollars each year in health care costs and the tragic loss of life. Embedding environmental safety messages in popular entertainment has become an increasingly effective means of raising awareness about the environment.

One of the early and most successful experiments in mixing entertainment and environmental education was a television special broadcast in 1977 called *The Great American Values Test*. Created by Milton and Sandra Ball Rokeach, two social scientists and experts on communication and belief change, the program was designed to persuade the viewing audience to self-reflect on the values of equality and a world of beauty, motivating viewers to increase the importance that they placed on those two values. The Rokeaches applied belief system theory to develop the program, postulating that long-term behavior change would best be induced by first changing values, facilitated through a process of self-reflection (Rokeach, 1973). They theorized that, if people knew how important a clean and safe environment was to those around them, and saw that they did not value the environment as highly as others did, they would be motivated to become more environmentally concerned and active.

In order to test their theory, they decided to simulcast a one-hour television special in the tri-city area of northern Washington state. This experiment took place in the days before cable television took root and when ABC, CBS, and NBC dominated television broadcasting. All three major networks broadcast the program so that if you lived in that area and watched television you were likely to see the program, which was hosted by Ed Asner and provided viewers with information about how much people in their area valued the environment. *The Great American Values Test* was highly effective in promoting the targeted values. Those who watched the program not only increased their value of a clean and healthy environment, but also increased their donations to environmental causes after watching the program (Ball-Rokeach, Rokeach, and Grube, 1984).

In the NBC comedy series *My Two Dads,* noted earlier, Joey Harris, one of the main characters in the series, was revealed as a dedicated environmentalist. Joey's environmental activism even landed him in jail on one episode, a storyline promoted by a Hollywood lobby group called the Environmental Media Association. Noting the popular series' ability to address social issues such as irresponsible drinking and polluting of the environment, producer David Steven Simon explained, "We can create consciousness and prompt activity" (Stevenson, 1990).

Another pro-environmental television program was Animal Planet's *Crocodile Hunter,* which attracted a large international audience of young viewers through the magnetic personality of its entertaining host, Steve Irwin. Parasocial interaction and identification with Irwin increased support for wildlife conservation, even after his tragic death by a stingray (Brown, 2010).

In film, perhaps the most recognizable pro-environmental entertainment production is the Hollywood movie *Erin Brockovich.* Based on a true story about a young woman who dared to take on the corporate powerhouse that controlled the town in which she lived, the film dramatizes the tragic effects of environmental irresponsibility. Played by actress Julia Roberts, who won an academy award nomination for her role, Ms. Brockevich becomes a hero for standing up for the rights of those whose lives have been destroyed by chemical wastes. Although no formal research on the film has been published, identification with Julia Roberts, a high-profile leading actress, likely helped to raise the environmental concerns of the films' viewers.

These are but a few of the many examples in which popular media has been used to effectively promote pro-environmental attitudes beliefs and behavior. Most of these efforts, for example, the several pro-environmental films produced by Disney, have not been studied. What is clear is that the entertainment media can strongly influence how we value our environment.

Promoting Care for Children with Disabilities

The nation of Nepal, the small country to the north of India and a favorite destination for Himalayan mountain climbers, has nearly 30 million people, most of them very poor. Estimates of the number of Nepalis with disabilities range from 5 to 10 percent of the population, or 1.5–3.0 million people (Boyce and Paterson, 2002). The average family size in Nepal is 6.6 people; therefore, many Nepali households are directly affected by someone with a disability – either a family member or a close relative. Only 4.9 percent of Nepal's budget is allocated for health care and virtually none is provided for those with disabilities (Boyce and Paterson, 2002). Most disabled persons in Nepal have little or no access to rehabilitation.

One of the powerful means for changing attitudes toward the handicapped in Nepal is through television. Television is an integral piece of household furniture in many Nepali homes. Where electricity is available in the country, among approximately 80 percent of the population, practically every house has at least one television set. Affluent families usually possess one or more television sets. In many homes, the television stays on from the moment one family member wakes up until the last family member goes to bed. It is the most popular form of entertainment for many families, occupying many hours in the lives of Nepali children.

In 2007, Nepal began airing *Khushi Ko Sansar (Happy World)*. *Khushi Ko Sansar (KKS)* is the Nepali version of the Hindi program, *Khushi Ki Duniya (Happy World* in Hindi*)*, a 30-minute weekly children's TV show produced by the Christian Broadcasting Network in India. *KKS* is now one of the top-rated programs in Nepal. In India, the program's producers received more than 20,000 letters from audience members in 2007 (Strong, 2008). The program features biblical stories with music, song, dance, and brightly colored amusing sets appealing to children. Lessons taught during the program cover topics such as speaking no evil, sowing and reaping, using things properly (not being destructive with others' property, books, household items, tools, and school items), choosing good role models, good health practices, honesty, not stealing, friendship, respect for their elders, and other subjects relevant to a child's character development.

In addition to these topics, some shows contain specific educational elements which discuss persons with disabilities. They explore the lives of deaf people, blind people, physically and mentally disabled people, accident victims who are now in wheelchairs or use other walking aids, autism, and other health concerns. These shows are intended to educate children about disabilities so they understand the importance of respecting those different from themselves, showing the importance of everyone's right to dignity in life. They emphasize how every person has worth and value and that someone with a disability can live almost as normal a life as can a nondisabled person.

In 2008, a study of the effects of involvement with *Khushi Ko Sansar (Happy World)* was conducted. Pretest and posttest survey data from 357 Nepali children from seven communities in the country were analyzed. Results indicated that children role modeled the prosocial beliefs of the program's star character, Kush (Strong and Brown, 2011). As was expected, media exposure increased identification and was effective in changing the thinking and perceptions of children toward people with disabilities, primarily through two means: (1) creating an increased sense of positive beliefs about with people with disabilities, and (2) increasing more positive intended behavior toward those with disabilities (Strong and Brown, 2011). Overall, findings of this study are encouraging and optimistic with regards to the use of an entertainment-education television program to promote positive attitudes and favorable treatment of people with disabilities.

Promoting Hearing Safety

In 2008, the Netherlands' Center for Media and Health designed, created, produced, and implemented a sound effects campaign to raise awareness of the need to use earplugs to protect against permanent hearing loss brought about by repeated exposure to loud music in bars, clubs, and discothèques. The campaign featured a web-based E-E drama mini-series called *Sound*, a media campaign called *Go Out and Plug In*, and extensive formative and summative research on the campaign effects. The innovative Internet-based campaign attracted media attention which prompted a discussion about hearing loss on the floor of the Dutch Parliament in 2009. Bouman (2010) reported that *Sound*, the internet soap series, effectively captivated the attention of the targeted audience, frequent attendees of clubs and discothèques in the 16–30 year old age group, and is now becoming a model for future webisodes

Conceptual and Theoretical Evolution of Entertainment-Education

In their summary of many decades of entertainment-education programs, Sood, Menard, and Witte (2004) document their conceptual and theoretical foundations. Prominent among the more than two dozen theories identified is Bandura's (1977, 1986) social learning theory and theory of self-efficacy (Bandura, 1997), Rogers' (2003) diffusion of innovations theory, Jung's (1970) theory of archetypes and the collective unconscious, and several behavior change models offered by McGuire (1989), Prochaska and colleagues (Prochaska *et al.*, 1994; Prochaska and Velicer, 1997), Piotrow and colleagues (Piotrow *et al.*, 1992), and Soul City (2000).

Tufte (2005) argues that these theories of behavior change, used in the first and second generations of entertainment-education practice, are now giving way to a third generation of entertainment-education initiatives that draw on theories of empowerment, structural change, dialogue, social justice, and collective action. Emerging uses of entertainment-education for health promotion confirm Tufte's assessment. Two examples of these new third generation initiatives are the Famina Health Information Project (HIP) in Tanzania and the Kwanda Project in South Africa.

Founded by Dr. Minou Fuglesang in 1999 with support from the Swedish International Development Cooperation Agency (Sida), Femina HIP provides a multimedia platform designed to empower youth to promote healthy lifestyles, sexual health, HIV/AIDS prevention, gender equality, and citizen engagement within their local communities. Through two popular magazines, a television talk show, radio programs, and booklets, the project is engaging millions of Tanzanians annually in public dialogue about sexual practices and empowering youth to create their own media to facilitate further dialogue (Thorfinn and Bagger, 2010).

The Kwanda Project was created by the Soul City Institute in South Africa in collaboration with the Department of Social Development and the South Africa Broadcasting Corporation. The project features a reality television program called *Kwanda,* a dramatic community make-over show in which five teams of young people work across the country to make their communities look better, work better, and feel better (Soul City, 2010). The program encourages youth and community leaders to build shelters for children, start soup kitchens, volunteer to serve in clinics and schools, and establish neighborhood watches. Social change in Kwanda is portrayed as a grass roots community-centered initiative.

Conclusion

In summary, entertainment-education initiatives to promote health and change health beliefs and practices are being implemented throughout the world through numerous forms of media and popular culture. Producers of these programs are drawing from a number of communication and social change theories and concepts, including perceived realism, perceived similarity, cultural proximity, agenda-setting, social learning, parasocial interaction, identification, empowerment, and dialogue. Research indicates that audience members who become more emotionally and psychologically involved with media personas, both real celebrities and fictional characters, will more likely adopt the health beliefs and behavior modeled by those personas.

Future research is needed to further explore processes of involvement incorporating other theoretical perspectives such as transportation theory and exploration of celebrity worship. More theoretical development is needed to understand how these various processes relate to each other and how communication scholars can more effectively measure them. The use of entertainment media for health education and development will no doubt continue to become an increasingly important global health endeavor. More nonprofit organizations and research centers, including Johns Hopkins University's Center for Communication Programs, the Norman Lear Center at the University of Southern California, the Netherlands Center for Media and Health, the Centers for Disease Control, the BBC World Service Trust, South Africa's Soul City Institute for Health, Population Media Center in Vermont, Population Communications International in New York, Minga in Peru, Encuentros in Nicaragua, and Twaweza Communications in Kenya, are applying the entertainment-education communication strategy in dozens of health initiatives throughout the world. The more health communication professionals and scholars understand about the power of entertainment to persuade and teach, the more it can be harnessed to improve health globally and to contribute toward a better quality of life for the world's communities.

References

Abdulla, R.A. (2004). Entertainment-education in the Middle East: Lessons from the Egyptian oral rehydration therapy campaign. In A. Singhal, M. J. Cody, E. N. Rogers, and M. Sabido (Eds.), *Entertainment-Education and Social Change* (pp 301–320). Mahwah, NJ: Lawrence Erlbaum Publishers.

Advocates for Youth. (1998). *The use of mainstream media to encourage social responsibility: The international experience.* Menlo Park, CA: Kaiser Family Foundation.

Bae, H.-S., Brown, W. J., and Kang, S. (2010). Social influence of a religious hero: The late Cardinal Stephen Kim Sou-hwan's impact on cornea donation and volunteerism. *Journal of Health Communication, 16*, 1–17.

Ball-Rokeach, S., Rokeach, M., and Grube, J. (1984). *The Great American Value Test.* New York: Free Press.

Bandura, A. (1977). *Social learning theory.* Englewood Cliffs, NJ: Prentice Hall.

Bandura, A. (1986). *Social Foundations of Thoughts and Action: A Social Cognitive Theory.* Englewood Cliffs, NJ: Prentice Hall.

Bandura, A. (1997). *Self-Efficacy: The Exercise of Control.* New York: W.H. Freeman and Company.

Basil, M. D. (1996). Identification as a mediator of celebrity effects. *Journal of Broadcasting and Electronic Media, 40*, 478–495.

Beck, V. (2004). Working with daytime and prime-time television shows in the United States to promote health. In A. Singhal, M. J. Cody, E. M. Rogers, and M. Sabido (Eds.), *Entertainment-education and social change: History, research, and practice* (pp. 207–224). Mahwah, NJ: Lawrence Erlbaum Associates.

Bentley, E. (1967). *The life of drama.* New York: Atheneum.

Bouman, M. P. A. (2010, September 20). *Report on entertainment-education activities in the Netherlands.* Retrieved from http://www.media-health.nl/news.html

Boyce, W., and Paterson, J. (2002). Community based rehabilitation for children in Nepal. Retrieved from http://www.aifo.it/old_sito/english/apdrj/January%202002%20Selected %20Readings%20CBR%20II.pdf#page=58

Brown, W. J. (1991). An AIDS prevention campaign: Effects on attitudes, beliefs, and communication behavior. *American Behavioral Scientist, 34*, 666–687.

Brown, W. J. (2009). Mediated influence of Pope John Paul II. *Journal of Communication and Religion, 32*(2), 33–62.

Brown, W. J. (2010). Steve Irwin's influence on wildlife conservation. *Journal of Communication, 60*, 73–93.

Brown, W. J., and Basil, M. D. (1995). Media celebrities and public health: responses to "Magic" Johnson's HIV disclosure and its impact on AIDS risk and high-risk behaviors. *Health Communication, 7*, 345–371.

Brown, W. J., Basil, M. D., and Bocarnea, M. C. (2003a). Social influence of an international celebrity: Responses to the death of Princess Diana. *Journal of Communication, 53*, 587–605.

Brown, W. J., Basil, M. D., and Bocarnea, M. C. (2003b). The influence of famous athletes on health beliefs and practices: Mark McGwire, child abuse prevention, and androstenedione. *Journal of Health Communication, 8*, 41–57.

Brown, W. J., and de Matviuk, M. A. C. (2010). Sports celebrities and public health: Diego Maradona's influence on drug use prevention. *Journal of Health Communication, 15*, 358–373.

Brown, W. J., Kiruswa, S. L., and Fraser, B. (2003). Promoting HIV/AIDS prevention through soap operas: Tanzania's experience with *Maisha. Communicare, 22*, 90–111.

Buenting, D. K. (2007). Exploring audience involvement with Yellow Card and its promotion of sexual responsibility among African youth. Doctoral Dissertation, Regent University, Virginia Beach, VA.

Buenting, D. K., and Brown, W. J. (2009). Exploring audience involvement with Yellow Card and its promotion of sexual responsibility among African youth. Paper presented to the International and Intercultural Communication Division of the National Communication Association for presentation at the 95th annual convention, November 12–15.

Burch, E. (2002). Media literacy, cultural proximity and TV aesthetics: Why India soap operas work in Nepal and the Hindu diaspora. *Media, Culture and Society, 24,* 571–579.

Busselle, R., and Bilindzic, H. (2008). Fictionality and perceived realism in experiencing stories: A model of narrative comprehension and engagement. *Communication Theory, 18,* 255–280.

Busselle, R., Ryabovolova, A., and Wilson, B. (2004). Ruining a good story: Cultivation, perceived realism and narrative. *Communications, 29,* 365–378.

Calvert, S. L., Kotler, J., Murray, W. *et al.* (2002). Children's online reports about educational and informational television programs. In S. L. Calvert, A. B. Jordan, and R. R. Cocking (Eds.), *Children in the Digital Age: Influences of Electronic Media on Development* (pp. 165–182). Westport, CT: Praeger.

Cambridge, V. (1992). Radio soap operas: The Jamaican experience 1958–1989. *Studies in Latin American Popular Culture II,* 93–109.

Church, C. A., and Geller, J. (1989). *Lights! camera! action! Promoting family planning with TV, video, and film.* Population Reports, J-38. Baltimore, MD: Johns Hopkins University, Population Information Program.

Clacherty, G., and Kushlick, A. (2004). Meeting the challenge of research with very young children: A practical outline of methodologies used in the formative research and pre-testing of the Takalani Sesame HIV and AIDS television and radio programmes. Paper presented to the Fourth International Entertainment-Education Conference, September 26–30, Cape Town. Retrieved from http://www.comminit.com/africa/edutainment/ edutainmentEE4/ edutainment-30.html

Cohen, J. (2001). Defining identification: A theoretical look at the identification of audiences with media characters. *Mass Communication and Society, 4,* 245–264.

Cole, T., and Leets, L. (1999). Attachment styles and intimate television viewing: Insecurely forming relationships in a parasocial way. *Journal of Personal and Social Relationships, 16,* 494–511.

Dejong, W., and Winsten, J. A. (1990). *The Harvard alcohol project: A demonstration project to promote the use of the "designated driver."* Cambridge, MA: Harvard School of Public Health, Harvard University.

Fraser, B. P., and Brown, W. J. (2002). Media, celebrities, and social influence: Identification with Elvis Presley. *Mass Communication and Society, 5,* 185–208.

Galavotti, C., Pappas-DeLuca, K. A., and Lansky, A. (2001). Modeling and reinforcement to combat HIV: The MARCH approach to behavior change. *American Journal of Public Health, 91,* 1602–1607.

Gilluly, R. H. and Moore, S. H. (1986). Radio – Spreading the word on family planning. *Population Reports Journal,* 853–886.

Green, M. C. (2004). Transportation into narrative worlds: The role of prior knowledge and perceived realism. *Discourse Processes, 38,* 247–266.

Hazzard, M., and Cambridge, V. (1988). Socio-drama as an applied technique for development communication in the Caribbean: Specialized content and narrative structure in the radio drama of Elaine Perkins in Jamaica. Paper presented to the Caribbean and Latin American Studies Conference, Guadelope, French West Indies.

Hoffner, C., and Buchanan, M. (2005). Young adults' wishful identification with television characters: The role of perceived similarity and character attributes. *Media Psychology, 7,* 325–351.

Horton, D., and Wohl, R. R. (1956). Mass communication and para-social interaction. *Psychiatry, 19,* 215–229.

Human Sciences Research Council. (2005). *HIV risk exposure among young children: A study of 2–9 year olds served by public health facilities in the Free State, South Africa.* Cape Town, South Africa: HSRC Press.

Japhet, G., and Goldstein, S. (1997). Soul City experience. *Integration, 53,* 10–11.

Jung, C. G. (1970). *Archetypes and the collective unconscious.* Buenos Aires: Ed. Paidos.

Jung, C. G. (1981). *The Collected Works of C.G. Jung, Vol. 9, Part 1: The Archetypes and the Collective Unconscious,* 2nd edn. Princeton, NJ: Princeton University Press.

Kean, L. G., and Albada, K. F. (2003). The relationship between college students schema regarding alcohol use, their television viewing patterns, and their previous experience with alcohol. *Health Communication, 15,* 277–298.

Kelman, H. C. (1961). Processes of opinion change. *Public Opinion Quarterly, 25,* 57–78.

Krugman, H. E. (1965). The impact of television advertising: Learning without involvement. *Public Opinion Quarterly, 29,* 349–356.

La Pastina, A. C., and Straubhaar, J. D. (2005). Multiple proximities between television genres and audiences. *Gazette, 67,* 271–288.

Levy, M. R. (1979). Watching TV news as para-social interaction. *Journal of Broadcasting, 23,* 69–80.

Ligaga, D. (2005). Narrativising development in radio drama: Tradition and realism in the Kenyan radio play Ushikwapo Shikamama. *Social Identities, 11,* 131–145.

London, A. J. (2005). Justice and the human development approach to international research. *Hastings Center Report, 35,* 24–37.

MacLean, P. D. (1973). *A triune concept of the brain and behavior.* Toronto, Ontario: University of Toronto Press.

Mazrui, A. and Kitsao, J. (1988, June). *A formative survey of Ushikwapo Shikimana.* Nairobi, Kenya: National Council for Population and Development.

McCombs, M. (2005). A look at agenda-setting: Past, present and future. *Journalism Studies, 6,* 543–557.

McCombs, M. E., and Shaw, D. L. (1993). The evolution of agenda-setting research: Twenty-five years in the marketplace of ideas. *Journal of Communication, 43,* 58–67.

McGuire, W. J. (1989). Theoretical foundations of campaigns. In R. E. Rice and C. K. Atkin (Eds.), *Public communication campaigns,* 2nd edn. (pp. 43–65). Newbury Park, CA: Sage.

Nariman, H. N. (1993). *Soap operas for social change: Toward a methodology for entertainment-education television.* Westport, CT: Praeger.

Norman Lear Center (2010). Hollywood, Health and Society Sentinel Awards. Retrieved from http://www.learcenter.org/html/projects/?cm=hhs

Perkins, E. (2000). *Proceedings from the 4ᵗʰ Entertainment-Education for Social Change Conference* (pp. 34–35). Gouda, Netherlands: Center for Media and Health.

Piotrow, P. T., Kincaid, D. L., Hindin, M. J. *et al.* (1992). Changing men's attitudes and behavior: The Zimbabwe male motivation project. *Studies in Family Planning, 23,* 365–375.

Piotrow, P. T., Rimon, J. G., Winnard, K. *et al.* (1990). Mass media family planning promotion in three Nigerian cities. *Studies in Family Planning, 21,* 265–274.

Poindexter, D. (2004). A history of entertainment-education, 1958–2000. In A. Singhal, M. Cody, E. Rogers, and M. Sabido (Eds.), *Entertainment-Education and Social Change: History, Research and Practice* (pp. 21–36). London: Lawrence Erlbaum Associates.

Population Communication International (2005). Kenya – *Ushikwapo Shikamana*. Retrieved from http://www.population.org/programs_ushikwapo_kenya.shtml

Prochaska, J. O., and Velicer, W. F. (1997). The transtheoretical model of health behavior change. *American Journal of Health Promotion, 12*, 38–48.

Prochaska, J. O., Velicer, W. F., Rossi, J. *et al.* (1994). Stages of change and decisional balance for 12 problem behaviors. *Health Psychology, 13*, 30–46.

Rassool, R. (2009). One love... One partner. *SafAIDS News, 15*(3), 1–5.

Riber, John. (1992). Synopsis of the film *Sonamoni* (*Golden Pearl*). Columbia, MD: Development through Self-Reliance, Inc.

Risopatron, F., and Spain, P. L. (1980). Reaching the poor: Human sexuality education in Costa Rica. *Journal of Communication, 30*, 81–89.

Rokeach, M. (1973). *The nature of human values.* New York: The Free Press.

Rogers, E. M. (2003). *Diffusion of innovations*, 5th edn. New York: The Free Press.

Rogers, E. M., and Dearing, J. W. (1993). The anatomy of agenda-setting research. *Journal of Communication, 43*(2), 68–85.

Rogers, E. M., Vaughan, P. W., Swalehe, R. A. *et al.* (1999). Effects of an entertainment-education radio soap opera on family planning behavior in Tanzania. *Studies in Family Planning, 30*, 193–211.

Rubin, A., and McHugh, M. P. (1987). Development of parasocial interaction relationships. *Journal of Broadcasting and Electronic Media, 31*, 279–292.

Rubin, A. M., and Perse, E. M. (1987). Audience activity and soap opera involvement: A uses and effects investigation. *Human Communication Research, 14*, 246–268.

Rubin, A. M., Perse, E. M., and Powell, R. A. (1985). Loneliness, parasocial interaction, and local television news viewing. *Human Communication Research, 12*, 155–180.

Sabido, M. (1981). *Towards the social use of soap operas.* Mexico City, Mexico: Institute for Communication Research.

Sawyer, J. (2002, December 1). Soap operas are proving helpful in informing public. *St. Louis Post-Dispatch*, B-1, 34.

Sharf, B. F., and Freimuth, V. S. (1993). The construction of illness on entertainment television: Coping with cancer on *Thirtysomething. Health Communication, 5*, 141–160.

Singhal, A. (2005). Entertainment-education: A communication strategy for HIV prevention. *University of Western Cape's Papers in Education, 3*, 40–49.

Singhal, A., Njogu, K., Bouman, M. and Elías, E. (2006). Entertainment-education and health promotion: A cross-continental journey. In A. Singhal and J. W. Dearing (Eds.), *Communication of Innovations: A Journey with Ev Rogers* (pp. 199–229). Thousand Oaks, CA: Sage Publications.

Singhal, A., Obregon, R., and Rogers, E. M. (1994). Reconstructing the story of "Simplemente Maria," the most popular *telenovela* in Latin America of all time. *Gazette, 54*(1), 1–16.

Singhal, A. and Rogers, E. M., (1988). Television soap operas for development in India. *Gazette, 41*(3), 109–126.

Singhal, A., and Rogers, E. M. (1989). Educating through television. *Populi,16*(2), 39–47.

Singhal, A., and Rogers, E. M. (1999). *Entertainment Education: A Communication Strategy for Social Change.* Mahwah, NJ: Lawrence Erlbaum.

Singhal, A. and Rogers, E. M., (2004). The status of entertainment-education worldwide. In A. Singhal, M. J. Cody, E. M. Rogers, and M. Sabido (Eds.), *Entertainment Education and Social Change: History, Research, and Practice* (pp. 3–20). Mahwah, NJ: Lawrence Erlbaum.

Singhal, A., Rogers, E. M., and Brown, W. J. (1993a). Entertainment *telenovelas* for development: Lessons learned. In A. Fadul (Ed.), *Serial fiction in TV: The Latin American Telenovelas* (pp. 149–165). Sao Paulo: Nucleo de Pesquisa de Telenovelas, UCA-USP.

Singhal, A., Rogers, E. M., and Brown, W. J. (1993b). Harnessing the potential of entertainment-education telenovelas. *Gazette, 51,* 1–18.

Singhal, A., and Udornpim, K. (1997). Cultural shareability, archetypes and television soaps: *Oshindrome* in Thailand. *Gazette, 59,* 171–188.

Sood, S., Menard, T., and Witte, K. (2004). The theory behind entertainment-education. In A. Singhal, M. Cody, E. Rogers, and M. Sabido (Eds.), *Entertainment Education and Social Change*. Mahwah, NJ: Lawrence Erlbaum Associates.

Soul City (2000). *Soul City 4 impact evaluation: AIDS*. Retrieved from http://www.soulcity.org.za/research/evaluations/soul-city-series-4/impact-on-aids

Soul City (2010). Kwanda, communities with soul. Retrieved from http://www.soulcity.org.za/projects/kwanda/overview

Stevenson, R. W. (1990, May 27). Television; ... And now a message from an advocacy group. *New York Times*. Retrieved from http://www.nytimes.com/1990/05/27/arts/television-and-now-a-message-from-an-advocacy-group.html

Stone, C. (1986). First national survey on "Naseberry Street" programme. Unpublished manuscript. Mona: University of the West Indies.

Straubhaar, J. D. (1991). Beyond media imperialism: Asymmetrical interdependence and cultural proximity. *Critical Studies in Mass Communication, 8,* 39–59.

Strong, D. A. (2008). Audience involvement with "Kushi Ko Sansar," a children's TV show in Nepal: An entertainment-education initiative promoting positive attitudes and actions toward people with disabilities. Unpublished doctoral dissertation, Regent University, Virginia Beach, VA.

Strong, D. A., and Brown, W. J. (2011). Effects of a children's entertainment-education television program in Nepal on beliefs and behavior toward people with disabilities. *Disability, CBR, and Inclusive Development, 22*(2), 22–37.

Televisa's Institute of Communication Research (1981). Toward the social use of soap operas. Paper presented at the International Institute of Communication, Strasbourg, France.

Thorfinn, J., and Bagger, A. K. (2010). Femina HIP Youth Conference 2010: From life skills to livelihoods – promoting entrepreneurship education in schools. Retrieved January 10, 2011, from http://www.feminahip.or.tz/fileadmin/pics/research/Femina_HIP_Youth_Conference_2010__final_report.pdf

Trepte, S. (2008). The intercultural perspective: Cultural proximity as a key factor of television success. *De Gruyter Reference Global Journal, 33,* 1–25.

Tufte, T. (2005). Entertainment-education in development communication – Between marketing behaviours and empowering people. In O. Hemer and T. Tufte (Eds.), *Media and glocal change: Rethinking communication for development* (pp. 159–174). Gothenburg: Nordicom

Usdin, S., Singhal, A., Shongwe, T. *et al.* (2004). No short cuts in entertainment-education: Designing soul city step-by-step. In A. Singhal, M. J. Cody, E. M. Rogers, and M. Sabido (Eds.), *Entertainment-Education and Social Change: History, Research, and Practice* (pp. 153–176). Mahwah, NJ: Lawrence Erlbaum.

Vaughan, P. W., Rogers, E. M., Singhal, A., and Swalehe, R. M. (2000). Entertainment-education and HIV/AIDS prevention: A field experiment in Tanzania. *Journal of Health Communication, 5* (supplement), 81–100.

Vidmar, N., and Rokeach, M. (1974). Archie Bunker's bigotry: A study in selection perception and exposure. *Journal of Communication, 24,* 36–47.

Wallack, L., Grube, J. W., Madden, P. A., and Breed,W. (1990). Portrayals of alcohol on prime-time television. *Journal of Studies on Alcohol, 51,* 428–437.

White, M. (1991). NCDDP: The completion of an initial phase. *Diarrheal Control Newsletter, 13,* 1.

Winsten, J. A. (1994). Promoting designated drivers: The Harvard alcohol project. *American Journal of Preventive Medicine, 10* (supplement 1), 11–14.

Winsten, J. A., and DeJong, W. (2001). The designated driver campaign. In R. E. Rice and C. Atkin (Eds.), *Public communication campaigns,* 3rd ed. (pp. 290–294). Newbury Park, CA: Sage Publications.

World Health Organisation (2010). *UNAIDS global facts and figures.* Retrieved October 22, 2010, from http://data.unaids.org/pub/FactSheet/2009/20091124_FS_global_en.pdf

7

Interpersonal Health Communication
An Ecological Perspective

Rukhsana Ahmed

Introduction

Rahima is a 25-year-old poor married woman who lives with her husband, two young children, and mother-in-law, in Bahadurpur village in the district of Jessore, Bangladesh. With no formal education, she works as a housemaid to support her family. Thirty weeks pregnant with high blood pressure, Rahima does not seek formal health care on a regular basis because the nearest Upazila Health Complex (sub district hospital) and district hospital are between 5 and 10 kilometres away from her home. Because of a complication in the second trimester of her pregnancy, Rahima's family took her to the district hospital, but, due to poor road conditions and transportation facilities, travel time and the costs of health care services increased. In the absence of information about other health and social care services, Rahima seeks health care services from unqualified village doctors and spiritual healers, who are available within close proximity to her home. Overriding doctor's recommendation to deliver in the hospital, as Rahima is approaching the time for labor, her family have decided to use traditional birth attendants and/or home delivery.

The above scenario, though not exhaustive, illustrates how a person's interpersonal health communication interactions are affected by his or her social contexts, which, in turn, can have an effect on health beliefs, attitude, behavior, and even outcomes. I begin with a discussion of the ecological perspective (Bronfenbrenner, 1977, 1979; McLeroy *et al.*, 1988; Stokols, 1992, 1996; Street, 2003) to help guide this chapter, which focuses on the intersections of interpersonal communication and health and health care in global contexts. I then provide a brief conceptualization of the key terms I shall be using, before presenting an overview of existing research in interpersonal health communication, discussing theoretical concepts, models, and developments relevant to the study of interpersonal communication in the health care context, and analyzing how theory informs

The Handbook of Global Health Communication, First Edition. Edited by Rafael Obregon and Silvio Waisbord.

research and practice. Next, I review various topics related to the interpersonal health communication process, its context, and its form in order to illuminate how interpersonal interactions in health contexts influence people's health and health care experiences. In doing so, although I review a wide range of scholarly literature, I do not present an exhaustive review of extant scholarship on interpersonal health communication. Rather, I survey studies that are particularly informative to elucidate the importance of interpersonal health communication in global contexts with an emphasis on developing countries. I then present and discuss case studies that illustrate innovative lines of research and programmatic experiences related to the role of interpersonal communication in health promotion and planning in developing countries. I conclude with pertinent questions for future research and debate.

An Ecological Perspective

I approach this chapter from an ecological perspective that, generally, accounts for inter-relationships between individuals and their environments. Interpersonal communication in health care is very complex, being shaped by a set of interrelated social contexts. The ecological perspective, also known as the social ecological model (McLeroy *et al.*,1988), provides a useful framework for examining the multiple contexts, including organizational, political-legal, media, cultural environments (Street, 2003), and other external influences, that can enable, or act as barriers to, interpersonal health communication exchanges between patients, health care providers, families, and others.

While ecology had its roots within the biological sciences "and refers to the interrelations between organisms and their environments" (p. 466), the ecological perspective in social science has evolved from advances in the fields of sociology, geography, psychology, health, education, political science, economics (Boss *et al.*, 2004, p. 466), and communication (Street, 2003).

Bronfenbrenner's (1977, 1979) ecological model of human development focuses on the context of the system of relationships that forms an individual's environment. Bronfenbrenner divided different aspects of the environment that influences human development into a set of nested systems – the micro, meso, exo, and macrosystems. The microsystem represents the relationship between individuals and their immediate environment, including family, home, school, peer groups, neighborhood, and workplace. The mesosystem represents the relationship between interconnected microsystems in which individuals participate. For example, the connections between home and school or between school and workplace. The exosystem represents social contexts in which individuals are not active participants but embedded, and thus which indirectly influence their development. Parent's work environments and the members of the extended family are examples of exosystem influences on a child's development. The macrosystem represents the overarching cultural values, beliefs, customs, and laws of a society that impact individual development. Ethnicity, religion, sexual orientation, political views are examples of macrosystem concepts (Berns, 2010). Lastly, the chronosystem encompasses the dimension of time as it relates to individuals' environments and their experiences in life, and includes elements, "such as changes over the life course in family structure, socioeconomic status, employment, place of residence, or the degree of hecticness and ability in everyday life" (Bronfenbrenner, 1993, p. 40). From Bronfenbrenner's developmental perspective, the dynamic interaction within and between the systems is constant and changing.

McLeroy, Bibeau, Steckler, and Glanz's (1988) ecological model for health promotion views health behavior as being influenced by intrapersonal factors (e.g., knowledge, attitude, behavior, self-concept), interpersonal processes (e.g., family, works groups, friends), institutional factors (e.g., social institutions), community factors (e.g., informal networks), and public policy (e.g., laws and policies). Accordingly, the model focuses attention on designing health promotion interventions aimed at changing these five individual and social environmental factors to the extent that they encourage, maintain, and reinforce unhealthy behaviors. For example, with regard to health promotion programs addressing drug and alcohol abuse, interventions at the intrapersonal level may include educational and mentoring programs, and peer counseling to bring about individual changes in drug- and alcohol-related knowledge, attitude, behavior, and skills. Interventions at the interpersonal level can include family support network programs and peer support groups to target social norms and social influences on drug and alcohol use. Interventions at the institutional level can involve professional associations, religious institutions, and local neighborhood organizations helping to garner social support for and adopt, implement, and institutionalize drug and alcohol abuse prevention programs. Interventions at the community level can bring in local voluntary agencies, neighborhoods, personal friendship networks, and health promotion consortiums to help coordinate community concerns, heighten community awareness, influence local health policies and expenditure with respect to drug- and alcohol-related problems. Interventions at the policy level can include raising public awareness about drug and alcohol related policies, organize coalition to support policy relate issues, and promoting public input into policy making process. Therefore, an ecological perspective on health promotion "assumes that appropriate changes in the social environment will produce change in individuals, and that the support of individuals in the population is essential for implementing environmental changes" (McLeroy et al., 1988, p. 351).

Street's (2003) ecological model of communication in medical encounters focuses on how communication in medical interactions is influenced by interpersonal (e.g., health care provider–patient interaction), organizational (e.g., the size of the health care facility), media (e.g., telemedicine), political-legal (e.g., malpractice litigation), and cultural contexts (e.g., race/ethnicity) within which they are situated. According to Street, it is the interpersonal context within which the medical encounter "is most fundamentally embedded" (2003, p. 64). Street's model provides a useful framework that accounts for a variety of interrelated social contexts that affect health care provider–patient interaction. Specifically, he highlights the interplay of predispositional influences (e.g., communication style, self-concept including personality), cognitive-affective influences (e.g., goals, perception of partner, communicative strategies), and partner's communication influences (e.g., conversational contributions, including asking questions, and communicative action, including the obligation to answer) that shapes health care provider–patient interactions further impacted by the organizational, media, political-legal, and cultural contexts within which they take place. Hence, Street called for a contextual approach to ground analysis of medical encounters in the settings in which they are embedded.

Communication scholars have applied Street's (2003) ecological perspective of communication in medical encounters to study issues related to interpersonal communication in health care. Moore, Wright, and Bernard (2009) tested Street's ecological perspective to examine the influence of sociocognitive variables on patient satisfaction with the health care system. Specifically, using structural equation modeling, the study assessed patient self-efficacy, nonverbal affirming behavior frequency on the part of the physician, patient wait time, perceptions of physician credibility, patient satisfaction with the physician, and health care system satisfaction overall, in order to investigate the relationship of these elements to satisfaction with the health delivery system. Although the findings provided no direct relationship between patient satisfaction with physicians and health care system satisfaction, they did reveal support for the possible influence of patient wait time and perceptions of physicians' nonverbal behavior on perceptions of physician credibility, satisfaction with physicians, and satisfaction with the health delivery system. Hence, the findings lend partial support to Street's "ecological perspective of communication to help explain the interrelationships between patients and various features of health-care environments" (2009, p. 285).

Drawing on Street's (2003) ecological model and focusing on how the media context impacts health care provider-patient relationship, Quick (2009) investigated the role of television viewing in cultivating patients' predispositions about real-world doctors. Specifically, the study applied cultivation theory to investigate the role of viewing *Grey's Anatomy* on patients' perceptions of medical doctors' courage and how that perception was associated with patient satisfaction. The survey findings indicated that heavy viewers of *Grey's Anatomy* perceived the program to be credible, and this credibility led them to perceive medical doctors as courageous, and this perceived courageousness led them to be more satisfied with their medical doctors. Although this study did not set out to test the ecological model, it "provided a testable theoretical framework to bolster Street's (2003) ecological model" and "a better understanding about the process by which the media infiltrates patients' predispositions about doctors in general" (Quick, 2009, p. 53).

Against the above backdrop, I argue for an ecological perspective to study interpersonal health communication, especially in the context of developing countries that bear a heavy burden of disease (World Bank, 1993, 2006). Many of these disease burdens and associated risk factors such as heart disease, cancer, and the use of tobacco, are behavior-oriented (Haider and Rogers, 2005). As such, interactions "among health, behavior, and communication is important in the context of the global burden of disease," which "is a product of interwoven demographic, economic, political, social, religious, and environmental factors" (Haider and Rogers, 2005, p. xxvii). While existing theories and models of health behavior change – such as the health belief model, theory of reasoned action, social cognitive theory, diffusion of innovation, and social marketing – champion individualism and focus on individual psychology, "which may be effective and meaningful in a western context, have lesser relevance in self-effacing cultures of Asia, Africa, Latin America, and the Caribbean," where "family and community are more central to the construction of health and well-being than the individual" (Airhihenbuwa and Obregon,

2000, p. 9), an ecological perspective provides a framework not only to focus on individual health behavior, but also to identify the multiple factors that influence that behavior. Informed by the works of Bronfenbrenner (1977, 1979), McLeroy *et al.* (1988), and Street (2003), an ecological perspective can explain interpersonal interactions that occur at multiple levels – individual, institutional, community, and policy – within the larger social environment. An ecological perspective also allows researchers to examine the various social contexts – organizational, media, political-legal, and cultural – that influence interpersonal health communication. A key concept of the perspective is embeddedness, in which each level and/or context functions within the operation of another level and/or context.

Key Terms

In this section, I conceptualize key terms such as health communication, interpersonal communication, and interpersonal health communication to help contextualize my approach to the study of the intersections of interpersonal communication and health and health care in global contexts. In doing so, I recognize the diversity of perspectives that abounds.

Health communication is the study of the interactions among various participants in the health care process, the dissemination of health- related messages and messaging by individuals, groups, and/or mass media to other individuals, organizations, and/or the general public, and the interpretation of these messages (Jackson and Duffy, 1998; Kreps and Thornton, 1984; Ray and Donohew, 1990; Thomas, 2006). Thomas, Fine, and Ibrahim (2004) argued that "factors such as belief systems, religious and cultural values, life experiences, and group identity act as powerful filters" through which health information is communicated (p. 2050). In this sense, health communication is negotiated in relation to context, experience, and culture.

Interpersonal communication refers to the process of information exchange by which two individuals "negotiate meanings, identity, and relationships" (Braithwaite and Baxter, 2008, p. 4).

Interpersonal health communication lies at the intersection of interpersonal communication and health communication. It focuses on how interpersonal communication shapes people's health and medical encounters, and how, in turn, people's health and medical encounters shape communication and relationship dynamics.

Overview of Interpersonal Health Communication Scholarship

Interpersonal communication is deeply woven into our daily life. Our everyday interactions in the health context play a significant role in our emotional and physical well-being (Cline, 2003). The interpersonal communication perspective has been a dominant area of research in health communication. Thompson and Parrot (2002) provided a comprehensive review of interpersonal communication research in the health care context. The review is roughly divided into descriptive studies that provide "descriptions of various communicative processes [information exchange between physicians and patients, length of interactions] observed in the medical context" and studies of the outcome of communication focusing on communication skills and training, the coding of provider–patient interaction, nonverbal aspects of communication, disclosure, language, diversity, control, prevention, and theoretical perspectives as these issues operate within the health care context (p. 681).

Either one-on-one or involving a small group, interpersonal interaction in the health care context occurs between different interactants and includes, for example, physician–patient communication, communication between patient and other health care professionals, communication between health care providers and patients' families, and communication between different health care professionals (Berry, 2007). These interactions are shaped by the contexts in which they occur and the conditions that surround them. For example, when faced with terminal medical conditions, patients, their families, caregivers, and health care providers are put in a situation that can be very stressful and emotionally draining; thus, the type of illness can influence health care interactions. Brashers and Goldsmith (2009) shed light on the important role of communication in health-related contexts. More specifically, they situate provider–patient interaction, patient identity management, and personal relationships within larger social, cultural, and economic conditions that shape health and illness experiences.

With the globalization of the world, society is becoming more and more diverse. Race, ethnicity, language, religion, gender, age, socioeconomic status, religion, culture, and many other factors interact with each other and have important implications for human communication. The complexities that multiculturalism brings into medical settings raise many new challenges to effective and satisfactory interpersonal communication in health care encounters. Thus, effective interpersonal communication about health is not an easy task. This difficulty is evident in the continued growth in health communication research to better understand the process through which communication shapes health and medical encounters and vice versa.

The growing diversity across North America denotes the importance of understanding, raising awareness, and accommodating the unique health care needs of culturally diverse people who often face challenges caused by culture, language, and knowledge barriers. Over the past two decades, there has been considerable growth in health communication scholarship to better understand the role of culture in shaping people's health beliefs, attitudes, behaviors, and experiences. The concern as to how health care professionals and practitioners can meet the health care needs of a diverse population seems to correspond to attempts aimed at developing culturally appropriate ways to enhance the quality of health care for culturally diverse communities by improving communication through education, advocacy, and research.

In recognition of how health communication research intersects with cultural dimensions, theoretical and practical approaches such as cultural competence, patient-centered care, and community participation, have gained important focus for improving the quality of health and health care delivery. A proliferation of cultural competence education programs across medical schools can be witnessed. For example, over 90 percent of US medical schools have integrated cultural competence training into their curriculum

(Boutin-Foster, Foster, and Konopasek, 2008). However, Boutin-Foster, Foster, and Konopasek (2008) highlight an important challenge that still remains when teaching cultural competence: learners' lack of awareness of their own cultural background. In response to the complexity of achieving cultural competence in health care, studies continue to look at issues of perceived cultural competence as they intersect with patient gender to examine how gender differences in patients' perceptions and expectations may influence the clinical encounter (Ahmed and Bates, 2007). Although no patient gender difference was revealed, the study found that cultural competence in health care does not exclude gender sensitivity because, regardless of gender, patients recognized the value of physicians' cultural awareness, awareness of cross-cultural differences, and adaptation to patients' cultural plurality in the context of physician–patient interactions. Studies also examine the relationship between patients' ethnocentric views and their perceptions of physicians' cultural competence in health care interactions (Ahmed and Bates, 2010). Cautioning that culturally competent care is not identical to patient-centered care, the findings challenge the often simplistic notions of patient-centered care to resolve health disparities. It was found that a more ethnocentric patient was less likely to recognize the physician as adapting to the cultural and linguistic dimensions of cultural competence, while a less ethnocentric patient was more likely to perceive the physician as accommodating cultural and linguistic differences in care. The findings also suggested that a patient with higher levels of ethnocentrism might find physicians as less patient-centered.

In the context of global health communication programs, emphasizing the role of communication in the implementation of Integrated Management of Childhood Illness (IMCI) at the health service level in Latin America, Obregon (2005) argued that, "effective communication between health professionals and parents and caretakers of children is critical to ensure adequate and effective care both at health centers and at home" (p. 256). In an examination of polio communication efforts in India and Pakistan between 2000 and 2007, Obregon *et al.* (2009) found that the integration of innovative and intensive interpersonal communication and social mobilization strategies, gender and culturally sensitive interventions, engagement of community and religious leaders, mass/folk media, and political advocacy gained access to the unreached poorest and marginalized populations in challenging socio-economic environments.

Theoretical Concepts, Models, and Developments

The emergence of theories, models, and frameworks has impacted the knowledge base of interpersonal communication in the health care context. A theory/framework/model is created when related constructs and concepts are combined to form a unit (Frankish, Lovato, and Poureslami, 2007). Airhihenbuwa and Obregon (2000) argued that, "theories, models, or frameworks are designed to guide the implementation and evaluation of programs along certain processes that are believed to yield an expected outcome" (p. 9). The study of health communication is simultaneously social scientific, humanistic, and professional in orientation. This interdisciplinarity allows health communication scholarship to connect and build upon many ideas of inquiry. Thompson and Parrott (2002) celebrated the copious efforts at theory building by current research on interpersonal communication in the health care context. This chapter highlights some of the underlying theories, models, and frameworks to understand and study interpersonal communication in the health care context (for a detailed list of theoretical perspectives, see Thompson and Parrott, 2002). Baxter and Braithwaite (2008) categorized interpersonal communication theories under three broad approaches – individually centered, discourse- or interaction-centered, and relationship-centered. The individually centered theories of interpersonal communication focus "on understanding how individuals plan, produce, and process interpersonal messages," discourse or interaction centered theories of interpersonal communication focus "on understanding interpersonal communication as a message or a joint action behaviorally enacted between persons," and relationship centered theories of interpersonal communication focus "on understanding the role of communication in developing, sustaining, and terminating social and personal relationships, including friendships, dating relationships, romantic relationships, and cohabiting relationships" (Baxter and Braithwaite, 2008, p. 5). In the following, I will highlight those theories that have been applied to the health care context. It should be noted that, due to space limitations, I do not discuss the details of these theories but rather bring to light some of their applications.

Cegala and Waldron's (1992) context-based model of communication competence has been applied to analyze physician-patient communication (McNeilis, 2001, 2002) and study competence in the delivery of bad news (Gillotti, Thompson, and McNeilis, 2002). From a dyadic perspective, communication accommodation theory has been applied to study doctor–patient encounters and patient–health professional interactions (Street, 1991; Watson and Gallois, 1998, 1999) and parents' perception of nurse–parent communication in the neonatal intensive care unit environment (Jones, Woodhouse, and Rowe, 2007). Babrow's (1992) problematic integration theory has been applied to study communication about end-of-life issues (Hines *et al.*, 2001); supportive communication for breast cancer patients (Repass and Matusitz, 2010); and Man-to-Man prostate cancer support groups (Arlington, 2010). Brashers' (2001a) uncertainty management theory has been applied to study the processes of communication and the management of uncertainty for people living with chronic illness such as HIV/ AIDS (Brashers, 2001b; Brashers, Goldsmith, and Hsieh, 2002; Brashers *et al.*, 2000; Brashers *et al.*, 2006; Brashers *et al.*, 2001). Social exchange theory has been applied to study patient-provider communication during medical encounters (Roter and Hall, 1991) and client–nurse interaction in the context of maternal–child home visits (Byrd, 2006). The relational model of health communication competence has been applied to lay caregivers of patients with Alzheimer's disease (Weathers, Query, and Kreps, 2010; Query and Kreps, 1996). Facework and politeness theory has been applied to study nursing interactions (Spiers, 1998) and pharmacist–physician interaction (Lambert, 1996).

Since the 1990s, the appeal of narratives has taken a substantive turn towards the pathologized body and chronic illness experiences (Gwyn, 2002). Scholars have underscored the importance of a narrative approach to study patient–physician discourse (Sharf, 1990); the value of socially shared health-related narratives (Sharf and Vanderford, 2003); and the intersections of health narratives and interpersonal relationships (Harter, Japp, and Beck, 2005). It is through telling and hearing stories that human beings have always come to understand their experiences. By situating narrative in real life settings, people seek to make "meaning" from their experiences of illness. However, as Harter, Japp, and Beck (2005) argued, narrative theory allows not only canonical stories but also disruptive understanding of health related issues. In other words, narrative can be messy too, a fact that has important implications for interpersonal health communication.

Integrating cultural contexts into health communication research has been important from both theoretical and applied standpoints. Scholars have developed communication frameworks grounded in culture (Airhihenbuwa and Obregon, 2000) and culture-centered understandings of health communication processes (Dutta, 2008). Airhihenbuwa and Obregon (2000) raised questions regarding the global relevance of commonly used theories and models that are based on individual psychology to inform HIV/AIDS prevention messages, and underlined the need to develop theories and models that take into consideration cultural contexts. In order to understand "the complexity of the context within which an individual is a part," the authors advocated for a contextual approach, especially cultural contexts, over individual theories and models in HIV/AIDS communication (pp. 9–10).

An emerging approach to health communication, "the culture-centered approach primarily focuses on understanding health meanings and experiences in marginalized settings" (Dutta, 2008, p. 4). It offers an opportunity to examine communication in traditional health interventions and the dominant value systems, and thereby to question the inherent biases in thinking about health and health promotion in communities. With regard to interpersonal health communication, the culture-centered approach offers a framework to examine physician–patient relationships, conceptualizes ways in which culture may inform such relationships, and explores alternative ways of health and healing (Dutta, 2008). Dutta (2010) urged critical health communication scholars to:

> continue to explore co-constructive processes through partnerships with local communities that seek to bring about transformations in local, national, and global structures by fundamentally attending to the agency of individuals and collectives living at the margins to define their own problems and participate in processes of change to address these problems (pp. 538–539).

Hence, interrogating health communication theorizing and application that operates "on the basis of West-centric universals" (Dutta, 2010, p. 535), creates alternative discursive spaces for marginalized cultural voices in health care and co-construction of alternate health communication theorizing (Dutta, 2008; Dutta, 2010; Dutta and Zoller, 2008).

Theory Informing Research and Practice

As Airhihenbuwa and Obregon (2000) argued, "Theories, models, or frameworks are designed to guide the implementation and evaluation of programs along certain processes that are believed to yield an expected outcome" (p. 9). According to Thompson (1994), "research or theory in a specific setting can help expand our understanding of communication in general" (p. 715). In the last 40 years, students and scholars in communication have studied health issues to help understand and improve health care. Although the field of health communication is fragmented, Thompson (1994) explained that the field began a "movement" towards theory building (p. 715). Recognizing the importance of theoretically informed work, Babrow and Mattson (2003) argued that "theoretical sense-making processes and practices not only construct understandings but justify belief in or perception of the reasonableness of the emerging, elaborated constructions" (p. 37).

Studies have underscored the direct link between health care provider-receiver communicative patterns and health behaviors and outcomes (Betancourt, 2003; Betancourt, Carrillo, and Green, 1999; Brown, Stewart, and Ryan, 2003; Hall, 1993; Howell, Koren and Tinsley, 1990; King, 1991; Korsch and Negrete, 1972; Langer, 1999; Liptak, Hulka, and Cassel, 1977; Ong *et al.*, 1995; Pendleton, 1982; Roter, 1989; Roter and Flores, 2000; Stewart, 1995; Street, 2001; Stewart *et al.*, 1999; Street, 1989; Street and Wiemann, 1987; Thompson, 1994; Woolley, Kane, Hughes, and Wright, 1978). Although Street (2003) acknowledged the line of research on provider-patient communication, he expressed his concern for the lack of effort "to develop and test theoretical models of the processes underlying these interactions" (p. 63).

Almost two decades ago, Thompson (1994) noted that "most of the research on interpersonal communication in health care is still atheoretical" (p. 716) and, that after 13 years, "we are still not close to a theory of health communication" (Thompson and Parrott, 2002, p. 709). Nonetheless, research on interpersonal communication in health care over the years has witnessed sustained efforts towards "theoretical offerings" (Thompson and Parrott, 2002, p. 709). For example, Street (2003) has employed an ecological perspective to study communication in medical encounters. Thompson and Parrott (2002) advocated for an ecological model as "most promising" for future health communication research and theory building (p. 710).

Topic Areas of Interpersonal Health Communication: Processes, Contexts, and Forms

In the following section I highlight some topic areas of interpersonal health communication according to processes (e.g., social support), contexts (e.g., family), and forms (e.g., computer-mediated) of communication (Braithwaite and Baxter, 2008).

Models of physician–patient communication

Emanuel and Emanuel (1992) developed four models of the physician–patient relationship – the paternalistic, informative, interpretive, and deliberative models. In a paternalistic model, the physician assumes an authoritative role, prescribing treatment for patients who are expected to adhere to it without question. This model undermines patient autonomy. In contrast, in an informative model the physician discloses all the information concerning the diagnosis and intervention options to the patient, but leaves the patient alone with the treatment decision placing him or her "in an unrealistically autonomous role" (p. 4). In an interpretive model, the physician acts as a counselor providing patients with all relevant medical information and helping to elucidate and articulate their values to determine medical interventions that will best realize those values. The physician in this model concerns himself or herself with more than just the patient's health-related values, but also with the patient's aspirations and commitments. In a deliberative model, the physician acts as a friend or teacher focusing on certain health-related values and engaging in moral deliberation with the patient to determine medical interventions that will best fit the patient's overall medical condition. In this model, the focus on only health-related values leads to other values that are also important to the decision making process being discounted.

Although Emanuel and Emanuel considered the deliberative model to be the ideal physician–patient relationship, they rightly argued that different physician–patient relationship models may work under different clinical circumstances. While some patients and cultural groups may prefer a paternalistic physician–patient relationship, others do better with the informative model. For example, in a population-based study, Levinson, Kao, Kuby, and Thisted (2004) found wide variation among people's preferences regarding participation in clinical decision making – e.g., reliance on physician for information about their condition, leaving final treatment decisions up to the physician. Consequently, the authors concluded that physicians and health care organizations should "assess individual patient preferences and tailor care accordingly" (p. 531). Similarly, given the variety of patient preferences in treatment decisions in terms of deferring decision to physicians, discussing treatment options with family members, Clarke, Hall, and Rosencrance (2004) advocated against any single model of physician–patient interaction, and urged physicians simply to ask patients about their preferred mode of interaction for medical information and decision-making.

Physician–patient Communication

For over 30 years, physician–patient communication has been a focal area of research in the field of health communication, and the medical, nursing, and allied health disciplines (for reviews, see Ong *et al.*, 1995; Rao *et al.*, 2007; Rorter, Hall, and Katz, 1988). Studies (Beckman and Frankel, 1984; Marvel, Epstein, Flowers, and Beckman, 1999) revealed that, on average, just 18 to 30 seconds into medical interviews, physicians interrupted patients, and only a small percentage of patients were allowed to complete their initial descriptions of their concerns. Studies also reveal that effective physician–patient communication can result in an improvement in patient safety, adherence to treatment, and health outcomes, reduced medical malpractice costs, and greater job satisfaction for physicians – indeed, that it can increase patient satisfaction across the continuum of healthcare (Brown, Stewart, and Ryan, 2003). Hence, communication is a key aspect in the physician–patient relationship because it allows the creation and preservation of good interpersonal relationships, exchange of information, and shared medical decision making (Ong *et al.*, 1995). Although the physician–patient relationship is an important determinant of quality health care, and this relationship is built on "trust" and "empathy," which comes from effective communication and interaction between doctors and patients (Berry, 2007), from an ecological perspective, physician–patient relationships are impacted by the organizational, media, political-legal, and cultural contexts within which they take place (Street, 2003).

With regard to the communication dynamics of physicians and patients, Cegala, Street, and Clinch (2007) underscored patients' communicative participation in a primary care medical interview and found that their style of participation greatly influenced the extent and type of information physicians provided. During medical encounters, physicians and patients mutually influence each other (Makoul, 1998). Highlighting the importance of examining physician and patient roles in empathic communication during medical encounters, Bylund and Makoul (2005) argued that patients who create positive empathic opportunities may elicit more empathic responses from physicians.

Patient–provider Communication

Patient–provider communication across the continuum of healthcare is an important and complex aspect of interpersonal health communication. The patient–provider relationship becomes more complex, however, when "the healthcare provider, rather than the patient, is the more powerful actor in clinical encounters" (Smedley, Stith, and Nelson, 2002, p. 12). Patients in a clinic often expect physicians to follow the biomedical approach and focus on diagnosis and treatment (Lebel, 2003). Providers' beliefs, attitudes, behaviors, and expectations are likely to be reinforced in a medical encounter when particular patient groups assume the role of obeying and cooperating with the providers. As Kim and colleagues' (2000) study found, Chinese patients were less willing to actively participate in medical encounters than their American counterparts.

Growing ethnic-minority population groups bring unique needs to health care interactions that may result from cultural differences between care provider and receiver (Berger, 1998; Betancourt, 2003, 2004). Sparks and Villagran (2010) identified certain cultural factors such as differences in patient–provider communication as consequences of patients' racial and ethnic backgrounds, language barriers, fatalistic beliefs about illness and disease, gender-based roles, and power differences between patients and providers, that affect patient–provider communication. These cultural differences between patients and providers pose further barriers to optimum health and health care delivery.

Cline and McKenzie (1998) moved beyond overt cultural categorization to also include covert personal attributes that place health care providers and receivers at two different ends of the health care spectrum. Differences in cultural values and beliefs between the health care provider and the receiver account for many misunderstandings in health interactions (Cline and McKenzie, 1998). When such differences are not accommodated, poor health outcomes arise.

Thus, provider–patient communication is an important component relating to racial/ethnic health disparities (Cegala and Post, 2006). Patient communication skills training helps promote patient participation in medical interviews, which, in turn, helps promote important health outcomes such as patient adherence. Cegala and Post argued for concerted efforts to determine ways to improve the effectiveness of patient communication interventions with racial and ethnic minorities because such interventions "for both patients and clinicians can enhance patient-centered care and have the potential to reduce racial and ethnic health care inequities" (p. 863).

Murphy and Gryboski (2005) underscored a strong relationship between the quality of client-provider interactions through courtesy and responsiveness to clients' needs and the adoption, effective use, and continuation of modern family planning methods, as well as client satisfaction.

Outcome of physician–patient communication

Scholars should take an interpersonal communication perspective to understanding the key factors that influence physician–patient interactions and their outcomes. Brown, Stewart, and Ryan (2003) indicated that various dimensions of patient–provider interaction impact patient satisfaction, adherence to treatment regimens, and health outcomes. The findings from various researches should "inform curriculum development at the undergraduate, postgraduate, and continuing educational levels, allowing clinician skills and attributions to be backed by strong evidence" (p. 154).

Perloff *et al.* (2006) argued that culturally sensitive doctor–patient communication has important implications for health care outcomes.

Communication with vulnerable patient populations

Nussbaum, Ragan, and Whaley (2003) identified children, the elderly, and women, as three underrepresented populations in the context of health communication research, especially as regards provider–patient interactions. Family members are often the major decision makers for pediatric, elderly, and incapacitated patients, thus these communicative dynamics are important for relationship building, reducing fear, and enhancing trust in provider–patient interactions (Berry 2007; Pagano, 2010). Drawing on a study of eight hospitals from across the United States that had demonstrated a commitment to providing patient-centered communication with culturally and linguistically diverse patient populations, Wynia and Matiasek (2006) listed promising practices including "having passionate champions to advocate for communication programs; collecting information on patient needs; engaging communities; developing a diverse and skilled workforce; involving patients; spreading awareness of cultural diversity; providing effective language assistance services; addressing low health literacy; and tracking performance over time." (p. v).

Patient-centered communication

Patient-centered communication (PCC) – focused on patients' needs, values, and wishes – is considered as essential for quality health care (Committee on Quality Health Care in America, 2001; Epstein, Franks, Fiscella, Shields, Meldrum, Kravitz, and Duberstein, 2005; Epstein, Mauksch, Carroll, and Jaén, 2008; Mead and Bower, 2000). Although improvement in patient adherence, trust, and satisfaction are associated with PCC (Mead and Bower, 2000; Fiscella, Meldrum, Franks, *et al.*, 2004), gaps exist in understanding PCC and problems exist in measuring it (Epstein *et al.*, 2005). Although many scholars treat "patient-centeredness," "patient-centered care," and "PCC" synonymously, these three constructs are not the same. For example, focusing on patient–physician interactions, Epstein *et al.* (2005) offered an operational definition of PCC that includes the patient's perspective, the psychosocial context, shared understanding, and sharing power and responsibility.

Although PCC advances patient-centeredness, the complexity of the multifaceted construct of PCC is further complicated by a lack of agreement about the definition of patient-centeredness (Mead and Bower, 2000; Epstein *et al.*, 2005). For example, patient-centeredness and cultural competence are two fundamental approaches to improving the quality of health care. Exploring the historical evolution of these concepts, Beach, Saha, and Cooper (2006) presented and compared various models of patient-centeredness and cultural competence at both the interpersonal and health care system levels. The authors explained that, although patient-centeredness (e.g., "broadly focused on the specific needs of people") and cultural competence (e.g., "historically focused on the specific needs of people and communities of color") are distinct approaches to improve the quality of health care, they "may look fairly similar in practice" (p. 13).

However, in their study of the relationship between patients' ethnocentric views (the assumption that one's group is superior to other groups) and their perceptions of physicians' cultural competence in health care interactions, Ahmed and Bates (2010) found that patients did not experience patient-centeredness and cultural competence similarly in practice; rather, depending on their level of ethnocentrism, patients appeared to perceive these care tactics as more or less preferable. Hence, in view of the effort to provide patient-centered care and to value communicating effectively with patients (Epstein *et al.*, 2008), because patients' active participation during medical interviews influences physicians' use of a patient-centered style of communication (Cegala and Post, 2009), PCC is not a unified construct, but a "multifaceted construct, the components of which each advances the values of patient-centeredness in a different way" (Epstein *et al.*, 2005, p. 1525).

Provider–patient communication skills training

Effective communication between health care providers and patients can be beneficial for all the parties involved in the health care process. Communicative skill development is an important area of focus in health communication. Cegala and Broz (2003) provided reviews of existing research into communication skills of providers and patient communication skills training. Given the dyadic nature of the medical encounter, it is of the utmost importance that clear and credible health information is accessible to everyone. Accordingly, Cegala and Broz not only emphasized the need for health care professionals to be trained to deliver health services to health care receivers as effectively and humanely as possible, but also advocated patient communication skills training. As Berry (2007) noted, "most complaints about doctors concern poor communication and failure to listen, rather than competence or more technical aspects of consultations" (p. 112). Human communication is the primary tool for delivering health care services to people, and research shows that communication between health care providers and receivers needs improvement.

Terry (2000) studied how physicians could educate patients so as to help improve patient satisfaction with care and patients' experience of physician–patient communication. He found an increase in satisfaction with care for patients who received self-care information from their physicians as compared to patients who did not receive such information. Although health care provider training in communication skills has long received attention in scholarly efforts (Thompson and Parrott, 2002), it is only recently that communication skills training for patients has been developed (Cegala *et al.*, 2000; Cegala and Broz, 2003; Cegala *et al.*, 2004). Cegala *et al.* (2000) found that patient-centered communication is more often present in the medical encounter when the patient has received skills training than when the patient did not receive such training. These encounters also show a more active role played by the patient in information seeking and giving. Cegala and Broz (2003) argued that when both the provider and the patient receive communication skills training there is a strongly positive effect on both interactants.

Family communication and health

Communicating about health within families can take various forms from initial disclosure of health information or illness (Smith *et al.*, 2004) to social support for the patient and the patient's family (Mallinger, Griggs, and Shields, 2006). Although most patients are likely to communicate with family members about their health and the provider's findings, recommendations, and decision making, families have their own unique attributes and communication styles: for example, some families like to share everything, while the members of some families want their independence.

Given the high concordance of health behaviors within families (Kristeller *et al.*, 1996), "open communication is likely to be of particular importance in the family setting, as the family is frequently a primary source of support" (Mallinger, Griggs, and Shields, 2006, p. 355). Efforts to enhance productive communication between patients and their family members may help women cope with and overcome the challenges of breast cancer survivorship.

Harris *et al.* (2009) highlighted the importance of understanding the complex process of family communication during the cancer experience in order to improve communication processes within the family, supporting families as caregivers, and improving patient outcomes. Conversely, Zhang and Siminoff (2003) found that growing patient–caregiver discord about care and treatment resulting from increasing stress of late-stage cancer led to avoidance of family communication. It was further revealed that lack of family communication was contingent upon the difficult subject matter inherent in late-stage cancer. This study underscores the importance of studying specific illness conditions that impact family communication patterns to identify ways to improve patient–caregiver communication for appropriate care for patients.

In light of the importance of family discussion as an important communication process in increasing the rates of family consent regarding organ donation, Smith *et al.* (2004) examined the relationship between willingness to communicate with family about organ donation and other variables associated with organ donation. The findings revealed that being willing to communicate about organ donation with one's family is related to prior thought and intent to sign an organ donor card, to perceiving organ donation messages as credible, and to feeling relatively low anxiety after reading organ donation messages.

Morgan and Miller (2001) examined the effect of knowledge, attitudes, and values on willingness to communicate about organ donation to family members. They found that the quality of discussions between the potential donor and his/her family depends on how well the donor is able to address vital issues regarding donation.

Polk (2005) studied the role of communication in family caregiving for patients with Alzheimer's Dementia (AD). Interview findings revealed that caregivers were more confident in their ability to make attributions regarding their loved ones' pleasurable as opposed to their nonpleasurable experiences. Because caregivers were uncertain about the extent to which loved ones' behaviors were dictated by AD, they tended to lose patience, get frustrated, and then feel bad because of responding negatively; they used humor as a coping mechanism to connect to loved ones. Caregivers used knowledge of loved ones and resources such as books, support groups, online resources, and distractions (caregiver-initiated activities) to manage uncertainty and increase confidence in their attributions resulting from communicative interactions. This study underscores the importance of looking at family caregiver stress and alleviating those stressors to enhance the caregiver relationship and ensure that patients receive proper care.

Interpersonal health communication and culture

Health and healing are constructed and reproduced in different cultural contexts. Case studies of cultural difficulty in health communication demonstrate that cultural difference includes factors beyond speaking different languages. Geist-Martin, Ray, and Sharf (2003), for example, used narratives from different cultural perspectives to reflect the complexities of health communication and to demonstrate that the cultural complexities of communicating health must go beyond finding translatable words for meaning to be shared. Using HIV/AIDS as a case study, they described five layers of meanings in physician–patient communication to provide "insight regarding the complex and multiple meanings that people bring to their relationships and to their conversations about AIDS" (p. 72). Because there may be differences in ideological, sociopolitical, institutional/professional, ethnocultural/familial, and interpersonal layers of meaning, accounting for semantic meaning is not enough.

Herselman (1996) argued that accuracy in doctor–patient communication is often challenged in a multicultural clinical context. By looking at the communication process between a group of Xhosa-speaking patients and their western medical practitioners in South Africa, Herselman identified barriers to effective communication in a multicultural clinical setting. These barriers included, sociocultural differences between doctor and patient (e.g., class, status, roles, perceptions of health and illness), language difficulty, defensiveness among patients (e.g., patients' discomfort in the clinical setting), psychosocial factors (e.g., politeness and submissiveness of Xhosa-speaking people), and the doctor–patient relationship (e.g., discernible racial and associated political differences between doctors and patients). Herselman concluded that both doctors and patients have a role in increasing communication efficacy in multicultural health care contexts.

In a qualitative study that gathered information from focus group discussions and in-depth qualitative interviews of rural Kenyan men and women, Muturi (2005) examined the social–cultural factors that influence Kenyan people's sexual behavior and practices. She highlighted the discrepancy between awareness and behavioral change among people of reproductive age. The study focused on rural women who suffer the most from reproductive illness. The role of men is also taken into account as they play important roles in reproductive health issues. Muturi drew from the theoretical framework of Grunig's model of excellence in communication that emphasizes understanding and relationship building between programs and their audiences. The findings of the study showed that lack of understanding of communicative messages among rural Kenyans overrides their awareness of sexually transmitted diseases, including HIV/AIDS. The author argued that cultural beliefs, values, and norms affect people's reproductive health decisions. Unfortunately, these sociocultural factors, however, had not been addressed by reproductive health communication programs. The author concluded that building a relationship between communicators and target audience through dialogues and two-way symmetrical communication is essential for HIV/AIDS health communication programs.

Naploes-Springer and colleagues (2005) identified key domains of cultural competence from the perspective of African-Americans, Latinos, and non-Latino Whites. The cultural factors that influenced the quality of medical encounters of these ethnically and linguistically diverse patients included sensitivity to complementary/alternative medicine, health insurance-based discrimination, social class-based discrimination, ethnic concordance of physician and patient, age-based discrimination, physicians' acceptance of the role of spirituality, family, and ethnicity-based discrimination, language issues, and immigration status.

Social support and health

Social interactions play an important role in the health and illness of individuals. Albrecht and Goldsmith (2003) reviewed existing literature dealing with the impact of supportive communication on health and illness. More specifically, the authors briefly traced the history of the conceptual foundations of social support as communication and provided a summary of research on social support and social networks and their impact on individual's health and illness. According to Albrecht and Adelman (1987), "social support is a communication process where the recipient and the provider mutually influence each other to reduce uncertainty about the situation, themselves, each other, and the relationship" (p. 38). Albrecht and Goldsmith also highlighted ethical considerations in supportive communication for health and healing. The prevalence of new technologies such as the Internet offers many alternative ways of providing/receiving social support in face-to-face interaction. However, Albrecht and Goldsmith cautioned that "computer mediated support groups may suffer from unregulated negative or critical messages, provide inaccurate information, and decrease involvement in more multiplex face-to-face relationships" (p. 276).

Existing literature documents the physical and psychological benefits of receiving social support. In health settings, providing/receiving social support is an indispensable component of communication. Apker and Ray (2003) brought to our attention the communicative processes of stress, burn-out, and social support in efforts to provide an understanding of health care organizations and their members. More specifically, the authors examined the impact of social support on job stress in health care organizations and found that "healthcare work is inherently stressful" (p. 348). They discussed issues of managed care, role changes, emotional labor, and home/work conflict as sources of job stress for health care professionals.

DiMatteo (2004) conducted a meta-analysis of empirical research from 1948 to 2001 on the association of social support and patient adherence to medical regimens, and underscored the importance of social support to the enhancement of adherence.

Telemedicine

Although basic persuasion strategies such as advertising and information campaigns are pertinent to health communication through the mass media, "the recent proliferation of new communication technologies ... has the potential to revolutionize health campaigns" (Salmon and Atkin, 2003, p. 468). For example, the Internet plays an important role in providing increasing information regarding different aspects of prevention, health promotion, and treatment for patients, their families, and health care providers. Turner (2003) provided a review of telemedicine in the context of the clinical practice of patient care. By defining telemedicine, documenting its history, and discussing the barriers to its implementation and applications, she underscored telemedicine as a means of bridging gaps in health care access.

Albrecht and Goldsmith (2003) highlighted ethical considerations in supportive communication for health and healing. The prevalence of new technologies such as the Internet offers many alternative ways of providing/receiving social support to face-to-face interaction. However, Albrecht and Goldsmith (2003) cautioned that "computer mediated support groups may suffer from unregulated negative or critical messages, provide inaccurate information, and decrease involvement in more multiplex face-to-face relationships" (p. 276).

Cases of Interpersonal Communication in Health Promotion and Planning

In this section, four case studies are discussed using an ecological perspective to illustrate innovative lines of research and programmatic experiences related to the role of interpersonal communication in health promotion and planning in developing countries.

Operation Lighthouse

Operation Lighthouse (OPL) was a five-year (2001–2005) HIV/AIDS/STI intervention program in India, funded by the US Agency for International Development (USAID) and implemented by the Population Services International (PSI). This comprehensive program adopted various integrated approaches, including interpersonal and mass media communication, advocacy, and service provision strategies that targeted HIV/AIDS high risk groups in 12 major port communities across India (PSI, 2004a, 2005). According to 2006 estimates, India has 2 million to 3.1 million people living with HIV infection (WHO, 2007a). India is home to the third largest population of HIV-infected individuals in the world (UNICEF, n.d.). The prevalence of HIV infection in the country is higher among vulnerable groups, including people who inject drugs, truckers, migrant laborers, commercial sex workers, and men who have sex with men (PSI, 2004a; WHO, 2007a). While 85.6 percent of HIV infections in India occur through sexual transmission (UNICEF, n.d.), open discussion about sex, safer sex practices, and HIV/AIDS still remains taboo (PSI, 2004a). Hence, the high risk of HIV acquisition among vulnerable groups in the absence of accurate knowledge and awareness about HIV/AIDS/STI.

Against this backdrop, Operation Lighthouse developed intensive interpersonal communication (IPC) interventions to decrease the spread of the HIV/AIDS epidemic among vulnerable groups. OPL focused on four desired behavior change outcomes: reducing the number of nonregular sex partners; increasing condom use with nonregular sex partners; increasing the treatment of sexually transmitted infections (STIs); and increasing the use of Voluntary Counseling and Testing (VCT) services (PSI, 2004a). In order to motivate hard-to-reach high-risk groups to adopt preventive behavior, trained OPL interpersonal communicators conducted one-to-one and one-to-group IPC sessions by engaging groups in discussions and activities to help address barriers to healthy behavior, focus on increasing risk perceptions, and improve skills and self-efficacy (PSI, 2004a, 2005). In addition to inspiring positive behavior change, OPL combined the powerful tool of IPC with complementary targeted mass media campaigns – TV and radio messaging, newspaper coverage, street theater, posters, billboards – and service promotion to persuade individuals to go for VCT and to seek STI treatment in order to bring about HIV/AIDS preventive behavior change among high-risk men (PSI, 2004a, 2005).

Considering the geographic, cultural, and linguistic diversity of India, Operation Lighthouse built a series of formative assessments, as well as continual qualitative and quantitative assessments, monitoring, and evaluation into their program design. The aim was to find out barriers to safer sexual behavior, develop appropriate and innovative messages, track exposure, attitudes, and behaviors, and to fine-tune and scale up HIV/AIDS interventions among high risk groups (PSI, 2004a, 2005). Thus, from an ecological perspective, Operation Lighthouse tailored its HIV/AIDS/STI intervention strategies to suit particular behaviors and population groups in the Indian context, for example, by successfully commencing targeted communication activities in 12 major port communities, increasing condom access in areas of high-risk behavior, creating mobile or conveniently located VCT facilities for vulnerable populations, and developing and disseminating mass media campaigns targeted at men in Mumbai, which has a high concentration of HIV/AIDS (PSI, 2003). According to data between 2002 and 2004, OPL's intensive IPC interventions coupled with mass media campaigns and health care service promotion produced improvements in attitudes and knowledge about HIV/AIDS, and increased personal risk perception among high risk men (PSI, 2005).

Nigeria's "Make We Talk" program

The Promoting Sexual and Reproductive Health and HIV/AIDS Reduction (PSRHH) program in Nigeria, also known as "Make We Talk," was a was a seven-year HIV/AIDS/STI intervention program that began in 2002 in Nigeria. "Make We Talk" was developed and implemented through collaboration between the United Kingdom's Department for International Development (DFID), the Society for Family Health (SFH), ActionAid International Nigeria (AAIN), and Population Services International (PSI) (AIDSMark, n.d.; PSI, 2004b; SFH, n.d.).

The most populous country in sub-Saharan Africa, Nigeria has the largest number of people living with HIV/AIDS in Africa (UNAIDS, 201; USAID, 2010). According to 2007 estimates, 2,980,000 people in Nigeria are living with HIV/AIDS (USAID, 2010). Although significant regional and gender variations in HIV prevalence exist, especially with most-at-risk populations being disproportionately affected, including female sex workers, men who have sex with men, injecting drug users, and brothel-based sex workers (USAID, 2010), HIV is firmly established in the Nigerian general population on account of risky behaviors being practiced in a fair number of communities and spots throughout the country putting sub-populations at higher risk of infection (SFH, n.d.).

Against such a backdrop, "Make We Talk" developed a sustainable behavior change model that integrated interpersonal outreach with participatory, rights-based community work and mass media to optimize HIV/AIDS prevention activities (AIDSMark, n.d.; PSI, 2004b). The program worked with civil society, community-based and faith-based organizations, and peer educators to help increase knowledge and awareness of ways to prevent HIV infection and adopt safer sexual and reproductive health practices among key target populations, including female sex workers, male and female youths, uniformed service men, and transport workers (SFH, n.d.).

In phases, "Make We Talk" implemented diverse and participatory IPC activities in pilot and control intervention sites the success of which provided the rationale to scale-up successful interventions into additional sites (PSI, 2004b).

Peer education activities were at the core of IPC efforts to facilitate behavior change among key target populations. Carefully selected peer educators – youth, sex workers, and other groups throughout Nigeria – were trained to communicate clearly and persuasively with fellow peers, exercise good interpersonal skills, be nonjudgmental and respectful to peers and persons living with HIV and AIDS, and conduct parent–child communication workshops (SFH, n.d.). The PSRHH interventions employed the Peer Education Plus (PEP) model which centered on peer education, but integrated community-based organizations and engagement with influencers (e.g., people who are not members of a given high-risk group, but may have close associations or regular contact with target groups in work or social settings) into a single unified program to cater to different communities to ensure positive behavior change (SFH, n.d.).

From an ecological perspective, "Make We Talk" adopted a comprehensive approach to designing and implementing interventions that engaged different community target groups to meet, discuss, and carry out activities, more particularly IPC interactions to create an enabling environment for behavior change. "Make We Talk" has been implemented in over 400 communities throughout Nigeria. Some of its notable achievements include:

- Reduction in indiscriminate sex;
- Use of condom for safe sex;
- Voluntary counseling and testing of HIV/AIDs test (SFH, n.d.).

The *Know Yourself* adolescent reproductive health communication program

The Bangladesh Center for Communication Programs (BCCP) has come forward with behavior change communication programs that involve a combination of individual, interpersonal, mass media, and community-based approaches, to educate the public about significant health issues. *Know Yourself* is an adolescent reproductive health (ARH) communication program to promote adolescent reproductive health in Bangladesh. Although adolescents form a significant part of the Bangladesh population, their reproductive health needs are often compromised partly because of the social and cultural norms and values that restrict open discussion regarding reproductive health issues and because of the lack of awareness about adolescents' need for reproductive health services (BCCP, 2005a, 2005b, 2006). This lack of adequate ARH care is a growing concern in Bangladesh, especially when the country's adolescent population (aged 15–24) is projected to reach an estimated 35 million in 2020 from about 28 million in 2000 (Barkat and Majid, 2003). Due to their unmet needs for reproductive health information and services, adolescents in Bangladesh remain susceptible to various reproductive health problems (Barkat and Majid, 2003; BCCP, 2005a, 2005b).

Against such a backdrop, with guidance from a national ARH Working Group, technical assistance from the Johns Hopkins Bloomberg School of Public Health/Center for Communication Programs (CCP) under the Health Communication Partnership (HCP), and funding from the United States Agency for International Development (USAID), BCCP developed the *Know Yourself* ARH program (2002 –2007) to give adolescents in Bangladesh the information and skills necessary to help them engage in positive reproductive health behaviors (BCCP, 2004, 2005a, 2005b, 2006). The program involved an integrated approach to promoting ARH developed through extensive formative research conducted with adolescents, parents, teachers, service providers, community members, researchers, writers, media personnel, programmers, and trainers, ensuring a participatory process at all stages from program design and materials development to pre-testing and production (BCCP, 2005a, 2005b, 2006). Utilizing multiple channels and approaches, such as mass media, community participation through NGOs and youth groups, and interpersonal communication and counseling with service providers, the program aimed at creating an open environment to dialogue about ARH issues and foster positive health-seeking behavior (BCCP, 2005a, 2006). As part of the larger *Know Yourself* ARH program, the *Nijeke Jano* or *Know Yourself* toolkit consisted of innovative multimedia, interactive methods including a series of four educational and entertaining videos, four corresponding facilitator's guides, question and answer booklets, and comic books related to reproductive health issues. The aim was to encourage adolescents to seek more information and discuss health issues including puberty, sexuality, unwanted pregnancy, HIV/AIDS, STIs, and marriage and family health.

Information regarding ARH is quite often fraught with deeply held cultural beliefs about sex, parenting, and the gender and sexual roles ascribed to males and females. In view of the strong presence and important role of family structure in the lives of adolescents in Bangladesh, yet the lack of family communication about reproductive health issues, the emphasis was placed on interpersonal communication about reproductive health issues with parents or older family members (BCCP, 2006). The *Know Yourself* toolkit also facilitated interpersonal communication with peers about reproductive health issues, given that adolescents are more likely to discuss RH issues with peer groups, and thus trained peer educators on RH issues (BCCP, 2006; Bhuiya *et al.*, 2004). In 2004, BCCP's *Know Yourself* received a global media award for best combined media effort (Shahjahan, Khan, and Haque, 2005). Periodic assessments provided considerable evidence that the *Know Yourself* program increased adolescent knowledge and stimulated parent–adolescent communication about reproductive health issues in Bangladesh (BCCP, 2004, 2005a, 2005b, 2006).

Thus, from an ecological perspective, the *Know Yourself* toolkit employed a range of culturally sensitive strategies to address underlying beliefs that may manifest as barriers to communicate about reproductive health issues.

The Hazipur eHealth Center

The Hazipur eHealth Centre is an initiative to grant people in Hazipur village in the District of Magura, Bangladesh, access to easy and effective health care services from their own location via information and communication technologies (ICTs), such as computers, the Internet, and mobile phones. Against the backdrop of a remote and resource-poor environment, the Hazipur eHealth Centre coordinates technology-enabled interpersonal interactions between a team of health care professionals, including paramedic staff, medical doctors and specialists, and patients to improve health care for rural populations.

Bangladesh is one of the most crowded and poorest countries in the world. It has a total population of 162,221,000 (WHO, 2011), 40 percent of whom are living below the poverty line (CIA, 2010). In recent times Bangladesh has experienced steady improvement in the health status of its population, particularly progress in reducing infant, maternal, and under-five mortality rates and increasing life expectancy at birth; yet, this progress is often uneven and health inequalities are present between different social groups and geographical regions (WHO, 2007b).

Although the health care system in Bangladesh consists of a variety of public and private sector initiatives, there is striking imbalance between rural and urban distribution of health care professionals (Werner, 2009; WHO Bangladesh, 2010; World Bank, 2005). Additionally, utilization of available services by rural people is comparatively low because of financial constraints, poor transport facilities, infrastructural inadequacies, social distance between client and provider, quality of health care services, and gender sensitivity (Ahmed *et al.*, 2006; Hossen and Westhues, 2010, 2011; Werner, 2009). As a result, many people resort to traditional healers, homeopathic practitioners, village doctors, and paramedical personnel to seek immediate medical help (Rashid, Akrarn, and Standing, 2011).

As a case in point, the situation in Hazipur village is no exception. Local people rely heavily on village doctors for their general health care. Only a handful of villagers can actually visit the district health complex or private medical practitioner, and most other patients:

* Have to depend on village doctors for a long time at the cost of aggravating their illness;
* End up wasting time and paying lots of money because of lack of knowledge about appropriate medical specialists in the capital city Dhaka;
* Have less access to the district health complex or a private medical practitioner owing to transportation and attendant problem (this applies especially to female patients);
* Discontinue medicine because of cost (Ahmed, Islam, and Khan, 2009).

Against this backdrop, the Hazipur eHealth Center was established. One local trained paramedic is on duty there for three days a week. The paramedic electronically records patient case history and, in case of emergency, discusses the case with the medical doctor in Magura by sharing patient data by email or waiting for the doctor's arrival in the village. Once a week, the medical doctor from Magura examines and treats patients at the eHealth Center. The organized case history helps the doctor communicate more easily with patients. In case of emergency, the medical doctor prescribes patients clinical tests and the e-Health Center sends the test reports electronically to the specialist doctor in Dhaka. From their own location, village patients can get medical suggestions from the specialist in Dhaka via teleconference or videoconference. In some instances, depending on the patient's condition, further tests and examinations may be required, and the patient may be recommended to visit the specialist in Dhaka (Ahmed, Islam, and Khan, 2009). Thus, by reducing costs for patients, these technology-enabled services help make health care possible and affordable to poor villagers in Hazipur. The eHealth Centre also facilitates technology-enabled interpersonal interactions between patients and a team of health care professionals to help build an inclusive health care system deemed necessary for improving health care for rural populations.

From an ecological perspective, the Hazipur eHealth Center illustrates how interpersonal interactions between a team of health care professionals and patients that occur within a media context, and are facilitated by ICTs, can reinforce the United Nations Foundations' recognition of the potential of ICTs and mobile communications to improve healthcare services even in some of the most remote and resource-poor environments (Vital Wave Consulting, 2009).

Conclusions

From an ecological perspective, the case studies discussed above identified and considered the social factors that influence health beliefs, attitude, behavior, and even outcomes at the individual, family, community, and policy levels, in planning the communication initiatives and interventions (Waisbord, 2005). While Airhihenbuwa and Obregon

(2000) argued that, "decisions about preventing HIV/AIDS are based on cultural norms that often mediate individual decisions in ways that individuals may not always realize" and that those decisions "are based on emotion and thus may not follow any pre-established pattern of decision making advanced in most of the theories and models" (p. 12), the same argument holds true for interpersonal health communication issues. Rahima's story at the beginning of this chapter is a case in point. Rahima's apparent nonadherence to proper medical treatment and reliance on an unlicensed health provider is influenced by multiple factors at the individual (e.g., unawareness of the severity of the condition, level of education, motivation, socioeconomic status), social (e.g., family influence, cultural background, access to social support networks), physical (e.g., geography, accommodation, public transport), and policy (e.g., workplace policies, health policies) levels. Thus, from an ecological perspective, efforts to change Rahima's health behavior should be designed based on an understanding of the interrelationships between herself and her social contexts.

Indeed, effective communication is one of the most crucial considerations in the health care context. Too often the problem is not just health-related, but communication-related. A while back Thompson (1994) highlighted a "lack of time spent on communication in health care encounters as well as lack of emphasis on relational factors during this communication" (p. 715).

Still, in the current literature there is less focus on the health care provider and patient dyads and communication patterns, and more focus on outcome. However, in the context of interpersonal health communication in global contexts with an emphasis on developing countries, the problem is more complex. The health gap between the rich and the poor across developing countries highlights the importance of social determinants of health, identified as income and social status, social support networks, education, employment and working conditions, social and physical environments, biology and genetic endowment, personal health practices and coping skills, healthy child development, health services, gender, and culture (National Collaborating Centers for Public Health, 2008; WHO Commission on Social Determinants of Health, 2007). These social determinants of health affect all aspects of one's development and impact one's ability to achieve optimum health potential in myriad ways.

These unique challenges make interpersonal health communication in global contexts a rich and interesting area that needs more exploration – an understanding of medical interaction from the interpersonal communication perspective and its contextualization in larger social contexts. A future research agenda in this area begs greater integration of an ecological perspective and the various topic areas discussed in this chapter. For example, with the rapid development of information and communication technologies, new opportunities are arising to the delivery of health services in developing countries (Epstein and Vernaci, 1998), and as "telemedicine applications develop, so do opportunities for communication research" (Turner (2003, p. 527). According to Turner, "The very practice of telemedicine makes the communication between health care providers and their patients problematic" (p. 532). Yet, most of the telemedicine research literature has focused on the technological ability to the exclusion of the shifting communicative context, the interpersonal dynamics among telemedicine participants. Accordingly, among other aspects, future research in interpersonal health communication can look into questions as to the effects of telemedicine on provider–patient communication; the building of rapport; whether people are likely to agree to the treatment; the communication strategies that need to be used to overcome communication barriers; and the implications of service quality for health behavior.

References

Ahmed, N. U., Alam, M. M., Sultana, F. *et al.* (2006). Reaching the unreachable: Barriers of the poorest to accessing NGO healthcare services in Bangladesh. *Journal of Health, Population and Nutrition, 24*(4), 456–466.

Ahmed, R. and Bates, B. R. (2007). Patient gender differences in patients' perceptions of physicians' cultural competence in health care interactions. *Women's Health and Urban Life: An International and Interdisciplinary Journal, VI*(2), 58–80.

Ahmed, R. and Bates, B. R. (2010). Patients' ethnocentric views and patients' perceptions of physicians' cultural competence in health care interactions. *Intercultural Communication Studies, 19*(2), 111–127.

Ahmed, R., Islam, D., and Khan, Z. H. (2009, October). A case study of the Hazipur eHealth-mHealth System: A developing country perspective. Poster presented at the 16th Canadian Conference on International Health, Ottawa, ON, Canada, Crowne Plaza Hotel.

AIDSMark (n. d.). Case study: Nigeria's "Make We Talk" program. Retrieved March 25, 2011, from http://www.aidsmark.org/ipc_en/nigeria.html

Airhihenbuwa, C. O., Makinwa, B., and Obregon, R. (2000).Toward a new communication framework for HIV/AIDS. *Journal of Health Communication, 5* (supplement), 101–111.

Albrecht, T. L., and Adelman, M. B. (1987). *Communicating Social Support.* Newbury Park, CA: Sage Publications.

Albrecht, T. L., and Goldsmith, D. J. (2003). Social support, social networks, and health. In T. L. Thompson, A. M. Dorsey, K. I. Miller, and R. Parrott (Eds.), *Handbook of Health Communication* (pp. 263–284). Mahwah, NJ: Lawrence Erlbaum Associates.

Apker, J., and Ray, E.B. (2003). Stress and social support in health care organizations. In T. L. Thomson, A. M. Dorsely, K. I. Miller, and R. Parrott (Eds.), *Handbook of Health Communication* (pp. 347–368). Mahwah, NJ: Lawrence Erlbaum Associates.

Arrington, M. I. (2010). Theorizing about social support and health communication in a prostate cancer support group. *Journal of Psychosocial Oncology, 28*(3), 260–268.

Babrow, A. S. (1992). Communication and problematic integration: Understanding diverging probability and value, ambiguity, ambivalence, and impossibility. *Communication Theory, 2*(2), 95–130.

Babrow, A. S., and Mattson, M. (2003). Theorizing about health communication. In T. L. Thomson, A. M. Dorsely, K. I. Miller, and R. Parrott (Eds.), *Handbook of Health Communication* (pp. 35–61). Mahwah, NJ: Lawrence Erlbaum Associates.

Barkat, A. and Majid, M. (2003). *Adolescent Reproductive Health in Bangladesh: Status, Policies, Programs, and Issues.* A policy report for USAID. Retrieved from http://www.policyproject.com/pubs/countryreports/ARH_Bangladesh.pdf

Baxter, L. A., and Braithwaite, D. O. (2008). *Engaging Theories in Interpersonal Communication: Multiple Perspectives.* Thousand Oaks, CA: Sage.

BCCP (Bangladesh Center for Communications Programs) (2004). Annual report, 2003–2004. Dhaka, Bangladesh: BCCP.

BCCP (Bangladesh Center for Communications Programs) (2005a). Focused community assessment of adolescent reproductive health communication program: A baseline survey. Dhaka, Bangladesh: BCCP.

BCCP (Bangladesh Center for Communications Programs) (2005b). Adolescent reproductive health communication: Communication midline assessment 2004. Dhaka, Bangladesh: BCCP.

BCCP (Bangladesh Center for Communications Programs) (2006).Bangladesh ARH focused community assessment final report. Dhaka, Bangladesh: BCCP.

Beach, M. C., Saha, S., and Cooper, L. A. (October 2006). *The Role and Relationship of Cultural Competence and Patient-Centeredness in Health Care Quality*, vol. 36. The Commonwealth Fund. New York, NY.

Beckman, H. B. and Frankel, R. M. (1984). The effect of physician behaviour on the collection of data. *Annals of Internal Medicine, 101*(5), 692–696.

Berger, T. J. (1998). Culture and ethnicity in clinical care. *Archives of Internal medicine, 159* (12), 2085–2090.

Berns, R. M. (2010). *Child, family, school, community: Socialization and support.* Belmont, CA: Wadsworth, Cengage Learning.

Berry, D. (2007). *Health communication: Theory and practice.* New York, NY: Open University Press.

Betancourt, J. R. (2003). Cross-cultural medical education: Conceptual approaches and frameworks for evaluation. *Academic Medicine, 78*(6), 560–569.

Betancourt, J. R. (2004). Becoming a physician: Cultural competence? Marginal or mainstream movement? *The New England Journal of Medicine, 351*, 953–955.

Betancourt, J. R., Carrillo, J. E., and Green, A. R. (1999). Hypertension in multicultural and minority populations: Linking communication to compliance. *Current Hypertension Reports, 1*, 482–488.

Bhuiya, I., Rob, U. Chowdhury, A. H. *et al.* (2004). Improving reproductive health of adolescents in Bangladesh. Dhaka, Bangladesh: Population Council.

Boutin-Foster, C., Foster, J. C., and Konopasek, L. (2008). Viewpoint: Physician know thyself: The professional culture of medicine as a framework for teaching cultural competence. *Academic Medicine, 83*, 106–111.

Braithwaite, D. O., and Baxter, L. A. (2008). Introduction: meta-theory and theory in interpersonal communication research. In L. A. Baxter and D. O. Braithwaite (Eds.), *Engaging theories in interpersonal communication: Multiple perspectives* (pp. 1–18). Thousand Oaks, CA: Sage Publications.

Brashers, D. E. (2001a). Communication and uncertainty management. *Journal of Communication, 51*(3), 477–497.

Brashers, D. E. (2001b). HIV and uncertainty: Managing treatment decision making. *Focus: A Guide to AIDS Research, 16*(9), 5–6.

Brashers, D. E., and Goldsmith, D. J. (Eds.) (2009). *Communicating to Manage Health and Illness.* New York: Routledge.

Brashers, D. E., Goldsmith, D. J., and Hsieh, E. (2002). Information seeking and avoiding in health contexts. *Human Communication Research, 28*(2), 258–271.

Brashers, D. E., Haas, S. M., Klingle, R. S., and Neidig, J. L. (2000). Collective AIDS activism and individual's perceived self-advocacy in physician-patient communication. *Human Communication Research, 26*(3), 372–402.

Brashers, D. E., Hsieh, E., Neidig, J. L., and Reynolds, N. R. (2006). Managing uncertainty about illness: Health care providers as credible authorities. In R. M. Dailey and B. A. Le Poire (Eds.), Applied interpersonal communication matters (pp. 219–240). New York: Peter Lang.

Brashers, D. E., Neidig, J. L., Dobbs, L. K. *et al.* (2001). Transitions and challenges: Revival and uncertainty for persons living with HIV and AIDS. In S.G. Funk, E. M. Tornquist, J. Leeman *et al.* (Eds.), *Key aspects of preventing and managing chronic illness* (pp. 141–160). New York: Springer.

Bronfenbrenner, U. (1977). Toward an experimental ecology of human development. *American Psychology, 32,* 515–531.

Bronfenbrenner, U. (1979). *The ecology of human development: Experiments by nature and design.* Cambridge, MA: Harvard University Press.

Bronfenbrenner, U. (1979). Ecological models of human development. In M. Gauvain and M. Cole (Eds.), *Readings on the Development of Children* (2nd ed.). NY: Freeman.

Brown, J. B., Stewart, M., and Ryan, B. L. (2003). Outcomes of patient–provider interaction. In T. L. Thompson, A. M. Dorsey, K. I. Miller, and R. Parrot (Eds.), *Handbook of Health Communication* (pp. 141–161). London: Lawrence Erlbaum Associates.

Bylund, C. L., and Makoul, G. (2005). Examining empathy in medical encounters: An observational study using the empathic communication coding system. *Health Communication, 18*(2), 123–140.

Byrd, M. E. (2006). Social exchange as a framework for client–nurse interaction during public health nursing maternal-child home visits. *Public Health Nursing 23*(3), 271–276.

Cegala, D. J., and Broz, S. L. (2003). Provider and patient communication skills training. In T. L. Thompson, A. M. Dorsey, K. I. Miller, and R. Parrott (Eds.), *Handbook of Health Communication* (pp. 95–119). Mahwah, NJ: Lawrence Erlbaum Associates.

Cegala, D. J., Gade, C., Broz, S. L., and McClure, L. (2004). Physicians' and patients' perceptions of patients' communication competence in a primary care medical interview. *Health Communication, 16*(3), 289–304.

Cegala, D. J., McClure, L., Marinelli, T. M., and Post, D. M. (2000). The effects of communication skills training on patients' participation during medical interviews. *Patient Education and Counseling, 41,* 209–222.

Cegala, D. J., and Post, D. M. (2006). On addressing racial and ethnic health disparities: The potential role of patient communication skills interventions. *American Behavioral Scientist, 49*(6), 853–867.

Cegala, D. J., and Post, D. M. (2009). The impact of patients' participation on physicians' patient-centered communication. *Patient Education and Counseling, 77*(2), 202–208.

Cegala, D. J., Street, R. L., Jr., and Clinch, C. R. (2007). The impact of patient participation on physicians' information provision during a primary care medical interview. *Health Communication, 21*(2), 177–185.

Cegala, D. J., and Waldron, V. R. (1992). A study of the relationship between communication performance and conversation participants' thoughts. *Communication Studies, 43,* 105–125.

CIA (2011). The World Factbook: Bangladesh population below poverty line. Retrieved from https://www.cia.gov/library/publications/the-world-factbook/fields/2046.html

Clarke, G., Hall, R. T., and Rosencrance, G. (2004). Physician–patient relations: No more models. *The American Journal of Bioethics, 4*(2), W16–W19.

Cline, R. J. (2003). Everyday interpersonal communication and health. In T. L. Thompson, A. M. Dorsey, K. I. Miller, and R. Parrot (Eds.), *Handbook of Health Communication* (pp. 285–311). London: Lawrence Erlbaum Associates.

Cline, R. J., and McKenzie, N. J. (1998). The many cultures of health care: Difference, dominance, and distance in physician–patient communication. In L. D. Jackson and Bernard K. Duffy (Eds.), *Health Communication Research: A Guide to Development and Directions* (pp. 57–74). Westport, CT: Greenwood Press.

Committee on Quality of Health Care in America. (2001). *Crossing the Quality Chasm: A New Health System for the 21st Century.* Washington, DC: National Academies Press.

DiMatteo, M. R. (2004). Social support and patient adherence to medical treatment: A meta-analysis. *Health Psychology, 23*(2), 207–218.

Dutta, M. J. (2008). *Communicating Health: A Culture-Centered Approach.* Cambridge: Polity Press.

Dutta, M., and Zoller, H. (2008). Theoretical foundations: Interpretive, critical and cultural approaches to health communication. In H. Zoller and M. Dutta (Eds.), *Emerging Perspectives in Health Communication: Interpretive, Critical and Cultural Approaches* (pp. 1–27). Mahwah, NJ: Lawrence Erlbaum Associates.

Emanuel, E. J., and Emanuel, L. L. (1992). Four models of the physician–patient relationship. *Journal of the American Medical Association, 267*, 2221–2226.

Epstein, R. M., Franks, P., Fiscella, K. *et al.* (2005). Measuring patient-centered communication in patient–physician consultations: Theoretical and practical issues. *Social Science and Medicine,61*(7), 1516–1528.

Epstein, R. M., Mauksch, L., Carroll, J., and Jaén, C. R. (2008). "Have you really addressed your patient's concerns?" *Family Practice Management, 15*(3), 35–40.

Epstein, D., and Vernaci, R. L. (1998). Telemedicine meets the global village. *Perspectives in Health, 3*(1).

Fiscella, K., Meldrum S., Franks, P. *et al.* (2004). Patient trust: Is it related to patient-centered behavior of primary care physicians? *Medical Care, 42*, 1049–1055.

Frankish J., Lovato C., and Poureslami, I. (2007). Models, theories and principles of health promotion in multicultural populations: Revisiting their use of multicultural populations. In R. Huff and M. Kline (Eds.), *Promoting Health in Multicultural Populations: A Handbook for Practitioners* (2nd ed.) (pp. 57–101). Thousand Oaks, CA: Sage.

Geist-Martin, P., Ray, E. B., and Sharf, B. F. (2003). Understanding health in cultural communities. In P. Geist-Martin, E. B. Ray, and B. F. Sharf (Eds.), *Communicating Health: Personal, Cultural, and Political Complexities* (pp. 54–94). Belmont, CA: Wadsworth/Thomson Learning.

Gillotti, C., Thompson, T. L., and McNeils, K. (2002). Communicative competence in the delivery of bad news. *Social Science and Medicine, 54*(7), 1011–1023.

Gwyn, R. (2002). *Communicating Health and Illness.* London, Thousand Oaks: Sage Publications.

Haider, M., and Rogers, E. M. (2005). Introduction: An overview of health communication – Utility, value, and challenges. In M. Haider (Ed.), *Global public health communication: Challenges, perspectives, and strategies* (pp. xxvii–xxxvii). Sudbury, Massachusetts: Jones and Bartlett Publishers.

Harris, J., Bowen, D. J., Badr, H. *et al.* (2009). Family communication during the cancer experience. *Journal of Health Communication 14*(Supplement 1), 76–84.

Harter, L. M., Japp, P. M., and Beck, C. S. (2005). Vital problematics of narrative theorizing about health and healing. In L. M. Harter, P. M. Japp, and C. S. Beck (Eds.), *Narrative, Health, and Healing: Communication Theory, Research, and Practice* (pp. 7–30). Mahwah, NJ: Lawrence Erlbaum Associates.

Herselman, S. (1996). Some problems in health communication in a multicultural clinical setting: A South African experience. *Health Communication, 8*(2), 153–170.

Hines, S. C., Babrow, A. S., Badzek, L., and Moss, A. (2001). From coping with life to coping with death: Problematic integration for the seriously ill elderly. *Health Communication, 13*(3), 327–342.

Hossen, A. and Westhues, A. (2010). A socially excluded space: Restrictions on access to health care for older women in rural Bangladesh. *Qualitative Health Research, 20*(9), 1192–1201.

Hossen, A. and Westhues, A. (2011). Rural women's access to health care in Bangladesh: Swimming against the tide? Social Work in Public Health. *Social Work in Public Health, 26*(2), 1–16.

Howell-Koren, P. R., and Tinsley, B. J. (1990). The relationships among maternal health beliefs, pediatrician–mother communication, and maternal satisfaction with well-infant care. *Health Communication, 2,* 233–253.

Jackson, L. D., and Duffy, B. K. (Eds). (1998). *Health Communication Research: A Guide to Developments and Directions.* Westport, CT: Greenwood.

Jones. L., Woodhouse, D., and Rowe, J. (2007). Effective nurse–parent communication: A study of parents' perceptions in the NICU environment. *Patient Education and Counseling 69*(1–3), 206–212.

Kim, S., Kingle, R. S., Sharkey, W. F. *et al.* (2000). A test of a cultural model of patients' motivation for verbal communication in patient–doctor interactions. *Communication Monograph, 67,* 262–283.

King, P. E. (1991). Communication, anxiety, and the management of postoperative pain. *Health Communication, 3,* 127–138.

Korsch, B. M., and Negrete, V. (1972). Doctor–patient communication. *Scientific American, 227,* 66–74.

Kreps, G. L. and Thornton, B. C. (1984). *Health Communication: Theory and Practice.* New York, NY: Longman Inc.

Kristeller, J. L., Hebert, J., Edmiston, K. *et al.,* (1996). Attitudes towards risk factor behavior of relatives of cancer patients. *Preventative Medicine, 25,* 162–169.

Lambert, B. L. (1996). Face and politeness in pharmacist–physician interaction. *Social Science and Medicine, 43*(8), 1189–1198.

Langer, N. (1999). Culturally competent professionals in therapeutic alliances enhance patient compliance. *Journal of Health Care for the Poor and Underserved, 10*(1), 19–26.

Lebel, J. (2003). *Health: An Ecosystem Approach.* Ottawa: International Development Research Centre.

Levinson, W., Kao, W., Kuby, A., and Thisted, R. A. (2005). Not all patients want to participate in decision making: A national study of public preferences. *Journal of General Internal Medicine, 20*(6), 531–535.

Liptak, G. S. Hulka, B. S., and Cassel, J. C. (1977). Effectiveness of physician–mother interaction during infancy. *Pediatrics, 60,* 186–192.

Makoul, G. (1998). Perpetuating passivity: Reliance and reciprocal determinism in physician-patient interaction. *Journal of Health Communication, 3*(3), 233–259.

Mallinger, J. B., Griggs, J. J., and Shields, C. G. (2006). Family communication and mental health after breast cancer. *European Journal of Cancer Care, 15*(4), 355–361.

Marvel, M., Epstein, R., Flowers, K., and Beckham, H. (1999). Soliciting the patient's agenda: Have we improved? *Journal of the American Medical Association, 281*(3), 283–287.

McLeroy, K. R., Bibeau, D., Steckler, A., and Glanz, K. (1988). An ecological perspective on health promotion programs. *Health Education Behavior, 15*(4), 4351–4377.

McNeils, K. (2001). Analyzing communication competence in medical consultations. *Health Communication, 13*(1), 5–18.

McNeils, K. (2002). Assessing communication competence in the primary care medical interview. *Communication Studies, 53*(4), 400–428.

Mead, N., and Bowe, P. (2000). Patient-centredness: A conceptual framework and review of the empirical literature. *Social Science and Medicine, 51*(7), 1087–1110.

Moore, S. D., Wright, K. B., and Bernard, D. R. (2009). Influences on health delivery system satisfaction: A partial test of the ecological model. *Health Communication, 24*(4), 285–294.

Muturi, N. W. (2005). Communication for HIV/AIDS prevention in Kenya: Social-cultural considerations. *Journal of Health Communication International Perspectives, 10*(1), 77–98.

Nápoles-Springer, A. M., Santoyo, J., Houston, K. *et al.* (2005). Patients' perceptions of cultural factors affecting the quality of their medical encounters. *Health Expectations, 8*(1), 4–17.

National Collaborating Centers for Public Health. (2008). Social determinants of health fact sheet. Retrieved from http://www.nccph.ca/docs/DoH_eng_PRESS_M.pdf

Nussbaum, J. F., Ragan, S., and Whaley, B. (2003). Children, older adults, and women: Impact on provider–patient interaction. In T. Thompson, A. Dorsey, K. Miller, & R. Parrot (Eds.), *The Handbook of Health Communication* (pp. 183–204). Mahwah, NJ: Lawrence Erlbaum.

Obregon, R. (2000). The role of communication in the integrated management of childhood illness: Progress, lessons learned, and challenges in Latin America. In M. Haider (Ed.), *Global Public Health Communication: Challenges, Perspectives, and Strategies.* (pp. 255–274). Sudbury, MA: Jones and Bartlett Publishers.

Obregon, R., Chitnis, K., Morry, C. *et al.* (2009). Achieving polio eradication: A review of health communication evidence and lessons learned in India and Pakistan. *Bulletin of the World Health Organisation, 87*, 624–630.

Ong, L. M. L., De Haes, C. J. M., Hoos, A. M., and Lammes, F. B. (1995). Doctor–patient communication: A review of the literature. *Social Science Medicine, 40*, 903–918.

Pagano, M. P. (2010). *Interactive Case Studies in Health Communication.* Sudbury, MA: Jones and Bartlett Publishers.

Pendleton, D. (1983). Doctor–patient communication: A review. In D. Pendleton and J. Hasler (Eds.), *Doctor–Patient Communication.* New York: Academic Press.

Perloff, R. M., Bonder, B., Ray, E. B., and Siminoff, L. A. (2006). Doctor–patient communication, cultural competence, and minority health: Theoretical and empirical perspectives. *American Behavioral Scientist, 49*(6), 835–852.

PSI (Population Services International) (2003).The Balbir Pasha story: An innovative approach to reducing HIV/AIDS prevalence through targeted mass media communications in Mumbai, India. Retrieved from http://pdf.usaid.gov/pdf_docs/PNADE789.pdf

PSI (Population Services International) (2004a). Nigeria. Retrieved from http://www.aidsmark. org/resources/pdfs/cp-nigeria.pdf

PSI (Population Services International) (2004b). Breaking barriers: An integrated approach to targeted interpersonal communications description, analysis and priorities 2002–2004. Retrieved from http://aidsmark.org/intervention/IBCC-casestudy.pdf

PSI (Population Services International) (2005). India's Operation Lighthouse: Breaking the mold on traditional HIV/AIDS behavior change approaches. Retrieved from http://pdf.usaid. gov/pdf_docs/PDACG074.pdf

Query, J. L., and Kreps, G. L. (1996). Testing a relational model of health communication competence among caregivers for individuals with Alzheimer's disease. *Journal of Health Psychology, 1*(3), 335–352.

Quick, B. (2009). The effects of viewing *Grey's Anatomy* on perceptions of doctors and patient satisfaction. *Journal of Broadcasting and Electronic Media, 53*(1), 38–55.

Rao, J. K., Anderson, L. A., Inui, T. S., and Frankel, R. M. (2007). Communication interventions make a difference in conversations between physicians and patients: a systematic review of the evidence. *Medical Care, 45*(4), 340–349.

Rashid, S. F. Akrarn, O., and Standing, H. (2011). The sexual and reproductive health care market in Bangladesh: Where do poor women go? *Reproductive Health Matters, 19*(37), 21–31.

Ray, E. B., and Donohew, L. (Ed.) (1990). *Communication and Health: Systems and Applications.* Hillside, NJ: Lawrence Erlbaum Associates.

Repass, M., and Matusitz, J. (2010). Problematic integration theory: Implications of supportive communication for breast cancer patients. *Health Care for Women International, 31*(5), 402–420.

Roter, D. L. (1989). Which facets of communication have strong effects on outcome: A meta-analysis. In M. Stewart, & D. Roter (Eds.), *Communicating with medical patients* (pp. 183–196). Newbury Park, CA: Sage Publications.

Roter, D. L. (2000). The enduring and evolving nature of the patient–physician relationship. *Patient Education and Counseling, 39*(1), 5–15.

Roter, D. L., and Hall, J. A. (1991). Health education theory: An application to the process of patient–provider communication. *Health Education Research,6*(2), 185–194.

Roter, D. L., Hall, J. A., and Katz, N. R. (1988). Patient–physician communication: A descriptive summary of the literature. *Patient Education and Counseling, 12,* 99–119.

Salmon, C. T., and Atkin, C. (2003). Using media campaigns for health promotion. In T. L. Thompson, A. M. Dorsey, K. I. Miller, and R. L. Parrott (Eds.), *Handbook of Health Communication* (pp. 449–472). Mahwah, NJ: Lawrence Erlbaum Associates.

Shahjahan, M., Khan, Y., and Haque, S. (2005). The "Know Yourself" adolescent reproductive health communication programme in Bangladesh. *Journal of Development Communication. 16*(2), 35–47.

Sharf, B. F. (1990). Physician–patient communication as interpersonal rhetoric: A narrative approach. *Health Communication, 2*(4), 217–231.

Sharf, B. F., and Vanderford, M. L. (2003). Social narratives and the construction of health. In T. L. Thompson, A. M. Dorsey, K. I. Miller, and R. L. Parrott (Eds.), *Handbook of Health Communication* (pp. 9–34). Mahwah, NJ: Lawrence Erlbaum Associates.

Smedley, B. D., Stith, A. Y., and Nelson, A. R. (Eds.). (2002). Unequal treatment: Confronting racial and ethnic disparities in health care. Washington, DC: National Academy Press.

Smith, S.W., Kopfman, J. E., Lindsey, L. L. *et al.* (2004). Encouraging family discussion on the decision to donate organs: The role of the willingness to communicate scale. *Health Commununication, 16*(3), 333–346.

Society for Family Health (SFH). (n. d.). Enhancing lives. *Newsletter of the Society for Family Health* (inaugural issue). Retrieved from http://www.sfhnigeria.org/Enhancing%20 Lives%20Newsletter%20(Inaugural%20Issue)%20SINGLES.pdf

Spiers, J. A. (1998). The use of face work and politeness theory. *Qualitative Health Research, 8*(1), 25–47.

Stewart, M. (1995). Effective physician–patient communication and health outcomes: A review. *Canadian Medical Association Journal, 152,* 1423–1433.

Stewart, M., Brown, J. B., Boon, H. *et al.* (1999). Evidence on patient–doctor communication. *Cancer Prevention Control, 3,* 25–30.

Stokols, D. (1992). Establishing and maintaining healthy environments: Toward a social Ecology of health promotion, *American Psychologist, 4*(1), 6–22.

Stokols, D. (1996). Translating social ecological theory into guidelines for community health promotion. *American Journal of Health Promotion, 10*(4), 282–298.

Street, R. L., Jr. (1989). Patient's satisfaction with dentists' communicative style. *Health Communication, 1,* 137–154.

Street, R. L., Jr. (1991). Accommodation in medical consultations. In H. Giles, J. Coupland, and N. Coupland (Eds.), *Contexts of Accommodation: Developments in Applied Sociolinguistics* (pp. 131–156). Cambridge: Cambridge University Press.

Street, R. L., Jr. (2001). Active patients as powerful communicators. In W. P. Robinson and H Giles (Eds.), *The New Handbook of Language and Social Psychology* (pp. 541–560). Chichester, England: Wiley.

Street, R. L., Jr. (2003).Communicating in medical encounters: An ecological perspective. In T. L. Thompson, A. M. Dorsey, K. I. Miller, and R. L. Parrott (Eds.), *Handbook of Health Communication* (pp. 449–472). Mahwah, NJ: Lawrence Erlbaum Associates.

Street, R.L., Jr., and Wiemann, J. M. (1987). Patient satisfaction with physician interpersonal involvement, expressiveness, and dominance. *Communication Yearbook*, *10*, 591–612.

Terry, P. E. (2000). The physician's role in educating patients. *Journal of Family Practice*, *49*, 314–318.

Thomas, R. K. (2006). *Health communication*. New York, NY: Springer.

Thomas, S. B., Fine, M. J., and Ibrahim, S. A. (2004). Health disparities: The importance of culture and health communication. *American Journal of Public Health*, *94*, 2050.

Thompson, T. L. (1994). Interpersonal communication and health care. In M. L. Knapp and G. R. Miller (Eds.), *Handbook of interpersonal communication* (2nd edn.) (pp. 696–725). Thousand Oaks, CA: Sage Publications.

Thompson, T. L., and Parrot, R. (2002). Interpersonal communication and healthcare. In M. L. Knapp and J. A. Daly (Eds.), *Handbook of Interpersonal Communication* (3rd ed.) (pp. 680–725). Thousand Oaks, CA: Sage Publications.

Turner, J. W. (2003). Telemedicine: Expanding health care into virtual environments. In T. L. Thompson, A. M. Dorsey, K. I. Miller, and R. Parrott (Eds.), *Handbook of Health Communication* (pp. 515–535). Mahwah, NJ: Lawrence Erlbaum Associates.

UNAIDS (Joint United Nations Programme on HIV/AIDS) (2010). *Nigeria. AIDS plus MDGs: synergies that serve people*. UNAIDS. Retrieved from http://www.unaids.org/en/Regionscountries/Countries/Nigeria/

UNICEF (United Nations Children's Fund) (n.d.). UNICEF. *HIV/AIDS*. Retrieved from http://www.unicef.org/india/hiv_aids.html

USAID (United States Agency for International Development) (2010). *Nigeria: HIV/AIDS Health Profile*. USAID. Retrieved from http://www.usaid.gov/our_work/global_health/aids/Countries/africa/nigeria.pdf

Vital Wave Consulting. (2009). *mHealth for development: The opportunity of mobile technology for healthcare in the developing world*. Washington, DC and Newbury, UK: UN Foundation–Vodafone Foundation Partnership. Retrieved from http://www.vitalwaveconsulting.com/pdf/mHealth.pdf

Waisbord, S. (2005). Linking communication for campaign and routine immunization: In need of a bifocal view. In M. Haider (Ed.), *Global Public Health Communication: Challenges, Perspectives, and Strategies*. (pp. 275–290). Sudbury, MA: Jones and Bartlett Publishers.

Watson, B. M. and Gallois, C. (1998). Nurturing communication by health professionals toward patients: A communication accommodation theory approach. *Health communication*, *10* (4), 343–355.

Watson, B. M. and Gallois, C. (1999).Communication accommodation between patients and health professionals: Themes and strategies in satisfying and unsatisfying encounters. *International Journal of Applied Linguistics*, *9*(2), 167–180.

Weathers, M., Query, J. L., and Kreps, G. L. (2010). A multivariate test of communication competence, social support, and coping among Hispanic lay caregivers for loved ones with Alzheimer's disease: An extension of the Relational Health Communication Competence Model. *Journal of Participative Medicine*, *2*, e14. Retrieved from http://www.jopm.org/evidence/research/2010/12/05/a-multivariate-test-of-communication-competence-social-support-and-coping-among-hispanic-lay-caregivers-for-loved-ones-with-alzheimers-disease-an-extension-of-the-relational-health-communication/

Werner, W. J. (2009). Micro-insurance in Bangladesh: Risk protection for the poor? *Journal of Health, Population and Nutrition*, *27*(4), 563–573.

WHO (World Health Organisation) (2007a). *2.5 Million People in India Living with HIV, according to New Estimates*. WHO. Retrieved from http://www.who.int/mediacentre/news/releases/2007/pr37/en/index.html

WHO (World Health Organisation) (2007b). *Health System in Bangladesh*. WHO. Retrieved from http://www.searo.who.int/LinkFiles/Bangladesh_CountryHealthSystemProfile-Bangladesh-Jan2005.pdf

WHO (World Health Organisation) (2008). Health system in Bangladesh. Retrieved from http://www.whoban.org/health_system_bangladesh.html

WHO (World Health Organisation) (2011). Bangladesh: Health profile. Retrieved from http://www.who.int/gho/countries/bgd.pdf

WHO (World Health Organisation, Bangladesh (2010). Health system in Bangladesh. Retrieved from http://ban.searo.who.int/en/Section25.htm

WHO Commission on Social Determinants of Health (2007). *Health Equity: From Root Causes to Fair Outcomes*. Retrieved from http://whqlibdoc.who.int/publications/2007/interim_statement_eng.pdf

Woolley, F. R., Kane, R. L., Hughes, C. C., and Wright, D. D. (1978). The effects of doctor–patient communication on satisfaction and outcome of care. *Social Science and Medicine, 12*, 123–128.

World Bank (1993). *World Development Report 1993: Investing in Health*. Washington, DC: World Bank.

World Bank (2005). *World Development Report 2006: Equity and Development*. Washington, DC: World Bank.

World Bank (2006). *Global Burden of Disease and Risk Factors*. Washington, DC: World Bank.

Wynia, M., and Matiasek, J. (August 2006). *Promising practices for patient-centered communication with vulnerable populations: Examples from eight hospitals*. (Volume: 32). The Commonwealth Fund. New York, NY: Retrieved from http://www.commonwealthfund.org/Publications/Fund-Reports/2006/Aug/Promising-Practices-for-Patient-Centered-Communication-with-Vulnerable-Populations–Examples-from-Ei.aspx

Zhang, A. Z. and Siminoff, L. A. (2003). The role of the family in treatment decision making by patients with cancer. *Oncology Nursing Forum, 30*(6), 1022–1028.

8

Community Health and Social Mobilization

Catherine Campbell and Kerry Scott

Introduction

This chapter examines the role of community mobilization in creating opportunities for improved health in marginalized communities. There is strong evidence that various forms of marginalization through interlocking social inequalities have negative impacts on health (WHO, 2008). Both globally and within particular countries and contexts, it is generally those with the most limited access to economic and political power who are the unhealthiest. Redistributive social policies – which increase peoples' access to economic resources and social and political recognition – are often seen as a necessary condition for narrowing the health gap between rich and poor and improving the health of groups who have limited access to social power in particular contexts, including women, children, the elderly, the poor, those of lower caste or social class, and the disabled.

However, social elites seldom voluntarily give up economic or political power in the absence of assertive and vociferous demands from less powerful groups. Unfortunately, the very people who must provide this assertive and vociferous "push from below" often have limited opportunities and resources to do so. Moreover, poverty and other forms of marginalization often foster a sense of disempowerment and fatalism among the excluded. Before members of socially excluded groups are able to demand substantive changes in the unequal social relations that undermine their health, they need to come to see themselves as active agents capable of improving their lives and increasing their control over their health and well-being (Gaventa and Cornwall, 2001). They also need to build alliances with more powerful social groupings who are willing and able to support their struggle for a better life (Gillies, 1998).

Didactic information-based health communication programs have repeatedly failed to improve health in many settings, and there has been a growing recognition of the

The Handbook of Global Health Communication, First Edition. Edited by Rafael Obregon and Silvio Waisbord.

need to involve communities in efforts to improve their health (Campbell, 2003; Stephens, 2009). This is particularly the case in the most marginalized contexts in which ill-health is most likely to flourish. Community involvement necessitates a shift away from approaches that try to *persuade* individuals to change risky health behaviors through strategies such as the provision of information about health risks, in favor of approaches that seek to create "health-enabling social environments" which enable and support the possibility of individual behavior change (Tawil, Verster, and O'Reilly, 1995). Community mobilization is a central pillar of efforts to create such healthy community contexts.

This chapter is framed within our theory of transformative communication, which maps the psychosocial pathways between community mobilization and health. We define community mobilization in terms of (1) the intertwined strategies of grassroots participation in health and social development efforts ("participation") and (2) the building of alliances between communities and more powerful groups ("partnerships"). More particularly, our theory of transformative communication explains how participation and partnerships open up new networks and opportunities for the forms of communication most likely to take forward struggles to create healthier social settings (Campbell and Cornish, 2010; Campbell and Scott, 2010). We will argue that participation and partnerships provide opportunities for new and empowering forms of communication through which marginalized people can work collectively to (1) develop a greater sense of individual and collective health-related agency; (2) develop strategies through which they might act to improve their health; and also (3) gain the attention of more powerful people outside their community who have the power to engage in "top-down" efforts to accommodate their demands.

Despite often clothing themselves in the politically correct rhetoric of "community-led structural interventions" (interventions through which communities are mobilized to tackle the structural drivers of ill-health), most existing community mobilization programs devote much of their energy to the *subjective* empowerment of poor people to take control over their health, paying less attention to the *objective* conditions that make this unlikely. Such programs work to build poor people's health-related knowledge and skills and to develop their "voice" – their ability to articulate their health-related needs and demands in a confident and forceful manner. Such programs often assume that, once the socially excluded are "empowered" in this way, they will automatically be able to gain the attention of more powerful social actors and groups. However, this is often not the case.

Elsewhere we have argued that there is an urgent need for community mobilization approaches to pay attention not only to the *subjective* empowerment of marginalized people, but also to the parallel need to create situations in which powerful people are willing to listen to the demands of the poor and take action to create the *objective* social changes which might be needed to increase their opportunities for health (Campbell, Cornish, Scott, and Gibbs, 2010). This chapter discusses the twin challenges of building community capacity and "voice," as well as facilitating the development of receptive and supportive social environments. To illustrate these processes we provide case studies of various forms of transformative communication seeking to promote maternal health in India.

Theoretical framework

We define health communication as any attempt to improve peoples' health through facilitating health-enhancing behavior change, the appropriate accessing of health-related services and support, the development of health-enabling social capital, collective action to tackle obstacles to health, and the development of health-related social policy.

Drawing on Paulo Freire's (1970, 1973) distinction between "extension" and "conscientization" we distinguish between "technical communication" (the one-way flow of skills and information from outside experts to poor communities) and "transformative communication" (Campbell and Cornish, 2010). The latter involves dialogue and exchange between experts and communities where each group is seen as having an equally important contribution to make in identifying and naming community problems, and formulating plans to tackle them. In the health field, professionals are often able to offer important biomedical and technical expertise. Communities are able to offer expertise about the extent to which medical and technical knowledge and services resonate with their own understandings of their needs and interests, and about how they might adapt, or make best use of, such skills and services. They are experts on the extent to which formal health services are most likely to interface with pre-existing indigenous responses to health promotion and care. Communities can also identify obstacles that would need to be overcome for them to derive optimal benefit from externally derived skills and services. Tackling such obstacles might involve wider political and economic changes. Communities may need to engage not only with health professionals, but also with a wider range of political and economic actors, to ensure that their needs and concerns are given attention by policy makers and appropriate political and economic actors and agencies whose decisions impact on their opportunities for health – a point taken up below.

Evolution of health communication: From social cognition to community mobilization

Historically, health communication was driven by "social cognition" models of behavior, which viewed human beings as rational actors, capable of making sensible choices on the basis of sound information. Proponents of social cognition models sought to promote individual behavior change by changing factors such as peoples' health-related knowledge, attitudes, or perceived self-efficacy. They used didactic communication strategies, which sought to transmit information from health experts to laypeople. However, a generation of program evaluations suggest that information-based health communication approaches have had a limited impact on the behavior of their audiences (Ogden, 2007). Information is often a weak determinant of behavior change, particularly amongst marginalized social groups whose freedom to control their behavior may be limited by wider social conditions such as poverty or gender.

Against this background, there is a growing move away from information provision in favor of community strengthening, social participation, and partnership/alliance-building approaches. These approaches provide opportunities for types of transformative communication that seek not only to educate people about health risks, but also to facilitate the types of social relationships most likely to empower them to resist the impacts of unhealthy social influences (Wallack, 2003). Rather than treating people as empty vessels that can be filled by health information, transformative communication seeks to change the contexts in which people live by facilitating forms of communication through which people can evaluate and adjust their understandings of the world and their behavior within it.

A growing body of evidence shows that various forms of grassroots participation have the potential to exert a powerful positive influence on health and well-being in particular settings (Rappaport, 1987; Kawachi, *et al.*, 1996; Baum, 1999). These include community engagement in health-related activities such as health service user groups and health promotion programs. These also include general community-strengthening activities such as voluntary associations, local civic and political groups, and informal networks of friends, neighbors, or family. In addition to providing the intrinsically health-enhancing benefits of social support (Berkman, 1984), social participation is health-enhancing because it links people into communication networks that provide opportunities for health-enhancing forms of transformative communication. This communication enables people to construct more empowering and positive understandings of themselves, their place in the world, and the future, which form the starting point for improved health, as discussed further below.

This move by health communicators away from the provision of information and towards a focus on the role of community mobilization in generating both networks and processes of transformative communication is in line with developments in critical social cognition studies, which highlight the role of dialogue in human thought and decision making. Billig (1996) argues that human thinking takes the form of a constant process of debate or argument and counterargument which we engage in both internally and when interacting with others. In his account of "the thinking society," Billig argues that people are constantly engaged, individually or collectively, in a process of weighing up different points of view. They continually evaluate new sources of knowledge both in terms of pre-existing assumptions, habits, custom, ideology, and tradition, and also in terms of the often contradictory motivations that influence their behavior as they move from one social setting to the next.

Health-related behaviors are not simply the result of individual knowledge and skills imparted to passive audiences by active health communicators. They are nested within complex social structures in which people collectively appropriate and construct new meanings, identities, and behavioral possibilities from one moment to the next in response to the challenges they face in their lives. For this reason, effective health communication needs to facilitate situations that constitute a microcosm of "the thinking society" through encouraging target communities to participate in the processes of dialogue and debate in which social identities and associated behavioral possibilities are created and recreated. Community mobilization succeeds as a health promotion strategy to the extent that it creates opportunities for such dialogue.

Communication and social identity

It is through communication and dialogue that we construct and negotiate the social identities, or "recipes for living," that drive our actions and shape our health and well-being. The symbolic interactionist perspective (Mead, 1934) emphasizes the role of social interaction and dialogue in constructing the social identities that influence the collectively negotiated "recipes for living" that drive our behavior. These identities are often associated with our position within hierarchical social groups. Health communication is effective to the extent that it provides opportunities for people to renegotiate their social identities in health-enhancing and empowering ways. It can serve as the first step in wider community efforts to create health-enabling social settings through participation and partnerships. To improve their health, people need to engage in critical reflection and dialogue, develop new insights into the ways unequal social relations limit their health and life chances, and brainstorm strategies to resist these negative impacts. They also need to build alliances with more powerful groups to assist them in meeting these goals.

Challenging disabling forms of "power-knowledge"

Within unequal societies, there is an overwhelming tendency for unequal power relations to perpetuate themselves, with communicative possibilities and outcomes tending to reinforce the position of dominant social groups in the vast majority of social interactions. One mechanism through which this happens is that marginalized social groupings become trapped in self-limiting forms of what Foucault (1980) termed "power-knowledge" – understandings of one's place in the world, and of one's potential for action – that often lead to fatalism and passivity.

In principle, the exertion of power always goes hand in hand with the possibility of resistance (Foucault, 1980). Foucault speaks of the "micro-capillarity" of power. Rather than being a monolithic force, power operates through a complex array of "meticulous rituals" (Foucault, 1975). Since communication is a key medium through which the meticulous rituals of power are continually enacted and re-enacted, the possibility always exists that groups of marginalized actors may develop the insight and confidence to refuse to engage in communicative styles and acts that undermine or disempower them. Key to this process of refusal is reformulating their social identities and sense of place in the world in ways that challenge the negative social relations that compromise their dignity and well-being (Cornish, 2006; Howarth, 2006). The task confronting health communicators concerned with challenging the social hierarchies that lead to health inequalities is to provide "transformative social spaces" for the development of such resistance.

Transformative social spaces

How can the types of social spaces most conducive to empowering dialogue best be characterized? Fraser (1990) argues that, in unequal societies, the public sphere tends to be dominated by the privileged elites, providing limited space for historically marginalized groups (women, the poor, ethnic minorities) to exert influence. Marginalized groups tend to lack the confidence, skills and social legitimacy to advance their needs and interests. For this reason, she posits the concept of "counter-publics," which are safe separate spaces in which marginalized groups can retreat to develop and "rehearse" the types of critical arguments they will eventually take into the dominant public sphere to challenge the power of dominant groupings and demand their share of symbolic and material social power.

What psychosocial processes need to take place within these "counter-public" spaces to best equip marginalized groups to make effective demands for social recognition? Paulo Freire (1973) answers this question with his concepts of dialogical critical thinking and praxis, through which people are able to reflect on and transform their existing understandings of themselves and their place in the world, and act to improve their life circumstances. It is through such reflection that excluded groups are able to deconstruct their existing self-limiting knowledge and develop understandings of how their taken-for-granted assumptions are shaped by oppressive power relations and by world views that support the interests of the dominant social classes (Vaughan, 2010).

Such reflection informs the development of new ways of making sense of the world, and more empowering understandings of the possibilities of alternative social relationships. Ideally, participatory dialogue also leads to an enhanced sense of confidence in one's ability to change one's social circumstances, as well as the identification of existing individual and group strengths, skills, and capacities to contribute to the fight for social change. Identification of strengths and skills is part and parcel of the collective formulation of feasible action plans to challenge limiting social relations. Finally, effective dialogue leads to the identification of potential support networks that marginalized communities can draw on to enable them to put these action plans into practice.

The role of strategic alliances

This latter point is based on the insight that marginalized groupings are often not able to tackle the social settings that undermine their health without significant assistance – referred to as "strategic alliances" by Spivak (1988) – from outsiders who have the economic and political power to assist them in achieving their goals. Bourdieu (1986) argues that limited access to social capital (which he defines as durable networks of socially advantageous intergroup relationships) is a key factor in perpetuating poverty and other forms of social disadvantage, hindering people from improving their life circumstances. Facilitating the development of "bridging social capital" – linking health-vulnerable communities to outside actors and agencies with the power and inclination to support them in improving their health, well-being, and life chances – needs to be a central aspect of any health communication program. A key challenge currently facing health communicators is to develop better understandings of how communication strategies can (1) facilitate links between marginalized communities and powerful and supportive outsiders (e.g. health professionals, political leaders and policy makers, powerful economic actors, various local, national and global networks of support), and (2) persuade these powerful actors to take poor peoples' needs seriously.

The need for multilevel strategies

Below we look at different strategies that public health experts have used to contribute to the overall challenge of facilitating widespread and effective transformative communication (where the marginalized develop the voice to assert their needs and the powerful are willing to listen) in relation to maternal mortality in India. There is no single "magic bullet" solution to tackling this challenge; maternal mortality in India is rooted in complex overlapping and mutually reinforcing hierarchies shaped by culture, history, gender, age, and poverty in the wider context of a country characterized by dramatic social inequalities. Neither can the impacts of complex and interlocking social inequalities be countered in sustainable ways in the types of short-term, one-off public health interventions so attractive to many national governments and international funding agencies forever in search of quick-fix solutions to complex social problems. The challenge of empowering poor and highly marginalized women to take control over their health is a long-term one that needs to be pursued at multiple levels – building skills within local communities, creating opportunities for local communities to communicate their needs to more powerful agencies that deliver services and shape policy, and creating wider national and global contexts that are receptive to the voices and needs of the poor and marginalized.

Each strategy discussed below operates at one of these three levels, making a particular contribution to the multilevel challenge of implementing the ideals of transformative communication in real life social contexts. Focusing on the challenges of improving maternal health in India, the first strategy we discuss, peer-to-peer communication, is an approach that trains and incentivizes women to serve as health advocates within their local communities. Such an approach potentially makes a vital contribution to building women's critical understandings of obstacles to health and how they might act to tackle them. We then look at strategies which seek to communicate such enhanced critical understandings beyond the local community context. We look at efforts to mobilize poor women in various forms of grassroots social activism to pressure local and national government actors to provide them with better health services. Finally we look at wider and more top-down health advocacy efforts by national and global health actors to put maternal health on the agenda of politicians and policy at the national and global levels.

Case Study: Tackling Maternal Mortality in India

Above we have outlined our theory of transformative communication, drawing on the concepts of dialogue, critical thinking, counter-publics and strategic alliances. This theory maps out the social psychological processes underlying our argument that efforts to empower marginalized communities to take control over their health need to build both (1) the voice of the marginalized; and (2) receptive social environments. We concluded that such complex goals are most likely to result from multiple, multilevel strategies. We now turn to the challenge of maternal mortality in India to illustrate the range of health communication strategies currently being implemented to tackle this problem at the local, regional, national and global levels.

Reducing maternal mortality (MM) by 75 percent between 1990 and 2015 is Millennium Development Goal (MDG) number five. However, the global maternal mortality rate (MMR) has fallen at a rate of just 1 percent per year between 1990 and 2005, making MDG5 the goal that has made the least progress and is most likely to fall short (Sen, 2009). A 5.5 percent annual rate of decline is needed to get back on track with the MDG, which will require an investment of US$12 billion per year (Women Deliver, 2010).

According to United Nations agencies, there are approximately 117,000 maternal deaths in India each year, which amounts to almost one quarter of worldwide maternal deaths (UNFPA, 2007). At about 300 deaths per 100,000 live births, India's maternal mortality rate (MMR) is higher than that of China (45), Sri Lanka (56), Brazil (110), Egypt (130) and even Namibia (210) (Hunt, 2007a). Over the past 20 years, quite a lot of effort has been put into Safe Motherhood initiatives in India. There is recent evidence that these efforts are seeing some success: India's MMR has been declining at an annual rate of about 4.0 percent since the beginning of the MDG period (Hogan *et al.*, 2010) and most reproductive health indicators are slowly improving. However, the country is still not on track to reach its MDG target. Half of all women still do not complete three antenatal care visits, half of all births are still not attended by a health professional and only 42 percent of women receive postnatal care within two months of delivery (Vora *et al.*, 2009).

Moreover, India's overall maternal mortality rate fails to reflect the severity of the problem in specific less developed regions of the country, and among subpopulations of less educated women and lower-caste women. In particular, India's northern states have very high rates of fertility and maternal mortality while India's southern states have indicators on a par with middle-income countries (Vora *et al.*, 2009). The MMR in Uttar Pradesh is 517 (MoHFW, 2008a) and in Rajasthan 445 (MoHFW 2008b), while unofficial estimates of the disparities are higher still, suggesting for instance that the MMR may be up to 898 in some parts of Jharkhand (Hunt, 2007b). Only 18 percent of illiterate women had institutional deliveries while 89 percent of women with 12 or more years of education did (NFHS3 2007). The vast variation in maternal health across India reflects the immense differences in female social status, literacy and empowerment between regions, castes and religions.

Maternal mortality is only a portion of the larger issue of ill-health associated with reproduction; while there are over half a million maternal deaths worldwide per year, an estimated 50 million women suffer from short- and long-term pregnancy-related morbidities such as fistula, weakness due to undernutrition and hemorrhaging, cervical tears, infections, incontinence, or nerve damage (WHO, 2005).

In this chapter we take up the case study of maternal health in India in order to illustrate the ways in which health communication strategies have been engaged to address a social issue through building the voice of the marginalized and creating receptive social environments among more powerful actors. We now examine three types of health communication initiatives that have been put into place to tackle MM in India and globally.

The first initiative is an example of peer-to-peer communication. The ASHA program is a community health worker initiative that involves engaging communities, in particular rural women, around health issues with a particular emphasis on reproductive health. The second initiative is the maternal health program spearheaded by an Indian health activist organization called SAHAYOG's maternal health program. This program seeks to build the voice of marginalized women to assert their right to reproductive health and develops partnerships to support collective action at the local, state, national, and international levels. And the third initiative focuses on broader global health advocacy through the International Initiative on Maternal Mortality and Human Rights (IIMMHR).

Initiative one: The ASHA program as peer-to-peer communication

The Accredited Social Health Activist (ASHA) program is a community health worker program and a central component of the Indian government's National Rural Health Mission (NRHM). The Indian government has committed to training and supporting one ASHA for every 1000 rural people across the country (MoHFW 2005). ASHAs are rural women trained to promote health amongst their peers through education, delivering basic care and encouraging increased involvement in health care programs and biomedical services.

Their tasks include encouraging women to register pregnancies and visit the health center, escorting people to the primary health center (PHC) as needed, bringing children to immunization clinics, encouraging family planning, treating basic illness and injury with first aid and medicine, keeping demographic records, and improving village sanitation. ASHAs are also to hold information meetings and raise awareness on issues including women's health, disease, social determinants of health, nutrition, and sanitation as well as to serve as counselors on adolescent and female sexual and reproductive health issues.

ASHAs receive remuneration for specific health outcomes. For example, ASHAs receive Rs. 150 for each child completing an immunization session and Rs. 150 for each individual who undergoes surgical sterilization. Under a parallel government program called Janani Suraksha Yojana (JSY), rural woman who choose to give in a health center rather than at home receives Rs. 1400; if an ASHA is involved in facilitating this institutional birth she receives Rs. 600.

We now move on to discussing the ways in which the ASHA program engages – and fails to engage – transformative communication as a mechanism to successful community mobilization. As discussed above, marginalized people (i.e. rural women) require several psycho-social elements in order to take control over their health, including information and skills, social spaces for critical dialogue about how to improve their health, increased sense of health-related agency and a sense of solidarity with similar others. To what extent does the ASHA program facilitate these elements?

Our discussion draws from Scott and Shanker's (2010) case study of the ASHA program in the rural north Indian state of Uttarakhand. While the findings are not necessarily generalizable to other areas of the country it offers a valuable study of the potential of this program to serve as a transformative communicative strategy.

In some ways, the program is going well in Uttarakhand; immunization rates have risen from 45 percent in 2002–2004 before the program began to 63 percent in 2007–2008 and the percentage of women who received three or more antenatal checkups (ANCs) went from 21 percent to 34 percent over the same period (MoHFW 2008c). Many ASHAs and health workers spoke glowingly of the program, with ASHAs saying that they enjoy talking to community members and that the position has increased their status in the community.

However, the health status – and social status more generally – of women in the region is still extremely poor. The gender- and age-dominated social order greatly limits the potential for women to access health services, eat well, and control their reproductive health. Gender inequality and far-reaching male privilege are deeply entrenched in society with, for instance, the birth of boy babies being seen as a cause for celebration while the birth of girls goes largely unremarked. Women are fed less than men with wives eating only after the husband and in-laws have eaten. Young women are often treated very poorly when they marry into their husband's home, especially by mothers-in-law. These mothers-in-law frequently draw on their culturally defined role as "guardians of tradition" and are strongly opposed to biomedical conceptualizations of health and health services.

In Scott and Shanker's case study, many women coped in this situation through constructing their identities as sacrificial, hard-working, and responsible, in contrast to the stereotype held by many women of men as violent drunkards who neglect their families. On the one hand, this served as a source of positive social identity, enabling them to cope with their difficult daily lives and take pride in the very sacrifices that harmed their health. On the other hand, it tended to undermine their personal health and autonomy, as well as limiting their capacity to assert their health needs.

Even within this unpromising context, there was evidence that ASHAs played a positive role in facilitating genuine dialogue about the relative benefits of biomedical and traditional approaches to childbirth. They were able to use their "insider knowledge" of their communities to develop convincing reasons why women should access formal health care, for example, by demystifying the health center through discussing their experiences there. In that sense they certainly succeeded in our criteria of generating knowledge, dialogue/critical thinking, and solidarity. However in relation to building health-enabling agency their efforts were constrained by several problematic structural features of the program, discussed next. Moreover, the program itself greatly curtailed any potential for government policy makers to become more receptive to the demands of rural women.

The greatest programmatic limitation to the ASHAs' capacity to use transformative communication to mobilize communities was the outcome-based payment method. This payment system rewards ASHAs only for tasks linked to specific vertical programs (JSY, malaria control, surgical sterilization, etc.) and, since ASHAs are very poor, they understandably seek to maximize earnings through concentrating their efforts on these narrow remunerated initiatives. ASHAs need the financial flexibility to perform health education and promotion activities and the financial security to work as activists accountable to their communities rather than to the health care center staff who pay their remuneration. This form of payment often led to mistrust and hostility between ASHAs and other community members. Furthermore, their preoccupation with encouraging service use limited the extent to which they developed their potential role as trusted community advocate.

Another central institutional barrier is that ASHAs are frequently affiliated with sorely understaffed and underequipped health centers that are unable to stay open 24 hours a day – a very significant problem when they are being promoted as a place to give birth. ASHAs, in order to keep their jobs and receive remuneration, must try to encourage people to use the local health center. By tasking ASHAs with promoting underequipped health centers as places to give birth, the government aligns them with the health system, not the community. Rather than acting as cultural mediators seeking to improve the fit between government services and community needs, community members see their ASHAs promoting services that do not necessarily serve them. Once an ASHA's advice to go to the clinic proves unsound due to the limited institutional support, she loses face in the community and people are less likely to trust her on other matters.

The public health care system is a highly unreceptive social environment for listening to marginalized women about their needs – ASHAs included. ASHAs are restricted to implementing top-down instructions from health authorities. As a result there are no opportunities for them to feed their insider knowledge about obstacles to service access back to service managers. For instance, ASHAs have a far more nuanced understanding of local resistance to institutional birth than health care workers (i.e., that lay people recognize that the clinics are poorly equipped and thus frequently not worth using; that mothers-in-law often insist on home births; that there is a preference for traditional birth attendants; and that hospitals disrupt traditional birth practices such as giving new mothers separate meals and privacy for 11 days). If medical professionals accessed these insights they could develop a safe birth environment that meets the needs of women and their families and addresses the considerable practical concerns of the local people. Unfortunately, these insights go untapped because health professionals are not receptive to ASHA knowledge, instead limiting their interactions with ASHAs to giving them directions.

Initiative two: Grassroots social activism through SAHAYOG

SAHAYOG is an extremely successful gender equity and women's health rights advocacy NGO based in the north Indian state of Uttar Pradesh (UP). This organization specifically seeks to both build the voice of marginalized groups and create receptive environments for these voices to be heard at the state, national, and international policy level. They have five broad areas of work: maternal health and rights (which we will focus on); work with men and boys; violence against women; youth sexual and reproductive health rights; and gender equity. SAHAYOG's efforts focus on developing the voice of marginalized communities (women, dalit, nonliterate, youth, rural, and minorities) and advocating for change at the state, national, and international levels. They work with communities to enable them to participate in decision making that affects their lives and to become effective advocates for the issues that most concern them. Partnerships are central to their operation; over their 18 years they have developed strong working relationships with national and international health and women's rights advocacy groups as well as local NGOs to build capacities of marginalized people, monitor government programs and gather information to use for advocacy (Dasgupta, 2008).

Our discussion will focus on their maternal health and rights program. Within this program, SAHAYOG seeks to increase women's access to and control over maternal health services through advocacy and monitoring. They engage in evidence-based policy advocacy with state actors, donors and the media, and monitor the quality of reproductive health programs to promote women's reproductive rights.

A main component of their work is to create "rights consciousness" among the rights holders (in this case low-income low-literacy women) and a corresponding "sense of accountability" among the duty bearers (including the health bureaucracy and political actors) (Dasgupta, 2008). In addition the program seeks to understand the maternal health situation in the villages and determine reasons for poor maternal health indicators and experiences. This is done through research, monitoring, and case documentation.

Capacity-building programs with marginalized women, communities, and local rights organizations engage participatory processes of dialogue, critical questioning and confidence building (Freire, 1973). In this way, SAHAYOG uses training sessions and workshops to build the capacity of rural women and partner organizations to carry out effective advocacy, monitoring, research, and case documentation around maternal health and rights issues. This capacity building involves empowering participants, usually rural women, by teaching them about maternal health and their entitlements under the NRHM. They have, for instance, trained traditional birth attendants on maternal health issues and safe childbirth using a participatory curriculum. The workshops then move on to discuss and plan how to claim these entitlements. SAHAYOG has trained field researchers on how to select cases of denial of maternal health rights, conduct in-depth interviews for case documentation, and document these cases. They have also worked with middle-level NGO workers and members of the UP grassroots women's health rights forum Mahila Swasthya Adhikar Manch (MSAM) to develop their advocacy skills, for instance, teaching them how to liaise with the media and plan and execute targeted women's health rights campaigns at the state level (IIMMHR, 2009a).

Their efforts have met with great successes. For instance, they have partnered with MSAM and seen membership grow from a few hundred rural women in 2007 to over 8000 at present across eight districts. In 2007 they worked with MSAM to run a one-week cross-district maternal rights awareness campaign, which culminated in the women writing a letter to the chief medical officer. This campaign resulted in many concrete improvements to women's health services including the appointment of doctors in all health centers where previously there had been none, the opening of five subcenters, and the development of delivery facilities in a community health center. Rather than trying to set up parallel health structures, SAHAYOG emphasizes the importance of holding the government health system accountable. They have thus organized district-level monitoring sessions, helped women mobilize to demand their JSY payments (see ASHA section, above), and demanded that the government conduct an audit of maternal deaths in their region (Dasgupta, 2008).

SAHAYOG is extremely active at the national level and has played an important role in getting and keeping maternal mortality on the national political agenda throughout the 2000s. In their study of the role of various multileveled health communication and health advocacy strategies that are currently driving forward the maternal mortality agenda in India, Shiffman and Ved (2007) point out how several streams of influence must converge in order to build a receptive social environment in which powerful national-level social actors are most likely to support the development of policy and action to improve maternal health. SAHAYOG has proven adept at facilitating many of these processes. To begin building political concern, Shiffman and Ved argue, the problem must be named and comprehensive research must prove its significance, two key areas where SAHAYOG has contributed, for example, through their collaborative and participatory studies Access to Maternal Health Services for Women Workers in the Unorganized Sector and National Study on Maternal Health and Institutional Delivery.

Alongside naming and research, Shiffman and Ved suggest that high profile national and international events must package the issue and bring it to the attention of national policy makers. In the case of MM, several events in the early 2000s, including a White Ribbon Alliance march to the Taj Mahal – a monument built in memory of a woman who died in childbirth – and the 2005 World Health Day (hosted by India), which happened to have maternal health as a key theme, packaged MM as a key development issue. Consensus building between senior government officials, donor agencies, NGOs and civil society is another vital element to building a receptive national-level environment; SAHAYOG is involved in organizing dialogue between the government and civil society and participating in policy meetings such as the Civil Society Dialogue on Maternal Mortality in India with the UN Special Rapporteur on the Right to Health. India launched the "Reproductive and Child Health II" policy and National Rural Health Mission, both of which had an unprecedentedly strong government involvement in design and funding and which SAHAYOG has played an important role in monitoring through the Healthwatch Forum. The convergence of several streams of influence that resulted in India's national level focus on maternal health has required the efforts of many groups; SAHAYOG has been a strong player.

At the international level, SAHAYOG is a part of the International Initiative on Maternal Mortality and Human Rights (discussed next), a South Asian partnership on maternal health and reproductive rights, and an initiative to tracing the regulation, distribution and consumption of pharmaceuticals in South Asia.

Initiative three: International advocacy through IIMMHR

The International Initiative on Maternal Mortality and Human Rights (IIMMHR) is a partnership of international, regional, and national civil society organizations committed to a comprehensive human rights approach to maternal mortality (IIMMHR, 2009a). This collaboration calls for greater political will to reduce maternal mortality, greater resources dedicated to this end, and more and better accountability mechanisms to ensure that women's right to maternal health becomes a reality. The initiative was launched in October 2007 during the Women Deliver Conference in London by six international organizations in the health and human rights fields: the Averting Maternal Death and Disability Program of the Mailman School of Public Health, Columbia University; CARE; the Center for Reproductive Rights; Family Care International; Physicians for Human Rights; and the UN Special Rapporteur on the Right to the Highest Attainable Standard of Health (Paul Hunt). SAHAYOG (discussed above), is one of the thirteen steering committee members, responsible for the governance of the Initiative and for advancing its goals and objectives.

IIMMHR takes a human rights approach to maternal health. This approach is central to fostering receptive environments at the level of international and national policy. A human rights approach frames maternal deaths not as "unfortunate" occurrences invoking pity or guilt but as a direct violation of rights indicating an unacceptable failure at the global, national, and local levels. The human rights approach demands accountability from governments and places women's rights and gender equity at the center of government responses to reproductive rights and health issues (IIMMHR, 2009b).

IIMMHR is engaged in many interlocking activities to keep maternal mortality on the international agenda. They produce publications such as global reports on maternal mortality and toolkits for advocates; support three field projects; provide print resources on MM and human rights; organize and participate in international discussions on women's rights (such as the UN Human Rights Commission); and work with their steering committee members (particularly the Center for Reproductive Rights) to engage legal processes to hold governments accountable. For example, IIMMHR worked to get the UN Human Rights Council to officially recognize maternal mortality as a human rights issue in 2009, enabling activists to push governments for greater accountability (IIMMHR, 2009c). Their three field projects (Voices from the Ground in India is linked to SAHAYOG, Right to care in Kenya and No Woman Behind in Peru) increase their understanding of how to integrate human rights ideas and approaches into maternal mortality work at national, subnational and local levels.

Conclusion

In this chapter we have looked at various multilevel communication strategies, ranging from programs to promote small-scale critical awareness and health-related action within and by local communities, to larger-scale alliance building at the regional, national, and international levels. We have used the notion of "transformative communication" to explain the social psychological processes by which the health of marginalized groups might be enhanced through community mobilization (participation and partnerships). Ideally, these strategies have the potential to contribute to the interlocking challenges of building the "voice" of the poor and marginalized, and facilitating the development of "receptive social environments" in which more powerful groups are willing to hear this voice, and take their needs seriously.

To what extent do these very different health communication approaches have the potential to succeed in tackling the drivers of maternal mortality in India, namely women's limited access to knowledge, health services, and human rights and a national and international failure to take women's health rights seriously? We have assessed the potential of these strategies to develop the voice of marginalized people through mobilizing them to take control over their own health and participate in collective action and create more receptive social environments among powerful actors to listen and respond to the demands of the poor at the national and global levels. The ASHA program has some scope to develop transformative social spaces in which the women most vulnerable to maternal ill-health can critically assess their current practices, learn about their entitlements, and potentially develop a sense of solidarity. However, we have showed that the program is limited by a rigid hierarchy, a weak public health care system, and a remuneration system that curtails the capacity for ASHAs to perform as anything more than mouthpieces of the government health care system, certainly not as health activists.

We presented SAHAYOG as a very effective approach to building up both the voice of the poor, through capacity building, rights-based education, government lobbying, and participatory research, and receptive social environments, by engaging in dialogue with the government, providing information, and monitoring programs. Finally we discussed the contribution of IIMMHR. This organization accepts that it is not enough simply to "empower the poor" to take control over their health, in the absence of wider changes to the social relations that place their health at risk. Without the efforts of powerful agents at the national and international levels, poor people cannot bring about significant social changes. IIMMHR puts its energies into pressurizing powerful national and international agents to accept the role that they need to play in making improved maternal health possible.

Through our case studies we have sought to illustrate various multilevel ways in which health communicators are working to build both the voice of women at risk as well as a receptive social environment where powerful people are willing to listen to them. These efforts take many forms including promoting various forms of dialogue, critical thinking, transformative social spaces and strategic alliance building.

As we have emphasized, there is no single "magic bullet" communications strategy that can alone tackle large-scale health problems, rooted in overlapping systems of inequality and discrimination (in our case study varying combinations of age, gender, class, and poverty). Such problems need to be addressed through a multilevel series of approaches, pulling in a wide range of actors and agencies and multiple levels. Much work remains to be done in driving the maternal health agenda forward, both in India and globally, but many strategies exist that have potential to contributing to the ongoing challenge of making maternal health a universal reality.

Acknowledgments

Thanks to Flora Cornish for discussion of many of the points above.

References

Baum, F. (1999). Social capital: Is it good for your health? *Journal of Epidemiology and Community Health, 53*, 195–196.

Berkman, L. (1984). Assessing the physical health effects of social networks and social support. *Annual Review of Public Health, 5*, 413–432.

Billig, M. (1996). *Arguing and Thinking*. Cambridge: Cambridge University Press.

Bourdieu, P. (1986). The forms of capital. In J. Richardson (Ed.), *Handbook of Theory and Research for the Sociology of Education* (pp. 241–258). New York: Greenwood Press.

Campbell, C. (2003). *Letting Them Die: Why HIV/AIDS Prevention Programmes Often Fail*. Bloomington, IN: Indiana University Press.

Campbell, C. and Cornish, F. (2011). How can community health programmes build enabling environments for transformative communication? Experiences from India and South Africa. *AIDS and Behavior*. DOI: 10.1007/s10461-011-9966-2.

Campbell, C., Cornish, F., Gibbs, A., and Scott, K. (2010). Heeding the push from below: How do social movements persuade the rich to listen to the poor? *Journal of Health Psychology* 15(7), 962–971.

Campbell, C., and Scott, K. (2010). Mediated health communication: from information to social change. In D. Hook, B. Franks, and M. Bauer (Eds.), *Social Psychology of communication*. Basingstoke, UK: Palgrave.

Cornish, F. (2006). Challenging the stigma of sex work in India. *Journal of Community and Applied Social Psychology, 16,* 462–471.

Dasgupta, J. (2008). *SAHAYOG Sixteenth Annual Report*. Lucknow: SAHAYOG.

Foucault, M. (1975). *Discipline and Punish: The Birth of the Prison*. New York: Random House.

Foucault, M. (1980). *Power/knowledge*. New York: Pantheon Books.

Fraser, N. (1990). Rethinking the public sphere: A contribution to the critique of actually existing democracy. *Social Text, 25*(26), 56–80.

Freire, P. (1970). *Pedagogy of the Oppressed*. New York: Herder and Herder.

Freire, P. (1973). *Education for Critical Consciousness*. New York: Continuum.

Gaventa, J., and Cornwall, A. (2001). Power and Knowledge. In P. Reason, and H. Bradbury (Eds.), *Handbook of Action Research* (pp. 71–82). London: Sage.

Gillies, P. (1998). Effectiveness of alliances and partnerships for health promotion. *Health Promotion International, 13*(2), 99–120.

Hogan, M., Foreman, K., Naghavi, M. *et al.* (2010). Maternal mortality for 181 countries, 1980–2008: A systematic analysis of progress towards Millennium Development Goal 5. *The Lancet 375*(9726), 1609–1623.

Howarth, C. (2006). Race as stigma: Positioning the stigmatised as agents, not objects. *Journal of Community and Applied Social Psychology, 16*(6), 442–451.

Hunt, P. (2007a, December 3). *Oral Remarks to the Press in Delhi, India*. Retrieved from The UN Special Rapporteur on the Right to the Highest Attainable Standard of Health: Hunt, Paul. (2007a).h, http://www.essex.ac.uk/human_rights_centre/research/rth/

Hunt, P. (2007b, December 1). *Civil Society Meeting with UN Special Rapporteur on the Right to Health, Delhi December 1, 2007 from a report by Prasanta Tripathy, EKJUT*. Cited in Center for Reproductive Rights, letter to the Committee on Economic, Social and Cultural Rights, Re: Supplementary Information on India. Retrieved from http://www2.ohchr.org/english/bodies/cescr/docs/info-ngos/CFRRIndia40.pdf

IIMMHR (International Initiative on Maternal Mortality and Human Rights) (2009a). Voices from the Ground. Women users' analysis of maternal health policy. SAHAYOG, Retrieved from http://righttomaternalhealth.org/project/voices-from-the-ground

IIMMHR (International Initiative on Maternal Mortality and Human Rights) (2009b). About us, brochure. Retrieved from http://righttomaternalhealth.org/sites/iimmhr.civicactions.net/files/MMHR%20brochure%20revised.pdf

IIMMHR (International Initiative on Maternal Mortality and Human Rights) (2009c). Fact sheet: UN Human Rights Council Resolution on Maternal Mortality. Retrieved from http://righttomaternalhealth.org/hrc-resolution

Kawachi, I., Colditz, G., Ascherio, A., *et al.* (1996). A prospective study of social networks in relation to total mortality and cardiovascular disease in men in the USA. *Journal of Epidemiology and Community Health, 50*(3), 245–251.

Mead, G. (1934). *Mind, Self, and Society*. Chicago: University of Chicago Press.

MoHFW (Ministry of Health and Family Welfare) (2005). *Mission Document*. Retrieved from National Rural Health Mission: http://mohfw.nic.in/NRHM/Documents/NRHM%20Mission%20Document.pdf

MoHFW (2008a, March). *Uttar Pradesh*. Retrieved June 22, 2010, from http://www.mohfw.nic.in/NRHM/State%20Files/up.htm

MoHFW (2008b). *Rajasthan*. Retrieved June 19, 2010, from Health Indicators: http://mohfw.nic.in/NRHM/State%20Files/raj.htm

MoHFW (2008c). *District level household and facility survey III: Fact Sheet Uttarakhand*. Retrieved January 10, 2010, from International Institute for Population Science, Deemed University, Mumbai: http://nrhm-mis.nic.in/ui/reports/dlhsiii/UTTRAKHAND/STATE%20FACT%20SHEET/Uttarkhand-body.pdf

NFHS3 (National Family Health Survey 3) (2007). *V. I. Chapter 8. Maternal health*. Mumbai: International Institute for Population Sciences.

Ogden, J. (2007). *Health Psychology: A Textbook*. Buckingham: Open University Press.

Rappaport, J. (1987). Terms of Empowerment/Exemplars of Prevention: Toward a Theory for Community Psychology. *American Journal of Community Psychology, 15*(2), 121–148.

Scott, K. and Shanker, S. (2010). Tying their hands? Institutional Obstacles to the success of the ASHA community health worker program in rural north India. *AIDS Care* 22 (Supplement 2): 1606–1612.

Sen, G. (2009). Health inequalities: Gendered puzzles and conundrums. The 10th Annual Sol Levine Lecture on Society and Health, October 6, 2008. *Social Science and Medicine, 69*, 1006–1009.

Shiffman, J. and Ved, R. (2007). The state of political priority for safe motherhood in India. *BJOG*, 114, 785–790.

Spivak, G. (1988). Can the subaltern speak? In C. Nelson, and L. Grossberg (Eds.), *Marxism and the Interpretation of Culture* (pp. 271–313). Urbana/Chicago: University of Illinois Press.

Stephens, C. (2009). *Health Promotion: A Psycho-Social Approach*. Maidenhead: Open University Press.

Tawil, O., Verster, A., and O'Reilly, K. (1995). Enabling approaches for HIV/AIDS prevention: Can we modify the environment and minimise the risk? *AIDS, 9*, 1299–1306.

UNFPA (United Nations Population Fund) (2007, October 12). *Maternal Mortality Declining in Middle Income Countries*. Retrieved June 19, 2010, from Joint Press Release: http://www.unfpa.org/news/news/cfm?ID=1042

Vaughan, C. (2010). Dialogue, critical consciousness and praxis. In D. Hook, B. Franks, and M. Bauer (Eds.), *Social Psychology of Communication*. Basingstoke: Palgrave.

Vora, K., Mavalankar, D., Ramani, K. *et al.* (2009). Maternal Health Situation in India: A Case Study. *Journal of Health, Population and Nutrition, 27*(2), 184–201.

Wallack, L. (2003). The role of mass media in creating social capital: A new dirction in for public health. In R. Hofrichter (Ed.), *Health and Social Justice: Politics, Ideology, and Inequity in the Distribution of Disease* (594–625). San Francisco: Jossey-Bass.

WHO (2005). *The World Health Report 2005: Make Every Mother and Child Count*. Geneva: World Health Organisation.

WHO (2008). *Closing the Gap in a Generation: Health Equity through Action on the Social Determinants of Health*. Geneva: Commission on Social Determinants of Health.

Women Deliver (2010, June 5). *Maternal Health Conference Examines Progress, Challenges; Pushes Donors Toward US$12 Billion*. Retrieved from News: http://www.womendeliver.org/updates/entry/maternal-health-conference-examines-progress-challenges-pushes-donors-towar/

9

Health, News, and Media Information

Jesus Arroyave

Introduction

Information about health from media and news outlets has become essential in Western societies. Various studies have shown that people are more often exposed to health information through the mass media than through traditional sources of information, such as physicians or health facilities (Cho, 2006; Montgomery, 1990; Wyn, 1994). In fact, it is not unusual for the media to bolster dialogue between physician and patient (Newport, 2002), or become a topic of conversation among their audience, which further highlights the important role they play as a source of information about health issues (Parrott, 1996).

Although abundant health information is available through the media, numerous studies have shown that such information is not necessarily adequate for the audience to be thoroughly informed or to make educated decisions about their health (Frost, Frank, and Maiback, 1997; Hoffman-Goetz and Friedman, 2005; Rothblum, 1999; Signorielli, 1993; Vargas and de Pyssler, 1999). Over the past three decades, research on health-related issues in the media also has shown that information is deceptive (Frost, Frank, and Maibach, 1997; Heeter, Perlstadt, and Greenberg, 1984; Kennedy and Bero, 1999), inaccurate (Gerlach, Marino, and Hoffman-Goetz, 1997; Signorielli, 1993; Carlson, Li, and Holm, 1997), contradictory (Gannon and Stevens, 1998; Hoffman-Goetz and MacDonald, 1999), alarmist (Oxman, Guyatt, Cook, *et al.*, 1993; Moynihan *et al.*, 2000), incomplete (Tsao, 1997; Deary *et al.*, 1998; Sandvik, 1999; Kline, 1996), and outdated (Turow and Coe, 1985). Given these limitations, news coverage of health might create false perceptions and mislead the public about many health topics (Rothblum, 1999; Vargas and de Pyssler, 1999; Wilson and Blackhurst, 1999). Likewise, scholars have warned of several challenges in the way that coverage of health news is approached,

The Handbook of Global Health Communication, First Edition. Edited by Rafael Obregon and Silvio Waisbord.
© 2012 John Wiley & Sons, Inc. Published 2012 by John Wiley & Sons, Inc.

the type of sources that are used, and the ideology that they promote or reproduce, which have implications for the quality of information that the audience receives (Kline, 2003; Tanner, 2004).

The aim of this chapter is to offer a critical review of news media coverage of health. The sociology of news production offers valuable analytical insights for studying trends and characteristics of health coverage in the news media, for it addresses various factors that shape health information. In this chapter, news is conceived as the product of a socially constructed reality. Heider (2008), for instance, asserts that the day's news is a result of many policies, decisions, and circumstances. It is a social process, in part institutional culture, in part human dynamics. As a part of the sociology of news framework, one of the main assumptions of this chapter is that the dynamics of news production shape the content of health news, which, in turn, limits the quality of health information.

This chapter is organized as follows. The first section briefly discusses the analytical framework of the chapter. The second discusses findings and arguments in the literature using the four-level framework of the *hierarchy of influences model* (Reese, 2008). The discussion section offers an analytical summary of the findings and recommendations for improving health news coverage. The intention is not to offer a comprehensive survey of health news coverage, but rather to produce a critical assessment of news media coverage of health issues, and make sense of some of the practices that may impact the quality of health information in the news.

Conceptual Framework and Methodological Considerations

Understanding how health news is constructed and reported is critically important. As Wallack *et al.* (1999) have emphasized, health communicators must monitor the media in order to understand how health issues are portrayed and/or ignored, what aspects are emphasized, and what solutions are offered. This information is crucial to how audiences learn about health and understand certain health problems. Given the large amount of health information available through media outlets, many of which are advertisements or commercials, people might be persuaded to follow incorrect or incomplete healthcare suggestions instead of consulting professional resources.

Furthermore, the agenda-setting function of news media also plays an important role, as media can promote the discussion of certain health topics by placing them on the public agenda over others. In this case, how health issues are portrayed or approached in the media may either facilitate the development of favorable public opinions or incite negative sentiments regarding related public health policies. Indeed, news media have often in the past served as the catalyst for bringing key health issues requiring action to public attention.

Studies suggest that news media and media content influence audience cognition, attitudes, and behavior in regards to health (Collins *et al.*, 2005; Finnegan and Viswanath, 2002; Singhal and Rogers, 2002) and public policy. Misconceptions about disease and health may lead to inappropriate personal actions. Furthermore, when the media ignore a health issue, it may cause delays in the implementation of important public policy that could have a positive impact on public health. Therefore, it is important not only to analyze media content, as we have done in the past, but to go even further and try to understand the dynamics that produced such content. By understanding the motivations and pressures that led to the construction of health-related news, it is possible to develop a better understanding of the type of health care-related information presented by the media.

Most of the public might think the process of newspaper or newscast production is straightforward and simple: a journalist covers a specific topic, writes about it or produces a news story, and hands it over to the editor. However, as Heider (2008) explains, there are several forces, factors, and considerations that surround decisions about news production each day in every news organization. Whereas early interest in mass media research focused on content and effects, sociological perspectives have shifted their focus to organizational dynamics and structural conditions that affect news production (Hirsh, 1972; Tuchman, 1978; Gitlin, 1980). A series of key articles and a book have set the stage for what Whitney and Ettema (2006) call the "rediscovery" of mass communicators. As Whitney and Ettema (2006, p. 158) explain,

> This rediscovery of mass communicators among sociologists and political scientists was a rediscovery of old questions – but new answers. Beginning in the 1970s, "the limited effects model" – the idea that media had little influence on public opinion as articulated in Katz and Lazarsfeld's (1955) *Personal Influence* and Klapper's (1960) *Effects of Mass Communication* – was overturned in favor of models such as agenda-setting that allocated far more sociopolitical power to the mass media. This made the question of how media content is produced more urgent and interesting.

Various organizational aspects and social forces that influence news production became the focus of several studies. As Reese (2008) states, research in the realm of media production "has begun to allow the field of communication to devote the same sustained research to the creation, control and shape of the mediated environment as it has to the effects on audiences of that environment" (p. 1).

Scholars have developed categories to analyze how the symbolic environment of news production is shaped or constructed. Drawing on Gans (1979) and Gitlin (1980), Reese (2008) proposes the *hierarchy of influences model* to understand how different factors shape media content. In this model, Reese (2008) suggests that content is influenced by the following factors: (1) media workers' socialization and attitudes; (2) media organizations and routines; (3) other social institutions and forces; and (4) ideological positions and maintaining the status quo. In a classic study, Shoemaker and Reese (1996) suggested 5 levels of analysis in the construction of news: individual, routines, organizational, extramedia (institutional), and ideological (sociocultural). However, Whitney and Ettema (2006) proposed three levels of analysis: individual, organizational, and institutional. While these levels vary depending on the scope of the approach, what is clear is that they all interact and influence one another (Reese, 2008).

Reese's four levels of analysis offer a helpful framework for understanding the coverage and construction of health news. While numerous studies have been conducted to understand how news media cover health issues (i.e., using framing as a guiding concept), and several studies have drawn on the hierarchy of influences model to analyze news coverage broadly, to our knowledge, coverage of health news has not been analyzed through Reese's model. In the next section, where possible, the findings related to health news coverage are critically assessed through the levels of the *hierarchy of influences model* (Reese, 2008). While different frameworks could be used in analyzing health news, using the sociology of news production framework makes it possible to better understand the dynamics that occur in newsrooms and help to shape the news in the way they are created.

The selection of the research articles and academic items that serve as the basis for this analysis included the following steps. First, I retrieved articles published in the past five years from key communication databases (i.e., Com-abstracts, Com-index, and Sage index) using the key words "health news," "medical coverage," and "health information." Articles that did not report on specific research or studies on news coverage of health issues or that did not focus on news media were not included. Second, relevant articles and book chapters that were cited in the journal articles reviewed were also identified and used for further analysis. In sum, approximately 30 journal articles and 10 book chapters and other academic writings were reviewed for this critical analysis.

The focus of the analysis is on health news and information produced by the news media, and on available content and textual analyses regarding health news coverage in newspapers, local and national TV newscasts, and magazines. The following section reports on the findings related to media and health news information using Reese's four levels of analysis. The findings section is structured as follows. First, a brief description of each level of the hierarchy of influences model is provided, followed by a summary of key issues that emerge in the analysis.

Findings

1. Content is influenced by media workers' socialization and attitudes.
According to Reese (2008), this is a communicator-centered approach that emphasizes the psychological factors impinging on an individual's work: professional, personal, and political. This category could be related to Whitney and Ettema's (2006) *individual level*, in which the essential research question is the role of individual consciousness in symbol production.

One of the theoretical concepts that helps to understand this first level of analysis is framing theory, which is directly linked to media worker's socialization and psychological factors. Framing has emerged as a particular theoretical construction to understand how journalists report about different issues. Bryant and Miron (2004) affirm that framing is one of the most widely used theoretical concepts to analyze news media. Reese (2001) states that framing is a process through which social actors use symbolic means to structure the social world. Gitlin (1980) defines frames as "the principles of selection, emphasis and presentation composed of little tacit theories about what exists, what happens, and what matters" (p. 6). Cappella and Jamieson (1997) suggest that the ideas of selection and salience imply that framing is a way to draw attention to certain features of an issue while minimizing attention to others. Pan (2008) states that framing cannot be completely reduced to the cognitive level: "Selecting what to include or emphasize in a new story is often ideologically motivated and politically charged; new text, regardless which frame structures it, is a physical embodiment of an ideology and is embedded with organizational and institutional rules and procedures of news production" (para. 3).

Journalists might frame health news in many ways, emphasizing certain aspects and minimizing others. The current literature on how health information is framed reveals that journalists cover health issues by emphasizing aspects such as the consequences of particular diseases (Slater *et al.*, 2008; Shih, Wijaya, and Brossard, 2008), causes and treatment (Cho, 2006), actions against the disease (Shih, Wijaya, and Brossard, 2008), and the severity of the problem (De Souza, 2007), aspects that might lead the audience to relate to a frame that primarily focuses on disease.

A common framing device in the news media is to approach a health story in a way that emphasizes the consequences of a health issue rather than its prevention. Slater *et al.*, (2008) found that, when lung cancer was covered, death was the primary topic more often than any other. As a consequence, the authors state, "this relatively greater emphasis on death for lung cancer seems to suggest a similarly greater likelihood that those who read stories on lung cancer would be made aware of its lethal nature" (p. 534).

In similar fashion, Slater *et al.*, (2008) also found that news stories relating to breast cancer put greater emphasis on information about causes and treatment than information about prevention. As the authors report,

> There is only moderate coverage of screening-early detection options, such as the use of mammograms, the PSA test, or colonoscopy. This is particularly unfortunate, given that prevention and screening behaviors are actionable, and coverage related to prevention and screening might well stimulate such behaviors among news consumers (p. 535).

As mentioned earlier, how news is framed might have consequences on how the audience views a particular issue. As Slater *et al.*, (2008, p. 535) remark, "the greater emphasis put on treatment and lesser emphasis put on detection, screening, and prevention suggests a public conceptualization of cancer as something to be addressed after it occurs, not before."

However, depending on the type of media, researchers have found that it is possible to find different frames in regard to cancer coverage. For instance, Cho (2006), after examining breast cancer coverage on TV networks, found that diagnostic methods and possible causes were the most framed issues in news media in the last three decades. Andsager and Powers (1999) found that cancer prevention was the most frequently covered issue in both news magazines and women's magazines. However, there were differences in the way each news media framed the story. Women's magazines were more likely to use personal stories as a frame, whereas newsmagazines emphasized the economic frame, focusing on aspects such as insurance cover and political issues.

Shih, Wijaya, and Brossard (2008), after analyzing 688 news stories relating to health epidemics such as mad cow disease, West Nile virus, and avian flu published in the *New York Times* over a 10-year period (1996–2005), found that the two most frequent frames used by journalist to construct their stories were the "action frame" and the "consequence frame." In the action frame, the story stresses any action(s) against the disease, including prevention, potential solutions, or strategies. In the consequences frames, the focus of the story is on the consequences of the diseases, such as human lives lost, the social impact, or the economic impact (cost).

According to Shih and colleagues (2008, p. 154), these findings have important consequences:

> The fact that some frames appeared consistently across diseases' coverage resonates with the argument that journalists tend to use the same themes for stories of similar nature (Bennett, 2001). The predominance of the action and consequence frames also suggests that journalists concentrate their attention on substantive aspects of epidemic hazards.

Health news comes to the public through the particular lens in which the journalist framed the story. News is a construction and is influenced by what journalists have been taught is news, the values that they absorb in newsrooms, and by what they believe should be the emphasis of the story.

De Souza (2007), after analyzing the two most widely circulated English newspapers in India for a period of 14 months, found that news related to HIV/AIDS was framed under three main categories: (1) severity of the problem, (2) cause and solution, and (3) beliefs about who is at risk. As regards the first frame, "a constant resource used to indicate the severity of the HIV/AIDS problem is the war metaphor" (p. 260). Examples of that metaphor used in headlines are "Media pledges to fight AIDS menace" (*Times of India*, January 12, 2005), "Children, main weapons in battle" (*The Hindu*, December 2, 2004), "India sitting on AIDS time-bomb" (*The Hindu*, September 17, 2004), and "It's a never-ending battle at the jaws of death" (*The Hindu*, March 8, 2004). De Souza (2007) concludes that,

> Terms such as *time-bomb, enemy,* and *killer disease* are constantly used to characterize the nature of the HIV/AIDS problem, while terms such as *battle, combat, defense,* and *line of defense* are used to describe the strategies required to manage the problem. The metaphor suggests that HIV/AIDS is a visible enemy that can be destroyed (p. 260).

Language helps us to recreate reality. When journalists and communicators select and create such strong metaphors, what may resonate in the audience is that HIV/AIDS problem is something extreme and complex that produces losses and many injuries, like a war. And, like war, the solution is far from simple and beyond most people.

In regard to the second frame, De Souza found that the media in India emphasize aspects such as the "decline of cultural values" and decry the influence of Western culture as the cause of the HIV/AIDS problem. An excerpt that illustrates such an approach is: "A doctor in the Banswada Area Hospital, Narasimha Rao felt that the youth were falling prey to so many ills due to the impact of Western culture" (*The Hindu*, December 12, 2004).

As regards solutions to this problem, reports on condom promotion and antiretroviral treatment therapy are found in the newspaper, however, they do not focus on prevention but rather on showcasing *government-led* initiatives to manage the HIV/AIDS problem. The frame of cause and solution reflects the divergent cultural values and beliefs that coexist in contemporary India. As De Souza concludes (2008, p. 262),

On the one hand, there is the firm belief and pride in modern tools used to control health risks as seen in ART promotion, but on the other hand there is an equal push to revert to traditional values as a means of controlling health risks, as seen in arguments for moral education, and actors contend with each other about these issues.

Examining the frame of risk groups, De Souza contends that children, poor women, and married women are portrayed as victims of the HIV/AIDS problem. In the case of poor children, they are victimized because they lack access to basic structural resources and this creates the possibility of a higher susceptibility to HIV. In the case of poor and married women, likewise, structural deprivation, oppressive social norms, a poorly enforced legal system, and gender inequality are factors that predispose them to HIV/AIDS. While De Souza praises the fact that the news includes structural factors that shape the susceptibility of women and children to the disease, she also contends that "the gratuitous narratives seem to serve only as a casual reminder to the reader that "others" exist in the country despite the economic advancements of recent years" (p. 265).

While it is possible to identify many other frames in which health news is presented, the examples shown above illustrate a key point in regards to media production. A particular illness or health issue could be framed in multiple ways. Journalists may emphasize aspects that make the story more attractive and in this way grab the attention of the reader. However, this does not mean that such an approach will help the audience to understand the health issue and provide a clear orientation on that particular health topic.

Effects of news framing

Frames play a key role in health coverage, not only in shaping public perception, but also in influencing public policy response. According to Nathanson (1999), there are many possible frames for health risks that contribute to accelerating the interest of people who promote policies in regards to specific health issues. When a health risk is framed in a way that suggests it could have a great impact on a defenseless public, it gains the attention of policy makers as well as social movements, who eventually push for action. Nathanson (1999) suggests that there are three possible frames for public health risks that may influence a public policy response. These are: (1) when the health risk is portrayed as having been acquired deliberately or involuntarily; (2) when it is portrayed as "universal (putting us all at risk) or as particular (only putting *them* at risk)"; (3) when it is portrayed as "arising from within the individual or from the environment" (p. 446). Thus, once a health risk is framed as involuntary, universal, or environmental, the stir created in public opinion may bring about a public policy that causes a reaction among economic or political groups. As Lawrence (2004), drawing on Nathanson (1999), concludes, the more an issue is framed in terms of an involuntary risk, universal risk, environmental risk, or knowingly created risk, the more likely it is that the environment will be conducive to *public policy solutions* that *burden powerful groups.*

This finding has enormous implications for the way the media frame health-related news. This can be clearly seen in the topics of obesity, alcohol use, smoking, and adolescent pregnancy. When these issues are conceived as a matter of individual responsibility and as affecting only a particular group, they are treated as conditions that individuals should solve by themselves.

This is the case for the alcohol-related products that sponsor the most important sports competitions in some Latin American countries. In Colombia, in the past, most liquor and beer companies sponsored soccer teams. Most of the billboards and stadium advertisements and the radio and television programs that broadcast the matches, heavily advertised alcohol as the natural product to consume while watching the game. On the field, the players wore jerseys with the logos of alcoholic products. What is more, the most important Colombian beer company paid the players in the Colombian national team to raise their hands after a goal in order to use the image for a commercial.

While consuming alcohol was framed as an individual behavior of adults who watch soccer matches at the stadium or on TV, the ambience and environment surrounding the game heavily stimulated the consumption of alcohol. Likewise, alcohol consumption was associated with fights between sports fans and other public order problems. A clear example of this situation is provided by the celebrations following a match between Argentina and Colombia in 1993 that the Colombian team won 5–0. After the celebration that weekend, 80 people were dead, predominately as a result of accidents and injuries preceded by high levels of alcohol consumption.

Violence in Colombian soccer stadiums, often associated with alcohol, resulted in injuries to fans and innocent bystanders. When this public health issue was framed as environmental and public, public policy was enacted to deal with it. Alcohol-related products and billboards and posters advertising alcohol were forbidden in the stadiums. Likewise, alcohol-related products are no longer allowed to sponsor soccer teams. However, alcohol products continue to be the main product sponsors on radio and television sports programs as well as in newspapers.

In the same fashion, Nathanson (1999) highlights the case of the tobacco industry in the United States. When tobacco became defined as an involuntary, environmental, and universal risk, there was fertile ground for tight regulation. The anti-tobacco movement won the regulatory battles, once the idea gained hold that the health dangers from tobacco do not merely stem from the voluntary choices of individuals who smoke.

As Lawrence (2004), drawing on Nathanson (1999), explains, anti-tobacco activists drew upon new scientific evidence to call attention to the health risks of secondhand smoke. This discovery powerfully reframed public discourse by overturning the libertarian defense of smoking – that smoking was something harmful only to those who willingly assumed the risk. Thus, nonsmokers became "innocent victims" of tobacco who acquired the risks of smoking *involuntarily*. The consequences of smoking potentially extended to *everyone* rather than just to smokers, and arose from a smoke-filled *environment*, not just from private, individual choice.

As far as obesity is concerned, Lawrence (2004) distinguished several frames for this health issue in the media. It has, for instance, been conceived as a biological disorder. If that is the case, the causes are beyond the individual and the solution rests on medical discovery. As Lawrence (2004) reports, one obesity researcher recently told a *New York Times* reporter, "I think we should do what we do for high blood pressure and high cholesterol.... We give them [overweight people] a tablet. It's not their fault. They're designed to get fat" (p. 62).

However, when the health issue is conceived and framed from an individualistic perspective, the tendency to assign the entire blame to the individual is strong. While in the United States there is clear evidence of an environment that promotes fast food and all kinds of saturated food, there is the tendency to blame individuals for their obesity problem because they are responsible for their weight. Lawrence (2004) points out that blaming the individual is commonplace in the American culture, not just with respect to obesity but also to health issues such as lung cancer, alcoholism, AIDS, gun-related injuries, and death.

In her study of obesity and how it is framed in American news media, Lawrence (2004) offers an interesting perspective for the analysis of public-health-related issues based on the frame theory. She identifies a continuum that goes from an individualizing frame pole to a systemic frame pole. Individualizing frames "limit the causes of a problem to particular individuals, often those who are afflicted with the problem" (p. 57). At the other end of the scale are the systemic frames that "broaden the focus, assigning responsibility to government, business, and larger social forces" (p. 57).

Lawrence (2004, p. 57) proposes that the way that an issue is framed determines the degree to which public attention and public policy can be exerted.

> The closer the overall pattern of public discourse moves toward the systemic end of the continuum, the more conducive the environment will be for creating public policies that burden powerful groups and hold political institutions responsible for addressing the problem. Defining a problem in individualized terms limits governmental responsibility for addressing it, while systemic frames invite governmental action.

This approach helps us to understand the importance of the frame theory with regard to any public health issue. As theorists highlight, frame theory asserts that journalists emphasize certain aspects and underplay others. This leads to stressing the importance of journalists being well-trained and clarifying which points of view should prevail when reporting health issues. Seeing a health issue as an individual problem may limit the solution of the problem to the individual. Approaching the issue by analyzing the structural causes and the contextual component may provide a more complete picture. In order to solve it, other actors such as the government, the media industry, and public policy need to be involved.

2. Content is influenced by media organizations and routines.

Reese (2008) states that this approach argues that content emerges directly from the way that media work is organized. The organizational routines within which an individual operates form a structure, constraining action while also enabling it.

Shoemaker and Reese (1996) define media organizations as social, formal, and usually economic entities that employ media workers to produce media content. In most cases, the main goal of these organizations is to generate profit, especially by targeting audiences that are attractive to advertisers. Nonetheless, factors such as the size of the media organization, the fact of being a member of a specific network, and the kind of ownership are also relevant to everyday journalistic decisions.

News routines

Lowrey (2008) defined news routines as repeated practices and forms that make it easier for journalists to accomplish tasks and ensure immediacy in an uncertain world, while working within production constraints. News routines are created in response to the limited resources of the news organization and the vast amount of raw material that can be made into news (Shoemaker and Reese, 1966). According to Shoemaker and Reese (1966), the job of these routines is to deliver, within time and space limitations, the most acceptable product to the consumer in the most efficient manner.

Typically, the routine which is most frequently used in the newsroom is that of relying on official sources. Studies regarding the most common sources quoted in news items show that over half the sources are government officials and the next largest group is made up of spokespersons for business and industries (Berkowitz and Beach, 1993; Gil, Arroyave, and Soruco, 2006; Comrie, 1999). Conversely, Soley (2008) asserts that, "Studies of news sources show that women, minorities, labor union representatives, and other less powerful groups are underrepresented compared to their number in the population." While this provides trustworthy status to the information being divulged to the public, it also reflects how the official voice has the power to shape the news agenda.

The characteristics of news related to health or medical issues pose certain challenges for news reporters. Due to the complex nature of medical and scientific information, health news reporting demands technical knowledge that is sometimes, owing to newsroom routines or the lack of specialization of a media professional, beyond the reporters who ordinarily cover health news. As a result, there are circumstances such as time constraints that lead most health journalists to rely on material from the scientific community or corporate industry, often in the form of press releases or public relations initiatives (Entwistle, 1995; Tanner, 2004). This excessive source dependency poses certain problems that sometimes translate into a lack of quality in the content of health information.

For instance, in a nationwide study conducted on local television health reporters, Tanner (2004) found that over 50 percent stated that they received most of their ideas from a "public relations spokesperson who personally contacted them with a story idea" (p. 356). Press releases were the second most popular manner in which journalists received ideas for health stories. In a similar fashion, Entwistle (1995) found that 86 percent of all medical stories began as a press releases from two medical journals, *The Lancet* or the *British Medical Journal*.

While excessively relying on one type of source tends to be problematic, the kind of sources journalists use poses another concern. They tend to prefer elite sources mostly. Literature about the topic reports that health news overemphasizes official sources such as government officials and health organizations, which prevents the audience from obtaining a broader perspective on a particular issue (Signorielli, 1993; Nelkin, 1995). Nelkin (1995) reported that the use of elite news sources prevented the audience from being exposed to other sources that might have a different view on the same issue. It seems that the polyphony of voices that allows the audience to have a wide range of approaches to and perspectives on a topic is not always present in health news coverage.

Because the nature of the job imposes strict deadlines and requirement to fill up a certain amount of space as part of their daily routine, journalists can be attracted to sources that are easily available and offer a translation of complex scientific health knowledge for a general audience. Likewise, a source with a recognized institutional background tends to eclipse other possible sources. This dependency may cause journalists not to question the information provided by the source. When working in the type of conditions that journalists do, a key source that helps solve informational issues is an asset that is worth keeping.

Likewise, news routines may affect the way health news is presented and portrayed in most media. While a particular health issue that emerges as news may be of interest to the audience because of its implications for them, owing to certain media routines, such as heavy reliance on attractive images in order to put news content across, this information may not be able to be presented because it does not fit with certain media. For instance, TV newscasts emphasize images that support the news. If there are none available or those that are available are hard to use, it is most likely that this information will not be presented. According to Slater (2008), after breast cancer, "the second-leading cancer in terms of attention in the news varies by medium: colon cancer is second in newspapers and prostate cancer is second in TV and magazines ... it may be that the visual emphasis of magazines and TV made colon cancer a less attractive candidate for coverage" (p. 534).

News values

News values is a category in the sociology of news production that allows us to understand why, among the myriads of issues available, certain topics are selected and others are ignored. According to McQuail (2005), three main factors influence selection, and they are organizational, genre-related, and sociocultural in nature. As regards the first, the selection of news depends on whether the event fits the machinery of selection and retransmission. Typically, this means that events that occur near the reporting facilities (i.e., cosmopolitan centers) are favored. Genre-related factors include a preference for news that fits audience expectation (i.e., consonance with past news) and can be placed within a familiar interpretative frame. Sociocultural influences relate to certain Western values that focus on individuals and involve an interest in the elite and also in negative, violent, and dramatic happenings. McQuail (2005) highlights values such as large-scale events, closeness to home, clarity of meaning, relevance, consonance, drama and action as the ones that prevail in most Western media (p. 310).

The concept of *news value* from the literature of news production may help us to understand why certain topics are neglected while others are overreported. In an analysis in 1999 and 2000 of the two most prestigious medical journals in Britain (*The Lancet* and the *British Medical Journal*) that serve as the basis for press releases that were subsequently reported in newspapers, Bartlett, Sterne, and Egger, (2002) found evidence for McQuail's assertion in regard to news selection. For instance, (1) journal articles reporting randomized controlled trails and observational studies were more likely to be press-released, but randomized trials were substantially less likely to be covered in the newspapers; (2) although good news and bad news were equally likely to be released to the press, bad news was more likely to appear in the newspapers; (3) research focusing on elderly people was proportionately represented in press releases, but ignored by the newspapers; (4) studies from the United Kingdom were more likely to be reported in the newspapers than studies from other industrialized countries. Studies from developing countries were practically ignored in the newspapers.

As Bartlett, Sterne, and Egger (2002, p. 84) concluded,

> We are concerned that many aspects of medical research are not well represented in newspapers. Randomized trials provided the strongest evidence in many situations, but are seldom regarded as newsworthy by journalists. Newspapers have a role to play in health care-for example, by explaining the importance of evidence from randomized controlled trial, dispelling the misconceptions and confusion that surround the concepts of randomized and equipoise.

Since the end of the 1970s, various studies have warned about problems in regard to media health coverage. For instance, a content analysis by Smith *et al.* (1972) of 130 hours of programming for a television network, found that major health problems such as cancer, heart disease, stroke, and hepatitis were practically ignored (Signorielli, 1990). In a similar fashion, Freimuth *et al.* (1984) and Greenberg, Freimuth, and Bratic (1979) reported that cancer was rarely the primary focus of a story in national newspapers. In Africa, Pratt, Ha, and Pratt (2002) found that among the five major infectious diseases mentioned in popular magazines and medical journals, only two diseases – HIV/AIDS and malaria – increased in coverage between 1981 and 1997, while the others were hardly covered by the press.

As McQuail (2005) explains, since lengthy explanations of health processes are not part of the machinery of selection and retransmission, research methods that are highly valued in the area of medical investigation such as randomized trials are practically ignored by journalists. Likewise, news that is consonant with past events or close to home is what prevails. Therefore, many other illnesses, health topics, important discoveries reported in other countries do not always fit the criteria for health values, and therefore are not publicized. Further, diseases that demand complex knowledge but do not fit within the frame of violent and dramatic events are less attractive for reporting. As a result, the public do not receive, or are not made aware of, this important information.

On the other hand, lack of training in the health and medical area may lead reporters to provide inaccurate information, even if they are reporting directly from scientific sources. For instance, Kline (2003) reports that of 113 citations of a scientific study on breast cancer and mammography in popular media articles, 60 were traceable to the original report. Of these 60, 42 contained content-based inaccuracies. Likewise, major health diseases reports in the media do not correspond with reality. As Cohen *et al.* (2008) found, "newspaper coverage overreported (relative to mortality rates) on breast cancer and underreported on lung, colon, and prostate cancers (pp. 433–434).

In a similar fashion, studies found that news about different health issues does not provide enough information to lead audiences to take particular actions in order to improve public health. In a content analysis of 15 years of coverage of organ donation in the leading television newscast, Quick *et al.* (2009) found that the three most important television networks in the United States rarely (less that 10 percent of content) cited ways to become a potential organ donor. Vargas and de Pyssler (1999) found that Latino publications rarely dealt with subjects such as disease prevention or public health.

A study by Lebow (1999) affirms that major US newspapers, when reporting on oral contraceptives, tend to report inconclusive studies that link oral contraceptives to breast cancer, ignoring overwhelming evidence in many studies showing that oral contraceptives do not increase the risk of breast cancer.

While mobilization of information is crucial when it comes to offering a course of action to the audience, the health advice given is often contradictory. African-American newspapers in the United States present stories that include not only personally mobilizing information when covering cancer stories, but also information that is locally relevant (Cohen *et al.*, 2008). This is not the case in other countries. For instance, Hoffman-Goetz and Friedman (2005) found that in Canada, in both ethnic minority magazines and general audience publications, few newspaper stories on cancer coverage contained mobilizing information to help the reader take action to reduce his or her risk.

Many of the problems mentioned above are associated with media organization and publication processes. Given the large amount of news that journalists handle and the limited time available to process it, inaccuracies and misconceptions can be found in the end product even when material is reported directly from scientific articles. Although journalists use elite sources to translate scientific findings into lay language, it is important to realize that these sources are not the only ones that may address a health issue. This tendency to use elite sources reveals a certain sociological environment in which the agendas of the government and well-known private health institutions prevail.

3. Content is influenced by other social institutions and forces

This approach finds the major impact on content located external to organizations and the communicator, namely in economic, political, and cultural forces (Reese, 2008). Scholars have coined terms such as events and pseudo-events to highlight how external forces may impact news content. "Pseudo-events" is a term coined by Boorstin (1961) and refers to "synthetic news." These are events that do not occur spontaneously but are planned with the purpose of getting media coverage. Scherer (2008) differentiates media events from pseudo-events on the basis of the ceremonious character of the latter. They are subject to media-related staging, to a mise-en-scène by the media for the viewers, to the telling of a story.

According to Scherer (2008), pseudo-events are staged to attract media attention and, therefore, most are strategic communication and public relations exercises. Their goal is to promote specific interests and needs, often those of the party that facilitates their production. For example, media events such as the Olympic Games and Academy Awards ceremonies are predictable for the media and are staged to gain the highest possible media interest. In both cases they are created with the ulterior motive of promoting specific aims and are not genuine "news" events.

As the evidence shows, different aspects of news production play a key role in the way health news is constructed. Official sources and pseudo-events in the form of press releases and public relations initiatives seem to carry a heavy weight in the information that permeates most newsrooms. While it is clear that official health organizations and big corporations such as pharmaceutical companies want to inform the public of any health discovery or scientific advance, it is also clear that journalists should play an active role in evaluating and validating the information that they receive from their sources.

Since public relations departments, press releases, and communication departments play an increasingly active role in newsrooms, it seems that journalists are assuming a passive role. As was previously discussed, press releases created and distributed by elite sources are the beginning of many health news stories, leading reporters to passively depend on them. For instance, Schwitzer (1992) found that 90 percent of medical stories originate from public relations sources.

Media scholars have coined a very interesting category to reflect this pervasive influence in most newsrooms, the *passive news discovery process*. Originally established by McManus (1990), it seems that this process plays a key role in directing the content and the kind of information that many news media outlets air or print. As Tanner (2004) explains, the passive news process suggests that "public relations and promotions from governments and big corporations may help build the public agenda by giving news professionals the information needed to cover a story with minimal costs to the news organizations" (p. 353).

As seen previously, the theory of news production states that pseudo-events are not genuine and respond to the particular interest of the party that facilitates the production. Given the increase in the importance of press releases, press conferences, and direct information from pharmaceutical and official health sources on the content of news media, this phenomenon deserves special attention with regard to the kind of information that is ultimately transmitted to the audience. There is a potential danger that this *passive news discovery process* will allow public and private sources to have direct influence on most newsrooms.

4. Content is a function of ideological positions and maintains the status quo

Reese (2008) emphasizes that the hegemony approach defines major influence on media content as pressure to support the status quo, i.e., to support the interests of those in power in society. According to this critical perspective, elite ideas tend to dominate and circulate widely in most social contexts.

Through different ideological mechanisms in every social system, there are different sectors close to power that tend to impose what critical scholars have called the dominant ideology. Most of the time, this ideology serves to reproduce and maintain the *status quo*. Mass media, as a part of the social system, serve as the vehicle by which this dominant position is divulged and spread. However, this hegemonic position is sometimes challenged, mostly by independent and alternative media.

Consequently, according to this approach, most health media information tends to reproduce the dominant health system ideology – in other words, the hegemonic position of the health system is the one that prevails in most media outlets. As a result, the *status quo* in this realm is rarely questioned. Likewise, findings that are reported from elite health sources are seldom challenged, which means that the audience predominantly receives one side of the story relating to health news.

The medical community, as part of the elite, exerts control over health information in most media outlets. As Gandy (1982) states, those in the health care industry to a large extent control the formulation of health policy through their ability to define problems, specify alternatives, and choose between benefits and costs. Corbett and Mori (1999) mention that, "the interdependencies between medicine, government, insurance companies, and private business reinforce the dominant ideology and the role of physicians as providers of medical information" (p. 230). Therefore, physicians and health researchers are considered natural sources in the realm of health information.

However, such elite sources tend to reproduce the dominant ideas of the health system. For instance, Fisher, Gandy, and Janus (1981), as reported by Corbett and Mori (1999), noted similarities during a 15-year period in peaks of news coverage about heart disease and peaks in the budget of the National Heart and Lung Institute. Likewise, Entwistle (1995), after interviewing medical journalists from the most important British newspapers, concluded that, "Medical correspondents on quality newspapers rely quite heavily on a few journals as sources of medical research news, so the publication policies of these journals largely determine the pool of information from which stories are selected." Logan (1991) reported that medicine media coverage implies support for the scientific and political agenda of the nation health care delivery system. This evidence led Corbett and Mori (1999) to conclude that "health coverage strongly resembles the priority of the medical community" (p. 231).

Discussion

News information and the media are one of the most important sources of health information in most Western countries. UNAIDS estimates that people receive about 70 percent of their information about health through the media (2004). Researchers have come to the conclusion that the quality of health information that people receive might affect what they think and believe about health, which, in turn, might lead them to take certain actions. Therefore, the quality of health information is crucial for the audience.

The aim of this chapter was to explore how media and news information cover and report health news. The analytical framework used for this chapter was the sociology of the news production, in particular the four levels of the hierarchy of influences model (Reese, 2008). By exploring different factors that surround the production of news it was possible to identify limitations, constraints, and key circumstances that affect and shape health news and how health news stories are constructed and delivered to the public. This section summarizes key findings and proposes some recommendations for further research and practice on coverage of health news.

In regard to *socialization and attitudes*, health news is framed from a broad variety of perspectives. For instance, how journalists report health issues may lead the audience to associate certain ideas with a particular disease. When the predominant frame for lung cancer is death, the audience may think that that is the only view of this disease (Slater, 2008). Likewise, from the perspective of effects, when the individualistic frame prevails with regard to public health issues such as tobacco, obesity, or alcohol consumption, the solution tends to focus on the individual and not on the society as a whole. Thus, health organizations that work with journalists and journalists themselves should be aware of the kind of frame that prevails when health news is reported, since it could leave a lasting impression.

As far as *media organizations and routines* are concerned, given the complex nature of journalism and the deadlines and time constraints under which most journalists work, inaccuracy, misreporting, and limited or local information are sometimes found in news content. Certain reporting practices and values that are common in most newsrooms may prevent the audience from obtaining accurate and important health information. Complex health research findings that demand technical knowledge and do not resemble dramatic events are not common in news media. Likewise, key international medical research is also excluded. The tendency to rely on the medical community leads journalists to not only become less autonomous but also to report what the elite community deem as important. These particularities of *media organization and news routines* interfere with the quality of health information that is published or aired in different media outlets.

This leads us to a discussion of the professionalism needed for health news production. Although it is clear that, because of the nature of their job, journalists may follow certain procedures and routines that are common in newsrooms and help them to resolve issues and conflicts and to meet deadlines, it is important to remember that media are a source of public information and have a social responsibility. A well-trained health journalist should work beyond the constraints and limitations imposed by news production practices and make autonomous decisions about the topics that he or she wants to report in order to provide the best and most accurate factual content for the audience.

Regarding *content influenced by other social institutions and forces,* pseudo-events such as press releases and press conferences seem to be vital to most health news. This *passive news discovery process* constitutes a tremendous challenge to health news reporters. It resembles the concept of agenda building, in which news media reflect and shape the priorities and points of view of government officials, elites, and decision makers. Nisbet (2008) critically argues that "media agendas tend to pay close attention only to the events, political figures and issues that favor the interest of elites and that fall within a narrow range of political perspectives" (para. 6).

When journalists assume a *passive role* in reporting health news, they are relinquishing a big responsibility to corporations and elite organizations. Although many of them work to protect and support actions that contribute to public health, there is no guarantee that all of them work for people's best interests instead of for their own. Likewise, not only does the habit of using elite and official sources prevent the audience from obtaining a broad perspective on health information, it also limits the details that the public deserves to see. Opportune and valuable health information could be crucial in enabling people to take the correct action regarding their own health.

This brings us to the final point – that *content is a function of ideological positions and maintains the status quo.* Most of the information that is transmitted to the audience is aligned with the interests of most elite sources. Accordingly, most health issues are related to medical aspects such as (1) hospital medicine, and research that is heavily sponsored by elite institutions, and (2) information disseminated by key health institutions through press releases. However, aspects such as structural causes of illness and the societal problems related to them are much less commonly covered in the health news. Since the media are conceived as a part of the social system, structural problems that affect the public and demand change are not disseminated.

While this study reveals the role that various factors play in affecting the quality of health news through different media outlets, more studies need to be done that draw on the hierarchy of influences model, particularly with regard to influences three and four. From a qualitative perspective, it is possible to explore some of the motivations of reporters covering certain health issues but not others. Through survey, the dynamics of newsrooms could be analyzed, identifying routines that journalists may internalize while working within a news organization. Both qualitative and quantitative analysis from the sociology of news production approach could be crucial for public health organizations. If people obtain information about health issues through journalists and media, it is beneficial for health organizations to work with news media by offering special support for journalists. This collaboration will guarantee better media coverage and presentation of health information as well as facilitate the development of important public health policies.

Citizens need quality health information that can help them make informed decisions and the right choices in regard to their own health, and news media play a key role in providing such quality information. By acknowledging that news is a socially constructed reality that is influenced by many forces and circumstances, a better understanding of how health news is reported emerges. Education, independence, autonomy, and aware-ness of their role in shaping public opinion and perspectives should be qualities that journalists strive to achieve when reporting health news.

References

Andsager, J. L. and Powers, A. (1999). Social or economic concerns: How news and women's magazines framed breast cancer in the 1990s. *Journalism and Mass Communication Quarterly*, *76*(3), 531–550.

Bartlett, C., Sterne, J. and Egger, M. (2002). What is newsworthy? Longitudinal study of the reporting of medical research in two British newspapers. *British Medical Journal* 325, 81–84.

Berkowitz, D. and Beach, D. (1993). Newspaper sources and news context: The role of routine news, conflict, and proximity. *Journalism Quarterly, 70*, 4–12.

Boorstin, D. J. (1961). *The Image, or What Happened to the American Dream*. London: Weidenfeld and Nicolson.

Bryant, J. and Miro, D. (2004). Theory and research in mass communication. *Journal of Communication, 54*(4), 662–704.

Cappella, J. N. and Jamieson, K. H. (1997). *The Spiral of Cynicism: The Press and the Public Good*. New York: Oxford University Press.

Carlson, E. S., Li, S., and Holm, K. (1997). An analysis of menopause in the popular press. *Health Care Woman International 18*(6), 557–564.

Cho, S. (2006). Network news coverage of breast cancer, 1974 to 2003. *Journalism and Mass Communication Quarterly, 83*(1), 116–130.

Cohen, E. L., Caburnay, C. A., Luke, D. A. *et al.* (2008). Cancer coverage in general-audience and black newspapers, *Health Communication, 23*(5), 427–435.

Collins, R. L., Marc N. E., Berry, S. H., Kanouse, D. E. and Hunter, S. (2003). Entertainment television as a healthy sex educator: The impact of condom efficacy information in an episode of Friends. *Pediatrics, 112*(5), 115–121.

Comrie, M. (1999). Television news and broadcast deregulation in New Zealand. *Journal of Communication, 49*(2), 42–53.

Corbett, J. B. and Mori, M. (1999). Medicine, media, and celebrities: News coverage of breast cancer, 1960–1995. *Journalism and Mass Communication Quarterly 76*(2), 229–249.

Deary I, J., Whiteman M. C., and Fowkes, F. G. (1998). Medical research and the popular media. *The Lancet 351*, 1726–1727.

De Souza, R. (2007). The Construction of HIV/AIDS in Indian newspapers: A frame analysis. *Health Communication, 21*(3), 257–266.

Entwistle, V. (1995). Reporting research in medical journals and newspapers. *British Medical Journal 310*(6984), 920–923.

Finnegan, J. R., and Viswanath, K. (2002). Communication theory and health behavior change. In K. Glanz, F. Lewis, and B. Rimer (Eds.), *Health Behavior and Health Education: Theory, Research and Practice* (pp. 361–388). San Francisco, CA: Jossey-Bass, Inc.

Fisher, J., Gandy, O., and Janus, N. (1981). The role of popular media in defining sickness and health. In E. G. McAnany, J. Schnitman, and N. Janus (Eds.), *Communication and Social Structure: Critical Studies in Mass Media Research* (pp. 240–262). New York: Praeger.

Freimuth, V. S., Greenberg, R. H., DeWitt, J., and Romano, R. M. (1984). Covering cancer: Newspapers and the public interest. *Journal of Communication, 34*, 62–73.

Frost, K., Frank, E., and Maibach, E. (1997). Relative risk in the news media: A quantification of misrepresentation. *American Journal of Public Health, 87*, 842–845.

Gandy, O. H. (1982). *Beyond Agenda-Setting: Information Subsidies and Public Policy.* Norwood, NJ: Ablex.

Gannon, L. and Stevens, J. (1998). Portraits of menopause in the mass media. *Women and Health, 27*(3), 1–15.

Gans, H. J. (1979). *Deciding What's News: A Study of CBS Evening News, NBC Nightly News, Newsweek and* Time. New York: Pantheon Books.

Gerlach, K. K., Marino, C., and Hoffman-Goetz, L. (1997). Cancer coverage in women's magazines: What information are women receiving? *Journal of Cancer Education, 12*(4), 240–244. In T. L. Thompson, A. Dorsey, K. I. Miller, R. Parrot (Eds.), *Handbook of Health Communication* (pp. 557–581). Mahwah, NJ: Lawrence Erlbaum Associates.

Gil, J., Arroyave, J., and Soruco, G. (2006). Covering Chávez in US media: How elite newspaper reports a controversial international figure. *Investigación y Desarrollo 14*(2), 240–267.

Gitlin, T. (1980). *The Whole World Is Watching: Mass Media in the Making and Unmaking of the New Left.* Berkeley, CA: University of California Press.

Greenberg, R., Freimuth, V. S., and Bratic, R. (1979). A content analytic study of newspaper coverage of cancer. In D. Nimmo (Ed.), *Communication Yearbook 3* (pp. 645–654). New Brunswick, NJ: Transaction Books.

Heeter, C., Perlstadt, H., and Greenberg, B. S. (1984). Health incidents, stages of illness and treatment on popular television programs. Paper presented at the annual convention of the International Communication Association. San Francisco, CA.

Heider, D. (2008). Construction of reality through the news. In W. Donsbach (Ed.), *The International Encyclopedia of Communication.* Oxford: Blackwell Publishing. Oxford: Blackwell Reference Online. Retrieved from http://www.blackwellreference.com/subscriber/tocnode?id=g9781405131995_yr2010_chunk_g97814051319958_ss129-1

Hirsch, P. M. (1972). Processing fads and fashions: An organization-set analysis of cultural industry systems. *American Journal of Sociology, 77*, 639–659.

Hoffman-Goetz, L. and Friedman, D. B. (2005). Disparities in coverage of cancer information in ethnic minority and mainstream print media. *Ethnicity and Disease, 15*, 332–340.

Hoffman-Goetz, L. and MacDonald, M. (1999). Cancer coverage in mass-circulating Canadian women's magazines. *Canadian Journal of Public Health, 90*, 55–59.

Katz, E. and Lazarsfeld, P. R. (1955). *Personal Influence.* New York: Cooper Square Publishers.

Kennedy, G. E., and Bero, L. A. (1999). Print media coverage of research on passive smoking. *Tobacco control,* 8(3), 254–260. In T. L. Thompson, A. Dorsey, K. I. Miller, and R. Parrot (Eds.), *Handbook of Health Communication* (pp. 557–581). Mahwah, NJ: Lawrence Erlbaum Associates.

Klapper, J. T. (1960). *Effects of Mass Communication.* New York: Free Press.

Kline, K. N. (1996). The drama of *in utero* drug exposure: Fetus takes first billing. In R. L. Parrot and C. M. Condit (Eds.), *Evaluating Women's Health Messages: A Resource Book* (pp. 61–75). Thousand Oaks, CA: Sage.

Kline, K. N. (2003). Popular media and health: Images, effects, and institutions. In T. Thompson, A. Dorsey, K. Miller, and R. Parrott (Eds.), *Handbook of Health Communication* (pp. 557–581). Mahwah, NJ: Lawrence Erlbaum Associates.

Lawrence, R. G. (2004). Framing obesity: The evolution of news discourse on a public health issue. *The Harvard International Journal of Press/Politics 9,* 56–75.

Lebow, M. A. (1999). The pill and the press: Reporting risk. *Obstetrics and Gynecology,* 93(3), 453–456.

Logan, R. A. (1991). Popularization versus secularization: Media coverage of health. In L. Wilkins and P. Patterson (Eds.), *Risky Business: Communicating Issues of Science, Risk, and Public Policy* (pp. 44–59). New York: Greenwood Press.

Lowrey, W. (2008). News routines. In W. Donsbach (Ed.), *The International Encyclopedia of Communication.* Oxford: Blackwell Reference Online. Retrieved from http://www.blackwellreference.com/subscriber/tocnode?id=g9781405131995_yr2010_chunk_g978140513199519_ss28-1

McManus, J. (1990). How local television learns what is news. *Journalism Quarterly* 67(4): 672–683.

McQuail, D. (2005). *Mass Communication Theory,* 5th edn. London: Sage.

Montgomery, K. C. (1990). Promoting health through entertainment television. In C.K. Atkin and L. Wallack (Eds.), *Mass Communication and Public Health: Complexities and Conflicts* (pp. 114–128). Newbury Park, CA: Sage.

Moynihan, R., Bero, L., Ross-Degnan, D. *et al.* (2000). Coverage by the news media of the benefits and risks of medications. *New England Journal of Medicine, 342,* 1645–1650.

Nathanson, C. A. (1999). Social movements as catalysts for policy change: The case of smoking and guns. *Journal of Health, Politics, and Law,* 24(3), 421–488.

Nelkin, D. (1995). *Selling Science. How the Press Covers Science and Technology.* New York: W. H. Freeman and Company.

Newport, F. (2002). *Americans Get Plenty of Health News on TV, But Tend Not To Trust It.* Princeton, NJ: The Gallup Organization. Retrieved from http://www.gallup.com/poll/6883/americans-get-plenty-health-news-tv-tend-trust.aspx

Nisbet. M. C. (2008). Agenda building. In W. Donsbach (Ed.), *The International Encyclopedia of Communication.* Oxford: Blackwell Reference Online. Retrieved from http://www.blackwellreference.com/subscriber/tocnode?id=g9781405131995_yr2010_chunk_g97814051319956_ss35-1

Oxman, A. D., Guyatt, G. H., Cook, D. J. *et al.* (1993). An index of scientific quality for health reports in the lay press. *Journal of Clinical Epidemiology, 46,* 987–1001.

Pan, Z. (2008). Framing of news. In W. Donsbach (Ed.), *The International Encyclopedia of Communication.* Oxford: Blackwell Reference Online. Retrieved from http://www.blackwellreference.com/subscriber/tocnode?id=g9781405131995_yr2010_chunk_g978140513199511_ss42-1

Parrott, R. (1996). Advocate or adversary? The self-reflexive roles of media message for health. *Critical studies in Mass Communication,* 13(3), 226–278.

Pratt, C. B., Ha, L., and Pratt, C. A. (2002). Setting the public agenda on major diseases in sub-Saharan Africa: African popular magazines and medical journals, 1981–1997. *Journal of Communication, 52*(4), 889–904.

Quick, B. L., Kim, D. K., and Meyer, K. (2009). A 15-year review of ABC, CBS, and NBC news coverage of organ donation: Implications for organ donation campaigns. *Health Communication, 24*(2), 137–145.

Reese, S. D. (2001). Prologue – Framing public life: A bridging model for media research. In S. D. Reese, O. H. Gandy, and A. E. Grant (Eds.), *Framing public life: Perspectives on media and our understanding of the social world* (pp. 7–31). Mahwah, NJ: Lawrence Erlbaum Associates.

Reese, S. D. (2008). Media production and content. In W. Donsbach (Ed.), *The International Encyclopedia of Communication*. Oxford: Blackwell Reference Online. Retrieved from http://www.blackwellreference.com/subscriber/tocnode?id=g9781405131995_yr2010_chunk_g978140513199518_ss49-1

Rothblum, E. M. (1999). Contradictions and confounds in coverage of obesity: Psychology journals, textbooks, and the media. *Journal of Social Issues, 55*(2), 335–469.

Sandvick, H. (1999). Health information and interaction on the internet: A survey of female urinary incontinence. *British Medical Journal, 319*(7201), 29–32.

Scherer, H. (2008). Media events and pseudo-events. In W. Donsbach (Ed.), *The International Encyclopedia of Communication*. Oxford: Blackwell Reference Online. Retrieved from http://www.blackwellreference.com/subscriber/tocnode?id=g9781405131995_yr2010_chunk_g978140513199518_ss36-1

Schwitzer, G. (1992). The magical medical media tour. *Journal of the American Medical Association 267*(14): 1969–1972.

Shih, T., Wijaya, R., and Brossard, D. (2008). Media coverage of public health epidemics: Linking framing and issue attention cycle toward an integrated theory of print news coverage of epidemics. *Mass Communication and Society, 11*(2), 141–160.

Signorielli, N. (1993). *Mass Media Images and Impact on Health: A Sourcebook*. Westport, CT: Greenwood.

Singhal, A., and Rogers, E. M. (2002). A theoretical agenda for entertainment education. *Communication theory, 12*, 117–135.

Shoemaker, P. and Reese, S. (1996). *Mediating the Message: Theories of Influences on Mass Media Content*, 2nd edn. White Plains, NY: Longman.

Slater, M. D., Long, M., Bettinghaus, E. P., and Reineke, J. B. (2008). News coverage of cancer in the United States: A national sample of newspapers, television, and magazines. *Journal of Health Communication. 13*(6), 523–537.

Smith, F. A., Trivax, G., Zuehlke, D. A. *et al.* (1972). Health information during a week of television. *New England Journal of Medicine, 286*(10), 516–520.

Soley, L. (2008). News sources. In W. Donsbach (Ed.), *The International Encyclopedia of Communication*. Oxford: Blackwell Reference Online. Retrieved from http://www.blackwellreference.com/subscriber/tocnode?id=g9781405131995_yr2010_chunk_g978140513199519_ss29-1

Tanner, A. (2004). Agenda building, source selection, and health news at local television stations: A nationwide survey of local television health reporters. *Science Communication 25*(4), 350–363.

Tsao, J. C. (1997). Informational and symbolic content of over-the-counter drug advertising on television. *Journal of Drug Education, 27*(2), 173–197.

Tuchman, G. (1978). *Making News: A Study in the Construction of Reality*. New York: The Free Press.

Turow, J. and Coe, L. (1985). Curing television ills: The portrayal of health care. *Journal of Health Communication, 35*(4), 36–51.

Vargas, L. C. and de Pyssler, B. J. (1999). U.S. Latino Newspapers as Health Communication Resources: A Content Analysis. *The Howard Journal of Communications 10*(3), 189–205.

Wallack, L., Woodruff, K., Dorfman, L., and Diaz, I. (1999). *News for a Change: An Advocate's Guide to Working with the Media.* Thousand Oaks, CA: Sage.

Whitney, D. C., and Ettema, J. M. (2006). Media production: Individuals, organizations and institutions. In A. N. Valdivia (Ed.), *A Companion to Media Studies.* Malden, MA: Blackwell Publishing.

Wilson, N. L., and Blackhurst, A. E. (1999). Food advertising and eating disorders: Marketing body dissatisfaction, the drive for thinness, and dieting in women's magazines. *Journal of Humanistic Counseling, Education and Development, 38*(2), 111–122.

Wyn, J. (1994). Young women and sexually transmitted diseases: The issues for public health. *Australian Journal of Public Health 18,* 32–39.

10

Using Complexity-Informed Communication Strategies to Address Complex Health Issues
The Case of Puntos de Encuentro, Nicaragua

Virginia Lacayo

Over the years, most development professionals and organizations that I have exchanged ideas with about social change agree that social change is a nonlinear, long-term, and often unpredictable process requiring efforts at multiple levels. However, most organizations continue to frame their strategies in measurable, cause–effect terms, as if their programs can be evaluated in isolation from other efforts, and can demonstrate effectiveness in the short term. This paradox characterizes the field of communication for social change.

For 12 years (1992 to 2004) I worked at a Nicaraguan NGO called *Puntos de Encuentro* ("Meeting Points" or "Common Grounds"), a feminist nonprofit organization that believes in the role of communication, research, and education in fostering social change. *Puntos de Encuentro* (Puntos hereafter) advocates an innovative approach to design communication strategies to promote social change, believing that "rather than seeking to change individual behavior, its work seeks to influence the social context in which individuals act and in which discussion about different aspects of daily life [public and private] occurs" (Bradshaw, Solórzano, and Bank, 2006, p. 1).

For the period 2002–2005, Puntos implemented the project "We Are Different, We Are Equal: Promoting a favorable environment for the prevention of the HIV epidemic" (SDSI II) combining actions for and with young people aiming to foster their capacity for preventing the infection. The project had two complementary strategies: a mass media component and a social mobilization one. Based on Puntos's conceptual framework that links the individual with the collective, the strategy focused on promoting the individual and collective capacity to enjoy a responsible sexuality, highlighting the importance of questioning gender norms and cultural beliefs about sexuality, stigma, and discrimination related to HIV/Aids.

The Handbook of Global Health Communication, First Edition. Edited by Rafael Obregon and Silvio Waisbord.

The objectives of SDSI II were: (1) to increase and personalize the level of risk perception of HIV infection among young people in their behavior in daily life; (2) to promote significant interpersonal communication with partners about issues of HIV, gender-based violence, and responsible sexuality; (3) to promote recourse and access to social and health services; (4) to question traditional social and gender norms in order to foster equity; (5) to reduce HIV-related stigma and discrimination; (6) to increase a sense of self-efficacy in the prevention of HIV infection and leading a responsible sexual life; and (7) to strengthen leadership capacities among young people and their organizations in order to increase their capacity for advocacy and social change (Puntos de Encuentro, 2002).

To this end, Puntos's overall strategy uses its weekly television social soap series *Sexto Sentido* [Sixth sense][1] as a launching pad for a multimedia, multilevel communication for social change strategy called *Somos Diferentes, Somos Iguales* [We Are Different, We Are Equal]. The strategy combines entertainment-education outcomes, youth leadership training, alliances between partners, and strengthening social movements to promote change in Nicaraguan society. The strategy has proven successful according several impact evaluations (D'Angelo and Welsh, 2006; Montoya *et al.*, 2004; Lynch, 2006) and has been validated by many national and international sectors.

In spite of its wide recognition as a cutting-edge organization,[2] Puntos has been struggling to frame and justify its outreach strategy theoretically.

Contradictions arise when organizations such as Puntos approach social change as a nonlinear, messy, *complex* problem while most donors, social scientists, and practitioners approach it as a predictable, linear process.

To understand the messy process of social change, I turn to complexity science, for it provides insights that are not so easily derivable from traditional, behavioral social science conceptions of social change. Complexity science includes the study of complex social phenomena, especially those that involve multiple interactions between various agents and actors over time, with less than predictable outcomes.

Complexity science is increasingly used as a framework to analyze complex interactions between various actors in systems such as stock markets, human bodies, forest ecosystems, manufacturing businesses, termite colonies, and hospitals (Plexus Institute, 1998a; Singhal, 2005, 2006). Since Puntos's strategy combines diverse approaches, methods, actors and media and it also operates in a complex system with numerous efforts and players interacting in various ways, I argue that complexity science is an adequate theoretical framework to analyze Puntos's communication approach to social change and its communication strategy to promote an enabling environment for HIV/AIDS prevention.

This exploratory analysis suggests that Puntos has inadvertently engaged with the ideas of complexity science to promote change in what it sees to be a complex world. However, Puntos also faces obstacles and challenges to operationalizing this complexity-based approach to its work and relationships, such as the lack of a shared approach (linear vs. nonlinear) between Puntos and its counterparts, the need to frame Puntos's projects in accordance with traditional approaches in order to get the funds needed for their implementation, and the pressure to evaluate those projects based on dominant indicators of "success".

This chapter also aims to invite development organizations, grant makers, and researchers to think outside the box about the complexity of social change processes and health communication interventions.

Background to Puntos de Encuentro

Puntos was formally established in 1991 as a feminist social change organization that worked in the realms of communication, research, and education, and was dedicated to promoting the individual and collective autonomy and empowerment of young people and women (Hernández and Campanile, 2000). Its institutional strategies have evolved over the past several years while its core goals have remained fairly consistent. Puntos' main goals are to: (1) promote social dialogue, influencing the issues discussed, the way those issues are discussed, and influencing who participates in the discussion; (2) link the personal and public spheres so that the analysis of personal experiences can feed and improve collective actions; (3) strengthen individual and organizational leadership capacities, especially those of women and youth; (4) promote movement building through the creation and strengthening of alliances between organizations and their collective actions; (5) promote formal and informal systems of social support for individual and collective actions; and (6) create and use its own mass media programming to influence public opinion, promote critical thinking, and promote attitude and behavioral change toward more equitable relationships (Bank, 1997; Puntos de Encuentro, 2006a[3]). As stated in Puntos's Conceptual Framework, "Social change must be a goal beyond achieving personal change and personal change must also be a goal for social movements. Our work at Puntos de Encuentro is to help people make the links and meet these challenges" (Puntos de Encuentro, 2004, p. 11).

In the case of SDSI II, Puntos acknowledged the well-known effectiveness of edutainment programs, especially when combined with and reinforced by social mobilization activities and the promotion of social networks around issues of sexual and reproductive health (Singhal and Rogers, 1999). The idea was then to influence collective processes – not just individual behavior – that facilitate and sustain the inequality in daily life relationships. According to this perspective, a social change strategy should aim to promote the participation and commitment of the diversity of social actors involved, the creation and strengthening of interpersonal and institutional supporting networks, the strengthening of individual and collective self-efficacy and the promotion of spaces and conditions needed for an open and well-informed dialogue and debate around issues related to sexuality, power relations, gender, etc. (Papa *et al.*, 2000).

Puntos started its communication activities by producing its own media outlets: a feminist magazine, a youth radio show, and then more integrated mass media campaigns to address social issues. However, according to Amy Bank (2002), former executive director of Puntos, SDSI evolved as a result of lessons learned by Puntos in its first 10 years of work in the area of communication for social change.

A turning point for Puntos's communication strategy was the creation of its television soap opera *Sexto Sentido* which became the centerpiece of its SDSI strategy. Entertainment-education formats such as television soap operas, given their rich multi-pronged narratives, represent effective means to address complex and interrelated issues (Singhal *et al.*, 2004). Bank (2002) argues that the engaging nature of mass media narratives assures audience popularity; emotional identification and role modeling that promotes efficacy; intertwined and ongoing storylines that allow complex and layered treatment of multiple themes (like sexual abuse and machismo, or abortion and the emergency contraception pill); long-term, repeated exposure to different aspects of the same theme; and other gains (see also Bandura, 1985; Singhal *et al.*, 2004). Further, Puntos's adoption of engaging television narratives is consistent with the value that complexity science places on story telling as a way to understand complex social problems. As Wheatley (1999) states "any process that encourages nonlinear thinking and intuition, and uses alternatives forms of expression such as drama, art, stories and pictures … leads us to new ways of comprehending" (p. 143).

Puntos's strategy in *Somos Diferentes, Somos Iguales (SDSI)* combines popular mass media appeal, ongoing coverage, and the environment-enabling benefits of television and radios shows: support of the local media; community mobilization and coordination alliances with over 200 organizations; training activities, interpersonal reinforcement mechanisms, and links with service delivery; ongoing monitoring and evaluation; and dissemination of the results (Bradshaw, Solórzano, and Bank, 2006; Bank, 2005).

So, how does Puntos's strategy work on the ground? Consider a young woman living in the northern Nicaragua who watches *Sexto Sentido* at the weekend on the national television station, then watches the repeat of the program on the local channel, and then listens, and calls in, to Puntos's radio show during a weekday to express her opinions and feelings on issues that concern her. Through the radio show and the billboards in her locality, she finds out about organizations that address those social issues, participates in their activities, and seeks needed services within her community. She has an opportunity to talk more about social issues that concern her with her classmates, especially when the casts of the *Sexto Sentido* radio and television programs visit her school. Finally, as a member of a youth organization, she participates in one or more of the workshops and/or camps lead by Puntos around the country. Here she will be involved in deeper discussions of the topic, and acquire skills and materials to address these issues back in her local community. Public opinion in the community, meanwhile, has a more favorable view of the social issues, given the coverage on national and local media and the collaborative effort of partner organizations on the ground.

"We believe the magic is in the mix", Bank concludes (2002, p. 4), "because then you have both individual AND social change catalysts operating simultaneously and over time. You get the benefits of both big scale and more concentrated face-to-face reinforcement at the local level. And, you can still do specific thematic campaigns for awareness raising. The result is that the synergy of the integrated whole is definitely more than the sum of the parts."

An Alternative Approach to Social Change

Communication for social change strategies that use entertainment-education (E-E) narrative formats (like television and radio soap operas) have become increasingly popular in Latin America, Africa, and Asia and have shown to be effective in educating people about sexual health, family planning, gender issues, and literacy (Singhal and Rogers, 1999). These strategies, however, subscribe to a behavioral change approach to promote health issues premised on the thesis that "over time the beliefs and behavior of individuals who share the same information will change and converge toward a state of 'greater cultural uniformity'" (see Kincaid, 2000).

According to Sara Bradshaw[4] (personal communication, September 4, 2006) the behavioral change models used by development agencies come from health organizations that primarily subscribe to cause–effect (linear) approaches to solve population problems. Many of them use evidence-based interventions – especially in the realm of public health – and/or are premised on Bandura's (1985) theories of social cognition, which suggests that individuals learn through watching the behavior of others, and this behavior may be adapted if it is seen to be "rewarded" or "punished."

However, there is value in understanding entertainment-education initiatives that have "not gone as well" – according to the accepted standards of "success" – as has been the case, for instance, for projects promoting gender equality that have produced contradictory results (Singhal and Rogers, 1999; Papa, Singhal, and Papa, 2006). Several E-E evaluations have suggested that it is very hard to asses the direct cause–effect relationship between the intervention and the evidence for change, especially when it comes to complex issues like domestic violence or HIV prevention (Usdin *et. al.*, 2006; Muirhead, Kumaranayake, and Watts, 2001; Bradshaw, Solórzano, and Bank, 2006).

In spite of this, the positive results demonstrated by impact evaluations of these strategies have created expectations of regularity and predictability about social change. This positivist approach leads us to think that there are "effective" ways to change societies. Many organizations (especially international aid organizations and foundations) use concepts as "best practices" to reinforce the idea that successful experiences in one setting can be replicated in different settings. This notion that what works in one place will work in other places privileges the importance of "outside experts" and reinforces beliefs that local organizations and communities need them in order to find the "right" solutions.

This linear approach to social change has been criticized by practitioners and scholars who share a more holistic and complex definition of social change as a process.[5] However, barring some exceptions, these criticisms have not translated into revamped field-based interventions (Bradshaw, Solórzano, and Bank, 2006).

Planning and evaluation are important to social change, but we need to open our minds to new ways to understand how social systems evolve. Wholeness matters. As complex adaptive systems, societies – made up of thinking, feeling, and believing people – are for the most part unpredictable and uncontrollable. They do not respond to general laws. Yet, while social change is complex and unpredictable, it is not at all unintelligible.

Simple, Complicated and Complex Problems: What Is Complexity Science?

As Glouberman and Zimmerman (2002, p. 6), note: for addressing simple problems – take cooking for instance – a recipe of various ingredients is essential. "It is often tested to assure easy replication without the need for any particular expertise. Recipes produce standardized products and the best recipes give good results every time."

To address complicated problems, like sending a rocket to the moon, formulae or recipes are critical and necessary, but are often not sufficient. Glouberman and Zimmerman (2002, p. 6) go on:

High levels of expertise in a variety of fields are necessary for success. Sending one rocket increases assurance that the next mission will be a success. In some critical ways, rockets are similar to each other and because of this there can be a relatively high degree of certainty of outcome.

Raising a child, on the other hand, is a complex problem. Here, formulae have a much more limited application. Raising one child provides experience but no assurance of success with the next. Although expertise can contribute to the process in valuable ways, it provides neither necessary nor sufficient conditions to assure success. To some extent this is because every child is unique and must be understood as an individual. As a result there is always some uncertainty of the outcome. The complexity of the process and the lack of certainty do not lead us to the conclusion that it is impossible to raise a child.

Complex problems, such as social change, disturb us "because their characteristics are not reducible to their constitutive parts. When solved, the solutions do not function as recipes, which can be applied to others like problems" (Glouberman and Zimmerman, 2002, p. 7). Complex problems are hard to predict and control; they are not linear, adaptable and heavily influenced by context. Yet, we deal with them as if they were complicated problems. Complexity science addresses aspects of living systems that are neglected or understated in traditional social change approaches.

Complex Adaptive Systems (CAS) are the units of study in complexity science. As explained in Plexus Institute (1998a, p. 6): All three terms "are each significant in the definition of a CAS: 'Complex' implies diversity – a great number of connections between a wide variety of elements. 'Adaptive' suggests the capacity to alter or change – the ability to learn from experience. A 'system' is a set of connected or interdependent things."

Complexity Science is not a single theory, it is a combination of various theories and concepts from different disciplines (biology, anthropology, economy, sociology, management, and others). Complexity science seeks to understand how complex adaptive systems work – the patterns of relationships within them, how they are sustained, how they self-organize, and how outcomes emerge – in a quest to answer some fundamental questions about living, adaptable, changeable systems (Papa, Singhal, and Papa, 2006). Contrary to the cause–effect Newtonian paradigm, complexity provides us with the opportunity to look at problems with multiple perspectives, studying the micro and macro issues, and understanding how they are interdependent. So, instead of describing how systems *should* behave, complexity science focuses the analysis on the interdependencies and interrelationships among its elements to describe how systems *actually* behave (Flynn, 2004).

Puntos and Complexity Science: Successes, Challenges, and Paradoxes

According to complexity theorists, all complex adaptive systems, such as organizations or communities, are governed by a few basic principles and share a number of linked attributes or proprieties. Understanding these principles could provide clues to designing and implementing interventions that evoke the natural quality of living systems to change and re-create themselves. The following sections will illustrate how Puntos's communication strategy incorporates some of these principles in their understanding and approach to social change.

Complexity science idea 1. Life is cluttered, full of paradoxes, and seldom is either/or: Breaking the rules of E-E with *Sexto Sentido* television

"As you study the world through a complexity lens you will be continually confronted with 'both-and' rather than 'either–or' thinking. The paradoxes of complexity are that both sides of many apparent contradictions are true" (Plexus, 1998a, p. 14). One of these paradoxes is that in any living system (people and communities), interdependence and independence co-exist. Life is complex and cluttered; issues should be considered and analyzed from all perspectives and in its complexity.

Complexity theorists also believe that the system changes when it "chooses" to be disturbed by information it receives and considers meaningful. It will only choose to be disturbed when the information provides a new meaning to the system. In other words, "the system becomes different because it understands the world differently" (Wheatley, 2005, p. 86). It is not just the intensity or frequency of the message that gets our attention; but mostly how meaningful the message is to us personally and our level of readiness to embrace change.

The key word here is "choice." People do not want to be bossed; they want information to make their own choices and decisions. That is where Puntos's strategy is fundamentally different from most other communication for behavioral change initiatives. First, instead of following the general advice "keep it short and simple," Puntos believes in making it "long and complicated." This orientation allows Puntos the opportunity to show how social issues are closely interrelated with each other, and how people often engage in contradictory behaviors.

Second, Puntos believes that people have the right to decide what they want. So, rather than presenting some forms of behavior as "good" behavior, or modeling the behavior as "socially desirable" or endorsed by particular donors, they promote the right of each individual to make informed decisions and take responsibility for the decisions they make. They do this by showing different alternatives to analyze and deal with different realities and issues.

Showing complex and contradictory behaviors, instead of stereotypical ones, doesn't make for a short-and-clear message – bad guys lose, and good guys win, but it allows audiences to reflect more deeply about their attitudes, behaviors, and options. It shows that people aren't bad or good, but often both. We all make mistakes and make bad decisions, but we can reflect on them, learn from them, and change. As Charlie Weinberg, one of the scriptwriting coordinators for *Sexto Sentido,* noted:

> Having a "bad" character that does not change or does not reflect on his/her acts in a series like *Sexto Sentido* is useless. For instance, Martha's husband – a 'macho' character who spends most of his time cheating on his wife without using a condom and refusing to use one with Martha – became HIV positive (and that is how Martha got infected) but he also ended up by looking for help and accepting responsibility. This way, *Sexto Sentido* shows that we all have the capacity to improve ourselves, to reflect, and to change into the kind of person we want to be. The "bad" character is not much use in a program where what we are primarily trying to show are the internal processes of reflection and the kind of decisions that lead us to our personal development" (Puntos de Encuentro, 2006b, p. 11).

So what matters most to Puntos is the reflective process that accompanies the mistakes and decisions taken by the characters. The kind of mistakes that *Sexto Sentido's* characters make are often the type of mistakes that real people make.

Puntos deliberately put on the national agenda the issues of the emergency contraception pill (also called "morning after pill"), HIV/AIDS among faithful married women, and abortion – not as an attempt to dictate people what to do or not to do, but to encourage them think for themselves and take responsibility for their decisions and actions.

Complexity idea 2. Free flow of diverse and meaningful information is essential for the system to evolve

In order to make decisions about their lives, people need to reflect on their condition. Bringing in diverse and meaningful information about alternatives is essential to this process. Providing information alone is far from being enough to achieve social change. Yet, complexity science suggests that the relationship the system has with information, particularly to new and status-quo-disturbing information, is essential for its evolution. (Wheatley, 1999).

Diversity and participation are key elements to promote the democratic and participatory change Puntos espouses. Diversity means not only having different voices on an issue, but also addressing issues that are generally considered taboo, or too sensitive to discuss. Participation means creating an environment so that everyone can feel comfortable sharing opinions and feelings. Mainstream ideas need to be questioned in a healthy debate, which is the environment created by Puntos's youth camps and interactive media such as its radio talk show and its women's magazine *La Boletina*.

Having its own media outlets gives Puntos the kind of autonomy it needs to promote dialogue and debate, and to provide a space for diverse and marginalized voices to be heard and legitimized. Having its own magazine and television and radio programs has allowed Puntos to broaden the public's access to diverse points of view. It also gives us Puntos a permanent space to share ideas and information without being tied to commercial considerations (Bank, 1997). This relative autonomy has also allowed Puntos to address diverse sensitive issues (e.g., abortion), that the commercial media do not cover because they clash with the dominant conservative ideology.

Complexity science advocates participation as being important for information to flow freely in the system so it can evolve. It is not just about what information is being shared, but who is sharing it. The wider the variety of people who share ideas, the greater the opportunity exists for new associations to form, and new patterns of meanings to propagate (Wheatley, 1999).

Vanesa Cortez, one of the radio producers at Puntos, explained: "Puntos's radio show *Sexto Sentido Radio* provides an ongoing space for teenagers and young adults to voice opinions and talk about their problems and concerns with other young people without the mediation of adult 'experts' disseminating advice" (personal communication, August 29, 2006). Puntos validates the wisdom and expertise people have concerning their own life, while consciously working to legitimize diverse and marginalized voices.

Puntos makes a point of taking "taboo" subjects out of the closet and getting them into the public agenda in order to destigmatize them and explain their relevance within a human development process based on equality and rights. At the same time, it pays careful attention to the language and structure of its arguments so that they have more of a chance to be accepted without their intent being "watered down." So, "instead of retreating on the issue for fear of rejection or even persecution [Puntos] decided to demystify it" (Bank, 2005, p. 1).

Puntos decided to address the topic of HIV during the last two seasons of *Sexto Sentido* (2004 to 2005), because it received numerous requests from young viewers to deal with this issue. Why? Amy Bank (2001, p. 9) explains:

> possibly because of a kind of nebulous perception of risk, of having heard about AIDS and knowing enough about it to know it's deadly, but not enough to know if it could affect them... but my hunch is that it was also a kind of code for saying: we want a "legitimate" way to talk about sex. Which is a code for saying: we want to talk about relationships and identity and self-esteem. Which is a code for saying: we want to TALK and feel connected, we need space to talk about our lives, all the things we experience and feel and want and fear that you're not supposed to talk about. The issue of HIV/AIDS can open up those spaces.

This illustrates the complexity of issues such as HIV/AIDS and gender-based violence and the multiple layers and perspectives that need to be addressed simultaneously.

The organization's purpose is not to create consensus around a topic, but to explore and be exposed to different points of view in a climate of respect and tolerance. Through the radio and television show, young people not only claim the right to have an opinion on issues and to make decisions about matters that affect their lives, the show also strengthens and legitimizes the voices of marginalized groups that are not active, or visible, in the mainstream public sphere. External evaluations of Puntos (Montoya *et al.*, 2004) suggest that this orientation of Puntos has positively influenced its audiences.

Sexto Sentido Radio motivated other young communicators to use the medium of radio to address social issues. Since 1992, when the radio show first aired, it gained iconic status in Nicaraguan broadcasting. Dozen of radios stations and young groups use it as a model to produce their own radio shows explains Hazel Jirón, coproducer of *Sexto Sentido Radio* (personal communication, August 29, 2006). Its recorded shows and scripts are in high demand. Young communicators draw upon its content or just simply rebroadcast the show on their own local station. Based on this groundswell of demand, Puntos launched workshops with young broadcast journalists to help them create their own productions, providing them technical and content advice. Puntos also launched, in alliance with 10 local radio stations, a Youth Radio Network that airs the *Sexto Sentido Radio* show live in 10 main cities of the country.

This multiplier effect – multiplied messages in multiple locations – contributes to the social change enterprise. As Wheatley (1999 states, "In nonlinear systems, iteration helps small differences grow into powerful and unpredictable effects" (p. 122). "When the system is far from equilibrium, singular or small influences can have enormous impact. It is not the law of large numbers or critical mass that creates change, but the presence of a small disturbance that gets into the system and is then amplified through the network." (p. 87).

Iteration is important. Ongoing debates around important issues, not only in Puntos's own media but in others as well, create a favorable public opinion toward discussing difficult topics. At the same time, the legitimization of such topics in the public sphere, contributes to the ground-based efforts of local organizations that work on those issues.

Complexity idea 3. The whole is greater than the sum of the parts, the quality of the relationships is more critical to the system than the quality of the individuals: Puntos's alliances for social change

In complex adaptive systems, the interacting agents are independent and interdependent at the same time. But, when an individual agent in the system changes, the system will change only if the change in the individuals affects the way agents relate to each other. Individual change per se is not enough to change the system. This way the entire system emerges from a dense pattern of interactions that reproduce themselves to create a new order. Wheatley (1999, p. 73) describes the world as "one divided not into different groups of objects or subjects but into different groups of connections. What is distinguishable and important is the kind of connections."

We see this frequently in team sports. The team with the best individual players can lose to a team of poorer players. The second team cannot rely on one or two stars but instead has to focus on creating outcomes that are beyond the talents of any one individual. They create outcomes based on the interrelationships between the players. This is not to dismiss individual excellence. It does suggest, however, that individual abilities are not a complete explanation of success or failure.

Puntos believes that social change results from both individual and collective change. Individual leadership is critical to push change forward, but Puntos also knows that social change won't happen without collective action. So, an essential part of Puntos's mission is to strengthen both individual and collective leadership (especially among women and the youth), and to improve the capacities of organizations to coordinate and implement collective actions by making alliances with each other.

In this sense, building and strengthening alliances is a key component of Puntos's work. Indeed, the strategy *Somos Diferentes, Somos Iguales (SDSI)* could not have been implemented without Puntos's long history of developing collaborative relationships with partner organizations as well as active involvement in Nicaragua's women and youth movements.

The continual exchange of material and information, the bilateral and multilateral support between Puntos, its allies, and other organizations strengthen the capacity of the social movements to make a deeper analysis of the political and social context, to improve their own performance and outcomes through feedback, to lobby for changes in existing policies and laws, and to implement nationwide campaigns and interventions.

The nationwide campaign on raising awareness about Law 230 (the domestic violence law) is a good example of such organizational synergy. During the first season of *Sexto Sentido TV*, Puntos carried out, in coordination with other organizations, a campaign designed to legitimize the view that violence is not a private issue. Law 230 was approved in 1996 but few Nicaraguan women knew about its existence, or how to apply it.

The television program portrayed the story of Elena, a girl dealing with an abusive father, who was trying to help her mother get out of this domestic situation while coping with their social and economical constraints. In addition, special vignettes were produced and aired at the end of *Sexto Sentido*'s episodes with the actress who portrays Elena talking about the issue, showing the informational pamphlet on Law 230 that had been produced, and telling viewers where they could seek more information and help. The content of the mass distribution pamphlet, which included guidance on how to identify a domestic violence situation, and what to do and where to go in case of violence, was discussed with participating organizations, and printing expenses were shared. Some 50,000 pamphlets were distributed through local organizations in Nicaragua, and the issue was also a central component of *Sexto Sentido Radio*'s programming during that season. The Law 230 campaign was coordinated with the Women's Network against Violence and 125 service providers all around the country. The national and local media in Nicaragua backed up the efforts by rebroadcasting the radio and television shows and/or publishing articles about the topic (Bank, 2003). Such coordination among organizations helped them to make the best of limited resources to put issues of their interest on the public agenda. Moreover, according to Evelyn Flores (personal communication, September 5, 2006), "these kinds of alliances help local media and small organizations to gain visibility and credibility, to de-centralize the resources that are usually held in the capital city, and allow them to access new resources and to improve their effectiveness."

The number and diversity of Puntos's allies increased the potential for emergent and self-organizing outcomes. The Law 230's campaign and the radio network are good examples of the outcomes that emerged from such alliance-based relationships.

Complexity idea 4. Planning the unpredictable: The challenges of detailed planning in a complex world

Every three years, all Puntos employees, from its Board of Directors to receptionists and drivers, come together to think about the next three years of work. Based on their understanding of social change as a complex process, they reflect about the society they want and the kind of contribution they can make to achieve it. At the end of this session, they return to their desks full of excitement and energy. That is when the problems begin. They need now to translate those complexity-based dreams into log frames, operational plans, activities, outcomes, and indicators.

The paradox here is that the collective dream is based on a complexity approach to social change, but the operative planning follows the "complicated" linear, step-by-step approach required by our donors and by the expectations of our collaborating partners. How one can reconcile the messy, unpredictable, and complex notion of social change with a short-term, cause-effect based schemata that can frame results as quantifiable and measurable?

Part of this frustrating process is the elaboration of the log frame, a format that asks you to plan your mission and goals in terms of actions, activities, outputs, outcomes, and measurable results. For instance when Puntos plans its youth leadership camps, it has to somehow "translate" its goals of "deconstructing the notion of oppression" and "creating new ways to relate with each other," "bringing people to the edge," "letting new directions emerge," and others into boxes that describe what and how many activities it will implement, how many participants it expects to attend, how it is going to reach them, what and how many materials are going to be distributed, how much it will cost, what the specific outcomes are predicted, and how it is going to measure them.

Although some planners would argue that a log frame is a guiding tool, not a straitjacket, the way the boxes are organized is linear, each one being connected to the other by arrows that show the cause–effect relationship between them (I will do this > this will happen > these will be the outcomes > and this is how I am going to measure them), forcing one to think in a linear way about one's "guiding tool." One can see Newtonian thinking etched on these log frames.

But does social reality work out that way? First, not all social processes are linear, meaning that not every action has a direct and single effect. Second, there are many unpredictable events that can influence one's strategy, and one should be flexible enough to change the strategy. Third, by detailing in advance how one is going to measure the expected outcomes, not only does one assume that these are going to be the exact outcomes and thus become predisposed to find them, but one also focuses one's attention on measuring them only, overlooking other important factors and contextual information. As Evelyn Flores (personal communication, September 5, 2006) from Puntos said, "We keep making the mistake of conferring too much prophetic capacity to the planning process, specially with five-year-long projects … and we make the same mistake over, and over…"

As Vanesa Cortez from the radio team also argues, "some great ideas have emerged from our ongoing exchange and coordination with other people and organizations.… If we had all that information from the beginning we would be able to include it in our plans, but we can not afford to lose an opportunity [to improve our work] just because we did not plan it that way… and that is what this [social change] is all about anyway" (personal communication, August 29, 2006).

At the end of each year, Puntos usually ends up achieving its initial expectations and often finishes the term by adding a number of extra activities and events to its originally stated plans. While this is usually applauded, Puntos staff members feel exhausted, acutely aware that the problem is not simply the lack of more detailed planning. In other words, planning in more detail will not make the challenge easier.

Complexity science recognizes the difficulty of planning everything in detail, especially when working within an unpredictable and constantly changing environment. Complexity science suggests that the best way to plan is by establishing minimum specifications and a general sense of direction, that is, describing the mission the organization is pursuing and a few basic principles on how the organization should get there. The organizational leadership should then allow appropriate autonomy for individuals to self-organize, adapting as time goes by to a continually changing context (Plexus Institute, 1998b, p. 3).

> You can never know exactly what will happen until you do it. So, allowing the flexibility of multiple approaches is a very reasonable thing to do …. When we do find ourselves in situations far from certainty and agreement, the management advice contained in this

[complexity] principle is to quit agonizing over it, quit trying to analyze it to certainty. Try several small experiments, reflect carefully on what happens and gradually shift time and attention toward those things that seem to be working the best – that is, let direction arise" (Plexus, 1998b. p. 9).

This complexity-based approach to planning is especially useful when the organization's mission is to promote changes in the environment and in the pattern of relationships between agents, rather than producing predetermined outcomes. This doesn't mean that social change organizations must not plan; it means they should change the way they plan (Glouberman and Zimmerman, 2002).

Measuring Processes: The Challenge of Impact Evaluations

Evaluations and impact assessments are another big challenge for Puntos. Because the evaluation process starts during the planning process, when the teams are establishing the activities, outcomes, and indicators, the evaluation methodologies have to respond to those indicators, which makes it difficult to take advantage of opportunities and unexpected changes that come along during the process of implementation, let alone other questions and issues not answered by the measurement of success of the predicted specific outcomes.

In trying to assess the impact of Puntos's strategy, the challenges have been many. For instance, the impact evaluation of the first phase of SDSI was affected, among other considerations, by financial issues. The survey questionnaire was administered only after the series had gone off air, meaning there was no baseline study for comparison. The survey questionnaire needed to be limited to two pages, which didn't allow many of the topics covered in the series to be addressed. Further, the questionnaire adopted a rather unusual format – of the same kind as quizzes found in magazines aimed at teenage girls where questions set up hypothetical situations – "what/how would you do/think/react if…" with multiple choice responses. This was done to make it suitable for administration to 13-year-olds, so that it would engage their interest and raise "sensitive" issues in such a way that would not upset them or their parents.

Despite the limitations of such research methods, they allowed Puntos to explore issues not usually addressed in survey research. As Amy Bank (2002, p. 4) explains: "the most exciting part has been to inventory and analyze the enormous variety of individual and collective change processes that have been sparked by this project, things that were not included in the original indicators we had developed, and that we definitely want to follow up on, thing that have to do with social cohesion, leadership, and the like." Yet such an orientation raised polemic discussions among experts. On the one hand, communication experts in the field criticized the methodology and thus the findings in terms of "scientific rigor," but, on the other, development professionals approached the findings in a different way, initiating debates around what the outcomes actually meant, what were the deeper issues, and the like.

The quantitative component of the evaluation of the second phase of *Somos Diferentes, Somos Iguales* was led by experts in research methods and conformed to international standards. This quantitative evaluation was complemented with qualitative methods that included data gathering from television viewers, radio listeners, and the local organizations that Puntos works with.

This second-phase assessment provided Puntos with the chance to discuss the outcomes of the initiative with greater authority. Puntos wants to position its work as different from work that follows linear and staged models of behavioural change as well as the participatory model of evaluation promoted by the Communication for Social Change Consortium (Parks *et al.*, 2005). While both provide valuable insights, neither alone is enough to explain the kind of changes that Puntos is promoting. "The former do not allow us to asses changes beyond the individual, that is, the changes in the environment; and the latter has the constraint of being applicable only to the local level, and our work cannot be delimited local boundaries [places and communities]. We need to build a paradigm that rather than reject one of the approaches, integrates both in a complementary and interdependent manner" (Irela Solórzano, personal communication, September 6, 2006).

But this is easier said than done. Puntos is still struggling with the challenge of developing more wholesome indicators and to more fully integrate the complementary qualitative components into its outcome analysis. Irela Solórzano (personal communication, September 6, 2006) states: "We need to gain external legitimation for our work, but we also wanted to have an opinion and to participate in the design [of the evaluation] to guarantee that it will be coherent with our vision and mission. The problem is we still haven't developed enough theoretical and methodological frameworks that allow us to offer effective alternatives. We need new indicators, but they can only be validated during the implementation and that affects the evaluation because it cannot be planned in detail at the beginning of the project."

Discussion and Final Thoughts

The present study aimed to lay out a theoretical framework for understanding Puntos's strategies for social change by drawing upon concepts of the new science of complexity. This exploratory analysis suggests that Puntos has inadvertently engaged with the ideas of complexity science to promote change in what it sees to be a complex world. However, Puntos also faces obstacles and challenges to operationalizing this complexity-based approach to its work and relationships.

First, while Puntos is planning its strategies in accordance with its notion of complex processes, most of its counterparts (the organizations and individuals with which it establishes partnerships) do not necessarily follow the same line of thinking and may believe in cause–effect strategies, measurable results, and different follow-up activities to achieve their own agendas and expectations.

Second, Puntos's sustainability still depends on development agencies' approval of funds to implement its projects. Most of these grant makers keep requesting Puntos to justify, plan, and evaluate its communication for social change strategies based on indicators and methods that have been legitimized as standards criteria of "success," but which, Puntos argues, are inadequate to respond to the vision and questions related to social change.

Third, an indicator-driven context for outcomes poses particular challenges for communication strategies such as *Somos Diferentes, Somos Iguales*. "As much as success stories may attract new converts to social communication strategies, the pressure to 'succeed' in traditional terms may also prevent innovation within the field, not only in terms of project design and implementation, but also in terms of evaluation. Those who do not conform to the standard evaluation framework, as was the case with the first series of *Sexto Sentido*, may be penalised in that their findings may be questioned in some quarter" (Bradshaw, Solórzano, and Bank, 2006, p. 24).

In other words, indicators of change in attitudes and behaviors are not enough. There is an urge to develop and legitimate new methodologies and indicators that can capture the complexity of social change processes. Evaluations are needed that explore the processes that lead to outcomes rather than focusing only on demonstrating those outcomes.

Certain social change initiatives are purposely promoting participatory communication for social change that involves the development of indicators that measure not only outcomes but also processes. The Rockefeller Foundation, Johns Hopkins University, UNICEF, and the Communication for Social Change Consortium have advocated participatory monitoring and evaluation in an attempt to bring attention to alternatives methods and indicators to evaluate development initiatives, especially those with a communication component (Parks, *et al.*, 2005; Singhal, 2001). Some alternative indicators to measure processes and other intangible outcomes have also been proposed. While such initiatives are getting more attention from practitioners and scholars, there is still a long way to go with grant makers before they will accept alternative methodologies, indicators, and data gathering processes as valid and legitimate.

Puntos agrees with these participatory initiatives about the need to understand not only how many or how much, but also the "hows" and "whys" of social change. In the same way, "Puntos's experience highlights the need to think further about what successful change looks like; both in terms of what is seen to be a 'success' and what is considered to be 'good' change" (Bradshaw, Solórzano, and Bank, 2006, p. 25). However, participatory methods are more useful to employ in interventions that can be easily localized (in a community, a territory, or a group), and also in situations that those affected and involved in the process of change can be reached and encouraged to participate in the planning, monitoring, and evaluation of the project. This is not the case with most large-scale interventions, including Puntos's own initiatives, where the boundaries are difficult to localize and where multiple media and partnerships make the assessment of the intervention even more challenging.

In the process of answering the main research questions of this paper, new questions were raised: How does Puntos's view of society and social change affect the patterns of relationship of the individuals, organizations, and communities with which Puntos interacts? How are complexity approaches affecting (or how might they affect) the way donors and development organizations plan their strategies and evaluate their impact? How can we facilitate, rather than control, the conditions to promote emergence and self-organizing processes, and what role should Puntos and other organizations play in this process? Where are traditional evaluation approaches and methodologies more appropriate, and where and how do complexity approaches add more value to innovate new strategies and research methods? And, finally, how can we improve our planning processes and methods if everything is context-related and everything is changing, including us? These are some of the questions that are not answered by this paper but worth exploring in further studies.

There is still much more to learn from, and understand about, complex adaptive systems and complexity science, as well as much more to understand about social change. Complexity science is still in development. Debates about complexity-based indicators and research and evaluation methods are strongly needed in order to be able to provide with better contributions to communication for social change strategies and interventions. However, complexity science applied to social change strategies (such as Puntos's) can open our mind, and help us to look for different ways to do things, ask different questions, get different answers, try different strategies; and better understand what does work and what doesn't in each context, but, most importantly, how and why social change happens. This is especially relevant when the issues we try to address are as complex as the HIV epidemic and other social and cultural related health issues.

Notes

1   The last episode was broadcast in Nicaragua in June 2005. Currently the series is being repeated in its entirety (80 episodes) on local TV stations around the country. As of August 2005, Centro America TV, a satellite station transmitted the show across the USA, and from September 2005 the programme has been shown on Costa Rican TV and Honduras. Puntos is in negotiations with Panamá, El Salvador, the Dominican Republic and Spain as to further transmissions. The programme is also now available on broadband on the Internet from the Puntos web page (in Spanish only).

2   Puntos's communication strategy and its *telenovela* for social change "*Sexto Sentido*" (Sixth Sense) have won international awards and recognition, including the "Freedom Award" at the Gay and Lesbian International Film Festival in Los Angeles 2002; the Hollywood "SHINE Awards" 2004, together with HBO (Home Box Office), for its excellence and its positive approach to sexual health and rights, among other things. The strategy "Somos Diferentes, Somos Iguales (SDSI)" has being highlighted by the IDB, UNIFEM, World Bank, USAID, UNFPA as a successful project in work with young in the world and its materials are being used and adapted in many Latin American countries.

3   While these institutional strategies are described in Puntos's constitutional document and grant proposals, the documents referred to explain the strategies further.

4   Sara Bradshaw, professor at Middlesex University, UK and long-time collaborator with Puntos, was part of the external team that designed, implemented, and analyzed the SDSI II impact evaluation.

5   For more on this debate see: Parks *et al.*, 2005; Figueroa *et al.*, 2002; and Singhal, 2001.

References

Bandura, A. (1985). *Social Foundations of Thought and Action*. Englewood Cliffs, NJ: Prentice-Hall.
Bank, A. (1997). Communication strategies for the empowerment of women and young people in Nicaragua: Some lessons learned. Presentation made at the Working Group Meeting of the

Health Development Policy Project on Communications Strategies. Washington, DC, December 10–11, 1997.

Bank, A. (2001). Grounding the debate. Presentation made at the Communication for Development Roundtable. Managua, November, 26.

Bank, A. (2002). Developing an integrated multi-media/multi-method approach for individual and social change around gender-based violence and sexual and reproductive health issues. Paper presented at the Technical Update of the Interagency Gender Working Group of USAID. Washington, DC, May 1.

Bank, A. (2003). *Somos Diferentes Somos Iguales*. Paper presented at USAID's Best Practices on Sexual and Reproductive Health meeting. Washington, July, 2002.

Bank, A. (2005). The magic is in the mix: Using a feminist soap opera to address the personal, the political and everything in-between. Presentation made at the 10th AWID International Forum in Bangkok, Thailand, 27 to 30 October. Puntos de Encuentro, Nicaragua.

Bradshaw, S., Solórzano, I. and Bank, A. (2006). Changing the nature of change: A nicaraguan feminist experience. Paper submitted to the World Congress on Communication for Development, Rome, Italy. October 2006.

D'Angelo, A. and Welsh, P. (2006). *Evaluación del Proyecto "Somos Diferentes, Somos Iguales: Fomentando un Entorno Favorable para la Prevención del VIH-Sida"* [Evaluation of the Project "We are different but equal: Promoting a favorable environment for the prevention of HIV/AIDS." (Puntos de Encuentro's external evaluation, final report). Managua, October.

Figueroa, M. E., Kincaid, D. L., Rani, M., and Lewis, G. (2002). *Communication for Social Change: An Integrated Model for Measuring the Process and Its Outcomes*. The Communication for Social Change Working Paper Series No. 1. New York: The Rockefeller Foundation.

Flynn, P. (2004). *Complexity Science Applied to Living Systems: Case Study to Inform Making Connections – Denver*. Paper prepared for the Piton Foundation, Denver, CO.

Glouberman, S. and Zimmerman, B. (2002). *Complicated and Complex Systems: What Would Successful Reform of Medicare Look Like?* Ottawa: Commission on the Future of Health Care in Canada. Retrieved from http://www.healthandeverything.org/fi les/Glouberman_E.pdf

Hernández, T. and Campanile, V. (2000). Feminism at work: A case study of transforming power relations in everyday life. In H. van Dam, A. Khadar and M. Valk (Eds.), *Institutionalizing Gender Equality: Commitment, Policy and Practice. A Global Source Book*. Gender, Society and Development series 4. Amsterdam: Royal Tropical Institute (KIT). Retrieved from http://www.kit.nl/net/KIT_Publicaties_output/ShowFile2.aspx?e=1307

Kincaid, D. L. (2000). *Change Characters to Change Audience Behavior*. Paper presented at the Third International Entertainment Education Conference for Social Change, September17–22, 2000, Arnhem and Amsterdam, The Netherlands.

Lynch, A. (2006). *A Whole Greater Than the Sum of Its Parts: Alliances for Change at Puntos de Encuentro*. Unpublished Master's Thesis, Institute of Development Studies, University of Sussex, Brighton, UK.

Montoya, O., Ulloa, K., Antillón, C., and Campos, R. A. (2004). *Componente Cualitativo del Estudio de Impacto del Proyecto "Somos Diferentes Somos Iguales" (SDSI). Primera Pase de Evaluación* [Qualitative component of the impact study of the Project "We are different but equal. First phase of evaluation]. (Puntos de Encuentro's external evaluation report). Managua, Nicaragua: Puentos de Encuentro.

Muirhead, D., Kumaranayake, L., and Watts, C. (2001). *Economically Evaluating the Fourth* Soul City *Series: Costs and Impact on HIV/AIDS and Violence against Women*. Report for Institute for Health and Development Communication/Soul City, South Africa, September 2001. Retrieved from http://www.soulcity.org.za/research/evaluations/soul-city-series-4/evaluation-cost-effectiveness/at_download/file

Papa, M. J., Singhal, A., Law, S. *et al.* (2000). Entertainment-education and social change: an analysis of parasocial interaction, social learning, collective efficacy, and paradoxical communication. *Journal of Communication, 50*(4), 31–55.

Papa, M. J., Singhal, A., and Papa, W. H. (2006). *Organizing for social change: A dialectic journey of theory and praxis.* New Delhi: SAGE Publications.

Parks, W., Grey-Felder, D., Hunt, J., and Byrne, A. (2005). *Who Measures Change? An Introduction to Participatory Monitoring and Evaluation of Communication for Social Change.* CFSC Consortium Inc. Retrieved from http://www.communicationforsocialchange.org/pdf/who_measures_change.pdf

Plexus Institute (1998a). *A Complexity Science Primer: What Is Complexity Science and Why Should I Learn about It?* Adapted from Zimmermann, B., Lindberg, C. and Plsek, P. (1998), *Edgeware: Lessons From Complexity Science for Health Care Leaders,* Dallas, TX: VHA Inc. Retrieved from http://www.plexusinstitute.com/Services/E-Library/

Plexus Institute (1998b). *Nine Emerging and Connected Organizational and Leadership Principles.* Adapted from Zimmermann, B., Lindberg, C. and Plsek, P. (1998), *Edgeware: Lessons From Complexity Science for Health Care Leaders,* Dallas, TX: VHA Inc. Retrieved February 12th, 2006 from Plexus Institute website: http://www.plexusinstitute.com/Services/E-Library/

Puntos de Encuentro (2002). *Proyecto SDSI 2002–2005 Fomentando un Entorno Favorable para la Prevención del VIH-SIDA* [SDSI Project 2002–2005 promoting an environment favorable to the prevention of HIV/AIDS]. Managua, Nicaragua: Puntos de Encuentro.

Puntos de Encuentro (2004). *Punto de Partida: Nuestros Conceptos Claves* [Point of departure: our key concepts]. Puntos de Encuentro's Conceptual framework. (Internal report), Managua, Nicaragua: Puentos de Encuentro.

Puntos de Encuentro (2006a). *Plan Estrategico Institucional 2006–2008* [Strategic institutional plan 2006–2008]. Managua, Nicaragua: Puntos de Encuentro.

Puntos de Encuentro (2006b). *Sistematización* [Systematization] (Institutional report). Managua, Nicaragua: Weinberg, Ch.

Singhal, A. (2001). *Facilitating Community Participation through Communication.* Submitted to GPP, Programme Division, UNICEF, New York. September, 2001. Retrieved from http://utminers.utep.edu/asinghal/Articles%20and%20Chapters/Singhal-UNICEF-Participation-Report.pdf

Singhal, A. (2005). The practice of medicine is in the interactions: A day with Robert A. Lindberg, M.D. *Stories: Complexity in Action.* Retrieved from http://www.plexusinstitute.com/services/stories/show.cfm?id=35

Singhal, A. (2006). Trust is the lubricant of organizational life: lessons from the life and career of Henri Lipmanowicz. *Deeper Learning 1*(1). Retrieved from Plexus Institute website, http://www.plexusinstitute.com/services/E-Library/show.cfm?id=367

Singhal, A., Cody, M., Rogers, E. M., and Sabido, M. (Eds.).(2004). *Entertainment-Education and Social Change: History, Research and Practice.* Mahwah, NJ: Lawrence Erlbaum Associates.

Singhal, A. and Rogers, E. M. (1999). *Entertainment-Education: A Communication Strategy for Social Change.* Mahwah, NJ: Lawrence Erlbaum Associates.

Usdin, S., Scheepers, E., Goldstein, S., and Japhet, G. (2006). Achieving social change on gender-based violence: A report on the impact evaluation of *Soul City*'s fourth series. *Social Science and Medicine, 61,* 2434–2445.

Wheatley, M. J. (1999). *Leadership and the New Science: Discovering Order in a Chaotic World,* 2nd edn. San Francisco, CA: Berrett-Koehler Publishers.

Wheatley, M. J. (2005). *Finding Our Way: Leadership for Uncertain Times.* San Francisco, CA: Berrett-Koehler Publishers.

11

Community Media, Health Communication, and Engagement
A Theoretical Matrix

Linje Manyozo

Introduction

This chapter critically examines an exploratory theoretical and methodological matrix propounded as an analytical facility for studying the integration of community media within health communication initiatives in developing world contexts. It argues that health communication has been largely informed by the empirical implementation of the diffusionist theoretical and methodological frameworks emerging from Western international public goods (IPG) industries such as the American Institutes for Research, Centers for Disease Control and Prevention, or Population Communication International–Media Impact. Employing community media within such a health communication framework conflicts with the epistemological foundations of such media, which center on empowerment, transformation, and the construction of history from below. This exposition scrutinizes the possibilities of a theoretical framework that transforms community media into a mediation facility for health development through strengthening social capital, social infrastructure, and social economy.

The chapter contends that a careful consideration of a marriage between community media and health communication within developing world contexts raises three difficult questions that cannot be answered by health communication theory (Coleman, 1998; Singhal and Rogers, 1999) nor community media theory (Bailey, Cammaerts, and Carpentier, 2007; Carpentier, Lie, and Servaes, 2003). These questions are: How can community media facilitate health communication and engagement? How should community media journalists work within developing world contexts? To what extent can community media build on indigenous knowledge in health communication and engagement? To answer these questions, this chapter has brought together three theoretical frameworks and one methodological trajectory, namely, community health development

The Handbook of Global Health Communication, First Edition. Edited by Rafael Obregon and Silvio Waisbord.
© 2012 John Wiley & Sons, Inc. Published 2012 by John Wiley & Sons, Inc.

(Ledwith, 2005; Taylor, Wilkinson, and Cheers, 2008), development journalism (Loo, 2009; Jamias, 1991), indigenous knowledge communication systems (Mundy and Compton, 1999; Pottier, 2003; Sillitoe, 2002), and participatory action research (Kamlongera, 2005). Community media could possibly then become an effective pathway for implementing health communication initiatives in the global south by mediating the praxes of participation, power and development.

Community Media

The strongest debates surrounding the rationale for community media emerged during the tenuous and confrontational negotiations around The International Commission for the Study of Communication Problems (ICSCP) and its Report (UNESCO, 1980). The third part of the Report raised five key problems that have contributed to global inequalities in the political economy of media and communications. These five problems are: huge flaws in communication (restrictive policies/regulations that hamper free flow, contribute to unidirectional and vertical flows and market dominance); dominance in communication contents (distortion of contents, cultural alienation, external influence); difficulties in the democratization of communication; problems in producing and circulating images of the world; and the conundrum over conceptualizing the public and public opinion (UNESCO, 1980).

It was, however, with respect to the problem of the democratization of communication that the need for community media was raised. The Report defines democratization of communication in terms of access and participation, conceiving it as communicative process in which the individual is an active participant, during which there is an increase in the messages being exchanged, and in which social representation in communication is consolidated (UNESCO, 1980). The Report also raises the key factors that determine such democratization in communication. These factors are: representation of the public in communication/media management and policy making; modernization of communication technologies; diversity and choice in communication content; the inclusion of marginalized groups in dominant communication channels; the space for alternative communications (UNESCO, 1980).

The Report then advocates the use of what it describes as alternative communications and counter-information, deliberately established to oppose institutionalized and official media and communication systems, their focus being on content and not the form (UNESCO, 1980). Here, three different social groups engaging in alternative communications are identified. The first group belongs to the radical opposition who produce counter-information to the dominant communication institutions, which are perceived as serving the interests of the dominant social groups. The second group belongs to community or local media movements who seek to actively involve audiences in media production and management. The third group belongs to civil society organizations (such as trade unions or social movements) that require communication networks to articulate their social, economic, or political struggles (UNESCO, 1980).

Probably building on these categorizations, Carpentier, Lie, and Servaes (2003) and Bailey, Cammaerts, and Carpentier (2007) would, many years later, posit a four-tiered framework for analyzing community media: community media that serve a community; community media as an alternative to mainstream media; community media that are linked to civil society; and community media as a rhizome. A major characteristic of all these kinds of community media is antagonism in which "community media can be seen as the condensation of the attempt to offer an alternative for a wide range of hegemonic discourses on communication, media, economics, organizational structures, politics and democracy" (Carpentier, Lie, and Servaes, 2003, p. 51). In fact, Rennie (2006) argues that community media are citizen-led and independent of the state and the market. Another key feature of such community media is the active involvement and participation of the communities that are served by them (Rennie, 2006).

This discussion contends that when factors such as health communication and underdevelopment are brought into the equation, the four-tiered theoretical framework propounded by Carpentier, Lie, and Servaes. (2003) and reiterated by Bailey, Cammaerts, and Carpentier (2007) does not elucidate the new functional challenges facing such media. This chapter is not a criticism of the four-tiered theoretical framework, which provides a comprehensive theory-informed analysis of the attributes and functions of community media. Far from it. In fact, it seeks to continue the building of the body of knowledge in community media theory by introducing a theoretical matrix that allows community media to meet the challenges of health communication in developing world contexts. The three theoretical and methodological frameworks in question are community health development, development journalism, and indigenous knowledge communication systems; all of them are linked together by the methodological adhesive of participatory action research.

Community Media and Health Communication

Discussions on the functional role of community media in health communication tend to focus on three key areas: dissemination of health information that originates from IPGs such as universities and research institutes; facilitation of linkages and communication networks between communities and service providers; and, more importantly, empowerment of communities to undertake rights-based and gender-sensitive approaches to community health development. This chapter builds on the communication for social change (CFSC) model to demonstrate that locating community media within and alongside health communication allows for a critical rethink of the notion of power. The CFSC model (Figueroa *et al.*, 2005, p. 5) describes a process where "community dialogue and collective action work together to produce social change in a community that improves the health and welfare of all of its members." From a CFSC perspective, the community media–health communication axis brings out three facets of power: power as the construction of development from below (a challenge to official development epistemology); power as collaborative decision making (that includes participation); and power as dialogue (based on local ways of speaking). Considered together, all these three ways of conceptualizing power constitute empowerment.

The first conceptualization of power deals with the construction of history from below, as is the case in community health development approaches in which communities are empowered to take the lead in identifying social determinants of health and propounding new directions in health service delivery in ways that challenge official development discourses while simultaneously meeting local aspirations. The second conceptualization of power, collaborative decision making, rests on organic intellectuals, who mobilize communities to think critically about local health challenges. Such an intellectual is Freire's (1972) educator, who, in this case, is the development journalist working within community media. The third conceptualization of power can be located within indigenous knowledge communication systems, in which the local and indigenous ways of speaking and knowing take centre stage in integrating the global within the local. Permeating all these three conceptualizations of power is participatory action research (PAR), a methodological facility that allows for both outsiders and insiders to collaboratively engage in a learning process so as to improve local livelihoods and well-being. As such, PAR is the methodological glue binding the three theoretical trajectories together.

Community Health Development: Mediating Health Development from Below

Debates on involving communities in health have usually been located within development theory and practice (Oakley and Kahssay, 1999). Their integration in health and well-being initiatives is recognition in itself that involving people in decision making in health service delivery creates healthier, stronger, and more livable communities (Ledwith, 2005; Taylor, Wilkinson, and Cheers, 2008). Governments and organizations have attempted to understand the institutional, structural, cultural, and ideological frameworks of communities as a platform for conceiving empowerment models that could increase social capital, community strength, and cohesion (Taylor, Wilkinson, and Cheers, 2008).

Community health development has been informed by three praxes, whose concepts need careful understanding: primary health care, community action for health, and community involvement in health. Primary Health Care (PHC) was conceptualized as a strategy of enabling people to seek better health locally, prevent disease and injury, and shape and manage their health environment (WHO, 1994). The 1978 *Alma Ata* Declaration on PHC highlighted the need for socially acceptable health care, meaning that well-being and healthy life cannot only be achieved by hospitals, medicine, and the availability of well-qualified professionals, but through general sanitation, health education, improved housing standards, nutrition, clean water, affordable and clean energy, and livable and safer communities (WHO, 1994). Community health has, therefore, become a social responsibility of the community.

By the late 1970s, community action for health appeared as a major strategy for achieving "health for all by the year 2000." The emphasis was on understanding public health policy as a health promotion action area (WHO, 1994). From the late 1980s, poverty, inequality, and marginalization were highlighted as major constraints preventing the achievement of sustainable PHC. PHC program reviews exposed the problematics of community participation in establishing wider determinants of health. The World Health

Organisation eventually developed *Guidelines for Rapid Participatory Appraisals to Assess Community Health Needs,* giving rise to the praxis of Community Involvement in Health Development (CIH).

CIH was a rebellion against the external delivery of health programs and services (Oakley and Kahssay, 1999). It was also a rejection of the sponsored and co-opted participation in which external agencies persuade people to expend their resources in return for some benefits. CIH now "involves both a commitment to promote better health with people and not merely for them" (Oakley and Kahssay, 1999, p. 8). Ratified by WHO's meeting in Yugoslavia in 1985, CIH relies on the involvement of communities in formulating decisions and actions affecting their health. It is believed this builds community esteem and responsibility, breaks local dependence, and ensures that health services appropriately meet local needs (Oakley and Kahssay, 1999). CIH acknowledges questions of power and grassroots decision making in achieving community health development.

In theory and practice, community health development has integrated all these three aforementioned praxes but added an aspect of radical community development (Ledwith, 2005). The radical approach to community development goes beyond the recommended best practices (in dealing with signs and symptoms of health inequalities) in order to address the fundamental causes of these health inequalities and marginalization (Ledwith, 2005). By doing this, community health development becomes radically transformative. The recognition within community health development has been that, on their own, health services cannot capacitate citizens and communities to achieve the maximum desired health status that meet their requisite well being requirements (Ledwith, 2005).

The challenge for community media, therefore, is not just to inform people of the best health practices, as posited in the media-centric health communication models originating from within Western IPG industries. Community media should go beyond mere health communications and rather aim to achieve community health engagement. Writing about community health engagement, Kilpatrick (2009) distinguishes between instrumental and empowerment approaches. Whereas instrumental engagement aims to employ community participation as an instrument/means to improve already extant health and social services, the empowerment engagement approach builds on social capital, social infrastructure, and social economy in the local community as a pathway towards eradicating the root causes of health inequalities (Kilpatrick, 2009; Taylor, Wilkinson, and Cheers, 2008).

Community health engagement has been defined as a strategic process involving communities in decisions that affect their health and well-being (NICE, 2008). This entails enabling people to participate in the planning and delivery of acceptable, relevant and appropriate health services (NICE, 2008). The communities in greater need of engagement processes comprise individuals and groups with severe and special health needs, those experiencing difficulties accessing health services, or people living in the most impoverished areas. Community engagement approaches ideally "help communities to work as equal partners or ... delegate some power to them, providing them with total control," in developing and implementing sustainable public health services (NICE, 2008, p. 6). From a community development perspective, engaging communities to improve health requires actual trust, delegation, and capacity being provided to communities in planning and designing the delivery and governance of health and well-being initiatives. The objective is to improve health literacy and the appropriateness, cost-effectiveness, sustainability, and the accessibility and uptake of health services (NICE, 2008).

What are the aspects of community health engagement that community media need to embrace when it comes to health communication? First, community health engagement challenges community media to focus on building and consolidating social capital and social infrastructure in the local community by getting involved in strengthening community cohesion through democratic leadership. Second, community media are being challenged to provide a mechanism for instrumental community engagement between the grassroots and service providers. This enables community media to function as a legitimate instrument of public consultation and collaboration that involves communities in making decisions on local health policy and service delivery. Third, community health engagement challenges community media to mediate and facilitate intracommunity engagement, that is, engagement within community groups. Community media then become effective facilitators and social lubricants that mediate development in ways that empower communities to make informed, clear, pragmatic, and socially acceptable decisions in relation to health challenges.

The praxis of community health development, therefore, provides important logistics for bringing the community into the decision-making process in health service delivery. Community media need to go beyond a merely informative role and become transformative. Rather than informing people and communities on best health practices, or linking communities to health service providers, community media need to be radically transformative in catalyzing communities to deal with the root causes of health inequalities. This means that community media represent the real interests of local communities rather than the short-term, organizational, and external subjective interests that often take a social work and philanthropic approach to community development. However, barriers to engagement still comprise hierarchical cultures within statutory organizations, top-down ideologies and approaches characterizing professional and institutional organizations, conflicting priorities and visions, inadequate community engagement skills for public service staff, and lack of knowledge of, and interest in, community engagement approaches (NICE, 2008).

Development Journalism: Mediating Collective Decision Making

The second conceptualization of power revolves around an organic educator as in development reporting, which is both a theory and practice that argues for an alternative approach to reporting development issues in ways that capture and engage with audiences proactively (Loo, 2009; Jamias, 1991). The emergence of this form of journalism can be traced back to South East Asia and the Indian subcontinent in the 1960s, when newspaper editors began to raise questions about the lack of effective and engaging coverage of development news in the national media. The pioneering work of the

Philippine Press Institute, Communication Foundation for Asia, and the *Hindustan Times* provided a theoretical springboard for the emergence and consolidation of the development journalism praxis. Initially concerned with economic reporting, development journalism would go beyond mere reporting of development news. It became a postcolonial strategy for circumventing and undermining the growing dominant corporate ownership of and influence on media systems and institutions, which is considered to be undermining journalistic professionalism (Loo, 2009).

Development journalism is the earliest of the strands and praxes that contributed to the emergence of the development communication paradigm. South East Asia again pioneered development communication; the aim in these early periods (1950s) was to find effective ways of communicating agricultural information to farming communities (Librero, 1985). Loo (2009) argues that the emergence of development journalism as a key development communication praxis was to address questions of knowledge management and dissemination, in which the subject matter experts were seen as the source of all knowledge and advice. Development journalism embraces the principles of community development by inventing a radical approach towards mediating knowledge brokering and exchange among journalists, expert scientists, and marginalized communities with the aim of improving livelihoods and bringing about development and social change (Librero, 1985; Loo, 2009).

The practice is driven by what Jamias (1991) describes as the people principle, thus the whole experience of capturing alternative voices and using them to report on development is motivated by the need to improve people's lives. Development journalism aims to drive development initiatives by, among other objectives, linking communities to service providers, analyzing complex economic and development information and data for rural and illiterate audiences, challenging audiences to raise questions about the roots of their poverty and marginalization, as well as strengthening grassroots decision-making structures through forging stronger cohesive communities.

These would be the values and ethos that the earliest development journalism experiments would embrace and advance. The community station, Radio DZLB, based at the University of the Philippines, College of Agriculture, went on air in 1964. The development journalism approach saw the radio allow community groups with special interests to produce and broadcast their own programs. On the other hand, professional broadcasters and agriculture scientists introduced agricultural radio schools known as *School on the Air*. Radio DZLB was established as an experimental rural radio network that would facilitate the scaling out and scaling up of knowledge and technology that was being generated by IPGs, especially the University of the Philippines. The Radio's approach to development journalism was packaged around the notion of rural educational broadcasting, which Librero (1985) defines as the use of participatory radio for nonformal education in promoting planned human development. This is done through helping people to "diagnose their problems and clarify their objectives so that they may be able to make wise decisions" (Librero, 1985, p. 1). Radio DZLB's rural educational broadcasters employed semi-structured, interactive, and ethnographic research methods to understand audience needs, prior to introducing new instructional and educational programming.

Following the DZLB development journalism experiment, other similar projects emerged in Indonesia, Malaysia, and India (Jamias, 1991). One such experiment was the Chhatera development journalism experiment in India, implemented between the 1960s and 1970s (Loo, 2009; Verghese, 1976, 2009). George Verghese (1976, 2009), the then editor of the *Hindustan Times* introduced this experiment as an attempt to highlight the daily struggles against poverty and underdevelopment encountered by a real impoverished community in Chhatera. The paper published fortnightly series of reports on development efforts in this small community with the aim of providing urban readers with a window on the reality of poverty and underdevelopment. Reflecting on the project itself, Verghese (2009) provides three key perspectives regarding development journalism, which might impact the role of community media in health communication within developing world contexts. First is that development journalism requires much effort from practitioners to develop a faithful readership/listenership. Urban audiences, advertisers, and corporate owners may even question the relevance of some of the articles and content. Second is that people assume the existential satisfaction of empowerment due to the ability of development journalism to connect their community to the outside world – the other, urban and privileged world that Verghese describes in the interview. Thirdly, development journalism is a form of education for journalists in that it increases their knowledge of a development issue and also sharpens their analytical capabilities, enabling them to take, what Verghese (2009) describes as a "more holistic view" of real life.

As if building on the lessons from the Radio DZLB and Chhatera village development journalism experiments, a community media project in Malawi was established exclusively to implement health communication projects in Mchinji District. *Mudzi Wathu* (Our Village) Community Radio Station, known as the "mouthpiece of the grassroots," was established in 2006 with logistical and financial support from USAID, American Institutes for Research, Radio Systems Incorporation, and a local NGO, the Creative Centre for Community Mobilization of Malawi (CRECCOM) (Chimutu, 2009).The establishment of the station was meant to consolidate an ongoing and broader donor-funded *In My Village Project* that was an HIV/AIDS communication project.

As part of the broader project, CRECCOM has been mobilizing communities to embrace abstinence and faithfulness, improve community support for education and care of orphans and vulnerable children, and build community support for those living with the virus (Chimutu, 2009). The community radio's introduction into the mobilization campaigns has involved two key strategies: health and general development communication programs being prepared by journalists in various formats; establishment of community-based radio listening clubs as local hubs for community development. While the general radio programs on HIV/AIDS provide audiences with information and knowledge, the radio clubs transform such dissemination into horizontal communication through holding group discussions after particular programs have been broadcast. Additionally, motivated by this group listenership, radio club members are engaged as frontline officers dealing with off-air community health development initiatives, such as micro-enterprise development to raise funding for supporting orphans and vulnerable children (Chimutu, 2009).

These examples of development journalism demonstrate that development journalists are more than reporters. Especially when working within community media, development journalists become community development workers and begin to function like frontline officers in rural development. In the case of community media, audiences are also transformed into journalists, since, through structures such as radio listening clubs, they also produce programs. In this case, development journalism becomes the shared communicative space that allows for the transformation of roles and responsibilities among journalists and their audiences. It is worth mentioning that questions have been raised over whether development journalism is an ideological apparatus for government propaganda (Gunaratne, 1996; Shafer, 1996). This concern has been posited in light of the repressive political contexts in which this interventionist model of journalism emerged. As a consequence, development reporters have avoided covering political issues, and instead preferred to cover issues pertaining to economic development, such as construction projects (road, bridges, schools), businesses, agriculture, and enterprise stories on economic development (Shafer, 1996).

Indigenous Knowledge Communication Systems: Mediating the Global and the Local

The third conceptualization of power is located in indigenous knowledge, which is also known as traditional or local knowledge, citizen science, or primitive epistemology (Sillitoe, 2002). Indigenous knowledge is conceptualized as a "unique formulation of knowledge coming from a range of sources rooted in local cultures, a dynamic and ever changing pastiche of past tradition and present invention with a view to the future" (Sillitoe, 2002, p. 113). Likewise, Pottier (2003, p. 4) describes local knowledge as "people's understanding of the social universe and also their rights." Similarly, the United Nations Environment Program (UNEP) web site describes indigenous knowledge as the way of knowing that an indigenous (local) community accumulates over generations of living in a particular environment, allowing them to sustain livelihoods and nurture their environment. UNEP (n.d.) notes that this knowledge goes beyond the abstract epistemological system governing the brokering and sustenance of such knowledge, and also encompasses the knowledge technologies and infrastructure, the skills, practices, and traditional regulatory mechanisms, the power structures and beliefs. These factors enable indigenous knowledges to be "rooted in a particular community and situated within broader cultural traditions" (UNEP, n.d.).

Therefore, indigenous knowledge is not generated, brokered, and sustained for the sake of it; it is rooted within the development of social cohesion and capital in that particular community. It constructs and explains questions of citizenship, identity, rights, law, policy, politics, economics, religion, and general well-being (Pottier, 2003; Sillitoe, 2002). Often postcolonial critiques have tended to criticize the missionaries, settlers, and colonizers for having failed to appreciate and understand the rules and systems governing the semiotics of indigenous knowledges. What is also forgotten is that indigenous knowledge systems are not homogenous. They are complex, plural, heterogeneous, and display some non-linguistic characteristics (Pottier, 2003).

This chapter, however, differentiates indigenous from local knowledges. All indigenous knowledge is local, as it evolves organically within a geographically conceived local time, space, context, and ecology. It is tied to the epistemological, spiritual, and religious belief system of a specific people, so that, even when a people with shared indigenous knowledge practices are separated by time and space, they still retain almost similar traditions and norms, though they might modify some aspects to respond to the geographical environment in which they are living. Religious practices of prayer are a good example.

Local knowledge, on the other hand, is not necessarily indigenous, it can also be scientific, evolving reactively and experientially in response to specific challenges a people are facing in a particular geographical location. It is not necessarily tied to a people's belief system. The building of the dyke system in the Netherlands is a case of local knowledge responding to problems of perennial floods. Building and using clay ovens as a method of conserving scarce firewood by people in arid or semi-arid zones could be considered as local knowledge responding to the problem of deforestation. So, whilst local knowledge reacts to certain environmental or social challenges and over time may become irrelevant once the challenges disappear, indigenous knowledge builds on years of accumulated experience and the passing down of that knowledge between generations, and is tied to the political economy of a people's belief infrastructure (Pottier, 2003; Sillitoe, 2002).

Epistemologically, indigenous knowledges are created, modified, used, and passed on down the generations through a series of overt and covert communicative practices and performances. Indigenous knowledge (IK) communication systems are the facilities that mediate indigenous knowledges. Thus IK communication systems do not exist on their own, or just for the sake of it. They perform a social function within an indigenous knowledge system, mostly related to the calendar of human life, from birth to death. Such communication systems function to generate, transfer, and share knowledge within that social system. Mundy and Compton (1999) observe that indigenous communications transmit technical information, entertain, pass on news, persuade, and announce important events and exchanges. IK communication systems, therefore, function to transmit information and share knowledge as well as facilitate the process of knowing itself – knowledge acquisition. Western systems and institutions have frequently approached IK systems with a modernization frame, conceiving them as unitary, unbounded, static, consensual, nonreflective, unscientific, and traditional (Pottier, 2003; Sillitoe, 2002). The Western assumption is that, on their own, indigenous systems are not capable of explaining and correcting socio-political phenomena, unless repackaged within the lens of Western modernity and science.

There exists a direct functional connection between IK communication systems and community media. IK communication systems often serve the social objectives of a particular community group; hence they are in themselves community media. Kamlongera et al. (1992) provide an example of *Gulewamkulu* initiation and *Vimbuza* therapeutic ceremonies in Malawi, in which IK communications and performances mediate a tenuous relationship between ritual and theater, the real and unreal, the global and the local. Referring to the *Gulewamkulu* initiation ceremony, which comprises the real initiation ceremony (for boys entering manhood) and the performance, Kamlongera et al. (1992) contend that indigenous knowledges serve educational, psychological, social, and aesthetic functions within African communities.

The educational function focuses on the instructive aspect, in which the performance masks provide advice on how to live and act in society. The names given to these masks and their respective *Gulewamkulu* characters entrench the specific human behaviors that are expected of the society. Kamlongera *et al.* (1992, p. 40) observe that the *Gulewamkulu* performance has "become a medium through which ideas of opposition to the normal world or of the distortion of accepted human and social values are expressed." In the end the *Gulewamkulu* characters become real in that they represent personalities and behaviors recognized by communities and social groups. Psychologically, *Gulewamkulu* performance provides an emotional window to let out the personality aspects that are sublimated by the society while claiming that the emotional outburst and expressions belong to the characters in the performance (Kamlongera *et al.*, 1992). Socially, Gulewamkulu performances provide an opportunity to meet new friends and make acquaintances. Aesthetically, the performances provide a sphere for communities to display their aesthetic skills in singing, dancing, and mimickry (Kamlongera *et al.*, 1992).

The differentiation between IK systems and IK communication systems challenges community media to augment the educational, aesthetic, psychological, and social functions of indigenous knowledge communication systems. As a performance, *Gulewamkulu* is very critical of oppressive social structures and often represents the real interests of the oppressed and marginalized. The challenge for community media is to have journalists with the relevant skills in engaging with indigenous knowledge systems and using them to capture the needs, aspirations, and dreams of those who are marginalized by an oppressive social structure. IK communication systems are completely different media and communication systems from the modern media systems extant within nation-states, and, as such, community media should serve the important function of mediating between the global and the local communication systems. Whereas modern theories of development consider indigenous knowledge systems very primitive and assume that they hold people back from achieving upward mobility, community media should mediate the educational attributes of the IK systems and contextualize them, especially in relation to health communication. Alongside or on the very periphery of Western-style health communications, IK communication systems rallied against multiple sexual partners, promiscuity, domestic violence, and other social evils.

In indigenous knowledge speech takes many forms, including riddles, proverbs and of course vulgarities (Mbembe, 2001; Zvomuya, 2011). In fact some of the indigenous knowledge instructions in public and community health employ seemingly sexualized language. This fact speaks against western-centric behavior change communications that assume that local cultures in the Global South are usually silent on sex and critical health issues. For example, an Igbo proverb in Nigeria says 'unless it dies young, the penis shall surely eat bearded meat' – which teachers societies the value of patience and that there 'is no point in rushing to indulge in sexual activities' (Zvomuya, 2011). In Malawi, the proverb 'The big headed one eventually fucked boiling water' has become more relevant in times of HIV/AIDS, in teaching the youth to listen to wise advice of the elderly to avoid contracting the virus (that's the fucking boiling water part). Vulgarity is therefore, at the very centre of indigenous knowledge-informed health communications in Africa and perhaps much of the Global South. But this vulgarity is functionally didactic. It must be pointed out however, that, when perceived from uncritical and dogmatic feminist perspectives, some of these didactic proverbs and instructions may seem paternalistic, chauvinistic and sexist. It is unfortunate that foreign religious institutions have played a huge part in discouraging most of these didactic indigenous knowledge communications on 'moral' grounds. The role of community media is to contextualize these local initiatives in relation to modern and global approaches to health communication. These three theoretical frameworks (community health development, development journalism, and indigenous knowledge communication systems) are tied together through the methodological string of participatory action research.

Participatory Action Research: Mediating the Three Theoretical Trajectories

Participatory Action Research (PAR) is a consultative research process that is half research and half pedagogy and aims to liberate and engage participants in the praxis of reflecting and learning so as to achieve planned social objectives. Kemmis and McTaggart (1988) conceive PAR as a method of inquiry that consultatively brings together social participants and engages them in a pedagogy that aims to enrich their own social practices. This exploratory facility revolves around four interdependent praxes: reflection, planning, action, and observation (Kemmis and McTaggart, 1988). PAR emerged as a postcolonial critique of dominant social research methods that often privileged the external researcher as a power holder, and in which the data collection process was solely extractive and for use by outsiders. Within developing world contexts, the PAR methodology has been employed using various action research strategies, such as theater for development (TfD) initiatives. TfD is a generic term that describes a group of methodologies in which theater, music, and drama are employed to sensitize communities to a particular development challenge and then empower them to act upon their collectively developed solutions. The PAR process in TfD takes place in five key steps, which are moments of encounter between the research team and local communities. These are establishing partnership, preliminary situation analysis, scenario and message development, rehearsal and performance, post-performance evaluation and engagement (Kamlongera, 2005).

The TfD model emerged as a form of community media largely due to three factors: the attempts by colonial governments to facilitate the modernization of people and communities using theater and drama; a recognition by colonial authorities that indigenous knowledge communication systems have positive social and educational functions; reactionary resistance by local communities to colonial attempts to develop indigenous cultures as part of the modernization project (Kamlongera, 2005). Within the colonial context TfD has often been involved in developing "social case dramas" to provide specific technical knowledge on social development issues (Kamlongera, 2005). For the newly independent African states, TfD has been a method of supplementing the mass media and communication systems that are still developing.

The theater for development education model has been strengthened by the work of Paulo Freire (1972), Augusto Boal (1993), and more recently, Ngugi wa Thiong'o (1986) and Chris Kamlongera (2005). The fundamental praxis of such theater is to engage communities in promoting collective action on social development. TfD as a praxis is located within problems of marginalization (social, economic, and political) and neocolonialism – the continued existence of colonialism despite the achievement of political independence. Emerging from the colonial attempts to develop indigenous people through the use of popular arts, African universities started experimenting with the same to provide a different kind of popular art form that would educate people about their situation (Kamlongera, 2005).

Whilst the work of Freire (1972) and Boal (1993) proved to be a theoretical springboard for the social uses of popular arts, African and South East Asian movements played a huge part in developing the theory and practice that would inform the use of popular arts as community media. There was the developmental theater movement (often conflated with the generic term, theater for development), whose work was enlightened by the emergent development communication paradigm from the Philippines and the United States. The establishment of the United Nations Development Programme's Communication Service in Thailand in the 1970s was an acknowledgement on the part of the international development community of the need to integrate communication as a critical component within development policy formulation. The theater for development movement would thus be greatly influenced by diffusionist models of communication. The movement and its various approaches would be roped in to play a huge part in the health, population, and rural development communication campaigns that organizations and governments would launch as part of the Integrated Rural Development Programs.

In this developmental theater model, external teams of action researchers (comprising university teachers and students, extension workers, and other subject matter specialists) go into a community, talk to villagers about local development challenges, and collect all this information to be used to prepare productions, which are then shown back to the community as surprise gifts. Though Kamlongera (2005) argues that the opening-up strategies during the actual performance, which involve inviting audience members to get involved in solving the onstage conflicts, often allow people to examine issues critically and talk about them even after the performance, there is not much evidence to support the level of concientization achieved. This diffusionist approach is very popular among government and development organizations working in media-based health and population communication campaigns. But such an approach offers little in terms of action, reflection, and transformation, and has, occasionally, been misconceived as a form of cultural imperialism.

Another important popular art movement was the protest theater movement that was championed by radicals like Ngugi wa Thiong'o (1986) and the various labor organizations in other parts of the world. The emphasis was to engage people in critically assessing their post-independence governments, a centre piece of Boal's concept of the poetics of the oppressed. This concept builds on Freirean notions of conscientization to advocate for a postcolonial theater that challenges people to understand the causes (not symptoms) of their marginalization (Boal, 1993). For Ngugi, popular theater was not just a space for entertaining or educating people, but a consultative conscientization initiative that allowed people to question what Mbembe (2001) describes as the vulgarity of the "autocrat" (in post-independence dictatorships) and his obscene banality of power. By doing this, popular theater assumed the role of community media (considering the appropriation of state broadcasters and other media by the post-independence nation-states). It thus provided a communicative space for challenging the illusion of independence as manifested by growing human rights abuses, corruption by politicians, political violence, lack of democracy, and growing rural poverty and urban unemployment (Mbembe, 2001). This movement of popular arts was often times banned by governments and its leaders were imprisoned or tortured (Ngugi wa Thiong'o, 1986).

The participatory action research aspect in these forms of popular theater is evident in the process leading up to the production. The central issues in PAR are action, reflection, and transformation. For example, in one of the many theater for development projects I have been involved in, the action research teams created drama around local development themes. In 2002, I was involved in a public health communication project at Ximba Primary School, outside Durban, South Africa. The objective of this action research initiative emanated from a situation analysis that I and a colleague from Swaziland carried out in relation to communities' gender-based allocation of domestic chores/jobs (Manyozo and Dlamini, 2002). This gender-based definition of "boys' jobs" or "girls' jobs," according to our analysis, disadvantaged girls and also affected their performance in school. Our health communication project was not intended to be a banking approach (Freire, 1972), but rather an action research exercise that would challenge young people to critically question how gender power relations affect the domestic economy in patriarchal communities (Manyozo and Dlamini, 2002).

With funding from the Johns Hopkins University Centre for Communications Programs, administered through the Centre for Culture, Communication, and Media Studies at the University of KwaZulu Natal, we approached Ximba Primary School for permission and partnership to carry out the project. The Department of Education in KwaZulu Natal eventually provided permission for the execution of the project. The process of action, learning, and reflection revolved around three specific aims, namely: establishing what the primary school kids understood as "men's jobs" and "women's jobs"; determining the prevalent attitudes and perceptions regarding the relationship between gender and household chores; and finally involving the pupils in producing a workshop play emerging from their participatory critical assessment of the gendered nature of the domestic economy (Manyozo and Dlamini, 2002).

This PAR project made use of three strategies to achieve these aims: preliminary field visits (to familiarize ourselves with local people, pupils and teachers); participatory forums (in which pupils would use arts and dialogue to question the social issues relating to gender allocation of domestic chores); and, collaborative development of plays and skits (Manyozo and Dlamini, 2002). The theoretical framework informing this study was entertainment-education (Coleman, 1998; Singhal and Rogers, 1999). Methodologically, the manual, *How to Make an Aids Play* produced by the Drama in Aids Education (DramAidE) Project provided a template that guided the PAR process leading to the creation of entertainment-education skits and dramas. The final performance comprised three short plays that raised questions about the gender division of labour in the home and how this affects the personal development of boys and girls as well as wider problems of discrimination in society. The challenge however, was that a one-off activity of this kind has limited impact. We believed, granted sufficient resources, we could have engaged the surrounding communities (Manyozo and Dlamini, 2002).

This theater for development project provides a theoretical illumination of what community media should normatively be in relation to health communication (though without being restricted to this role). Community media should not just be about educating and disseminating information that is of relevance to the community. In a conversation to Myles Horton, Freire (1990) regretted having written *Pedagogy of the Oppressed* (1972) before reading Gramsci. It is obvious that Freire was alluding to two Gramscian projects that he would dwell on in his later works: the formation of the organic intellectual (one allied to a particular ideological block); and the notion of power (as in hegemony). Community media should be actively involved as an organic intellectual in transformatively mediating power at the community level. This implies that community media should reflect the two contradictory roles of the organic and traditional intellectual. Whilst they are committed to the transformation of the community polity, the media should function as traditional intellectuals by objectively questioning the community-level exercise of power that oppresses and marginalizes. Participatory Action Research should become a philosophy driving community media-facilitated health and development initiatives. The methodology should involve local people in a continuous cycle of learning, reflection and action.

Afterthoughts: Community Media and Health Communication

The CFSC model allows for a strategic integration of community media within health communication at three levels: community health development (power as development from below); development journalism (power as collective decision making); and indigenous knowledge communication systems (power as the articulation of local ways of knowing and speaking). These three trajectories are linked by PAR, itself a pedagogical research methodology that allows communities and external stakeholders to reflect and learn together in local development initiatives. The diagram below elucidates this integration.

This chapter has argued that, whereas Bailey, Cammaerts, and Carpentier (2007) and Carpentier, Lie, and Servaes (2003) propounded a four-tiered theoretical framework for studying alternative and community media that defines, locates, and assigns attributes to different categories of alternative and community media, this discussion has shown that the framework requires a rethink and, of course, consolidation when questions of health communication and development are brought into the equation. The chapter has successfully argued that studying the community media–health communication–development nexus requires a theoretical facility that addresses questions of participation, power, and development. No one single theory can capture the challenge of answering the critical questions that arise within this confluence. The discussion has introduced the three theories of community health development, development journalism, and indigenous knowledge communication systems, which are linked together by the Participatory Action Research (PAR) methodology. Therefore, the examination has provided a diagnostic instrument for rethinking how community media need to be reoriented to meet the health communication and engagement needs of marginalized communities in particular.

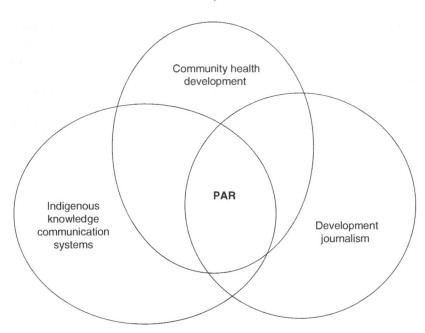

Figure 11.1 Integrating community media within health communication.

The responsibility of community media lies in establishing compromise interests during the critical processes of message development and stakeholder engagement. This chapter has therefore argued that, whereas health communication has been largely informed by the diffusionist theoretical and methodological frameworks emerging from the Western international public goods industries, the epistemological foundations of community media require reconsideration of the theoretical matrix that explains health communication in terms of community engagement and sustainable development. The discussion contends that a marriage between community media and health communication within developing world contexts is made possible by bringing together three theoretical frameworks and one methodological glue that allow one to make sense of participation, power, and development. Together the four frameworks enable community media to effectively mediate health and development issues in developing countries. The re-emergence of the radio listening club concept demonstrates that the challenge for community media is not just to provide and disseminate health information, but rather to act as a strategic instrument and sphere for local engagement.

References

Bailey, O., Cammaerts, B., and Carpentier, N. (2001). *Understanding Alternative Media.* Maidenhead: Open University Press.

Boal, A. (1993). *Theater of the Oppressed.* New York: Theater Communications Group.

Carpentier, N., Lie, R., and Servaes, J. (2003). Community media: muting the democratic media discourse? *Continuum: Journal of Media and Cultural Studies, 17*(1), 51–68.

Chimutu, P. (2009). Mudzi Wathu (Our Village) Community Radio Station, Malawi: Abidjan Power Point Presentation. Retrieved from http://www.comminit.com/en/node/304828/376

Coleman, P. (1998). Enter-educate: New word from Johns Hopkins. *Japanese Organization for International Cooperation in Family Planning, 15,* 28–31.

Figueroa, M. E., Kincaid, D. E., Rani, M., and Lewis, G. (2005). *Communication for Social Change: An Integrated Model for Measuring the Process and Its Outcomes.* Communication for Social Change Working Paper Series. New York: Rockefeller Foundation.

Freire, P. (1972). *Pedagogy of the Oppressed.* London: Penguin Books.

Freire, P. and Horton, M (1990). *We Make the Road by Walking: Conversations on Education and Social Change Between Myles Horton and Paulo Freire.* Edited by Brenda Bell, John Gaventa, and John Peters. Philadelphia: Temple University Press.

Gunaratne, S. (1996). Old wine in a new bottle: Public journalism movement in the United States and the erstwhile NWICO debate. Paper presented at the 20th General assembly, Scientific Conference of the International Association for Media and Communication Research, Sydney, August 18–22.

Jamias, J. (1991). *Writing for Development: Focus on Specialised Reporting Areas.* Laguna:UPLB College of Development Communication and the Foundation for Development and Communication.

Kamlongera, C., Nambote, M., Soko, B., and Timpunza-Mvula, E. (1992). *Kubvina: An Introduction to Malawian Dance and Theatre.* Zomba: Research and Publication Committee, University of Malawi.

Kamlongera, C. (2005). Theatre for development in Africa. In O. Hemer and T. Tufte (Eds.), *Media and Glocal Change: Rethinking Communication for Development* (pp. 435–452). Göteborg and Buenos Aires: NORDICOM and CLASCO.

Kemmis, S. and McTaggart, R. (1988). *The Action Research Planner.* Geelong, Victoria: Deakin University Press.

Kilpatrick, S. (2009). Multi-level rural community engagement in health. *Australian Journal of Rural Health, 17*(1), 39–44.

Ledwith, M. (2005). *Community Development: A Critical Appraisal.* Bristol: Polity Press.

Librero, F. (1985). *Rural Educational Broadcasting: A Philippine Experience.* Laguna: UPLB College of Agriculture.

Loo, E. (2009). *Best Practices of Journalism in Asia.* Singapore: Konrad-Adenauer-Stiftung.

Manyozo, L. and Dlamini, L. (2002). Challenges of collaborative play production on social issues: An entertainment-education project report on Ximba primary school participatory play-making. A Public Health Promotion Project report submitted to the Culture, Communication and Media Studies (CCMS), University of Natal, Durban. Retrieved from http://ccms.ukzn.ac.za/index.php?option=com_content&task=view&id=548&Itemid=70

Mbembe, A. (2001). *On the Postcolony.* Los Angeles and Berkeley: University of California Press.

Mundy, P. A. and Compton, J. L. (1999). Indigenous communication and indigenous knowledge. In D. C. Warren, L. J. Slikkerveer, and D. Brokensha (Eds.), *The Cultural Dimension of Development: Indigenous Knowledge Systems* (pp. 112–123). Intermediate Technology Publications, London.

Ngugi wa Thiong'o (1986). *Decolonising the Mind: The Politics of Language in African Literature.* London and Nairobi: James Currey and Heinemann Kenya.

NICE (2008). *Community Engagement to Improve Health.* London: National Institute for Health and Clinical Excellence.

Oakley, P. and Kahssay, H. M. (1999). *Community Involvement in Health Development: A Review of the Concept and Practice.* Geneva: World Health Organisation.

Pottier, J. (2003). Negotiating local knowledge: An introduction. In J. Pottier, P. Sillitoe and A. Bicker (Eds.). *Negotiating Local Knowledge: Identity and Power in Development.* London: Pluto.

Rennie, E. (2006). *Community Media: A Global Introduction*. Lanham, MD: Rowman and Littlefield.

Shafer, R. (1996). Journalists as reluctant interventionists: Comparing development and civic journalism. Paper Presented at the Conference of the Association for Education in Journalism and Mass Communication (AEJMC), Anaheim, California, August, 1996. Retrieved from http://list.msu.edu/cgi-bin/wa?A2=ind9612aandL=aejmcandP=4533

Sillitoe, P. (2002). Globalizing indigenous knowledge. In P. Sillitoe, A. Bicker and J. Pottier (Eds.), *Participating in Development: Approaches to Indigenous Knowledge* (pp. 108–138). London: Routledge.

Singhal, A. and Rogers, E. (1999). *Entertainment-Education: A Communication Strategy for Social Change*. Mahwah, NJ: Lawrence Erlbaum Associates.

Taylor, J., Wilkinson, D., and Cheers, B. (2008). *Working with Communities in Health and Human Services*. Oxford: Oxford University Press.

UNEP (n.d.). What is indigenous knowledge? Available at: http://www.unep.org/IK/Pages.asp?id=About%20IK

UNESCO (1980). *Many Voices One World: Communication and Society, Today and Tomorrow; Towards a New More Just and More Efficient World Information and Communication Order*. London, New York and Paris: Kogan Page and The International Commission for the Study of Communication Problems, UNESCO.

Verghese, G. (1976). *Project Chhatera: An Experiment in Development Journalism*. Occasional Paper Number 4. Singapore: Asian Mass Communication Research and Information Centre.

Verghese, B. (2009). Development journalism in Asia: Beware of cynicism, kindle hope. Transcribed interview conducted by Eric Loo. In E. Loo, *Best Practices of Journalism in Asia* (pp. 155–162). Singapore: Konrad-Adenauer-Stiftung.

WHO. (1994). *Health Promotion and Community Action for Health in Developing Countries*. Geneva: World Health Organisation.

Zvomuya, P. (2011). African culture uncensored. *The Mail and Guardian Online*. December 23. Retrieved from http://mg.co.za/article/2011-12-23-african-culture-uncensored.

12

Global E-health Communication

L. Suzanne Suggs and Scott C. Ratzan

Introduction

E-health affords many opportunities for the development of innovative and effective health communication practices that contribute to increased knowledge and improved health behaviors. E-health has evolved tremendously in the past decades and includes any transfer of health communication, services, surveillance, or treatment through the use of digital means (Eng, 2001; Haider, Ratzan, and Meltzer, 2009). In the early to mid 1990s e-health primarily consisted of didactic patient information web sites and tele-medicine, but later progressed to interactive and participant-centered approaches including web sites, blogs, wikis, mobile phones, email, video, and podcasts, and electronic medical records. While the struggle with taxonomy persisted for some time, documented by the numerous papers defining "e-health" and other related terms (i.e., Medicine 2.0, m-health, digital health), the progression beyond telemedicine and static web sites has resulted in an e-health evolution.

This chapter is not a review of best practices, as these are published elsewhere, nor is it a history lesson on the development of e-health. It is rather a discussion of where e-health communication is and where it is headed, why we must go there, and ideas on how we get there. Certainly, this cannot be accomplished by ignoring the past; we must first present some illustrative examples to show how this roadmap for the next generation of e-health communication evolved. Therefore, we start this chapter by briefly revisiting the development and promise of e-health and perspectives that framed the way we think of e-health. We then discuss e-health today, highlighting the public health need, and examples of innovative and simple solutions to meet the challenges of real world global public health needs. Next, we discuss the future of

The Handbook of Global Health Communication, First Edition. Edited by Rafael Obregon and Silvio Waisbord.
© 2012 John Wiley & Sons, Inc. Published 2012 by John Wiley & Sons, Inc.

e-health, as we see it, providing readers with a set of critical questions, checklists, and proposals for measuring our progress.

E-health: Past

It has been almost two decades since the Mosaic Web browser changed the way people could obtain information, which subsequently changed the way we thought about delivering and retrieving health communication. Electronic medical records, telemedicine, the World Wide Web, other technology channels, and programming abilities designed to reach more people with more efficacious interventions were new, interesting, innovative and gave us great optimism about the future of public health communication. E-health was seen as an alternative way to communicate health information and initial efforts focused on providing care remotely, sharing knowledge and data between providers, and creating opportunities for patients to talk with one another and with their doctor remotely. Using e-health to enhance health literacy, shared decision-making, and improve health outcomes became a reality (Barrera *et al.*, 2002; Eysenbach *et al.*, 2004; Gustafson *et al.*, 1999; Wantland *et al.*, 2004; Suggs, 2006; Ratzan, 2010a; Ratzan and Gilhooly, 2010).

E-health grew in virtually all areas of health communication and the amount of research increased dramatically. For instance, in December 2000, a search for the word "Internet" in PubMed yielded over 6,600 citations (Ratzan and Busquets, 2002) and the first meta-analysis of Web-based health programs highlighted a twelvefold increase for "Web-based therapies" in MEDLINE between 1996 and 2003 (Wantland *et al.*, 2004). Much of the literature touted the potential of technology to reach large numbers of people, in real time, where resources were absent or scarce, in addition to augmenting services and communication efforts in wealthier nations (Eysenbach, 2001; Fogg, 2003; Neuhauser and Kreps, 2003; Suggs, 2006; Haider, Ratzan, and Meltzer, 2009). E-health communication solutions were supported because of their capacity to adapt new technologies to the needs of providers, patients, consumers, and health systems, as well as the volume of health content available and the need to cut costs and expand access to services. Technology-based approaches showed promise to enhance active learning, to increase skills, motivation, and self-efficacy to perform a task or behavior, and to provide an environment for shared and informed decision making. Indeed, Wantland and colleagues' (2004) meta-analysis of Web-based behavior change initiatives found better behavior change outcomes for Web-based programs compared to off-line programs. These efforts also resulted in increased satisfaction with care, health outcome improvements, and, in some cases, contained costs (Glasgow *et al.*, 2004; Gustafson *et al.*, 1999; Wantland *et al.*, 2004). People liked communicating about health information in a digital way, as technology quickly became a more "normal" part of everyday life.

Health promotion, disease prevention, and self-management interventions were successfully being delivered using new technologies such as the Web, CD-Rom, the telephone, and hand-held computers (Suggs, 2006). Health care delivery could be provided through telephone, video, e-mail consultations, e-prescribing, claims processing, physician Web portals, and electronic medical records (EMRs) (Anderson and Stenzel, 2001). Delivering tailored communication by using appropriate content, visuals, and channels became possible and promising. Digital technologies were no longer only used to deliver communication; they were now being implemented to create individualized communication delivered through both traditional and technology channels.

While we witnessed a surge in activity regarding e-health, concerns about access, privacy, costs, culture, and loss of interpersonal communication persisted. In many parts of the world, enthusiasm for e-health was accompanied by caution. The digital divide (the gap between those with and those without access to computers, the Internet, or other digital technologies) was of great concern, with increasing digital access being a priority for governments and industry around the world. In the United States, the Healthy People 2010 objectives, a set of 10-year national goals published in 2000, made access to communication technology a priority, aiming for 80 percent of US homes to have Internet access (DHHS, 2000). Yet, in some parts of the world, home Internet access was never going to be realized, reinforcing concerns about the digital divide. Hence, low-cost, low-resource-intensive technologies (e.g., the telephone) were sought and prioritized. This is when the global focus began to shift from getting people to use the technology that others decided they should (e.g., many programs budgeted for home computers for entire populations) to using pervasive technologies.

As more people gained access to communication technologies, health communicators and other health professionals began to embrace using pervasive and other exiting technologies in new ways. As satisfaction with communicating through digital means and the ability to achieve positive outcomes using e-health channels became evident, the field of e-health was ready for the next generation of challenges and possibilities.

Present

Substantial progress has been made in providing digital access. In 2000, approximately 400 million people worldwide had access to the Internet. Today it is estimated that about 1.8–1.9 billion people are connected to the Web, distributed mainly in Asia, Europe, and North America, with an average penetration rate of 28.7 percent (Broadband Commission for Digital Development, 2010; Internet World Stats, 2010). The geographic areas with the biggest Internet penetration rates are North America (77%), followed by Australia and Oceania (61%), and Europe (58%). Latin America and the Caribbean (35%), the Middle-East (30%), Asia (22%), and Africa (11%), while lagging behind, are experiencing the largest annual growth.

Hence, when we think of e-health communication today, we can no longer speak of it as an alternative to "traditional" media providing the same communication but packaged through a different channel. Rather, we must view it as part of a necessary and integrated approach to health communication that is flexible; allowing the adaptability of content, dosage, timing, purpose, and channel (i.e., wikis, patient portals, Short Message Service (SMS), Multimedia Message Service (MMS), and social media (i.e., Facebook, MySpace, Twitter, Flicker, Youtube, Second Life). Today's e-health communication is not only about new technology or new media; it is about using new and traditional media in new ways. It is not about repackaging the same content for a different channel; it is about using the power of technology to deliver content in different ways, through multiple channels (video,

---

Box 12.1   E-health's impact on patients and providers

In the United States, e-health is helping people get care remotely and provides comfort to their families…

> We live in a community of 25,000 people in the rural state of South Dakota. The nearest infectious disease specialist is 3 hours away. My husband, who has stage 4 colon cancer, has benefitted from consultation with the infectious disease specialist via distance technology/video-conferencing at our local hospital. Without this form of e-health he would either have had to make a very difficult 6 hour round trip or had no consultation with this specialist.(K. Courtney, South Dakota, USA)

In Switzerland, Dr. A. Kick believes e-health has a positive impact on his practice and his patients…

> In our practice we don't use paper any more for the documentation of our medical records. Everything is written directly into the computer, so it is legible and immediately available in a well- structured form for any member of our team. My orders to the assistants are given only in a digitally written form directly by the task manager of the computer program, so documented and univocal to avoid communication errors. All test results (e.g. laboratory, ECG, X-rays) and reports enter instantly into the electronic file of the patient without further transcription errors. All these documents are well classified and can be searched without human power or time-consuming processes. I can confirm that the use of an electronic patient file, for us, saves money, time, manpower, is very efficient, and improves outcomes.
>
> I never was skeptical about using this kind of technology during medical consultation or communicating with patients. In fact, I couldn't work any longer without these very helpful electronic instruments. (Dr. med. A. Kick, Specialist FMH in internal medicine, Switzerland).

---

audio, SMS) tailored to individual needs and preferences. It's no longer just about health professionals reaching a broader audience with health information; it's about people being active participants, exchanging knowledge and experience, developing skills to make informed choices, reaching people where they are (e.g., through their phone), improving access to quality information and services, and improving communication.

Back in those early days of e-health communication research and practice, you could not talk about e-health without someone reminding you of the digital divide or raising concerns about privacy; concerns that, while important, reflected a lack of understanding about the reach and privacy of traditional communication channels. We were worried about the pitfalls of being "too connected," increasing health disparities between rich and poor, creating issues regarding who pays and how we reimburse for e-care, leaving people vulnerable to inaccurate online content, and having EMRs that were not transferrable to other systems. While we still do not have all the answers, major progress has been made. Today, the responsibility for health is becoming increasingly shared, with patients taking a more active interest in their own health care options, and diseases and illnesses are becoming increasingly self-managed. The amount of drugs administered, both prescription and nonprescription, doubled between 1995–1996 and 2004–2005. There also has been a decline in hospital stays since 2000 (Miron-Shatz, 2010). With improved access to health information (e.g., via the Internet and the mass media), along with a growing level of medical sophistication among lay persons, patients today are evolving rapidly into "health-competent consumers," taking an active role in their own health and health care, and demanding safe and more effective health care solutions. We now struggle with questions like:

- How do we ensure that people are health literate and can find, understand and act upon the communication we provide?
- How can we engage citizens and help facilitate their own, innate ability to help themselves when given the right tools, skills, and motivation?
- How do we best harness the capabilities and possibilities of a variety of communication technologies, including traditional ones such as the phone, to provide applications that are flexible, adaptable, sustainable, and cost effective?

And, then and perhaps most importantly,

- How do we develop systems that strike a perfect balance of didactic and interactive user-generated, tailored, quality communication?

These are important questions given the disease burden currently facing society.

The burden of disease

Noncommunicable (chronic) and communicable diseases are hitting populations and health systems hard. Chronic disease, in particular, is one of the top four risks threatening the planet, along with fiscal crises, unemployment, and underinvestment in infrastructures, according to the 2010 World Economic Forum Global Risks Report. These major risks share a potential for wider systemic impact and are strongly linked to a number of long-term global trends. Chronic diseases are now among the central risks that threaten the global economy and development over the next decade.

Between 2005 and 2015, income loss estimates (in international dollars) related to chronic disease are forecast to increase to $558 billion in China, $237 billion in India, $303 billion in Russia, $33 billion in the United Kingdom, and $49 billion in Brazil. Costs associated with poor mental health account for 2–3 percent of GDP.

This should be no surprise to those of us in the health field. Today roughly 60 percent of all deaths, 35 million people per year, result from chronic diseases. Almost 80 percent of deaths from chronic diseases occur in developing countries (WHO, 2009). Of the total global deaths from heart attack, stroke, diabetes, and asthma, 40 percent, or 15.8 million, are attributable to risk factors and would be considered premature deaths from preventable diseases/conditions. By 2030, 75 percent of all deaths worldwide will be from chronic diseases, unless preventive action is taken.

Box 12.2   Diabetes: A global health challenge

Diabetes is certain to be one of the most challenging health problems in the 21st century (International Diabetes Federation, 2007).

- By 2030, there will be 350 million people living with diabetes;
- Type 2 Diabetes Mellitus (T2DM) accounts for 85–95 percent of all cases;
- T2DM is associated with higher risk for heart disease, nerve and kidney damage, and stroke;
- Heart disease and stroke account for about 65 percent of deaths among people with diabetes;
- Diabetes is one of the most common non-communicable diseases globally;
- It is the fourth or fifth leading cause of death in most developed countries;
- Complications can be reduced or even prevented through individual lifestyle behavior change.

We know that we need to address the big four diseases: cardiovascular disease, cancers, diabetes, and chronic respiratory disease; the big four behavioral risk factors: tobacco use, unhealthy diets, physical inactivity, and the harmful use of alcohol; and the big four biological risk factors: raised blood pressure, raised cholesterol, raised blood sugar, and high body mass index. As much as 80 percent percent of heart disease, stroke, and type 2 diabetes, and 40 percent of cancers can be prevented through inexpensive and cost-effective interventions, such as controlling tobacco, encouraging appropriate and affordable diets, promoting physical activity, avoiding harmful alcohol use, and enabling health services for early detection.

However, to focus exclusively on chronic diseases would be a mistake. Communicable diseases, viruses, and neglected tropical diseases (NTDs), predominantly infectious parasitic diseases spread by insects or contaminated water and soil, prospering in poor and remote tropical settings, are a serious threat to individual health and society. It is estimated that more than 1 billion people suffer from a NTD (WHO, 2010). The emergence of new infectious diseases and the resurgence of diseases previously controlled by vaccination and treatment (e.g., malaria and smallpox) are creating important public health challenges (WHO, 2007).

To better understand the challenge and stakes of global health, we must address health and well-being as central and crucial to human, business, and social capital development.

The importance of promoting health literacy

Informed patients, health-competent consumers and citizens, are better able to make optimal economic health decisions, thus contributing to the reduction of unnecessary health care spending. The first step toward improving health literacy is helping individuals understand how they can stay healthy, get better, and live well with disease.

Health literate patients and consumers:

- have better treatment outcomes;
- are more likely to adopt and adhere to preventive regimes;
- seek necessary health care services because they know the warning signs of serious disease;
- follow instructions better and are less likely to misuse or abuse medicines;
- are not afraid to ask questions when they do not understand what a health care professional is saying or doing, which further reduces the risk of medical errors and increases adherence to recommendations.

In thinking about health literacy and e-health, the focus includes both improving patient and consumer health literacy as well as implementing a broader system change. As members of a holistic society, we must encourage efforts to advance general literacy and individual health literacy skills. As health professionals and members of health and health care systems, we must understand how well we communicate with patients and citizens. Recent trends in e-health communication give health consumers more control and power regarding how, what, and when they receive and provide information about health. Web technology pushed and continues to push the boundaries that health communication professionals used to control. Society's technological progress presents an opportunity for developing health literacy – advancing knowledge and skills while reducing complexity such that individuals and health providers can make appropriate decisions.

E-health goes social

Social media are changing the health communication landscape by providing accessible and uncomplicated methods to share and exchange knowledge, ideas, and experiences, establish linkages among users, and essentially redistribute power from a small number of corporate or government controlled outlets to the people who choose to participate.

Social media are "a group of Internet-based applications that build on the ideological and technological foundations of Web 2.0, and that allow the creation and exchange of user-generated content" (Kaplan and Haenlein, 2010, p. 61). In other words, social media are the social aspects of Web 2.0 applications: participation, openness, conversation, community, and connectedness (Mayfield, 2008).

Social media possess several characteristics that set them apart from other technologies and traditional media, but, at its foundation, it is unique because of its reliance on user-generated content. Social media are a global phenomenon that involves organizations and individuals in all markets regardless of economic, social, and cultural development. The Web is now composed of many social media applications such as blogs, wikis, video-sharing and photo-sharing sites, social networking sites (i.e. Facebook, MySpace, Flicker), portable phone applications and widgets and gadgets that connect content, people, and systems.

Today, social media platforms are used as sources of public health information, stages for behavior change campaigns, knowledge-sharing platforms, sites for patient organizing and advocacy, and places where providers and patients can interact. Social media provide a level of timeliness and oversight unlike traditional media sources. Just like years ago when you "had to have a web presence," today you must use social media in order to be perceived as "relevant," "cutting edge," and "reputable" in many cultures and contexts. Numerous organizations, patient groups, and governments across the globe are embracing social media for health communication purposes. Illustrative examples include the following.

- PatientsLikeMe is a social networking platform freely available for patients across the globe. It serves as a platform for patients to talk with one another about living with a disease, to get information about treatment options, clinical trials, lifestyle issues, to reduce barriers and concerns, and to communicate effectively with their health care providers. Patients can share questions, symptoms, current medication regimens, and their health history and status and seek advice and tips from other "patients like them."
- The FAN project (Family, Activity, and Nutrition), funded by the local Public Health Department (Canton Ticino) and Health Promotion Switzerland, is providing parents and their young children (ages 6–12) in Switzerland with weekly communication using an interactive Web 2.0 powered social media platform (using Wordpress) that allows users to share experiences, tips, and ideas, view skill-teaching videos, and receive tailored e-mails and SMS reinforcements to improve their diet and physical activity behaviors.
- FaceSpace is a program in Australia that uses Social Networking for communication about sexual health and safer sex to young people and men who have sex with men.
- The US Centers for Disease Control and Prevention (CDC) use social media "to provide users with access to credible, science-based health information when, where, and how [they] want it. A variety of social media tools are used to reinforce and personalize messages, reach new audiences, and build a communication infrastructure based on open information exchange" (CDC, 2009b). A mix of social networks, like MySpace, blogs, and mobile phones, are used for communication about H1N1 (swine flu), food contamination, colorectal cancer, HIV testing, breast cancer, and other important health topics.
- The World Health Organisation's 1000 cities, 1000 lives campaign uses social media to communicate about health inequalities in cities. The ultimate goal is to encourage representatives of local and national governments to develop policies to protect and promote health, across multiple sectors, including the environment, health, transport, education and urban planning. Specifically, *1000 cities* aims to open streets to health in public spaces, ideally by closing off portions of streets to motor vehicles and *1000 lives* aims to collect 1000 stories of urban health champions who have taken action and had a significant impact on health in their cities.

Social media allow opportunities for enhancing and supporting critical health literacy, by extending traditional communication behaviors to an "e" platform that is predicated on user-generated content. Estimates of social media use vary depending on the source and sampling procedures, but most indicate that social media are used by a lot of people. For example, recent estimates suggest that some 500 million people use Facebook,

400 million watch video online, 350 million read blogs and over 300 million visit friend's social network site profile (Parker, 2009; Zuckerberg, 2010). Given the rapid speed of social media development, there is no doubt that these data will be outdated by the time this chapter is published.

E-health goes mobile

M-health is the communication of health and provision of health related services via mobile technologies (Ratzan and Gilhooly, 2010). There is a growing body of evidence that mobile devices can advance progress in both advanced economies and some of the most remote and resource-poor environments. Access to mobile telephone subscriptions has increased dramatically over a short period of time. Today there are approximately 7 billion mobile phone subscriptions worldwide, up from approximately 740 million just 10 years ago (Broadband Commission for Digital Development, 2010). Nearly 85 percent of the world's population is now covered by wireless signals. In 2007, mobile phone access reached more than 40 percent of the population. Africa continues to have the highest growth, with a rate of 32 percent in 2006–2007, linking 28 percent of its population. Mobile devices could have considerable implications for health and social and economic development. For example, economic growth was positively and significantly influenced by mobile phone diffusion, with the impact being twice as large in developing countries (Wavermann, Meschi, and Fuss, 2005).

The adoption of mobile communication methods can be applied across the continuum of care in all areas of health, including prevention, management, treatment, and end of life care. M-health can increase the reach of health communication by going to people where they are. Like other e-channels, mobile devices have the ability to reach people with tailored messages and be complemented by print, radio, television, and the Internet. In a review of mobile health interventions using SMS, Fjeldsoe, Marshall, and Miller (2009) found that tailoring content and interactivity were important characteristics of effective mobile health interventions. M-health shows promise in a number of areas including: patient diagnostic and treatment support, health care provider training and communication support, remote patient data collection and monitoring, consumer and patient education and awareness, disease epidemic outbreak tracking, and compliance with treatment and care.

The following demonstration projects have shown encouraging results:

- *Consultation and Communication*: Nurse midwives in Dangme West, Ghana, used mobile phones to consult with their peers, supervisors, and other medical colleagues on complex cases. Mobile phones also helped patients to communicate with their health care providers saving travel time and resulting in quicker, more efficient health service delivery (Mechael and Dodowa Health Research Center, 2009).
- *Information on Prevention and Care*: An intervention called mDhil in India offers text messages in 40 characters or less, with information on various health topics not commonly discussed, and supports prevention and patient self-management efforts (Dolan, 2010).

- *Disease Surveillance*: In rural southern Tanzania the technology was used to gather infant mortality data (Shirima *et al.*, 2007).
- *Monitoring*: Mobile technology was used in Norway to transmit data from a diabetic child's glucometer to a parent's phone via text message, a system which appealed to both parents and children (Gammon *et al.*, 2005).

Mobile phones allow for SMS (text communication with a maximum of 160 characters) or MMS (images, videos, audio and rich text) to be sent to and received by subscribers, SMS is gaining the attention of health researchers and has been used effectively for promoting smoking cessation (Rodgers *et al.*, 2005), physical activity (Hurling *et al.*, 2007; Joo and Kim, 2007), and diet (Joo and Kim, 2007). SMS has been examined in clinical settings with patients living with Type 1 and Type 2 diabetes in South Korea (Kwon *et al.*, 2004; Kim, 2007), Scotland (Franklin *et al.*, 2006), Austria (Rami *et al.*, 2006; Kollman *et al.*, 2007), and Finland (Vahatalo *et al.*, 2004). A recent systematic review by Déglise, Suggs, and Odermatt (2011), found that some 98 mobile applications are being used for prevention, management, compliance, and surveillance activities in developing countries. These are low-cost applications, reaching large segments of the target populations.

Although the m-health field is in its early stages, there are indications that it is starting to transform health systems – demonstrating its potential for extending the reach of health information and services to remote populations and promoting a shift toward citizen-centered health care and well-being.

Some illustrative examples include:

- China: The *Cada project* sends patients living with diabetes messages about the disease, including recommendations for diet, weight, and physical activity. Additionally, patients can send in their glucose level data via SMS to their physicians (Cada Project, 2009).
- Philippines: The *Community Health Information and Tracking System* uses SMS for improving communication between remote practitioners and the hospital. (Marcelo, 2009).
- Rwanda: The treatment and research AIDS center project called *TRACnet* covers over 75 percent of the 340 clinics in Rwanda and 32,000 patients. Health workers track HIV/AIDS patients, diagnostic information, and the inventory count of antiretroviral treatment. They can also receive results of blood tests, drug recall SMS alerts, treatment guidelines, and training manuals on their mobile phones (Crampton, 2007).
- United Kingdom: Adult employees at UK worksites participating in a program called *MoveM8!* receive one e-mail per week, plus two reinforcing SMS per week encouraging them to be physically active. A sample message sent on a Friday afternoon: "Schedule your health & make time for physical activity. Tomorrow is the weekend… what activity will you be doing?" (Suggs, *et al.*, 2009).
- United States: TeamTADD, a volunteer youth group in Medford Massachusetts (an area outside Boston) developed the "I'm Allergic to Stupid Decisions" campaign. Youth in the area text "FACT," "ALTERNATIVE," or "EXCUSE" to the SMS

service short code (a five digit code that is, in essence, a "phone number") and receive targeted messages about the facts associated with underage drinking, alternative activities to drinking, and excuses to get them out of situations when there is pressure to drink. Just one of the hundreds of messages youth receive is "FACT: One drink can make you fail a breathalyzer test" (Suggs *et al.*, 2011).

• South Africa: In 2009, two nongovernmental organizations (Cell-Life and LifeLine) formed a partnership to extend the freely available National AIDS Hotline (NAHL) to mobile phone subscribers. The NAHL was available free of charge from landlines, but not from mobile lines. Patients and consumers can send a text message to the system and receive live feedback from counselors about HIV and AIDS, including modes of transmission, testing services, and living with AIDS. Conversations are tracked, so repeat users can pick up the conversation where they left off last time (de Tolly and Benjamin, 2011).

Some promising m-health applications are addressing some of the major burdens to health that were mentioned previously. However, maternal and child health issues are gaining much needed attention, as evidenced in the Millennium Development Goals (MDG5), and m-health is already playing an important role in improving outcomes.

Today, nearly 3.2 million stillbirths and four million neonatal deaths occur. An overwhelming 97 percent of the world's maternal, newborn, and child deaths are concentrated in poorer, high-fertility countries; mostly in sub-Saharan Africa and parts of South East Asia where the highest maternal, fetal, and neonatal mortality rates and the lowest use of hospitals for delivery or newborn care exist.

To date, potentially life-saving interventions have not yet diffused amongst societies that could help the mother, newborn, or infant. In most of the locations, there are limited resources, little to no electricity, a lack of clean water, poor transportation, and few trained health professionals or functional hospitals. Fewer than 50 percent of women deliver in hospitals. Many do not have trained or skilled birth attendants, and, even if they do, the birth process can be further complicated by illiteracy and numeracy challenges. As the 2015 deadline to achieve the Millennium Development Goals (MDGs) looms upon the global health community with uneven and limited progress, UN Secretary-General Ban Ki-moon launched a global effort on women's and children's health stating, "Of all the millennium goals, maternal health has advanced the least and it is a key to all the rest. That is why today we are putting women's health front and center in the push to meet the millennium development goals." (United Nations, 2010; see also Ratzen, 2010b).

Cases of m-health applications to reduce maternal morbidity and improve child health show promise for meeting these goals.

• Rwanda, which is ranked worst in the world in maternal mortality, is working to reduce its annual maternal deaths. Together with three UN organizations, Rwanda has set an ambitious goal of reducing maternal death by 75 percent by the year 2015. Citing long travel distances to health facilities as one of several serious obstacles for pregnant women receiving regular screening and early intervention, a system using mobile phones for rapid and timely health communication has been put in place.

The system, Rapid SMS, launched in 2009 and is credited for saving lives and reducing annual maternal deaths from 10 to zero in one hospital. Health workers equipped with mobile phones register pregnant women and follow them throughout their pregnancy using SMS. A text is sent to a hospital if urgent care, including for the birth of a child, is needed. Ambulances can be sent, reducing time to the hospital by hours (Holland, 2010).

- In the United States a national educational program of the National Healthy Mothers, Healthy Babies Coalition, called *Text4baby* was launched in 2010. It provides free SMS to subscribers and addressed a variety of topics appropriate throughout pregnancy and the baby's first year. Topics include immunization, nutrition, seasonal flu, prenatal care, emotional well-being, drugs and alcohol, labor and delivery, smoking cessation, breast feeding, mental health, birth defects prevention, oral health, car seat safety, exercise and fitness, developmental milestones, safe sleep, and family violence. After signing up, the subscriber receives one message per day for the first six days and then three messages a week. One such message is: "If a baby is under 3 months of age and has a fever of 104.1 degrees or above, a physician should be called."

Future

While it is worthwhile to strive to improve public health and increase health literacy, our best evidence confirms that no single intervention is sufficient. Development of a health-competent society that incorporates a seamless continuum of care is necessary from preconception to mortality. We have to understand how to enable healthy lifestyle behaviors associated with preventing or managing diabetes, cardiovascular disease, cancer, overweight, and obesity. We must improve maternal and child health and implement both preventative measures and tests for infections such as HIV, TB, and malaria. These are integral components requiring tailored interventions that reach people where they are and when they need it.

As previously mentioned, social media and m-health are growing rapidly and the number of users presented earlier in this chapter will quickly be outdated. What will not be outdated is the need for high-quality research that tests the role social media and related technologies actually play in advancing health literacy and improving health outcomes. Just as we once questioned the role of the Internet in facilitating health and changing health behaviors, we now have sparse data about the specific impact of social media on health outcomes. We must move beyond the "promise" of such channels and platforms and test what aspects work best, how people use social and mobile technologies, and what the associated outcomes are when compared with, or complemented by, other communication options. Undoubtedly, future use will benefit from a policy environment that recognizes the potential of social and mobile media, fosters increased understanding of how they influence health literacy and health-related behaviors, and promotes collaboration among health providers, researchers, patients, and consumers.

There is a need for a strategic and cooperative global framework in e-health, especially against the background of growing economic challenges. These challenges, relating to greater social diversity, economic inequalities, the need for sustainable growth and competitiveness, globalization, an aging population, and the impact of innovation and technological developments, are making their impact felt across the world. Systems and governments are setting up infrastructures, funding mechanisms, and defining measureable objectives for e-health progress.

The European Commission (EC) recently proposed a "Digital Agenda" that includes large-scale IT investments aimed at helping member countries address rising health care costs and aging populations (Bruce, 2010). The agenda involves a 10-year action plan where:

- By 2012, certain information from patient medical records can be accessed electronically among all 27-member states of the European Union,
- By 2015, pilot programs throughout the EU will eventually lead to all Europeans having secure, online access to their medical information,
- By 2020, there will be widespread deployment of telemedicine services.

To address the barriers to meeting the EC's goals, the agenda calls for: (1) establishing a single digital market for the entire EU; (2) improving interoperability; (3) improving the security and safety of the Internet; and (4) providing much faster Internet access to the public (Robinson, 2010).

The United States Department of Health and Human Services Healthy People 2020 Objectives for the Nation includes specific measurable objectives for Health Communication/Health Information Technology:

- Improving the health literacy of the population,
- Increasing the proportion of persons who report their health care provider always gives them information targeted for patients with low health literacy,
- Increase the proportion of persons who use electronic personal health management tools.

Additionally, the new *Health Reform: Patient Protection and Affordable Care Act* incorporates mandates and support for improved health literacy by:

- Awarding Wellness Program grants to small employers on the basis of: (1) health awareness; (2) employee engagement; (3) behavioral change; and (4) a supportive environment,
- Developing and producing decision aids or educational tools to reflect diverse levels of health literacy and cultural and education backgrounds,
- Awarding incentives for prevention of chronic diseases in Medicaid, with $100 million of grants to States to carry out initiatives,
- Providing access by Medicare beneficiaries to a comprehensive health risk assessment. Payment will also be made for a visit to a primary care provider to create a personalized prevention plan (DHHS, 2010).

The Broadband Commission for Digital Development recently proposed a set of recommendations and associated plan of action, "Broadband Inclusion for All", for meeting the

Millennium Development Goals. This was prepared for the United Nations Secretary General in 2010. "Broadband Inclusion for All" promotes greater access to fast Internet connections, with a goal of having 50 percent of the world's population connected to the Internet via broadband connection by 2015, stating "for every 10 percent increase in broadband penetration, we can expect an average of 1.3% growth in GDP." The plan outlines 10 steps:

1   Building global commitment to broadband inclusion for all by connecting broadband with the Millennium Development Goals and Knowledge Society priorities.
2   Maximizing social and economic stimulus with broadband inclusion for all via transformational change in health care, education, government, and environmental sustainability.
3   Addressing issues of convergent broadband networks toward an open, competitive, technology-neutral model, offering interconnection and interoperability at the national, regional, and global levels.
4   Developing the right conditions for broadband content and applications creation, diffusion, and distribution via an enabling environment based on trust and confidence for economic and social stability and prosperity.
5   Addressing the unique emerging and evolving cross-sector and cross-cutting implications of broadband inclusion for all, for both developed and developing economies and societies.
6   Accelerating access to broadband infrastructure and services for women and girls, to promote gender equality and social and economic development.
7   Supporting wider broadband inclusion for least developed countries and countries in special need and extending broadband access to rural and remote areas and vulnerable and disadvantaged groups.
8   Modeling, measuring, and monitoring relative targets and timelines for broadband inclusion, with the development of economic, social, and usage indicators appropriate to the broadband environment.
9   Building a global partnership for broadband development with concrete commitments, recognizing that the cross-sector and cross-cutting nature of broadband will take us beyond the MDG agenda.
10 Next steps for partnerships, with concrete coordination including innovative and multi-stakeholder follow-up mechanisms at the national, regional and global levels, including national broadband committees.

Recognizing the limited resources available for supporting health, greater innovation and efficiency are required in order to be optimally effective. Both the public and private sectors need to work together and synergistically maximize each other's strengths. For example, the public sector can learn from the private sector's ability to innovate, take risks, measure and achieve efficiencies of scale, address customer interests, and take optimal advantage of established distribution system knowledge. The private sector can take advantage of the demand for health care being generated by emerging economies. In many cases, in order to achieve successful partnerships, a dialogue will need to be fostered where one does not currently exist, and partnerships will need to be established based on mutual trust and respect.

Many of the private–public partnerships in m-health have been developed in relation to Millennium Development Goals 4, 5, and 6, (Child Health, Maternal Health, and HIV), where the deployment of mobile communication technologies are appropriate and efficient in delivering care and tracking results. Wireless applications connected to databases could enable efficient registration of pregnant women and those who have recently delivered, as well as their newborns. This information could be valuable in workforce planning and administration along the continuum of care. HIV prevention, surveillance, and testing communication can use mobile phones to send messages about the importance of condom use, testing, and transmission, to community members, infected individuals, and mothers. Indeed, in Déglise and colleagues' 2010 review of SMS applications in developing countries, HIV was the health topic targeted most frequently across interventions.

Several of the previously mentioned illustrative examples highlight current private–public partnerships:

- The *TRAcnet* project in Rwanda: Rwanda uses mobile with doctors and health workers and uses TRACnet to monitor and manage patients with HIV/AIDS. TRACnet is an electronic records system that can be uploaded to mobile phones. In Masaka it is being used to track and record the distribution of antiretroviral medications, ensure drug adherence, electronically create and submit patient reports, and access the most up-to-date information about HIV/AIDS care and treatment.
- The *Grameen Foundation* in Ghana: The Grameen Foundation has been developing, from a grant of the Bill and Melinda Gates Foundation, a platform for parental child health. That platform sends personalized messages about child health and routine immunization to pregnant women across Ghana. For the current project, Johnson and Johnson has extended a grant to the Grameen Foundation to integrate into this platform a clinical decision support capability that has been developed by the Robertson Research Institute. This will extend the capabilities of the platform to personalize the intervention based on the individual medical status of the user.
- *Text4baby* in the United States: The White House announced the first large-scale partnership of m-health with the launch of a free m-health service, Text4baby, that provides timely and expert health information through SMS text messages to pregnant women and to new mothers throughout their babies' first year. Text4baby was developed with BabyCenter, a Johnson and Johnson Company, and is a broad-based partnership, which includes federal, state and local governments, corporations, academic institutions, professional associations, tribal agencies, and non-profit organizations.

How do we measure our progress?

E-health technologies are changing the way we think about communicating health, tracking health, and providing health services, yet we have not developed and defined effective metrics to measure our progress. Ongoing debate over the applicability of conventional metrics and the lack of clearly defined best practices for measuring social and mobile technologies are certainly problems. We need carefully defined criteria that include: health behaviors, health literacy, health outcomes, reach, cost-benefit analysis, level of adaptability and flexibility, and sustainability metrics.

One parsimonious idea is to develop a scorecard to effectively demonstrate the varia-bles that contribute to ill health, chronic disease, and early death. Such a scorecard would allow individuals, as well as organizations and systems, to keep track of their health metrics and know when intervention is necessary. A scorecard could be developed at the individual, community, and country levels to assist decision makers in knowing their numbers, to prevent and detect disease and, when necessary, to manage chronic and infectious disease appropriately. Scorecards could be used for tracking surveillance efforts, education, training, environmental improvements, and outreach.

We could develop a scorecard with communication and health literacy principles:

> A scorecard could be designed as an understandable compilation of clinical and societal risk factors with clinical values so that individuals, providers, payers and policymakers can act upon such information with evidence-based informed decision-making and public policy (Ratzan, 2010c, p. 468).

This scorecard can take many shapes and sizes, dependent on the age of the population, access to services, the environment, education level, and regional demographics, among other variables. The WEF Global Agenda Council (2010) has called for a "Health and Well-being Footprint" that captures these variables on a global level. It is proposed to, "help measure the contribution of the public and private sectors and individual behaviors to health and well-being, to help identify opportunities to manage the causes of chronic diseases at the key levels of impact and to serve as a yardstick of progress in delivering change."

A scorecard will not address all causes of disease – in fact, as indicated with the four risk factors, (tobacco use, unhealthy diets, physical inactivity, and the harmful use of alcohol), we may only be addressing 60 percent of the disease. Yet, the cost of interven-tion and prevention of these risk factors is low. We cannot afford to do otherwise, as the risk to our society is so great that the health care spending required to ethically address the sequela of the risk factors will cripple the system, resulting in difficult ethical decisions with undesirable health outcomes for too many members of society.

Looking ahead

The spread of digital technology has created valuable channels to communicate with citizens, patients, caregivers, and health workers.

Potential opportunities include the ability to:

- Improve people's health literacy and health-related skills by educating them with engaging, personalized information and teaching them about healthy behaviors. This will complement other investments in health systems by creating appropriate demand for services and encouraging compliance. This can include simple voice and text informational messaging and reminders based on a basic personal record, emergency calls, data collection, check lists, and basic training for workers delivered electronically along with administrative workforce management and facilitation.

- Collect data from the field back into the health system. This could include registrations of pregnancy and childbirth, disease outbreaks, and other information gleaned electronically from underlying basic electronic medical records.
- Enhance formative and summative research and evaluation about the efficacy of programs, providing rapid feedback for results-based health programs through an efficient assessment, measurement, and evaluation based on data from the actual delivery of care.
- Create supporting applications for health workers that could help them manage their workload, communicate with a central clinic, receive training, or educate their patients and citizens. Over time, this could be extended to include a range of remote diagnostics connected to medical facilities and expertise by wireless technologies.

One of the promising areas could be to develop a standards-based, open architecture, interoperable system, (e.g., perhaps a platform), that could be used in support of many different programs across varying health areas. One key objective would be to reduce the fragmented nature of the investment in e-health across developing world programs. A standard platform would be offered with evidence-based communication strategies and components that organizations and programs could pick and choose from in support of their respective initiatives to improve health care.

Critical questions and suggestions

As communication technologies advance from an IEC (Information, Education and Communication) to an IHC (Interactive Health Communication) approach supplemented by m-health, diffusion could be further advanced with a coordinated, transparent, and integrated approach in health communication. A five-part process of parallel work streams is needed, with each area informing the others on the following dimensions:

- *Applying Interactive Communication Technologies (ICT) to Priority Needs*: In physical and virtual meetings of health and technology experts, we need to answer the question: How can ICT, especially mobile, assist in meeting the existing requirements of the health communication community?
- *Designing and Building System-Strengthening Solutions*: NGOs, government, and industry need to work with users and stakeholders to design the specific first ICT reference models to support global health and the accompanying content and policies. These need to be integrated, end-to-end systems along the continuum of care designed to scale. Key areas include: software for information sharing, content, diagnostic devices, and capacity building.
- *Measurement and Evaluation*: There needs to be a broad consensus reached on new measurement and evaluation approaches that will be possible in this future information-rich environment. Both the health-value chain and economics-value chain need to be measured.

Box 12.3   Checklist for building good e-health communication

Start by defining what problem you are addressing.

1   Get to know your audience.
   a.   What channels do they use (not just for health purposes)?
   b.   How do they use them?
   c.   How do they communicate about health?
   d.   What are their attitudes, knowledge, and current practices?
2   Let the purpose and audience drive the technology used, not your preferences.
3   Think about scalability. Start small, but with the big picture in mind.
4   Be relevant. Communication that is perceived as relevant to the user is more effective.
5   Embrace input and feedback, even when it is negative.
6   Let audiences contribute and become co-creators. You do not need to, nor should you, control everything.

- *Trial Deployments of System-Strengthening Solutions*: Projects need to be surveyed, and then partnerships need to be formed to contribute technology, financing, content, and/or time and expertise (local leadership, supporting work), to undertake the trial deployments of the new solutions, and to test them.
- *Communication*: Along the way, there needs to be far greater exposure and transparency of all of the above activities to global input and use, in addition to full coordination and information sharing. A virtual, interactive platform will serve this need best.

One idea would be to embrace the Maternal and Newborn m-health Initiative. This growing public and private partnership addresses the MDG 5 (reducing maternal mortality by 75 percent) in a science-based approach with priority setting, needs analysis, integrated design, measurement (including formative, operational, and summative research/evaluation), and integrated communication. This includes the m-health Alliance (hosted by the United Nations Foundation), the Partnership for Maternal, Newborn and Child Health, BRAC, the White Ribbon Alliance, PATH, the wireless industry, and other stakeholders. They share the goal of applying the benefits of modern information and communications technologies, especially mobile, to help achieve the Millennium Development Goals and strengthen country health systems, starting with MDG 5.

Successful e-health initiatives can best be developed with multidisciplinary input, creativity, collaboration, and partnership. It is through public–private partnerships or "public interest partnerships" that progress can be made. Ideally, it will be essential to:

- Integrate political realities, telecommunications core business expertise, and national telecommunications infrastructure, along with national health infrastructures and health priorities, to reach underserved and remote populations;

- Identify and evaluate health needs highlighted by the data gathering capacity of e-health, while leveraging resources to meet these needs;
- Understand and promote interactive health communication to enhance health literacy and facilitate appropriate health related behaviors; and
- Leverage and engage multiple stakeholders to construct innovative models that take into account the constraints of a country's health system and a community's purchasing power.

Conclusion

To address public health problems effectively, we must strive for a health-literate population. Effective solutions that are adaptable and flexible to a changing society are critical. The e-health evolution has been playing, and will continue to play, a critical, if not fundamental, role in these efforts.

In this light, future e-health applications should:

- embrace the social aspect of technology
- measure their process and outcomes
- be scalable
- be health literacy friendly, adapting to the needs of the audience
- be affordable and accessible
- allow for choice in terms of channel, timing, framing, and length
- be sustainable.

The practice of e-health communication has come a long way, yet there is still much more work to do. We no longer need studies that report the acceptance of technology based initiatives. Rather, we need to pay more attention to learning the best way to use such technology and the best way to provide relevant, tailored communication at a population wide level. We need to establish best practices for sharing resources, content, and systems, so that communities can learn and benefit from each other's successes and failures. We need scorecards to help us understand how we are doing. We need innovation. We need data. We need to think differently.

Chapter Summary

In this chapter on global e-health communication, we have provided an overview of past, present, and future efforts in digital health, including social and mobile health. Many more opportunities exist and many more solutions are currently in the planning stages. It is clear that there are numerous examples of practices, but we have major work to do in terms of evaluation, scalability, and sustainability. There is both a need, in alignment with the will of public and private sectors, to advance digital health in a manner that is beneficial for individuals, society, health systems, governments, and industry. We have presented a set of critical questions, a checklist for developing e-health applications and tools, and our thoughts on how we measure progress. We hope this chapter provides

Box 12.4   E-health resources

http://www.unfoundation.org/global-issues/technology/mhealth-alliance.html
http://www.mhealthalliance.org/
http://1000cities.who.int/
http://www.epgpatientdirect.org/social-media-directory.cfm/
http://www.patientslikeme.com/
http://www.ehealthinnovation.org/
http://www.pewinternet.org/
http://www.internetworldstats.com/
http://govhealthit.com/
http://www.ehealtheurope.net/
http://www.ihealthbeat.org/
http://www.healthnewsreview.org/
http://www.kff.org/

readers with evidence and also fodder for reflection about their own practices and research. The coming years will prove an exciting time for our field and those reading this text will help shape the future. The world of e-health may very well still be in its infancy. The breadth of academic analysis and planning combined with the creativity and careful planning of health practitioners, industry and government, the future, even the very near future, could bring a significant growth period for e-health, bringing new solutions to the forefront to improve global health.

References

Anderson, D. G. and Stenzel, C. (2001). Internet patient care applications in ambulatory care. *Journal of Ambulatory Care Management, 24*(4), 1–38.

Barrera, M., Glasgow, R., McKay, H. G. *et al.* (2002). Do Internet-based support interventions change perceptions of social support? An experimental trial of approaches for supporting diabetes self-management. *American Journal of Community Psychology, 30*(5), 637–654.

Broadband Commission for Digital Development (2010). *Inclusion for All*. Prepared for the U.N. Secretary General. Retrieved from http://www.broadbandcommission.org/Reports/Report_1.pdf

Bruce, S. (2010). EC puts health on digital agenda. *E-health Europe*. May 26. Retrieved from http://www.ehealtheurope.net/news/5938/ec_puts_health_on_digital_agenda

Cada Project (2009). Use Smartphones to promote diabetes self-management: Robust elderly in urban and rural China. Retrieved from http://www.cadaproject.com/index.php?pag=project.

CDC (Centers for Disease Control and Prevention) (2009). *Interactive Media \ CDC health marketing*. Retrieved from: http://www.cdc.gov/healthmarketing/ehm/interactive.html

Crampton, T. (2007). Cellphones open front in fight against disease. *The New York Times*. March 4. Retrieved from http://www.nytimes.com/2007/03/04/technology/04iht-wireless05.4787228.html

Déglise, C., Suggs, L. S., and Odermatt, P. (forthcoming, 2012). SMS for disease control in developing countries: A systematic review of mobile health applications. *Journal of Telemedicine and Telecare.*

de Tolly, K. and Benjamin, P. (2011). Mobile phones: Opening new channels for health communication. In S. Waisbord and R. Obregon, R. (Eds.), *Handbook of Global Health Communication.* Oxford: Wiley-Blackwell.

DHHS (Department of Health and Human Services) (2000). *Healthy People 2010.* Office of Disease Prevention and Health Promotion. Retrieved from http://www.healthypeople.gov/2010/

DHHS (Department of Health and Human Services) (2010a). *Healthy People 2020.* Office of Disease Prevention and Health Promotion. Retrieved from http://www.healthypeople.gov

DHHS (Department of Health and Human Services) (2010b). *Health Reform: Patient Protection and Affordable Care Act.* Retrieved from http://www.healthcare.gov/

Dolan, B. (2010). @mHI startup boasts 150K paying mHealth users. *Mobihealthnews,* February 3, 2010. Retrieved from http://mobihealthnews.com/6381/mhi-startup-boasts-150k-paying-mhealth-users/

Eng, T.R. (2001). *The e Health Landscape: A terrain map of emerging information and communication technologies in health and health care.* Princeton, NJ: Robert Wood Johnson Foundation.

Eysenbach, G. (2001). What is e-health? *Journal of Medical Internet Research, 3*(2), e20.

Eysenbach, G., Powell, J., Englesakis, M. *et al.* (2004). Health related virtual communities and electronic support groups: Systematic review of the effects of online peer to peer interactions. *British Medical Journal, 328*(7449), 1166–1170.

Fjeldsoe, B. S., Marshall, A. L., and Miller, Y. D. (2009). Behavior change interventions delivered by mobile telephone short-message service. *American Journal of Preventive Medicine, 36*(2), 165–173.

Fogg, B. J. (2003). *Persuasive Technology: Using Computers to Change What We Think and Do.* San Francisco, CA: Morgan Kaufmann Publishers.

Franklin, V., Waller, A., Pagliari, C., and Greene, S. (2006). A randomized controlled trial of SweetTalk, a text-messaging system to support young people with diabetes. *Diabetes Medicine, 23,* 1332–1338.

Gammon, D., Arsand, E., Walseth, O. A. *et al.* (2005). Parent–child interaction using a mobile and wireless system for blood glucose monitoring. *Journal of Medical Internet Research, 7*(5), e57.

Glasgow, R., Bull, S., Piette, J. and Steiner, J. (2004). Interactive behavior change technology: A partial solution to the competing demands for primary care. *American Journal of Preventive Medicine, 27*(2S), 80–87.

Gustafson, D. H., Hawkins, R., Boberg, E. *et al.* (1999). Impact of a patient-centered, computer-based health information support system. *American Journal of Preventive Medicine, 16*(1), 1–9.

Haider, M., Ratzan, S. C., and Meltzer, W. (2009). International innovations in health communication. In J. S. Parker and E. Thorson (Eds.), *Health Communication in the New Media Landscape* (pp. 373–394). New York: Springer Publishing Company.

Holland, H. (2010). Text messages save pregnant Rwandan women. Reuters. May 28. Retrieved from http://www.reuters.com/article/2010/05/28/us-rwanda-health-idUSTRE64R2CL20 100528

Hurling, R., Catt, M., De Boni, M. *et al.* (2007). Using Internet and mobile phone technology to deliver an automated physical activity program: Randomized controlled trial. *Journal of Medical Internet Research 9,* e7.

International Diabetes Federation, (2007). Diabetes fact and figures. Retrieved from http://www.diabetesatlas.org/

Internet World Stats (2010). Usage and population statistics (current as of June 30 2010). Retrieved from http://www.internetworldstats.com/stats.htm

Joo, N.and Kim, B. (2007). Mobile phone short message service messaging for behavior modification in a community-based weight control programme in Korea. *Journal of Telemedicine and Telecare 13*:416–420.

Kaplan, A. M. and Haenlein, M. (2010). Users of the world, unite! The challenges and opportunities of social media. *Business Horizons, 53*(1), 59–68.

Kim, H. (2007). A randomized controlled trial of a nurse short-message service by cellular phone for people with diabetes. *International Journal of Nursing Studies. 44*, 687–92.

Kollman, A., Riedl, M., Kastner, P. *et al.* (2007). Feasibility of a mobile phone-based data service for functional insulin treatment of Type 1 Diabetes Mellitus patients. *Journal of Medical Internet Research, 9*, e36.

Kwon, H., Cho, J., Kim, H. *et al.* (2004). Development of web-based diabetic patient management system using short message service (SMS). *Diabetes Research Clinical Practice. 66*, s133–s137.

Marcelo, A.B. (2009). Telehealth in developing countries: Perspectives from the Philippines. In R. Wootton, N. G. Patil, R. E. Scott, and K. Ho (Eds.), *Telehealth in the Developing World* (pp. 27–33). London: Royal Society of Medicine Press/IDRC.

Mayfield, A. (Ed.). (2008). *What is social media?* http://www.icrossing.co.uk/fileadmin/uploads/eBooks/What_is_Social_Media_iCrossing_ebook.pdf (v1.4 ed.) iCrossing

Mechael, P. N. and Dodowa Health Research Center (2009). *MoTECH: mHealth Ethnography Report*, for the Grameen Foundation. Retrieved from http://www.grameenfoundation.applab.org/uploads/Grameen_Foundation_FinalReport_3_.pdf

Miron-Shatz, T. (2010). *White paper: The Potential of a Health Scorecard for Promoting Health Literacy*. Health Literacy Action Metrics Workshop: Enhancing individual, systems, and policy maker quality performance. Retrieved from http://marketing.wharton.upenn.edu/documents/research/Miron-Shatz_Health_scorecards%20Working%20paper.pdf

Neuhauser, L. and Kreps, G. (2003). Rethinking communication in the e-healh era. *Journal of Health Psychology, 8*(1).7–23.

Parker, G. (2009). *Power to the people – social media tracker wave 4*, July 2009 Universal McCann. Retrieved from http://*universalmccann.bitecp.com/wave4/Wave4.pdf*

Rami, B., Popow, C., Horn, W. *et al.* (2006). Telemedicine support to improve glycemic control in adolescents with Type 1 Diabetes Mellitus. *European Journal of Pediatrics. 165*:701–705.

Ratzan, S. C. (2010a). Global health: The path forward. *Journal of Health Communication. 15*, 111–113.

Ratzan, S. C. (2010b). A call to action: The global effort on women's and children's health. *Journal of Health Communication, 15* (4), 355–357.

Ratzan, S. C. (2010c). Chronic disease: A risk we need to score. *Journal of Health Communication. 15*(5), 467–469.

Ratzan, S. C. and Busquets, M.I. (2002). The future of information technology for health in developing countries. In Bushko, R.G. (Ed.), *Future of Health Technology* (pp. 181–194). Amsterdam: IOS Press.

Ratzan, S. C. and Gilhooly, D. (2010). Innovative use of mobile phones and related technologies. In United Nations *Every Woman Every Child: Investing in Our Common Future*, Working Papers of the innovation Working Group – version 2. Retrieved from http://www.who.int/pmnch/activities/jointactionplan/100922_2_investing.pdf

Robinson, B. (2010). EU sets major investments in health IT, telemedicine. *Government Health IT*. May 27 Retrieved from http://www.govhealthit.com/news/eu-sets-major-investments-health-it-telemedicine

Rodgers, A., Corbett, T., Riddell, T. *et al.* (2005). Do u smoke after txt? Results of a randomized trial of smoking cessation using mobile phone text messaging. *Tobacco Control. 14,* 255–261.

Shirima, K., Mukasa, O., Schellenberg, J. A. *et al.* (2007). The use of personal digital assistants for data entry at the point of collection in a large household survey in southern Tanzania. *Emerging Themes in Epidemiology, 4*(5). Retrieved from http://www.ipti-malaria.org/LinkClick.aspx?fileticket=z0nrs0xWvio%3D&tabid=228

Suggs, L. S. (2006). A 10-year retrospective of research in new technologies for health communication. *Journal of Health Communication. 11*(1), 61–74.

Suggs, L. S., Blake, H., Lloyd, S., and Bardus, M. (2009). An individualised approach: MoveM8! E-mail and SMS physical activity communication in the workplace. Presentation at the British Association of Sport and Exercise Sciences (BASES) Annual Conference. Leeds, UK, September 1–3.

Suggs, L. S., Rots, G., Jacques, J., Vong, H., Mui, J., Reardon, B., and Team IA2SD. (2011). "I'm allergic to stupid decisions": An m-health campaign to reduce youth alcohol consumption. *Cases in Public Health Communication and Marketing. 5*:111–135.

United Nations (2010).The Secretary General: Remarks to the press: Launch of the joint effort on women's and children's health. April 14, 2020. Retrieved from http://www.un.org/sg/hf/Press_remarks.pdf

Vahatalo, M.A., Virtamo, H.E., Viikari, J.S., and Ronnemaa, T. (2004). Cellular phone transferred self blood glucose monitoring: prerequisites for positive outcome. *Practical Diabetes International. 21*:192–194.

Wantland, D. J., Portillo, C. J., Holzemer, W. L. *et al.* (2004). The effectiveness of web-based vs. non-web-based interventions: A meta-analysis of behavioral change outcomes. *Journal of Medical Internet Research, 6*(4), e40. Retrieved from http://www.jmir.org/2004/4/e40/

Wavermann, L., Meschi, M.,and Fuss, M. (2005). *The Impact of Telecoms on Economic Growth in DevelopingCountries.*Retrievedfromhttp://web.si.umich.edu/tprc/papers/2005/450/L%20Waverman-%20Telecoms%20Growth%20in%20Dev.%20Countries.pdf

WEF Global Agenda Council (2010). *Global Agenda Councils.* Retrieved from http://www.weforum.org/en/Communities/GlobalAgendaCouncils/index.htm

WHO (World Health Organisation) (2007). *The World Health Report 2007 – A Safer Future: Global Public Health Security in the 21st Century.* Retrieved from http://www.who.int/whr/2007/en/index.html

WHO (World Health Organisation) (2009). *Chronic Diseases and Health Promotion. Integrated Chronic Disease Prevention and Control.* Retrieved from http://www.who.int/chp/about/integrated_cd/en/index.html

WHO (World Health Organisation) (2010). *Neglected Tropical Diseases.* Retrieved from http://www.who.int/neglected_diseases/en/

Zuckerberg, M. (2010). *500 Million Stories.* Facebook. Retrieved from http://blog.facebook.com/blog.php?post=409753352130

13

Managing Fear to Promote Healthy Change

Merissa Ferrara, Anthony J. Roberto, and Kim Witte

"I'd rather my baby die than take that drug."

A woman stated this loudly at my first focus group of women in rural Namibia, reminding me that we were not in Kansas or even in the United States anymore and to proceed with culturally-sensitive caution. These are troubling words to hear from a pregnant woman regarding her unborn child for health researchers trying to promote a better future. Some people may ask why a mother would make such a comment when she could take medicine to prevent HIV being passed to her child during the birthing process. The answer is as simple as it is complex: fear. Fear can be a powerful motivator. Careful management of people's fear is essential to health promotion. Educators in developing countries face unique challenges; their target audiences often report high levels of fear on many issues (e.g., HIV/AIDS, STIs, malaria, stigma, infant deaths), yet feel solutions are implausible (i.e., no access, costly, stigma, against cultural beliefs). It is important to know of what the target population is afraid in order to design convincing, effective solutions to responsibly manage the fear.

The authors of this chapter have collectively amassed over 60 years of experience researching and constructing fear appeals on a range of topics in various countries. This chapter reviews the Extended Parallel Process Model (EPPM), presents examples of how EPPM can be an effective tool to promote healthy change, illustrates how scholars have extended the EPPM framework to include the presence of social threat and collective efficacy, discusses the challenges created when the target population reports high levels of pre-existing fear, and offers suggestions for future EPPM scholars trying to make a difference in global health outcomes.

The Handbook of Global Health Communication, First Edition. Edited by Rafael Obregon and Silvio Waisbord.

The Extended Parallel Process Model

The EPPM (Witte, 1992) is an integration and extension of the fear-as-acquired-drive model (Janis, 1967), the parallel process model (Leventhal, 1970), and protection motivation theory (Rogers, 1975). Though a review of these previous theoretical perspectives is beyond the scope of the current chapter, readers interested in learning more about these perspectives are referred to the original citations, or to overviews written by Witte (1992) and Witte, Meyer, and Martell (2001). What is worth noting here is that the principal difference between the EPPM and earlier fear appeal theories is that earlier theories focused solely upon individuals who adopted the recommended response after being exposed to a fear appeal message, and placed everyone else into the no-response category. According to the EPPM, however, the no-response category is actually comprised of two groups: those who truly had no response to the campaign; and, those who attempted to control their fear rather than react (change) in response to the actual danger, which is masked as no behavior change.

Before reviewing the EPPM (Witte, 1992) itself, it is necessary to define four key variables in this model (note, these definitions are taken or adapted from Roberto, Goodall, and Witte, 2009 or Witte, 1992):

- *Susceptibility*: Beliefs about one's risk of experiencing the threat; how likely is it that the threat will occur?
- *Severity*: Beliefs about the significance or magnitude of the threat; how serious are the short- or long-term consequences of the threat?
- *Response-efficacy*: Beliefs about the effectiveness of the recommended response; is the recommended behavior safe and effective?
- *Self-efficacy*: Beliefs about one's ability to perform the recommended response; does a person have the necessary skills and resources to engage in the recommended behavior?

Together, perceptions of susceptibility and severity combine to form an individual's overall level of *perceived threat*, while perceptions of response-efficacy and self-efficacy combine to make up an individual's overall level of *perceived efficacy*.

With this in mind, the EPPM predicts that perceived threat and efficacy combine to produce one of three possible reactions to a persuasive message. *No response* occurs when perceived threat is low. In this instance, a person does not perceive the existence of a personally relevant or serious threat, and therefore will not feel the need to pay attention or respond to the message. A *fear control* response occurs when perceived threat is high but perceived efficacy is low. Under such conditions, individuals will focus on reducing their degree of fear rather than focusing on the actual danger. Finally, a *danger control* response occurs when both perceived threat and perceived efficacy are high. Under these circumstances, individuals will think carefully about the recommended response and adapt their behavior in a way that reduces their actual danger. In sum, "perceived threat motivates action; perceived efficacy determines the nature of that action – specifically, whether people attempt to control the danger or

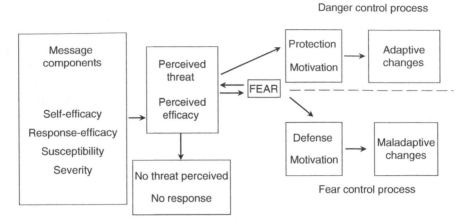

Figure 13.1   The Extended Parallel Process Model (Witte, 1992).
Source: Adapted from Witte (1992). Reprinted by permission of Taylor and Francis, Ltd. (http://www. informaworld.com).

control their fear. This critical point, when perceived efficacy exceeds perceived threat, is an important concept in the development of effective applied communication messages" (Witte and Roberto, 2009, p. 586). A visual representation of how perceived threat and efficacy combine to produce these three possible outcomes is included in Figure 13.1.

To illustrate the three possible outcomes mentioned previously, let us consider an entertainment-education intervention that Anthony Roberto (coauthor of this chapter) recently helped develop. By way of background, Singhal and Rogers (2004, p. 5) define *entertainment-education* as, "the process of purposefully designing and implementing a media message to both entertain and educate, in order to increase audience members' knowledge about an educational issue, create favorable attitudes, shift social norms, and change overt behavior." Though this and other traditional definitions and examples of entertainment-education all focus on efforts involving some form of media message, "today there exist multiple types of E-E [entertainment-education]" (Singhal and Rogers, 2004, p. 8), and "E-E comes in many different sizes and shapes" (Piotrow and de Fossard, 2004, p. 43). For example, numerous entertainment-education programs now involve *live* (i.e., non-mediated) theatrical performances (Glik *et al.*, 2002; Guttman, Gasser-Edelsburg, and Israelashvili, 2008; Singhal, 2004).

With this in mind, Roberto recently helped design a live musical theatrical performance based on the EPPM in an effort to increase early detection and treatment of breast cancer among women in rural Bangladesh. The goal of the intervention is to encourage Bangladeshi women with breast problems to go to a local health clinic for free breast cancer screening to prevent the threat of more advanced breast cancer or death. The following section illustrates the three paths a woman might take depending on her levels of perceived threat and efficacy after hearing the entertainment-education message.

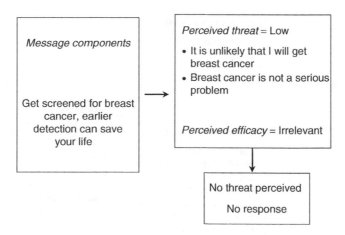

Figure 13.2   The Extended Parallel Process Model – low-threat example.

Low-threat path

No response will occur when perceived threat is low. That is, if a women does not believe that she is susceptible to breast cancer (e.g., "it is unlikely that I will get breast cancer"), or if she does not believe that breast cancer has severe consequences (e.g., "breast cancer is not a serious problem"), then she will not be motivated to pay attention to or respond to the message. Under such conditions she would not be motivated to engage in an appraisal of efficacy or, in this example, to get screened for breast cancer. As a reminder, both perceived susceptibility and perceived severity have to be high for one's appraisal of threat to be high. This path is represented visually in Figure 13.2.

High-threat/low-efficacy path

An individual will engage in *fear control* when perceived threat is high and perceived efficacy is low. That is, if a women believes that she is susceptible to breast cancer (e.g., "it is possible that I will get breast cancer") and believes that breast cancer has severe consequences (e.g., "breast cancer is a serious problem"), her level of perceived threat will be high, and she will be motivated to engage in the second appraisal of efficacy. However, if she does not believe the recommended response is effective (e.g., "getting screened is *not* an effective way to reduce the risk or seriousness of breast cancer"), or if she does not believe that she has the ability to engage in the recommended response (e.g., "I do *not* have the time or money to get screened for breast cancer"), her level of perceived efficacy will be low. Since being afraid is an uncomfortable state, she is likely to take steps to reduce the fear that do not necessarily decrease the actual danger. For example, she might ignore the information (i.e., *defensive avoidance*), refuse to believe that the health threat is real (i.e., *denial*), or view the message as trying to manipulate her and therefore reject it (i.e., *reactance*). As a reminder, both response-efficacy and self-efficacy must be high for one's appraisal of efficacy to be high. See Figure 13.3 for a visual representation of this path.

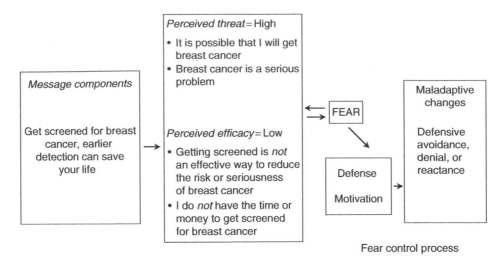

Figure 13.3 The Extended Parallel Process Model – high-threat/low-efficacy example.

High-threat/high-efficacy path

An individual will engage in *danger control* only when both perceived threat and perceived efficacy are high. In this case, the message will have accomplished all of its goals by convincing a woman both that a personally relevant and serious threat exists, and that an effective means to reduce the threat has been provided (e.g., high response-efficacy; "getting screened is an effective way to reduce the risk and seriousness of breast cancer") that she is able to perform (e.g., high self-efficacy; "I can make the time to go to the free clinic to get screened for breast cancer"). It is only when *both* perceived threat and perceived efficacy are high that a person will focus on potential solutions to the problem, which will likely lead to the recommended attitude or behavior change. The visual representation of this path can be found in Figure 13.4. Notably, this is the approach that was taken in the entertainment-education intervention created by Roberto. The performance was about 25 minutes long and included images and lyrics specifically designed to create or reinforce higher perceptions of susceptibility, severity, response-efficacy, and self-efficacy in an effort to increase the likelihood that Bangladeshi women with breast problems would follow the danger control path and go to the local health clinic for a free breast cancer screening.

In addition to the breast cancer entertainment-education program reviewed above, the EPPM has been used to guide numerous international health communication campaigns since it was first developed nearly two decades ago. For example, it has been used to guide family planning and HIV/AIDS prevention projects in Ethiopia (Belete, Girgre, and Witte, 2003; Witte, Girma, and Girgre, 2002–2003), Kenya (Witte *et al.*, 1998), Namibia (Smith, Downs, and Witte, 2007), Uganda (Mulogo *et al.*, 2006), India (Witte, *et al.*, 2003), and Zimbabwe (Chikombero, 2009), and among Mexican-Americans (Hubbell, 2006) and Mexican immigrants and Taiwanese students living in the United States (Murray-Johnson *et al.*, 2001). Information about and reviews of some of these and other interventions

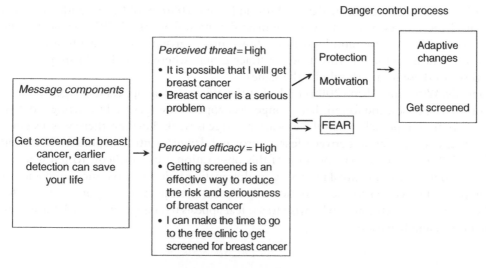

Figure 13.4   The Extended Parallel Process Model – high-threat/high-efficacy example.

guided by the EPPM can be found in Roberto (2004), Roberto Goodall, and Witte. (2009), Roberto, Murray-Johnson, and Witte (in press), and Witte and Roberto (2009).

Meta-analysis of the effects of fear appeal messages

Witte and Allen (2000) conducted a meta-analysis to determine "how people react (both perceptually and persuasively) to fear appeal messages" (p. 596). The meta-analysis included data from 96 published and unpublished studies overall, with ks for various analysis ranging from 8 to 51, and ns ranging from 1,348 to 12,735.

This meta-analysis looked primarily at the effects of various message features on perceptions. Results indicate that stronger fear appeal messages produced significantly greater fear, severity, and susceptibility. Similarly, messages with stronger efficacy components generated significantly greater response-efficacy and self-efficacy. Second, Witte and Allen (2000) assessed the main effects of various message features on three key dependent variables. The investigators found that messages including stronger fear, severity, susceptibility, response-efficacy, and self-efficacy components lead to attitudes, intentions, and behavior more strongly directed toward the recommended response.

Third, the authors next examined "danger control" processes by looking at the interaction effects between threat and efficacy using both the "additive model" and the EPPM. The additive model predicts that higher levels of threat and/or efficacy will produce greater attitudes, intentions, and behaviors (i.e., low threat/low efficacy < low threat/high efficacy = high threat/low efficacy < high threat/high efficacy). The EPPM, in contrast, predicts that the high-threat/high-efficacy group should have the highest mean, with the other three groups producing lower means that are similar to each other (i.e., low threat/low efficacy = low threat/high efficacy = high threat/low efficacy < high threat/high efficacy). It was concluded that while "both the additive model and the

EPPM model appear to fit the data" (Witte and Allen, 2000, p. 600), the additive model received the greatest support (with the main deviation from the EPPM being that the low-threat/high-efficacy and high-threat/low-efficacy groups were equal to each other but different from the low-threat/low-efficacy group, whereas the EPPM suggests that all three of these means should be the same).

Finally, Witte and Allen (2000) looked at the effects of fear appeal messages on "fear control" responses, and found that stronger fear appeal messages lead to stronger defensive responses, especially when the efficacy message is weak. Further, there was a significant negative correlation between fear control and danger control responses. Witte and Allen (2000) conclude that, because of this observation, "it is difficult to tell whether danger control or fear control processes are dominating unless one has measured and/or manipulated perceived efficacy" (p. 601). This conclusion provides important advice for researchers and practitioners who wish to use fear appeals to change individuals' attitudes, intentions, and behaviors.

The risk perception analysis framework

Rimal and Real's (2003) risk perception attitude (RPA) framework is derived from the predictions of the EPPM in that it "posits that efficacy beliefs moderate the relationship between risk perception and health outcomes" (Rimal *et al.*, 2009, p. 210). However, unlike the EPPM which conceptualizes perceptions of threat and efficacy as a property of a message, the RPA framework "conceptualizes risk perception as a property not of the message but rather of the individual" (Rimal and Real, 2003, p. 327). Specifically, the RPA framework categorizes individuals into one of four groups based on their current perceptions of threat and efficacy: (1) *responsive* – high risk and high efficacy, (2) avoidance – high risk and low efficacy, (3) proactive – low risk and high efficacy, and (4) indifference – low risk and low efficacy. Predictions about how individuals in each group are likely to behave mirror those of the EPPM model (e.g., individuals in the high risk/high efficacy responsive category should be most motivated to enact self-protective behaviors).

To illustrate using a recent global health example, Rimal *et al.* (2009) tested the key hypothesis of the RPA framework using two HIV/AIDS-prevention behaviors (i.e., use of condoms and remaining monogamous) in Malawi, which is located in southeastern Africa. Results were consistent with the RPA framework for one of the two variables under investigation. Specifically, "efficacy beliefs were found to moderate the relationship between risk perception and intentions to remain monogamous, but not between risk perceptions and intentions to use condoms" (p. 210). So, we again see the importance of efficacy perceptions in guiding or changing attitudes, intentions, and behaviors.

Extensions and Innovations

To return to the beginning of the chapter, a woman said she would rather her baby die than take HIV medicines such as Nevirapine and Zidovudine and formula (rather than breast) feed, each of which can significantly reduce the risk of transmitting HIV from

HIV positive mothers to their babies (McIntyre, 1998). For her, it was not a financial or access issue, nor was it an aversion to needles or hospitals. She spoke of being constantly fearful of AIDS, afraid that taking the drugs and using formula would make her and her baby social outcasts in the community. Her thoughts represent important considerations for health educators working with communities who have been immersed in a health topic like HIV/AIDS for almost two decades. When assessing people's personal efficacy, do they consider their social network? Should we move beyond individualistic health variables (i.e., condom use, getting tested) to see how we can help communities care for their orphans? Is it productive to further scare the already fearful? This chapter presents two innovative lines of research regarding HIV/AIDS in the country of Namibia that extend EPPM to address these important health questions.

Background and need

Namibia, which established its independence from South Africa in 1990, is located on the Western coastline of Southern Africa. Despite roughly 20 years of HIV health education campaigns, Namibia is struggling with an epidemic of HIV infection. It ranks fifth in the world for adult HIV prevalence (United Nations Economic Commission for Africa, 2008), and is one of seven countries that have HIV prevalence rates higher than 15 percent (UNICEF, 2007). Although estimates vary and precise figures are difficult to obtain, the Joint United Nations Program on HIV/AIDS (UNAIDS, 2010) estimates that approximately one in six (12.5% to 18.3%) of all 15- to 49-year-old Namibians are people living with HIV/AIDS (PLWHA), of which 69 percent are women. Adults are not the only ones affected by the AIDS epidemic in Namibia. As of 2010, 14,000 Namibian children (aged 0 to 14 years) are PLWHA and over 53,000 Namibian children (aged 17 or younger) reported being orphaned because of AIDS-related deaths of one or both of their parents (UNAIDS, 2010). HIV is the number one reason for hospitalization and the main cause of death in the country. Namibians have considerable intrinsic knowledge about the causes and consequences of the virus, as most reported having had at least one loved one die from the disease or had to care for children orphaned due to AIDS (Murray-Johnson *et al.*, 2004). HIV has ravaged Namibia. Those left are knowledgeable yet highly fearful of the disease; HIV positive parents worry what will happen to their children (Murray-Johnson *et al.*, 2004; Muthusamy, Levine, and Weber, 2009).

The social side of threat

Many public health campaigns concentrate on the adverse medical consequences of HIV/AIDS as a means to induce lifestyle change. These health scholars would suggest that, without feeling threatened by the consequences of HIV/AIDS (e.g., chronic and severe illness and death), the population at risk will not be sufficiently motivated into an alternative action. Health communication scholars have recently challenged this assumption. Smith, Ferrara, and Witte (2007) argued that perceptions of interpersonal networks can be used to motivate behavioral change. Viruses like HIV can incubate for years, so the social consequences of being ostracized within the community may be more salient and compelling than are the physical effects of an AIDS-related illness. HIV has inspired social responses of compassion and solidarity as well as anxiety, prejudice, and rejection/banishment of PLWHA (Frediksson and Kanabus, 2004). Some researchers have paid attention to its social context, given that it shapes and situates personal values, beliefs, and behaviors (e.g., Cohen, 2000; DeGraff, Bilsborrow, and Guilkey, 1997; Grady, Klepinger, Billy, and Tanfer, 1993; Maharaj and Cleland, 2004; Newman and Zimmerman, 2000), but behaviors such as caring for PLWHA or adopting orphaned children have been virtually unexplored in theory and research. In the study reviewed here, Smith, Ferrara, and Witte (2007) extended EPPM by incorporating stigma and collective efficacy. The research team interviewed 400 people living nearby a mission hospital in Andara, Namibia. They argued that potential caretakers assess the stigma associated with PLWHA in addition to their personal susceptibility to, and the seriousness of, HIV/AIDS when deciding whether to shelter an orphan or PLWHA. *Stigma* is a process of devaluation based on an undesirable or discrediting attribute or attributes that a person possesses. It derives from stereotypes or beliefs about the attributes used to characterize a group of people (e.g., all people with HIV are unclean, careless, immoral, promiscuous, etc.).

The social side of efficacy

While communities may be the root of stigma, they could also be the root of positive feelings like collective efficacy, a plausible social extension to efficacy. *Collective efficacy* refers to group members' confidence (or a group's confidence) in their group's abilities to attain their goals and accomplish desired tasks (Bandura, 1986). Smith, Ferrara, and Witte (2007) posited that a person evaluates his or her community's collective efficacy in supporting those affected by HIV in addition to his personal ability to resist social hostility when assessing his own level of personal efficacy. With greater confidence in the community's ability to mobilize resources to help people living with HIV, its members would report more willingness to help those living with HIV and their associated dependents, that is, their children. The process involves perceptions or beliefs that an effective collective action to address a social or public health predicament is achievable (Figueroa *et al.*, 2002). Members of communities with high (versus low) collective efficacy participate more in their sociocultural environments, secure and access more community resources, develop stronger networks of social support, and feel more personal empowerment (Baum, 1999; Dutta-Bergman, 2003; Rappaport, 1987; Repucci, Woolard, and Fried, 1999). Perceptions of group efficacy may carry more power than self-efficacy. Even if individual group members feel efficacy in their personal ability to help adopt an AIDS orphan, low collective efficacy may hinder community dialogue about AIDS orphans and collective actions to help or to adopt them, as well as persistence in performing collective activities when barriers arise (Figueroa *et al.*, 2002).

Interestingly Smith, Ferrara, and Witte (2007) found they could motivate people who do not feel physically threatened (neither serious nor severe for them) through stigma. The threat of stigma would motivate their intentions to provide care to those affected by HIV, as long as their efficacy perceptions also remained strong. The more that people who did not feel threatened by HIV sensed that their groups held a stigma about HIV as well as an ability to mobilize resources, the more they believed that they and their group members would adopt AIDS orphans. Personal stigma (but not self-efficacy to resist social pressure) predicted Namibian respondents' willingness to support people living with HIV. The more they held a personal stigma, the more they reported willingness to help people living with HIV.

The Smith, Ferrara, and Witte's study is unique in that it (1) extends EPPM beyond individualistic variables (self-efficacy, response efficacy, personal adoption of recommended response), (2) suggests that using stigma as a fear source results in some positive outcomes for the community, and (3) looks beyond the recommended medical response (i.e., adoption of condoms) to address the problem of whether a community would collectively house and care for orphans and PLWHA. While Smith, Ferrara, and Witte investigated collective variables, a second group of researchers sought to determine whether different levels of pre-existing fear impact EPPM.

Pre-existing fear

Muthusamy, Levine, and Weber (2009) investigated the role of fear-inducing message content in the high-fear category among Namibians. They thought it plausible that fear appeals may not be effective when trying to persuade people who are already highly afraid, so they conducted an experiment to explore this unique idea. A total of 434 undergraduate students from the University of Namibia were randomly assigned as participants into one of six experimental conditions. Efficacy and threat were varied in a 2 (high-efficacy, low-efficacy) × 2 (high-threat, low-threat) design with one control group (no message) and one high-self-efficacy-only group.

The messages were adapted from Witte (1992). The high- and low-threat messages entailed a classic message informing participants what HIV was and including a case study of a fictitious AIDS patient. The high-threat condition emphasized severity by using vivid language and showing graphic photographs of late-stage AIDS victims. In the low-threat condition story susceptibility and severity were minimized with neutral language about non-college-aged victims and innocuous photographs of clinical tests.

The efficacy conditions included a message about the effectiveness of condoms. Self-efficacy was increased by discussing the simplicity and benefits of condoms. Helpful responses to typical excuses partners give for not wanting to use condoms were included. Response efficacy was maximized by emphasizing that condoms, when used properly, substantially minimize the transmission of HIV.

The message type was tested to see how each impacted participants' attitudes toward condom use, intentions to use condoms, and safe sex behaviors.

Message design impact on threat

The majority of the Namibians sampled, even those in the no-message control condition, reported being "terrified" by HIV/AIDS. When they tried to induce even more threat with the experimental conditions, they were unsuccessful. The participant group that read the high-threat messages did not report significantly higher amounts of fear than the no-message control or the low-threat group. While the messages had been assessed as scary, they did little to make an already terrified group even more so. Interestingly, the threat content of the messages did somewhat reduce fear in the low-threat message condition. Because threat content did not increase fear, message threat levels had little effect on condom-related attitudes, intentions, and behaviors.

Message design impact on efficacy

Efficacy content of the message had little impact on attitudes and intentions, but had marginal impact on behavior. The efficacy messages were no more successful than the messages lacking efficacy content and the efficacy-only condition results did not substantially differ from the no-message control. Fascinatingly, Namibians who reported more perceived efficacy also tended to have more positive attitudes, intentions, and more frequent usage of condoms. It is possible that a more powerful efficacy message may be effective, though the authors wonder what that message may entail while maintaining factual accuracy.

Implications

Consistent with EPPM, because initial fear was already very high, messages designed to instil fear and messages offering efficacy content had little effect on attitudes, intentions, and behaviors. The most obvious implication of this study is that using fear appeals in the context of high pre-existing fear is likely unproductive (though it does not produce a boomerang effect). Muthuswamy, Levine, and Weber (2009, p. 339) posit that:

> when the extent and magnitude of a threat is so high that it crosses some threshold, fear messages do little to change fear levels or to achieving desired outcomes. Similarly, if the threat is very low or nonexistent, fear reduction is less likely to have much motivation force. Above and below these threshold points, the content of fear appeal might be irrelevant, but between the threshold points, it is likely that fear can be effectively induced to elicit desirable outcomes.

They caution that fear appeal messages in countries that have long been ravaged by HIV/AIDS may have lost their effectiveness. They do believe that fear appeals will have an impact in countries like India and China, where the spread of HIV/AIDS is comparatively new. Fear appeal messages in such countries may prove timely. The bottom line of this study – that scaring the already terrified did not improve health behaviors – clearly highlights the need to assess an audience's fear levels prior to launching a fear appeal campaign.

Conclusions

The EPPM has successfully altered thousands of people's health knowledge base, attitudes, and behaviors worldwide through the management of fear. It details the necessary components to build a strong campaign. Scholars have extended EPPM to include the concepts collective efficacy and stigma.

Health educators who discover they are dealing with high levels of pre-existing fear, however, may consider Muthswamy, Levine, and Weber's (2009) research and consider looking elsewhere in this book for a persuasive campaign design.

References

Bandura, A. (1986). *Social Foundations of Thought and Action: A Social Cognitive Theory.* Englewood Cliffs, NJ: Prentice Hall.

Baum, F. (1999). The role of social capital in health promotion: Australian perspectives. *Health Promotion Journal of Australia, 9,* 171–178.

Belete, S., Girgre, A., and Witte, K. (2003, March). *Summative Evaluation of "Journey of Life":
The Ethiopia Reproductive Health Communication Project.* Addis Ababa: Johns Hopkins Bloomberg School of Public Health/Center for Communication Programs and Ethiopia National Office of Population. Retrieved from http://www.popline.org/ics-wpd/mmc/media/treth4.pdf

Chikombero, M. (2009). Assessing the effectiveness and impact of televised HIV/AIDS public service announcements in Zimbabwe. Paper presented at the annual meeting of the International Communication Association, Sheraton New York, New York City. Retrieved from http://www.allacademic.com/meta/p11737_index.html

Cohen, B. (2000). Family planning programs, socioeconomic characteristics, and contraceptive use in Malawi. *World Development, 28,* 843–860.

DeGraff, D. S., Bilsborrow, R. E., and Guilkey, D. K. (1997). Community level determinants of contraceptive use in the Philippines: A structural analysis. *Demography, 34,* 385–398.

Dutta-Bergman, M. (2003). Demographic and psychographic antecedents of community participation: Applying a social marketing model. *Social Marketing Quarterly, 9,* 17–31.

Figueroa, M. E., Kincaid, L., Rani, M., and Lewis, G. (2002). *Communication for social change:
An integrated model for measuring the process and its outcomes.* Communication for Social Change Working Paper Series 1, Rockefeller Foundation, New York.

Fredriksson, J., and Kanabus, A. (2004). *HIV and AIDS: Stigma and discrimination* [Brochure]. Horsham, UK: Avert. See also http://www.avert.org/hiv-aids-stigma.htm

Glik, D., Nowak, G., Valente, T. *et al.* (2002). Youth performing arts entertainment-education for HIV/AIDS prevention and health promotion: Practice and research. *Journal of Health Communication, 7,* 39–57.

Grady, W. R., Klepinger, D. H., Billy, J. O. G., and Tanfer, K. (1993). Condom characteristics:
The perceptions and preferences of men in the United States. *Family Planning Perspectives, 25,* 67–73.

Guttman, N., Gesser-Edelsburg, A. and Israelashvili, M. (2008). The paradox of realism and "authenticity" in entertainment-education: A study of adolescents' views about anti-drug abuse dramas. *Health Communication, 23,* 128–141.

Hubbell, A. (2006). Mexican American women in a rural area and barriers to their ability to enact protective behaviors against breast cancer. *Health Communication, 8,* 35–44.

Janis, I. L. (1967). Effects of fear arousal on attitude change: Recent developments in theory and experimental research. In L. Berkowitz (Ed.), *Advances in experimental social psychology* (Vol. 3, pp. 166–225). New York: Academic Press.

Leventhal, H. (1970). Findings and theory in the study of fear communications. In L. Berkowitz (Ed.), *Advances in experimental social psychology* (Vol. 5, pp. 119–186). New York: Academic Press.

Maharaj, P., and Cleland, J. (2004). Condom use within marital and cohabitating partnerships. *Family Planning, 35*, 116–125.

McIntyre, J. (1998). *HIV in Pregnancy: A review*. Paper prepared for WHO and UNAIDS. Retrieved from http://data.unaids.org/publications/IRC-pub01/jc151-hiv-in-pregnancy_en.doc

Mulogo, E. M., Witte, K., Bajunirwe, F., *et al.* (2006). Birth plans: Influence on decisions about seeking assisted deliveries among rural communities in Uganda. *East African Medical Journal, 83*(3), 74–83.

Murray-Johnson L., Witte K., Liu W. Y.*et al.* (2001). Addressing cultural orientation in fear appeals: Promoting AIDS-protective behaviors among Hispanic immigrants and African-American adolescents, and American and Taiwanese college students. *Journal of Health Communication. 6*(4), 1–23.

Muthusamy, N. Levine, T., and Weber, R., (2009). Scaring the already scared: Some problems with HIV/AIDS fear appeals in Namibia. *Journal of Communication, 59*(2), 317–344.

Newman, P., and Zimmerman, M. (2000). Gender differences in HIV-related sexual risk behavior among urban African American youth: A multivariate approach. *AIDS Education and Prevention, 12*, 308–325.

Piotrow, P. T., and de Fossard, E. D. (2004). Entertainment-education as public health intervention. In A. Singhal, M. J. Cody, E. M. Rogers, and M. Sabido (Eds.), *Entertainment-education and social change: History, research, and practice* (pp. 39–60). Mahwah, NJ: Lawrence Erlbaum Associates.

Rappaport, J. (1987). Terms of empowerment/exemplars of prevention: Toward a theory of community psychology. *American Journal of Community Psychology, 15*, 121–148.

Repucci, N. D., Woolard, J. L., and Fried, C. S. (1999). Social, community, and preventive interventions. *Annual Review of Psychology, 50*, 387–418.

Rimal, R. N., Böse, K., Brown, J. *et al.* (2009). Extending the purview of the risk perception attitude framework: Findings from HIV/AIDS prevention research in Malawi. *Health Communication, 24*, 210–218.

Rimal, R. N. and Real, K. (2003). Perceived risk and efficacy beliefs as motivators of change: Use of the risk perception attitude (RPA) framework to understand health behaviors. *Human Communication Research, 29*, 370–399.

Roberto, A. J. (2004). Putting communication theory into practice: The extended parallel process model. *Communication Teacher, 18*, 38–43.

Roberto, A. J., Goodall, C. E., and Witte, K. (2009). Raising the alarm and calming fears: Perceived threat and efficacy during risk and crisis. In R. Heath and D. O'Hair (Eds.), *Handbook of risk and crisis communication* (pp. 287–303). Washington, DC: Routledge.

Roberto, A. J., Murray-Johnson, L., and Witte, K. (in press). International health communication campaigns in developing countries. In T. Thompson, R. Parrott, and J. Nussbaum (Eds.), *Handbook of Health Communication*. New York: Taylor and Francis.

Rogers, R. W. (1975). A protection motivation theory of fear appeals and attitude change. *Journal of Psychology, 91*, 93–114.

Singhal, A. (2004). Entertainment-education through participatory theater: Freirean strategies for empowering the oppressed. In A. Singhal, M. J. Cody, E. M. Rogers, and M. Sabido (Eds.), *Entertainment-Education and Social Change: History, Research, and Practice* (pp. 377–398). Mahwah, NJ: Lawrence Erlbaum Associates.

Singhal, A., and Rogers, E. M. (2004). The status of entertainment-education worldwide. In A. Singhal, M. J. Cody, E. M. Rogers, and M. Sabido (Eds.), *Entertainment-Education and Social Change: History, Research, and Practice* (pp. 3–20). Mahwah, NJ: Earlbaum.

Smith, R. A., Downs, E., and Witte, K. (2007). Drama theory and entertainment education: Exploring the effects of a radio drama on behavioral intentions to limit HIV transmission in Ethiopia. *Communication Monographs, 74,* 133–153.

Smith, R.A., Ferrara, M., and Witte, K (2007). *Social Sides of Health Risks. Health Communication, 21,* 55–64.

UNAIDS (United Nations Programme on HIV/AIDS) (2010). *The Global AIDS Epidemic.* Retrieved from http://www.unaids.org/documents/20101123 GlobalReport_em.pdf

UNICEF (United Nations Children's Fund) (2007, September). *Children and the Millennium Development Goals.* (ISBN: 978-92-806-4219-3). Retrieved from www.unicef.org/publications

United Nations Economic Commission for Africa (2008). *Securing our Future.* Retrieved from http://www.uneca.org/chga/report/CHGAReport.pdf

Witte, K. (1992). Putting the fear back into fear appeals: The extended parallel process model. *Communication Monographs, 59,* 329–349.

Witte, K., and Allen, M. (2000). A meta-analysis of fear appeals: Implications for effective public health campaigns. *Heath Education Behavior, 27,* 591–614.

Witte, K., Cameron, K. A., Lapinski, M. K., and Nzyuko, S. (1998). Evaluating HIV/AIDS prevention programs according to theory: A field project along the Trans-Africa highway in Kenya. *Journal of Health Communication, 4,* 345–363.

Witte, K., Girma, B., and Girgre, A. (2002–2003). Addressing the underlying mechanisms to HIV/AIDS preventive behaviors in Ethiopia. *International Quarterly of Community Health Education, 21,* 163–176.

Witte, K., Meyer, G., and Martell, D. (2001). *Effective Health Risk Messages: A Step-By-Step Guide.* Thousand Oaks, CA: Sage.

Witte, K., and Roberto, A. J. (2009). Fear appeals and public health: Managing fear and creating hope. In L. R. Frey and K. N. Cissna (Eds.), *Handbook of Applied Communication Research* (pp. 584–610). New York: Routledge.

Witte, K., Singhal, A., Muthuswamy, N., and Duff, D. (2003). *Compilation of Three Quantitative Reports Assessing Effects of Taru* [Report]. Athens: Ohio University.

14

Innovations in the Evaluation of Social Change Communication for HIV and AIDS

Ailish Byrne and Robin Vincent

This chapter[1] explores innovative approaches to evaluation that have the potential to strengthen assessment of the social dimensions of health and well-being. Our focus is their application in the HIV and AIDS fields where they remain relatively unknown, but the analysis has far wider relevance. As interest in addressing the social drivers of HIV grows, the concepts, theory, and practice of evaluation need strengthening to better cater to the complex, multifaceted, and unpredictable character of social change. Recognizing that social outcomes typically emerge and cannot be predetermined or planned in advance, significant questions are raised about the adequacy of traditional linear-model planning and evaluations.

The nature of social change poses serious challenges for its evaluation. These include the engagement of multiple actors and perspectives, the numerous factors that impact, complex and unpredictable "impact trajectories," power differentials, and differing evaluation expectations and needs. We are challenged to address dynamic and emerging relationships and networks between diverse development actors, and social processes rather than static structures. These characteristics demand more realistic expectations of evaluation, ones that emphasize *contribution* rather than attribution.

In this context we explore promising innovations in evaluation, drawing on theory and practice in participatory monitoring and evaluation, utilization focused evaluation, systems thinking, and complex systems approaches. Arguing that evaluation dynamics should match those of the system they are evaluating, we show how core social change principles of participation, equity, local ownership, and sustainability resonate strongly with evaluation approaches informed by systemic and complex systems thinking.

The approaches advocated pose significant challenges to existing organizational cultures, hierarchies and ways of working. They demand being open to change and to informed risk taking.

The Handbook of Global Health Communication, First Edition. Edited by Rafael Obregon and Silvio Waisbord.

Our aim is to spark critical reflection on current evaluation practice and to foster greater interest in and support for experimentation with viable alternatives that do justice to the inherent complexities of social change and social change communication processes. We wish to nurture support for innovators and for decision makers well positioned to make environments conducive to creative and more effective evaluation practice.

Introduction

There is growing concern to address the social drivers of HIV, but interventions and evaluation approaches that better cater to the complex and multiply caused issues like stigma and gender inequalities remain underdeveloped. Lasting social change results from multiple, interrelated, and interacting factors, and social outcomes are often emergent rather than planned. Some early successes in country responses to HIV, such as Uganda and Brazil, benefitted from widespread public communication, community mobilization, and a combination of contextual factors beyond the actions of health or development agencies (Low-Beer and Stoneburner, 2004; Vincent, 2006). This raises questions about the adequacy of traditional linear planning and evaluation approaches when addressing complex social change processes (Eoyang and Berkas, 1998; Rogers, 2008).

Sustainable, rights-based programming to reduce HIV risk and vulnerability requires addressing social and structural factors (UNAIDS, 2010). The causal pathways and impact trajectories of interventions to promote deeper social change relating to HIV and AIDS differ from those focusing on immediate aspects of awareness, knowledge, and behavior that have dominated programming to date (Woolcock, 2009). Yet evaluation approaches typically remain focused on short-term, project-oriented attribution.

Initiatives aimed at social change require programming that combines efforts at a range of levels and finds ways of achieving scale through aligning this range of interventions, and facilitating dialogue and feedback between them, toward common objectives (Burns, 2007a). To promote local-level initiative and action, district- and national-level interventions need to create an enabling environment, which includes addressing elements of social infrastructure and context which fuel vulnerability to HIV infection. Attributing cause in social life is "complex and contingent" (Byrne, 2002, p. 2) and public health and development approaches that capture and better address the complexities of social change are urgently needed. As we discuss, the confluence of learning from participatory communication and social research with emerging ideas from complexity science provides renewed impetus to address the challenges of facilitating and evaluating social change.

Many SCC planners and practitioners share concern that development agencies may not tackle change in ways appropriate and sophisticated enough for the change processes they are involved in. The evaluation of social change communication urgently needs strengthening to effectively demonstrate impact in a context where "structural" approaches are seen as vital to effective HIV "Combination" prevention, and where the importance of providing an enabling environment for community action is increasingly recognized UNAIDS, 2010). Although a variety of organizations are working to develop and evaluate SCC strategies, relatively few resources have been dedicated to the challenge. Consequently, in 2009 the SCC Working Group of UNAIDS and the CFSC Consortium, working with

---

Box 14.1   What is Social Change Communication (SCC)?

Social change communication, similar to Communication for Social Change (CFSC²), is recognized as a promising approach to address the social aspects of HIV, AIDS and other development issues (UNAIDS, 2007). Relevant to diverse contexts, it engages multiple and diverse stakeholders and initiatives, in recognition that social life is inherently complex. SCC appreciates that social life is dynamic, and that contextual factors significantly shape the outcomes of individual action and program interventions.

UNAIDS defines Social Change Communication (for AIDS) as "the strategic use of advocacy, communication and social mobilization to systematically facilitate and accelerate change in the underlying determinants of HIV risk, vulnerability and impact. It enables communities and national AIDS programs to tackle structural barriers to effective AIDS responses, such as gender inequality, violation of human rights and HIV-related stigma" (UNAIDS, 2011, p.21).

SCC is always one component of wider social change processes. It is widely understood as an umbrella term referring to processes, initiatives, and programs that may differ widely in specific objectives, audience and program components. But they are united by common underlying principles, including: working strategically and collaboratively at multiple levels; engaging multiple and diverse actors, particularly marginalized stakeholders; using diverse and complementary approaches and methods; explicitly addressing power dynamics that intensify vulnerability; catalyzing and nurturing sustainable social change; addressing the underlying drivers of social change; being firmly grounded in local contexts.

Panos, initiated a research process to identify ways of advancing the evaluation of social change communication efforts in relation to HIV programming.

This chapter stems from a longer report produced for UNAIDS in 2011. Deliberations from an expert group meeting in May 2009 have closely informed the substance and shape of both.[3]

We draw on theory and practice in participatory monitoring and evaluation, utilization focused evaluation (UFE), systems thinking, complex systems, and soft systems approaches, including related innovations of whole systems action research, Complex Adaptive Systems (CAS), and Social Network Analysis (SNA). These significant bodies of theory and practice are introduced to illustrate their potential to strengthen the evaluation of HIV programs that aim to address the social complexities of HIV and AIDS, and to inspire further application, adaptation, and creativity in evaluation approaches.

In the first section we highlight what addressing the social dimensions of HIV and AIDS requires and consider core challenges underlying the evaluation of social change processes. The second section briefly outlines evaluation questions critical to SCC and SC contexts, which will inform decisions about evaluation methodology and methods. The third considers the scope of evaluation in contexts of social change, with a focus on issues of causality and underlying theories of change. In the fourth section we briefly outline innovative approaches that could strengthen monitoring and evaluation (M&E) in the HIV and AIDS fields, and complement indicators. The final section outlines key principles of evaluation in social change contexts, to inspire the use of approaches more appropriate to the evaluation of social change and social change communication. Lastly we offer recommendations to progress related work and research, with the ultimate aim of consolidating learning in related areas and strengthening practice, to enhance impact.

Addressing the Social Dimensions of HIV and AIDS and Understanding Social Change

> HIV prevention must be able to deal with complexity: what makes the difference between a growing and a diminishing HIV epidemic is not merely net changes in individual behaviors, but dynamic shifts in sexual and social networks. Analytical tools need to be designed to capture these dynamics (Piot *et al.*, 2008, 853–854).

HIV initiatives and their evaluation are overwhelmingly dominated by interventions that target individuals and their behaviors, with very few targeting social, policy, or structural factors (Coates, Richter, and Caceres, 2008). Long-standing recognition of the need to address social context in HIV interventions[4] and dissatisfaction with the overly individual-focused theory and practice of HIV programming has fuelled contemporary concern to address the social drivers of HIV infection (Vincent, 2006) and renewed interest in the social vulnerabilities which mediate risk of HIV infection (Stillwaggon, 2006). The widely endorsed UNAIDS communication framework of 1999 highlighted the need to address five dimensions of context: culture, gender, spirituality, policy, and socioeconomic status. Yet, despite drawing on extensive regional involvement, it has failed to substantially change practice.

Addressing social and structural factors

The scale of the challenge of concerted multilevel programming is evident from recent discussions on "structural prevention" and attempts to address the social determinants of HIV.[5] Frameworks developed to understand structural factors tend to distinguish three levels: (1) *macro structural factors* – the social characteristics that impact on people's lives such as racism, sexism and discrimination; (2) *intermediate-level structural factors* of infrastructure and service availability, neighborhood characteristics, and local resources; and (3) individual *micro-level factors* of socially mediated knowledge and skills (see Rao Gupta *et al.*, 2008; Auerbach *et al.*, 2009).

Understanding social change

Despite important advances in understanding the significance of structural factors to HIV prevention, there remains a need to better conceptualize how social change happens and, in particular, the relationship between individual and social change and the range of "levels" identified in structural approaches to HIV prevention (Vincent 2009b). Critical social theory argues that individuals are always socially located and embedded, they are both shaped by and shape prevailing social norms and social practice. Thus, what is conceived as "individual behavior" is nested in a range of influences at different levels, which facilitate or constrain change at the individual level. To date, attempts to address social norms and social change in HIV have tended to treat social factors as either the aggregate of individual voluntaristic action, or as things that are intangible and impossible to pin down. Both views are inaccurate and result in insufficient attention to social context and the way individual and social practice is intimately intertwined. This false dualism is reflected in even relatively sophisticated frameworks developed to evaluate social change, which inadequately capture its complex and dynamic nature (e.g. Figueroa *et al.*, 2003).

In contrast, social movements and societal level mobilizations are illuminating for their role in responses to HIV. Broad social mobilizations and particularities of national context have together fuelled some relatively successful country responses to HIV and AIDS (e.g. Uganda, see Low-Beer and Stoneburner, 2004). In notable contrast to linear cause–effect models, the most widely known national success stories highlight how a combination of individual and social factors can converge in ongoing social change processes to fuel reductions in HIV infection. They point to the need to appreciate how multiple social factors interact over longer time frames to produce sustainable change. In such dynamic and context-specific scenarios, assumptions about replication need questioning and attempts to measure the effects of targeted interventions with prespecified, immediately measurable inputs and outcomes can produce misleading, narrow and short-lived results.

Critical Questions: Evaluation for What, for Whom, and Why?

Analysis of ways to better evaluate social change communication in the context of HIV interventions brings to the fore critical questions relating to dominant models of development and social change, HIV/AIDS programming, evaluation, and power, all of which have long fuelled important debates. Here we briefly highlight their implications in SCC contexts.

The need for greater demonstration of policy and program impact, and for evaluation approaches that better capture the essence and achievements of development efforts and promote learning, organizational development, and change, is widely recognized. To reconcile the objectives of demonstrating impact and promoting learning and change, it is necessary to address critical questions about what is prioritized in an evaluation, why, by whom and for whom (Guijt, 2007, 2008). Calls for more political – rather than technical – understandings of "accountability" that highlight issues of voice and justice are significant (Eyben, 2006).

Given this scenario, there is notable excitement about "new" approaches to the assessment of social change. Too often, critiques have focused narrowly on the merits or limitations of particular methods, and deeper, critical thinking about the fundamentals of assessment is neglected. What methods and tools are relevant will depend (implicitly or explicitly) on the interlinked aspects of program objectives, chosen strategy, theory of change, epistemology, and other factors, as discussed below. These "bigger picture" issues cannot be overlooked if the M&E of SCC is to be strengthened in ways consistent with the principles of SCC outlined above.

Evaluation does not occur in a vacuum. Despite prolific rhetoric about participation, partnership, and local ownership in development circles, the demands of externally imposed evaluations and indicators often serve to undermine these principles (Mowles, Stacey, and Griffin, 2008) and to strain development "partnerships" (Vincent and Byrne, 2006). The widespread use of external evaluators, justified by a desire for "objectivity," "independence," and quality, combined with dominant ideas about what counts as evidence, often precludes recognition of the value and validity of locally generated assessments (Chambers, 2008, p. 105). Yet questions of what evidence and whose evidence remain critical. We argue that evaluation should capture and "legitimize" the perspectives and achievements of key development actors (Byrne, 2008). Reflecting the core social change values embedded in the initiative being assessed has significant implications for evaluation approaches (Guijt, 2007).

To some extent, SCC evaluators will inevitably set different objectives, foci, and methods for evaluations because they are interested in different components or aspects of communication, social change, or both. As no practical evaluation can cover everything, prioritization is inevitable – based on practical resource issues, the theoretical and epistemological preferences of evaluators, managers, and donors, and other factors. Given that the essence of SCC is social, it is essential that evaluation choices made do not exclude features fundamental to social context and social life – including meanings, motivations, emergent social structures, historical events, and the dynamics of all of these in driving behavioral and social change. Yet these essential social features continue to receive inadequate attention and support in SCC evaluations. The following section discusses related issues and shares practical examples to illustrate how the evaluation of SCC can be made more appropriate and more effective.

Addressing Social Change: The Scope of Evaluation

Complex causality in social change

A key issue for SCC evaluation is where it is appropriate to expect a linear, one-way causal relationship between inputs and outputs; and where it is necessary to use models that presume complex, multidirectional, and thus less predictable causal relationships. In the first instance, with the use of experimental evaluation designs it is possible to show direct *attribution*. However when describing effects of a program that entails more complex, multidirectional processes, it is only realistic to speak of *contribution*. The dynamics of social change and the social aspects of HIV call for approaches to evaluation that reflect and appreciate the unpredictable, complex nature of lived realities and social change. Applying an experimental or quasi-experimental approach and seeking linear relationships in such contexts risks overextending attribution and prioritizing ease of measurement over content validity.

Despite widespread recognition of this reality in the social sciences and amongst development practitioners, until relatively recently the evaluation of development interventions has extensively focused on defining and confirming linear impact trajectories, aiming to establish clear, causal links between activities, outputs, outcomes, and impact. This explains the continued prevalence of *logical frameworks* (e.g. the Logical Framework Approach, or LFA). LFAs can help those involved think through program aims and processes and are useful for a "relatively narrow range of results-oriented management that is based on a simple logic model … where both staff activities and the results of those activities can be readily observed" (Rogers, 2008, p. 34). But their application, ethical and practical relevance has been consistently questioned when it comes to understanding social action (Prowse, 2007). In fields like SCC and HIV prevention, logic models, if used, should be complemented with approaches more suited to complex and dynamic situations.

Theories of change underlying development initiatives

How we conceptualise a social and organizational system has an impact on how we structure it and how we intervene in it … this is crucial material for evaluators to engage with" (Burns, 2007a: 188).

To consider the impact of social change communication and development interventions generally, we need to clarify and make explicit how we believe change happens in a particular context. This includes a clear picture of "success," of what we consider necessary preconditions for achieving and sustaining success, and of intermediate outcomes that indicate that change is happening. In other words, we need to make explicit our "theory of change" (Keystone Accountability, 2008). A theory of change is usefully defined as "an observational map to help practitioners … to read and thus navigate processes of social change" (Reeler, 2007, p. 2). Proponents of utilization focused evaluation (UFE, see Patton, 1997) and action research, among others, advocate a "grounded," inductive, and dynamic approach to theories of change, rather than assuming that a model of change developed in advance can be applied to different contexts.

Addressing the simple, complicated, and complex

Notions of simple, complicated, and complex are useful when considering evaluation methodologies. Stacey (2002) highlights a number of dimensions needed to understand change and related decision making, including outcomes, or what needs to happen to achieve and sustain change, identifying who can influence these outcomes, and the degree of certainty about an issue and level of agreement about it.[6] All these factors will inform appropriate decision making, ranging from "simple" decisions based on close agreement and certainty of outcomes, to "complex" decisions where there is little agreement or certainty about outcomes. In parallel, Westley, Zimmerman, and Patton (2007) suggest that simple, complicated, and complex problems all demand distinct responses.[7] Their example compares the "simple" baking of a cake – where following a recipe assures the same results every time, with the "complicated" sending of a rocket to the moon – where many detailed operations need to be carefully controlled to produce an exact outcome, and the "complex" raising of a child – where previous experience is important but no guarantee of success and outcomes are uncertain and negotiated.

HIV and AIDS prevention and treatment inevitably encompass a combination of simple, complicated, and complex problems and a range of complementary methods is needed to evaluate such scenarios. Two contrasting examples are revealing. A BBC Trust-sponsored campaign to promote condom use in India illustrates a relatively simple theory of change.[8] Assumptions are made about being close to certainty and agreement about the expected change, according to Stacey's dimensions. An M&E approach would probably seek to verify this assumption by measuring individual changes in audience knowledge, attitudes and practice, possibly using a control group. A linear, predictable trajectory of change is feasible, given the focus on individual-level outcomes and some consensus on the intervention and its likely efficacy.

In contrast, Puntos de Encuentro's approach focuses explicitly on influencing social context using a combination of media, edutainment programming, and youth empowerment training, and fostering links and networks between existing organizations and movements to catalyze social change. In Puntos's complexity-oriented approach, no single factor is perceived as being the cause of change. An evaluator would likely consider the extent to which different factors have *contributed* to changes in social norms and creating an enabling environment (Lacayo, Obregon, and Singhal, 2008). Here we are in the realm of complex social processes and decision making, where both the overall social complexity of many interrelated factors and additional political factors are significant.

We have argued that addressing the social aspects of HIV tends to fall in the area of complex decision making – where sociocultural, political, and organizational influences are all part of the context, and where longer-term, multilevel programs do not lend themselves to a linear theory of change. In this realm dominant approaches to evaluation reach their limits and need supplementing with methodologies better able to gauge effectiveness in the face of complexity. These broad distinctions can help identify and select elements of an overall evaluation framework appropriate to particular SCC contexts.

Evolving theories of change

Many practitioners and theorists argue that dynamic social contexts demand a flexible or evolving theory of change, to reflect deepening understanding and questions and issues that come to prominence over time (Mowles, Stacey, and Griffin, 2008; Eoyang and Berkas, 1998). Several approaches explored in the next section incorporate dynamic theories of change.

The scope of SCC evaluation for HIV programs

The fundamentals of social change and issues of causality discussed above call for approaches to SCC program evaluation which recognize that social processes are key to effective responses to HIV and AIDS, but that these are complex and we will never be able to fully grasp or predict them. Social change processes precede and will long outlive particular bounded "development" initiatives or programs, and particular programs cannot be meaningfully evaluated in isolation from their wider contexts, including the socio-cultural, political, economic and institutional environments within which they exist. This highlights how boundaries of an enquiry are critical – what or who is included or left out, and why.

In social change contexts, where limited agreement and lack of certainty about outcomes are commonplace, the partiality of any knowledge is evident. Researchers and evaluators should be explicit about their underlying objectives and values, so audiences know who has legitimized particular "knowledge" and "findings," and on what basis. We argue that the efforts and achievements of intended beneficiaries are central and should be captured and "legitimized" by evaluations. Developmental, learning-oriented evaluations can themselves reinforce processes of development and social change by fostering meaningful engagement and ownership. Yet numerous factors continue to inhibit this potential.

These issues are not new and many evaluators, development practitioners and researchers have already found effective ways of addressing them, as discussed below.

Innovative Approaches to Monitoring and Evaluation

Following discussion above on what the characteristics of social change, social aspects of HIV, and social change communication imply for evaluation, we turn now to approaches largely neglected in the HIV and AIDS fields, which promise more relevant and useful frameworks to address issues of social change. We argue that complexity-informed approaches have notable potential to deliver a richer and more comprehensive picture of change, one which includes the interconnectedness of living social change processes particularly pertinent to social aspects of HIV and AIDS. They resonate with the inclusive, learning and action-orientation of participatory M&E (Byrne *et al.*, 2005).

Notable literature and practice has embraced complex systems concepts for over 30 years. Experience in systems thinking and its application to development evaluation includes work on "whole systems action research" and "Complex Adaptive Systems." Systems-informed approaches emphasize the importance of local/insider participation, collective knowledge generation, and learning. We also consider another strand of work using complex systems concepts, Qualitative Comparative Analysis (QCA), which looks at the trajectory of social systems over the long term to identify particular social factors that may influence overall social outcomes. It provides broad pointers for policy that can guide social change in directions of greater equity and better health outcomes. We briefly outline related evaluation approaches including Utilization Focused Evaluation (UFE), Social Network Analysis (SNA), Outcome Mapping (OM), and Most Significant Change (MSC).

Systems thinking and systemic perspectives

Systems thinking shares many fundamentals with participatory monitoring and evaluation (PM&E), and shares with complexity approaches a focus on the bigger picture, interrelationships, and processes. Boundaries and the values they reflect are central considerations: "Boundaries … are judgments about worth. Defining boundaries is an essential part of systems work/inquiry/thinking" (Imam *et al.*, 2007 p. 6). As Imam *et al.* emphasize "value is contained in the relevance of the inquiry to those affected by it … Stakeholders are not passive players or mere informants – they are actively engaged in the critique about boundaries" (Imam *et al.*, 2007, p. 8). For evaluation this implies appreciating significant actors and factors in the wider, beyond-project context, highlighting the challenge of attributing impact. Importantly, systemic thinking "highlights dynamics that are not always visible through the scrutiny of individual interactions. This is crucial because outcomes (positive or negative) will often have more to do with the interrelationship between interacting interventions than the effect of any individual action. Understanding the wider system within which these emerge is crucial because action rarely impacts in a linear way" (Burns, 2007b, p. 182).

A systems-influenced evaluation explores assumptions about what constitutes "valid knowledge." Key questions include: Whose reality is being considered? Who is defining the situation and on what basis? How do you establish what is in or left out of the scope of work (i.e. which *interrelationships* are relevant)? How do you establish what standpoint to take (i.e. whose *perspectives* are relevant)? Who or what (ideas) benefit from these decisions and who or what is disadvantaged by them? (Williams, n. d.). See Midgley (2007), Checkland and Scholes (2004), and Burns (2007a, 2007b), for more on systemic thinking.

Complexity theory

Closely related to systems thinking, complexity theory has become influential across disciplines in recent years (Byrne, 1998; Ramalingam *et al.*, 2008). In "systems" where there are extensive interactions and feedback between constituent parts, complexity theory highlights the inadequacy of linear models of causality in predicting outcomes, as interactions in the system give rise to emergent properties that are qualitatively different from the character of the constituents of the system themselves. A defining characteristic of complexity thinking is overriding concern with social *processes* rather than social *structures*.

What do systems and complex systems approaches imply for evaluation?

Social change is often emergent and difficult to predict, dependent as it is on the dynamics of interdependent and interacting processes. This implies a shift from relying on certainties to estimating probabilities. The nonlinear causal pathways of social change and of interventions aimed at social factors require different approaches and expectations of the scope of evaluation. Qualitative changes in social life may result from apparently small changes, which combine and feed back to produce wider changes (popularly known as the "butterfly effect" or "tipping point"). This is critical for evaluations in complex systems of governance (Burns, 2007b).

As discussed above, how the boundaries of a particular intervention or system are defined has major implications for the kinds of change considered important and those tracked. Expanding the boundaries of an inquiry may alter who is legitimately considered a decision maker, who has valid knowledge, and who has a stake in the findings. Consequently boundary adjustment is significant and can bring in, or inhibit, a broader array of relevant perspectives (Midgley, 2007, p. 21).

Clearly many challenges posed by evaluating social change in HIV contexts resonate with systems approaches. Below we introduce some specific applications of systems and complexity approaches, while recognizing that triangulating diverse methods and perspectives helps achieve a fuller understanding of social change.

Whole Systems Action Research (WSAR)

From the rich literature and practice in the fields of Action Research and Participatory Action Research, we highlight Whole Systems Action Research, which synthesizes insights from complex systems approaches and proposes a way of addressing complex social issues. The approach facilitates community involvement in wider learning and change processes, to inform policy in a bottom-up manner. WSAR has framed large-scale evaluations in complex social and community contexts (Burns, 2007a).

WSAR combines parallel research and insight-generating processes with periodically bringing all stakeholders together in "large events," to review emerging data and identify systemic issues that resonate across the system. As significant issues are identified, they are addressed through exploratory action by groups of stakeholders directly involved with the issue. Subsequently, reflection and learning from these actions is fed back for review by wider stakeholder groups, in ongoing cycles of action and reflection. This approach has proven effective at unlocking complex social issues and systemic factors that are often missed and which defy easy resolution (Burns, 2007a, p. 23).

Beginning with locally grounded enquiry processes rather than preconceptions about "problems," and recognizing that understanding of issues will evolve over time and that boundaries of a system initially deemed relevant may also change, WSAR attends to the systemic nature of problems (Burns, 2007a). Like Complex Adaptive Systems introduced below, WSAR employs a flexible and emergent design which matches the emergent nature of the reality it seeks to evaluate.

WSAR holds great learning potential for large numbers of participants, as in the evaluation of the Welsh Assembly Governments "Communities First" program (2003–2006). Supporting 142 neighborhoods and various grant recipients, the action research became a hub through which learning about the complex multi-stakeholder and multi-community intervention was analyzed and acted upon. Insights from the field were linked to core decision-making processes through adaptation facilitated by the action research. Substantial changes were implemented within three years (Burns, 2007b, p. 191).

Complex Adaptive Systems (CAS)

Eoyang and Berkas' valuable insights into evaluating CAS are highly relevant to SC contexts: "As CASs, human systems are dynamic, entangled, scale independent, transformative and emergent. These characteristics challenge the basic assumptions of traditional evaluation methods. They necessitate new evaluation approaches that are as rich and varied as the human systems they are designed to assess" (Eoyang and Berkas, 1998, p. 16). The authors emphasize that such evaluation approaches should remain flexible and open to the emergent, subscribe to general and simple rules applicable to the whole system, and should match the dynamics of the system they are being applied to. In keeping with our ethos, Eoyang and Berkas share practical evaluation tools reflective of CAS, emphasizing that evaluation should be an appreciative "reinforcing rather than dampening feedback mechanism" (1998, p. 12).

Qualitative Comparative Analysis (QCA) – understanding complex cases

A different application of complexity theory takes a more macro view of the social factors which influence the overall character of particular societies. QCA uses social and behavioral survey data to examine trends and identify key social parameters that impact on the broad emergent character of social outcomes of a society over time (Byrne, 2002). To date the methods have been applied in relation to TB, housing, and social exclusion, but not to HIV trends. However, the potential to identify policy insights and data-relevant conclusions for action on a range of wider social determinants of health and social drivers of HIV, making use of widely available surveillance data, is notable. This could valuably complement existing modeling of epidemiological and behavioral surveys, which has been used to evaluate large HIV and AIDS programs.

Proponents of this method are careful to stress that the social factors identified in QCA are not determining, nor do they have easily predictable causal influence on social outcomes, since interaction with other factors and wider context is constant. The method does, however, provide pointers to broad social policies that can be seen to put limits on, and influence the character of, social change. In this vein, efforts may need to focus on investing in making environments more conducive to good health, well-being, and social capabilities, to create enabling contexts in which local action and initiative can independently flourish, rather than trying to control particular behaviors through direct programming (Vincent, 2009a).

Networks and Social Network Analysis (SNA)

The importance of networks and relationships to development is increasingly recognized. This is occurring within the context of growing interest in the dynamics of contemporary globalization and "the network society," which recognizes that much change and innovation happens through networks, often in an emergent, nonplanned way (Castells, 2000). It is a broad concept with extensive application.

As Davies argues, attending to networks of relationships and how these change over the course of an initiative seems a more relevant and tangible way of capturing influence and change, than more abstract processes of change reflected in the language and logic of the logical framework approach (Davies, 2003). Network perspectives are better able to capture multidirectional and reciprocal influences and causality that typify development initiatives: "Removing the one-directional nature of change leads us from thinking about a chain of events to a network of events, and from a chain of actors to a network of actors. Networks are found on all scales, within and between organizations, and can be formal and informal, visible and less so" (Davies, 2004, p. 134).

The strengths of network perspectives include their inclusiveness and that they can be described and analyzed at many scales. Valuable tools to describe and measure networks already exist and are supported by an extensive and growing body of relevant theory and research (Davies, 2004).

By making visible patterns of connections between stakeholders and how these change over time, network approaches can show, literally, lines of influence and power between groups and individuals and how these shift. Consequently, network approaches are useful to attend to shifts in power dynamics and relationships, aspects critical to social change and SCC. Rick Davies' 2009 paper explores potential uses, methods and tools of relevance, from the field of Social Network Analysis (SNA) and other related perspectives.

Outcome Mapping

Outcome Mapping (OM), now widely adopted, makes particular use of the network lens. In line with systems thinking, OM explicitly recognizes that no program operates in isolation from wider external factors, so we cannot plan or evaluate as if it did. That is to say, no single agency or group can realistically claim full credit for ultimate impact. Monitoring and evaluation in OM is focused around "boundary partners," or those individuals, groups, and organizations with whom the program interacts directly. The originality of the methodology is its explicit focus on changes in the behaviors, relationships, actions, and activities of boundary partners (Earl and Carden, 2002). While these outcomes enhance the possibility of development impacts, it is not a relationship of direct cause and effect.

Reflecting a more realistic and humble approach to evaluation, OM explicitly recognizes the contributions of multiple actors to large-scale and long-term change processes. It is "well suited to the complex functioning and long-term aspects of international development programs where outcomes are intermeshed and cannot be easily or usefully separated from each other" (Earl and Carden, 2002, p. 520). OM is a truly participatory and learning-oriented process, initially developed by the IDRC, Canada, and supported by high quality, easily accessed resources and an online forum.[9]

The above network-based approaches provide contrasting ways of representing change, from linear models to more social and networked "maps." They stem from different assumptions about what is significant and feasible in terms of impact, and highlight the relevance of underlying theories of change.

Other approaches

The Most Significant Change
The best-known story-based approach is the Most Significant Change (MSC) methodology, which today attracts notable international interest. The essence of MSC is enabling key stakeholders to tell, select, and learn from their own stories of change in ways that

help demonstrate impact. Transparency about why particular stories are selected by insiders results from guided discussion amongst key participants. MSC thereby helps to surface the assumptions and values of different stakeholder groups, fostering understanding and mutual learning through a dialogue process. It intentionally prioritizes group and/or organizational learning. The approach appeals to practitioners keen to prioritize often neglected but key voices, and to work more systematically with stories, to complement dominant M&E approaches (Davies and Dart, 2005). Much gray literature testifies to the strengths of MSC (e.g. India HIV/AIDS Alliance, 2010).

Community AIDS competence and community capacity

"AIDS competence" and community capacity approaches focus on developing key domains of capacity that may also be important dimensions for assessing social change (Campbell, Nair, and Maimane, 2007). The approaches involve a process of community dialogue and self-assessment of strengths and needs in responding to HIV and AIDS. They build understanding of broader social change needs and address wider sectoral development needs, mirroring the principles of SCC. In the interest of creating contexts conducive to effective HIV/AIDS management, Campbell and colleagues (2007) outline six strategies to foster "HIV-competent" communities: building knowledge and basic skills; creating social spaces for dialogue and critical thinking; promoting a sense of local ownership of the problem and incentives for action; emphasizing community strengths and resources; mobilizing existing formal and informal local networks; and building partnerships between marginalized communities and more powerful outside actors and agencies. These resonate significantly with SCC fundamentals.

Strengthening and complementing indicators

No discussion on the evaluation of SC and SCC would be complete without attention to indicators, given their prominence in practice. Here we pose questions to be considered before particular indicators are selected, including who should select indicators and how aspects of change not adequately captured by indicators can be better catered to.

It is important to appreciate that indicators are not neutral but always reflect particular values and priorities. Consequently, to secure legitimacy for any indicator, transparency about how and by whom it has been developed is essential. Checking "expert indicators" with various stakeholder groups facilitates the expression of different perceptions and priorities, which can be weighed according to relative importance in connection with selecting indicators (see Davies, 2008).

The widespread imposition of indicators fuels much frustration, given their often dubious value to program insiders. However, examples from practice illustrate more positive, dialogic ways of developing indicators in complex, evolving situations typical to SC and SCC. For examples of creative and participatory processes of indicator development among Canadian aboriginals, see Ramírez and Richardson (2005).

Our discussion of social change recognizes the importance of upstream social factors in creating enabling environments for ownership and action at local levels. It points to the need to move beyond HIV-specific indicators to ways of capturing broader social changes that underpin effective responses. Initiatives to develop "AIDS competence", for example, illustrate approaches which prioritize strengthening local capacity to act and adapt, to communicate with partners and other initiatives, and to identify common dimensions of capacity that may be useful for assessing social change. While indicators might be suitable to assess more simple aspects of programs and change processes, they need complementing with approaches more befitting SC and SCC, as discussed above. We have shown how insights from complexity and systems thinking, reflected in related methods and approaches, can strengthen evaluation in ways that foster accountability, learning and positive change. They befit situations where direct attribution is neither possible nor appropriate, and focus on relationships and broad social and contextual issues which can be important enabling or inhibiting factors in relation to social change and development processes.

Conclusions and Recommendations

The paper has explored a range of innovative approaches that hold promise for more effectively assessing the social dimensions of HIV and AIDS and involving those most affected by HIV in evaluation processes. Our focus has been the "complicated" and "complex" dimensions of social change and SCC, in recognition that "simple" aspects are generally well catered for by dominant approaches and methods. In HIV contexts, evaluation practice based on linear attribution is most applicable to clinical and individual-focused interventions, where causality is direct, interventions are short-term and relatively replicable (Bartos, 2009). The methodologies and methods we advocate are intended to *complement* current practice, to ensure that wider social context is appropriately addressed in HIV programming.

Exploration of the issues has led us to key guiding principles that can usefully inform the effective evaluation of social change in HIV contexts. Our recommendations broadly echo those of an expert group that has considered the challenges of assessing social change in depth, including the need to dialogue with donors about the bases of assessment and learning processes (Guijt, 2007).

Evaluation approaches should be consistent with the underlying values and principles of an initiative. Complex, emergent programs and processes require evolutionary evaluation designs able to embrace complexity. As social change processes inevitably encompass multiple, and at times conflicting, perspectives and voices, it is important that evaluations pay explicit attention to multiple perspectives, power relations, and ways of meaningfully involving people in assessing their own change. The ultimate value of any evaluation will depend on how it is used, and use is fostered by involving key stakeholders in evaluation processes.

Learning and "learning how to think evaluatively" (Patton, 1998), should lie at the heart of evaluation for social change, as exemplified in participatory approaches and "process use." Keeping processes of critical reflection, learning, and feedback alive is more important than being seduced by an apparent sense of control that particular planning tools might offer. Overprescription typically overwhelms rather than supports those involved, and stifles creativity, innovation and local ownership (Sibthorpe *et al.*, 2004, cited in Rogers, 2008, p. 43). Instead project plans and evaluations should be considered works in progress, appreciating that social complexity often demands evaluation based on a dynamic theory of change and that we need to remain open to the unexpected and the emergent. The approaches outlined above offer alternatives that broadly reflect these recommendations, as opposed to ideas of measurement based on prediction and control.

We need to let go of the notion of "best practice" and instead consider diverse and contextualized "better practice." Instead of seeking consensus on one standard M&E framework, we should seed and catalyze parallel and complementary evaluation approaches, in recognition of the value of methodological pluralism. There is also a need to reconsider assumptions about replication when contextual factors are critical, and to further explore notions of "scaling across" and "resonance." Instead of assumed scale-up, the focus shifts to learning from broadly comparable contexts, adapting and applying learning appropriately in particular contexts.

The above shifts will enable wide-ranging evidence to be gathered through diverse methods, emphasizing appropriateness to context over illusions of perfection. Diverse means are available to explore critical issues and challenges with different stakeholder groups (Keystone Accountability, 2008), and participatory communication including video, drama, and culturally informed expressions of issues can significantly strengthen traditional research and "evidence." Many systems and action research approaches value stories for their strengths in conveying rich detail in appealing, accessible ways.

Clarity about where direct cause–effect (linear mode) thinking and methods are appropriate and where they are not is essential and there needs to be greater modesty and realism about attributing impact to any one initiative. The distinctions between Simple, Complicated, and Complex may help identify where there is a need to employ approaches outlined above, to capture social change. This in turn has implications for expectations of attribution, appropriate time frames for evaluation and necessary resources.

Implications for funders, managers, and evaluators

How do we nurture the shifts in thinking and practice implied by the above evaluation principles? To meet the challenges posed and implement recommendations offered, there are significant implications for all key stakeholders.

Funders and commissioners, themselves part of complex webs of accountability, are called to "rethink the principles on which they base their models of evaluation and learning," to ensure greater consistency between espoused values and the evaluation approaches they use (Guijt, 2007, p. 52). Longer-term funding and programming is critical to social change initiatives, as is actively supporting flexibility and learning and nurturing sustainability. Donor practice needs to reflect a more realistic perspective on what types of change can occur in specified time periods, and appreciation of the need for consensus building between key actors, to ensure overall buy-in to an initiative and its results.

All senior stakeholders need to actively promote developments in concepts, methodologies and methods suited to the evaluation of complex social change. This implies supporting innovation and informed risk-taking, without guarantees. It demands active support for effective and sustainable capacity development in "alternative" M&E methodologies, at all levels. Managers and policy makers need to consider how to create and nurture organizational cultures that foster, rather than inhibit, meaningful participation in evaluations. Given the importance of local, contextual knowledge, insider experts and champions should be trusted, and funded beyond the life of specific projects.

Evaluation facilitators need to create safe spaces for honest reflection and learning, to ensure an effective strategy and conceptual clarity, foster a questioning approach, advocate for necessary resources and support and balance locally driven assessment with outsider insights.

To strengthen evaluation practice and build the evidence base, the gathering of case studies and inspiring examples of HIV initiatives that address social drivers should be supported, as should peer-learning and dialogue amongst innovators in social change evaluation, to help build a critical mass.

There is notable scope for further research into strengthening the evaluation of SC and SCC processes, and into ways of effectively supporting and sustaining such processes. Specific areas of focus might include: (1) how best to build on the learning from existing HIV initiatives that have attempted to address social dimensions of HIV; (2) how to strengthen the documentation of innovations in the field using diverse means; (3) how to gather and disseminate ideas, tools, games and stories that help teams deal with complex SC scenarios; (4) the strengths and weaknesses of diverse theories of change for SCC initiatives. Deeper understanding of the support, resources, and other requirements of related capacity development initiatives is needed, as is understanding of the most effective ways to convince senior decision makers to support these processes over time.

We need to be honest about the complexity and scale of the challenge posed by evaluating SCC programs. Demonstrating the impact of SC (or SCC) processes will never be quick or simple, yet evidence shows how numerous small and diverse actions and shifts, over time, help social movements reach a critical tipping point. The same could become true of evaluation thinking and practice and we need to strengthen alliances, support diverse initiatives, share innovations and foster learning in this interest. We can catalyze shifts in positive directions, using systematic insights and available methodological resources creatively. As Picciotto (2007, p. 520) notes

> a new paradigm has transformed the evaluation environment and raised the bar for the fledgling development evaluation profession. In the new century, development evaluation will have to be transformed and liberated from its current strictures to reach beyond aid, beyond projects, and beyond top-down approaches. It should be more comprehensive, more participatory, and better adapted to the felt needs of society.

We hope the questions raised and approaches advocated will help make evaluations more worthy of the social change communication processes they are part of. Ultimately, strengthened evaluation practice should reaffirm positive social change processes and help make service providers more accountable to the communities they serve.

Notes

1 This chapter is based on *Evaluating Social Change Communication for HIV/AIDS: New Directions*, produced by the Communication for Social Change Consortium (CFSCC), and published by UNAIDS (2011).

2 See www.communicationforsocialchange.org

3 At the Institute of Development Studies in Sussex. Thanks to Danny Burns, Rick Davies, Virginia Lacayo, and Ricardo Ramirez, coparticipants.

4 See http://www.unaids.org/html/pub/publications/ircpub01/jc335-commframew_en_pdf.pdf

5 Structural factors have traditionally been understood as enduring social influences rooted in more fundamental causes. In this paper we use the terms social and structural interchangeably. UNAIDS defines structural interventions as strategies that aim to alter the (social, cultural, political or economic) conditions that produce or impair health (UNAIDS, 2010).

6 Captured graphically in the Stacey Matrix, see Stacey (2002).

7 See the table on page 6 of Westley, Zimmerman, and Patton (2006).

8 http://www.bbc.co.uk/worldservice/trust/whatwedo/where/asia/india/2008/04/080806_india_gates_condomcondom_video.shtml

9 See http://www.idrc.ca/evaluation.

References

Auerbach, J., Parkhurst, J., Caceres, C., and Keller, K. (2009). *Addressing Social Drivers of HIV/AIDS: Some Conceptual, Methodological and Evidentiary Considerations.* Commissioned for Aids2031 Social Driver Working Group. Retrieved from http://www.aids2031.org/pdfs/aids2031%20social%20drivers%20paper%2024-auerbach%20et%20all.pdf

Bartos, M. (2009). Addressing the crisis of confidence in HIV prevention. Presentation at Think Tank on the Evaluation of HIV Prevention, Wilton Park, September 2–4.

Burns, D. (2007a). *Systemic Action Research: A Strategy for Whole System Change.* Bristol: The Policy Press.

Burns, D. (2007b). *Evaluation in Complex Governance Arenas: The Potential of Large System Action Research.* In B. Williams and I. Imam (Eds.), *Systems Concepts in Evaluation. An Expert Anthology* (pp. 181–195). Point Reyes, CA: Edge Press/American Evaluation Association.

Byrne, A. (2008). *Evaluating Social Change and Communication for Social Change: New Perspectives.* MAZI 17 (Nov 2008). New Jersey: CFSC Consortium. Retrieved from http://www.communicationforsocialchange.org/mazi-articles.php?id=385

Byrne, A., (Ed.) with Gray-Felder, D., Hunt, J., and Parks, W. (2005). *Measuring Change: A Guide to Participatory Monitoring and Evaluation of Communication for Social Change.* New Jersey: CFSC Consortium. Retrieved from http://www.communicationforsocialchange.org/pdf/measuring_change.pdf

Byrne, D. (1998). *Complexity Theory and the Social Sciences: An Introduction.* London: Routledge.

Byrne, D. (2002). *Interpreting Quantitative Data.* London: Sage Publications.

Campbell, C., Nair, Y., and Maimane, S. (2007). Building context that supports effective community responses to HIV/AIDS: A South African case study. *American Journal of Community Psychology, 39*(3–4), 347–363.

Castells, M. (2000). *The Rise of the Network Society*, 2nd edn. Oxford: Blackwell.

Chambers, R. (2008). *Revolutions in Development Enquiry.* London: Earthscan.

Checkland, P. and Scholes, J. (2004). *Soft Systems Methodology in Action*. Chichester: John Wiley and Sons.

Coates, T., Richter, L., and Caceres, C (2008). Behavioral strategies to reduce HIV transmission: How to make them work better (HIV prevention 3). Retrieved from http://www.who.int/ hiv/events/artprevention/coates.pdf

Davies, R. (2003). *Network Perspectives in the Evaluation of Development Interventions: More Than a Metaphor*. Retrieved from http://www.mande.co.uk/docs/nape.pdf

Davies, R. (2004). Scale, complexity and the representation of theories of change (Part II). *Evaluation 11*, 133–149.

Davies, R. (2008). *Weighted Checklists: A Participatory Means of Measuring Complex Change*. Retrieved from http://mande.co.uk/special-issues/weighted-checklists/

Davies, R. (2009). The use of social network analysis tools in the evaluation of social change communications. An input into the Background Conceptual Paper: *An Expanded M&E Framework for Social Change Communication*. New Jersey: CFSC Consortium. Retrieved from http:// www.communicationforsocialchange.org/pdfs/2nd%20draft%20the%20use%20of%20 social%20network%20analysis%20tools%20in%20the%20evaluation%20of%20social%20 change%20communications%20b.pdf

Davies, R. and Dart, J. (2005). *The Most Significant Change (MSC) Technique. A Guide to Its Use*. Retrieved from http://www.mande.co.uk/docs/MSCGuide.pdf

Earl, S. and Carden, F. (2002). Learning from complexity: The International Development Research Centre's experience with outcome mapping. *Development in Practice, 12*(3&4), 518–524.

Eoyang, G. and Berkas, T. (1998). *Evaluation in Complex Adaptive Systems*. Retrieved from http:// www.hsdinstitute.org/learn-more/library/articles/Evaluating-Performance-in-a-CAS.pdf

Eyben, R. (Ed.) (2006). *Relationships for Aid*. London: Earthscan.

Figueroa, M. E., Kincaid, D. L., Rani, M., and Lewis, G. (2002). *Communication For Social Change: An Integrated Model for Measuring the Process and Its Outcomes*. New York, Rockefeller Foundation. Retrieved from http://www.communicationforsocialchange.org/pdf/ socialchange.pdf

Guijt, I. (2007). *Assessing and Learning from Social Change: A Discussion Paper*. Brighton: IDS. Retrieved from http://www.ids.ac.uk/files/dmfile/ASClowresfinalversion.pdf

Guijt, I. (2008). *Critical Readings on Assessing and Learning for Social Change: A Review*. IDS Development Bibliography 21. Brighton: IDS. http://www.ids.ac.uk/UserFiles/File/ participation_team/Db21.pdf

Imam, I., LaGoy, A., and Williams, B. (2007). Introduction. In B. Williams and I. Imam (Eds.), *Systems Concepts in Evaluation. An Expert Anthology* (pp. 3–10). Point Reyes, CA: Edge Press/American Evaluation Association.

India HIV/AIDS Alliance (2010). *Stories of Significance. Understanding Change Through Community Voices and Articulations. A Report Based on an Evaluation of the Home and Community-Based Care and Support Programme for Children, CHANA, by Means of the "Most Significant Change" Technique*. New Delhi: HIV/AIDS Alliance. Retrieved from http:// www.aidsalliance.org/includes/Publication/Stories_of_significance.pdf

Keystone Accountability (2008). *Impact Planning, Assessment and Learning*. Retrieved from http://www.keystoneaccountability.org/sites/default/files/1%20IPAL%20overview%20 and%20service%20offering_0.pdf

Lacayo, V., Obregon, R., and Singhal, A. (2008). *Approaching social change as a complex problem in a world that treats it as a complicated one: the case of Puntos de Encuentro, Nicaragua*. *Investigación y Desarrollo, 16*(2), 126–159. Colombia: Universidad del Norte. Retrieved from http://redalyc.uaemex.mx/pdf/268/26816205.pdf

Low-Beer, D. and Stoneburner, R. (2004). Uganda and the challenge of HIV/AIDS. In N. Pou and A. Whiteside (Eds.), *The Political Economy of AIDS* (pp. 165–190). Aldershot: Ashgate Publishing.

Midgley, G. (2007). Systems thinking for evaluation. In B. Williams and I. Imam (Eds.), *Systems Concepts in Evaluation. An Expert Anthology* (pp. 11–34). Point Reyes, CA: Edge Press/ American Evaluation Association.

Mowles, C., Stacey, R., and Griffin, D. (2008). What Contribution can Insights from the Complexity Sciences make to the Theory and Practice of Development Management? *Journal of International Development 20*, 804–820.

Patton, M. Q. (1997). *Utilization-Focused Evaluation*, 3rd edn. Thousand Oaks, CA: Sage.

Patton, M. Q. (1998). Discovering process use. *Evaluation, 4*(2), 225–233.

Picciotto, R. (2007). The new environment for development evaluation. *American Journal of Evaluation, 28*(4), 509–521.

Piot, P., Bartos, M., Larson, H. *et al.* (2008). Coming to terms with complexity: A call to action for HIV prevention. *The Lancet, 372*, 845–859.

Prowse, M. (2007). *Aid Effectiveness: The Role of Qualitative Research in Impact Evaluation*. Background Note. London: ODI. Retrieved from http://www.odi.org.uk/resources/download/430.pdf

Ramalingam, B., Jones, H., with Reba, T. and Young, J. (2008). *Exploring the Science of Complexity: Ideas and Implications for Development and Humanitarian Efforts*. London: ODI.

Ramírez, R. and Richardson, D. (2005). Measuring the impact of telecommunication services on rural and remote communities. *Telecommunications Policy, 29*, 297–319.

Rao Gupta, G., Parkhurst, J., Ogden, J. A. *et al.* (2008). Structural approaches to HIV prevention. *The Lancet, 372*, 764–775.

Reeler, D. (2007). *A Three-fold Theory of Social Change and Implications for Practice, Planning, Monitoring and Evaluation*. South Africa: CDRA. Retrieved from http://www.cdra.org.za/articles/A%20Theory%20of%20Social%20Change%20by%20Doug%20Reeler.pdf

Rogers, P. (2008). Using programme theory to evaluate complicated and complex aspects of interventions. *Evaluation, 14*(1), 29–48.

Stacey, R. (2002). *Strategic Management and Organizational Dynamics: The Challenge of Complexity*, 3rd. edn. Harlow/New York: Prentice-Hall.

Stillwaggon, E. (2006). *AIDS and the Ecology of Poverty*. Oxford: Oxford University Press.

UNAIDS (2007). *Report of the UNAIDS Technical Consultation on Social Change Communication*. Geneva: UNAIDS.

UNAIDS (2010). *Combination HIV Prevention: Tailoring and Coordinating Behavioral, Structural and Biomedical Strategies to reduce NEW HIV Infections*. Geneva: UNAIDS.

UNAIDS (2011). UNAIDS Terminology Guidelines (January 2011). Retrieved from http://www.unaids.org/en/media/unaids/contentassets/documents/document/2011/jc1336_unaids_terminology_guide_en.pdf

Vincent, R. (2006). *Breaking Barriers: Effective Communication for HIV Prevention, Treatment, Care and Support by 2010*. London: Panos Institute.

Vincent, R. (2009a). Tackling the social complexities of HIV and AIDS: Understanding the social roots of the epidemic and learning from development in HIV communication. In C. Barrow, M. de Bruin, and R. Carr (Eds.), *Sexuality Social Exclusion and Human Rights: Vulnerability in the Caribbean Context of HIV* (pp.153–176). Kingston, Jamaica: Ian Randle.

Vincent, R. (2009b). Measuring social and structural change for HIV prevention: Background paper for UNAIDS HIV Prevention Think Tank, Wilton Park, Sussex, UK, September 2–4.

Vincent, R. and Byrne, A (2006). Enhancing learning in development partnerships. *Development in Practice, 16*(5). Retrieved from http://www.jstor.org/pss/4030035

Westley, F., Zimmerman, B., and Patton, M. (2006). *Getting to Maybe: How the World is Changed*. Toronto: Random House.

Williams, B. (n. d.). *Critical Systems Thinking and Boundaries*. Retrieved from http://www.bobwilliams.co.nz/Systems_Resources_files/CSH.pdf

Williams, B. and Imam, I. (Eds.) (2007). *Systems Concepts in Evaluation. An Expert Anthology*. Point Reyes, CA: Edge Press/American Evaluation Association.

Woolcock, M. (2009). Toward a plurality of methods in project evaluation: A contextualized approach to understanding impact trajectories and efficacy. *Journal of Development Effectiveness, 1*(1), 1–14.

Part III

Case Studies of Applied Theory and Innovation

15

Mobile Phones
Opening New Channels for Health Communication

Katherine de Tolly and Peter Benjamin

Mobile phones are becoming an increasingly "everyday" technology, in the sense that what was once a luxury item is relatively rapidly becoming something that most people own, even people in developing countries. This makes mobiles an appealing way of reaching people in health communications. As well as being another channel for communications, mobile phones also allow interaction and feedback that is not possible with conventional broadcasting.

Mobile presents exciting opportunities for health communication for a range of reasons: their growing ubiquity; the ability to reach poor people; the ability to reach people who may well not have access to other media; and the "personal" and private nature of mobile. Furthermore the use of mobile helps in measuring outcomes, which is important in health communications; we have to measure (and assess) our interventions to see if they are working, and how they can be improved.

There are a range of constraints to be considered in the use of mobiles for health communication, including: cost; literacy; constraints on content length; network coverage; phone sharing; variability in phone functionality; people's familiarity with the technology; and challenges around involving people in materials development.

In the remainder of this chapter, case studies illustrating the use of mobiles in health communications will be explored and up-and-coming projects will be briefly described.

The Scope of mHealth

Simply put, mhealth is the use of mobile phones for the provision of health services and information. Broadly, mhealth can be divided into two categories: interventions implemented within the health sector, and implementations that are aimed at the general

The Handbook of Global Health Communication, First Edition. Edited by Rafael Obregon and Silvio Waisbord.
© 2012 John Wiley & Sons, Inc. Published 2012 by John Wiley & Sons, Inc.

population (Mechael and Dodowa Health Research Center, 2009). Mhealth can be broken down more finely, with interventions classified in this way (Vital Wave, 2009):

- Education and awareness
- Remote data collection
- Remote monitoring
- Communication and training for health care workers
- Disease and epidemic outbreak tracking
- Diagnostics and treatment support.

Mechael *et al* (2010) use this typology for mhealth projects:

- Health promotion and disease prevention
- Data collection and disease surveillance
- Health information systems and point-of-care support
- Treatment compliance
- Emergency medical response.

The focus of this chapter is mhealth as used for health communication for development and social change, as opposed to mhealth as applied to health systems, data collection, treatment adherence, or emergency response. In the above typologies, the emphasis of this chapter is on "education and awareness" and "health promotion and disease prevention."

Mobile Phones – Global and Growing

Diverse, small mobile networks were in operation in the 1970s, and the 1980s saw the development of various standards that allowed for greater capacity on networks. These were still mutually incompatible, however, and in the late 80s work began in Europe on the GSM standard, which is still widely used today (Ling, 2004). Fast-forward to 2009, and global penetration of mobiles stood at 67 percent (4.6 billion mobile cellular subscriptions). By the end of 2009, the International Telecommunications Union estimates that in developing countries this figure stood at over 50 percent. Developing country mobile phone penetration has been growing exponentially, having more than doubled since 2005 (ITU, 2010). It is estimated that by 2012, half of those in remote areas of the world will have mobile phones (Vital Wave, 2009).

What does this mean?

Having started as high-end devices available only to wealthy businesspeople, mobiles are now everyday items that put communication in the pockets of people who were previously excluded from such services. Globally, mobiles have "leapfrogged" fixed-line telephony and since 2002 there have been more mobile than fixed-line subscribers; this is independent of factors such as gender, geographic area or income per capita (Kaplan, 2006).

It's important to bear in mind that mobiles enable far more than voice communication (though that is important in itself, for instance in summoning an ambulance). The range of technologies (e.g., SMS, USSD) embodied in mobiles is explored later in this chapter.

Opportunities presented by mobile

The sheer reach of mobiles can be a compelling reason to consider them in health communication. There are a range of other factors, however, that make them a potentially exciting communication medium:

Reaching poor people
Mobiles are no longer restricted to rich people. (Though income obviously does affect mobile ownership; for instance in South Africa, 31 percent of people in Living Standards Measurement (LSM) 1 use a mobile; 45 percent of LSM2, 53 percent of LSM3, and 60 percent of LSM4.) (Mobile Marketing Association of SA, 2009).

Interactivity
Mobiles present opportunities for two-way or interactive communication and dialogue, which can facilitate greater participation and engagement.

High penetration to cost ratio
Mobile can be a cost-effective way of reaching people, especially when compared to other media. For instance, TV penetration is very high in South Africa, as is mobile, but TV production and advertising costs can be much higher than creating a mobile campaign.

Reaching people anywhere
While obvious, mobility is an important characteristic of mobile phones – they allow health communication to occur in a wide range of locations. Getting messages to and from them does not rely on the person being in a fixed physical location (as it does with fixed-line telephony or TV).

Personal technology
The mobile phone is generally carried on the person, meaning that messages (e.g.,SMSs) are more likely to reach people than, say, communication that relies on their seeing a billboard message. Also, people often develop a "relationship" with their phone: "the mobile phone may represent one of the most "loved" and "personal" technologies" (Winchester, 2009).

Dealing with stigma and confidentiality
Mobiles can be useful where privacy is important (Atun and Soalen, 2006), for instance, where there is stigma associated with a disease. This is largely dependent, however, on the user having his or her own phone (not a shared phone).

Narrowcasting

As opposed to broadcasting, narrowcasting is where a message is targeted at the small population to whom the message should be relevant. If the demographics or interests of people are known, then mobile phones provide an easy way to reach this population (as would an email if they have the facility, or a normal letter if there is the time).

Ability to measure

Because mhealth communication is electronic, it is usually easy to measure outcomes, that is, how much services are being used (e.g., number of SMSs successfully delivered, number of subscriptions via please-call-me messages, number of cellbooks downloaded). Some technologies allow for even more detailed usage statistics. For instance, on USSD, mobisites, and MXit it is possible to see what "pages" have been viewed and thus what kinds of information are most in demand. Statistics on how often information is viewed or a service is used is not a measure of impact, but it is a good start in any monitoring or evaluation process.

One device, many uses

Mobiles facilitate both voice and text communication, the latter in a variety of ways. Not all phones have all these capabilities, though over time more phones will have more sophisticated functions.

Each of the ways of using mobiles outlined in Table 15.1 has advantages and disadvantages, and is appropriate in different contexts. In some cases, it might be necessary to use a variety of channels in order to reach a greater proportion of the target audience.

Constraints presented by the technology

With all the exciting potential that mobiles present for health communication, it is important to remember the very real constraints that exist; while the increasing ubiquity of mobiles makes them a very appealing way to try and reach people, these constraints can derail the use of mobiles for health communication. As noted by Mefalopulos (2008): "to avoid past mistakes, media and ICTs, powerful as they are, should always be considered as tools to be used within the context of the broader social and communication environment."

Cost

When using mobiles in developing country contexts, cost to the user is critical. For instance, in South Africa, sending an SMS costs around 10 US cents, so designing communication so that people have to SMS to take part, can seriously constrain uptake. The challenge with all the channels described in Table 15.1 is how to make services free or as close to free as possible for users.

Literacy

Reading of text on a mobile phone requires at least some level of literacy; careful assessment of a target market's literacy levels is thus necessary.

Table 15.1 Nonvoice ways mobiles can be used for information provision and interaction.

Channel	What is it?	Advantages	Disadvantages	Handset	Examples of use
Broadcast SMS	SMSs sent to a list of known numbers.	All phones can receive SMSs. Free for recipient in most countries. Can be scheduled (e.g., send at 9 a.m. every day).	SMSs limited to 160 characters each. Can send longer SMSs, but different phones treat multiples differently (e.g., with some the first SMS in a pair is received first; with others, the second is received first).	Any.	Announcements sent out for World AIDS Day. Reminders to take medication.
Interactive SMS	Person SMSs a keyword and gets information back through another SMS.	Everyone can use it. No fancy phone needed.	160 character limit/SMS. Person has to get keyword exactly right.	Any.	Find date, time, and venue of next meeting; find nearest clinic by SMSing postcode.
Please-call-me messages (PCM)	Person sends their number to another (usually to request a call back, e.g., if they don't have airtime).	Everyone can use it. No fancy phone needed. Free for the sender.	Person can at most send their name and number.	Any (works differently in different countries).	Subscribing to services (e.g., person can send a PCM to an advertised number to receive weekly health updates).
Text menus (USSD)	Way of transmitting text-based information over a mobile network. Basic text menus and info. Person can drill down to information.	Everyone can use it. No fancy phone needed.	130–182 characters/screen. Two-minute session then content disappears (though can SMS at end). Can be expensive (e.g., in South Africa 30 US cents for 2 minutes).	Any.	Directory-style information (e.g., organization's contact info, by department).

(Continued)

Table 15.1 (*cont'd*).

Channel	What is it?	Advantages	Disadvantages	Handset	Examples of use
Location-based services	The network knows where the mobile phone is. So information can be sent to people based on where they are. (Used via SMS and USSD).	Everyone can use it. No fancy phone needed.	Usually requires two-stage communications with user confirming that they want to give their position.	Any.	Find a local event or facility.
Instant Messaging chat applications (e.g., MXit)	Application for "instant messaging" text-chat and information "portals." Users must download application onto their phone that allows them to text-chat.	Very cheap to use. Interactive. 10 million South Africans and 2.8 million people internationally use it. Text-length restriction of 1,000 characters.	Old and cheap phones can't use it. Unlikely to reach older people. GPRS connection needed. Some association with pornography and abuse.	Java-enabled phone.	Text-based counseling and health information provision.
Mobisites	Sites designed for browsing via the Web on a mobile phone.	Can be cheap. No text-length restrictions. Can display colors, graphics, etc.	Costs vary greatly by country. Variable penetration of WAP-enabled phones in different countries.	Must be WAP-enabled.	Health information provision. Health quizzes.
Cellbook	Book that downloads via WAP to the phone.	Pretty cheap. No character restrictions.	Need to have WAP. Unfamiliar tech can be a barrier. Can be hard to find cellbook once on phone (usually under Games or Applications).	Must be WAP- and Java-enabled.	Treatment guidelines distributed to health workers.

Not everyone has a mobile phone

While mobile phones provide a means of reaching a large number of people (in most countries a majority), it must be remembered that there are a significant number of people who do not have access to this technology. Health communications that assume universal mobile phone usage will leave out the people who are likely to be the most disadvantaged – which can lead to a form of "double exclusion."

Content-length restrictions

Mobile screens are small, making reading large amounts of content difficult. Thus, while large amounts of content can be delivered to mobiles (e.g., via cellbook or WAP), we are not aware of any usability studies assessing how much information people can manage to read on the small screen.

   Also, certain of the channels listed in the table above also have inbuilt constraints on content, for instance 160 characters per SMS, or 130–182 characters per USSD screen. It takes a level of skill to put meaningful content into such a short space, and the use of nuanced language is severely constrained.

Languages' length

Character-length constraints are amplified where certain languages inherently use more characters. For instance, in South Africa, Xhosa (one of the official languages of the country) uses on average around 20 percent more characters than English.[1] These issues may be exacerbated with other languages: in SMS, non-Latin alphabets constrain SMS length to 70 characters (Guthery and Cronin, 2001).

Mobile phone network coverage and electricity grid

It cannot be assumed that mobile phones can be used anywhere in a country; sometimes networks do not penetrate into certain areas, and some areas do not have a reliable electricity supply to recharge phones. This means that while people may have phones, they might not always be able to use them. So health communications campaigns need to look at network and grid coverage in intended target areas and assess if the level of coverage is good enough to reach the intended audience.

Variability of phones

Not all phones have complete functionality. All phones can do voice calls, SMS, and USSD, but only some have Java and WAP (Internet capabilities). Hence, in designing a mobile communications campaign, an assessment needs to be made of the likely kinds of phones that the target audience has.

Phone sharing

Where mobiles are used for health communications that are of a very personal nature or involve sensitive topics, phone sharing needs to be considered. For instance, if messaging implies that the recipient is HIV-positive, this could cause problems if the phone is shared and an unintended recipient picks up the message. Where communication is user-initiated (e.g., visiting a mobisite), this issue falls away.

User familiarity with the technology

While SMS is familiar to most users, other technologies like USSD and cellbooks are not so familiar. This can be exacerbated by the age profile of the target market (as, generally, older people use fewer of the functions on their phones).

Usability

Many mobile phone applications are difficult to use for the inexperienced. Even for more experienced users, WAP, downloads, and instant messaging can be tricky. One reason for this is the lack of mobile phone standards between software – for example, when a file is downloaded through GPRS, it frequently requires searching in order to find it on the phone.

Participation of target communities

Participation is often seen as a critical component of successful communications for social change, and can involve stakeholders and target communities in problem definition, intervention design, materials development, and evaluation (see, for instance, Mefalopulos, 2008). If participatory approaches are to be used in message development, this can be particularly challenging on mobile as the technical constraints (such as character limitations) mean that it may be possible to have involvement in broader campaign development, but not in specific materials development. To illustrate: youth may easily be able to design posters or banners that they think might be effective in their neighborhood, but getting them to write the SMS texts for a campaign is not likely to be viable.

This constraint can be alleviated through piloting or testing mobile content and campaigns on the target audiences in order to refine messaging. In these pilots it is important, however, to try and separate out target audience reactions to the content/messaging and the technology. For instance, a campaign delivered via USSD might present problems not due to the content being presented, but to user difficulties with the technology.

Case Studies

This section discusses a range of case studies in mhealth communication. As mentioned at the start of this chapter, the emphasis is on mhealth communication projects, not projects where mobiles have been used to strengthen health systems, respond to emergencies, or collect data. The case studies below are ones for which documentation or studies could be found; no doubt there are a host of other initiatives, whether formal or informal, where projects have not been written up.

It is worth noting that in most of the case studies below, SMS was the mobile technology used. This could be because SMSs are usually free to the recipient (in the United States some pay to receive SMSs), and, importantly, they are a familiar technology. It is also possible to time SMSs (for instance for a particular time of day), and SMSs can be set up in advance (i.e., a schedule of SMSs can be set up to run for, say, a month). It will be interesting to review a similar list of case studies in five years' time to see if SMS is still the predominant channel used, or if, say, the mobile Web has become sufficiently widely used in developing countries to replace SMS as the dominant form of mobile-text communication.

SEXINFO: sexual health SMSs

The problem

San Francisco was experiencing rising rates of gonorrhea among heterosexual people, especially amongst African-American youth aged 15–19. According to Deb Levine, originator of the project, "In 2005, African American women in San Francisco had a rate of gonorrhea that was 12 times the rate of White women – a 69 percent increase from 2004" (Levine *et al.*, 2008).

The intervention

In 2006 Internet Sexuality Information Services (ISIS Inc), in partnership with the San Francisco Department of Public Health, developed an SMS-based service to give people access to information related to sexual health and relationships.

Focus groups were held to discuss the feasibility of the service, the messaging, and the marketing. A group of health agencies and community organizations helped identify culturally appropriate referral services and provided other guidance to the project. The service was marketed through a range of media such as bus shelters, pamphlets, and Internet banner advertising.

Users text the word "SEXINFO" to an advertised number and then receive a directory of codes to get answers and referral information on questions such as "what to do if your condom broke."

SEXINFO has since expanded to cover the whole of California. Youth SMS the word "HOOKUP" to a short number in order to subscribe to weekly SMSs containing educational information and referrals to free clinic services (Levine, 2009).

Outputs/outcomes

In its first 25 weeks, there were over 4,500 enquiries, and 2,500 of those led to accessing more information and referrals. At the time of writing, only preliminary evaluations have been done. Levine notes that "Of those who saw the ad [for the SEXINFO service], nearly 10 percent sent a text message to the SEXINFO service" and that of those who saw the advertisements, the fact that the service used mobile phones and SMS caught their attention (Levine *et al*, 2008).

In 2007 further surveying was done to assess the service that involved youth going out with a professional market researcher and a video camera to see how the service was being used. This led to the identification of usability problems with the service. Adjustments were made to the service that resulted in an increase of over 100 percent in effective usage of the service (i.e., usage where the person found information as opposed to giving up due to difficulties) (Kinkade and Verclas, 2008).

In its first three months, Hookup had 1,400 subscribers, with around 30 percent SMSing to get clinic referrals (Levine, 2009).

Lessons

Levine says that in her work in using technology in the area of sexual health, she has learnt that technology is always changing and that what's popular now can change very quickly (Levine, 2009). While she is referring to technology more broadly rather than just to mobile phones, this point should be borne in mind in mhealth communication. For instance, while mobile Internet usage is currently low in a country like South Africa at 11 percent (Mobile Marketing Association of South Africa, 2009), this number is likely to grow in the near future. Hence, services developed now should ideally be designed to migrate easily to being provided via the Internet on mobile.

She also recommends that one should "Use each form of technology for what it can do best. For instance, text messages are only 160 characters (2–3 sentences) – certainly better for referrals and reminders than unraveling complex sexuality issues." (Levine, 2009)

She advises that one's target audience should be involved in the design, implementation and evaluation of programs.

Lastly usability testing is important – a service can look good on paper, but users need to be observed using services in order to understand any potential problems, so that services can be adapted to work better.

Text to Change

The problem

The Uganda demographic and health survey of 2006 found that despite general awareness of HIV and AIDS, comprehensive knowledge of the disease was relatively low: 70 percent of women and 60 percent of men were found not to have comprehensive knowledge (AIC and TTC, 2009).

The intervention

Text to Change, a Dutch nongovernmental organization (NGO), partnered with Celtel, a Ugandan mobile network, and the local NGO AIDS Information Centre to run a pilot from February to April 2008 in the Mbarra region of Uganda, aiming to increase knowledge about AIDS and get people to test. An SMS-based multiple-choice quiz was advertised to 15,000 Celtel mobile subscribers.

Users were SMSd a question and when they gave a wrong answer, they would get a return SMS with the right answer. At the end of the quiz, they were sent an SMS encouraging them to go for HIV testing. Airtime was used as an incentive to participate in the quiz (Vital Wave, 2009).

Outputs/outcomes

The uptake rate of the quiz was high at around 17 percent: of the 15,000 Celtel subscribers who were SMSd about the quiz, 2,500 participated (Mechael, 2009). The quiz led to a 40 percent increase in the number of people coming to test: from 1,000 to 1,400 in a six -week period (Vital Wave, 2009).

Answers to quiz questions were analyzed to find information gaps. It was found that although there were high levels of knowledge about things like condom use, people did not think that HIV testing was accurate or anonymous (Vital Wave, 2009). Findings like this can be useful if fed into other programs so that messaging and interventions can be refined.

Lessons

This pilot project highlighted a range of lessons (Mechael *et al*, 2010; Vital Wave, 2009):

- The need for marketing, for instance through newspapers, billboards and radio.
- The importance of an introductory message that explains the service and guarantees anonymity.
- The need to keep programs short so that people don't lose interest.
- The need for assessment and technical improvements.
- Service provision in local languages to increase accessibility.
- The need to collaborate with other mhealth organizations to share things like software.

HIV counseling via instant messaging (IM) chat

The problem

South Africa had about 5.2 million people living with HIV and AIDS in 2009, more than any other country (Republic of South Africa, 2010). The government funds the National AIDS Helpline (NAHL), a 24-hour telephone counseling service that is free from a landline. However, only nine out of 100 South Africans have a landline (ITU, 2008), and HIV counseling does not lend itself to public telephones. Mobile penetration rates are high at around 90 percent (ITU, 2008), although voice calls to the NAHL from mobiles are charged at normal mobile rates.

The intervention

In 2009 Cell-Life, a South African NGO, partnered with LifeLine, the NGO that runs the NAHL, to look at how counseling could be made available to more people. It was decided to leverage the power of MXit, an IM application for mobile with over 19 million registered users South Africa. Counsellors were trained to provide counseling via a web-based IM application,[2] and counseling started at the beginning of September 2009. A small amount of advertising was done on MXit to publicize the service.

Outputs/outcomes

The project is in its early stages, with two hours of counseling provided four days per week. In this limited time (around 720 counseling hours provided in 140 sessions) there have been:

- Almost 8,900 conversations.
- Almost one million messages in those conversations.

(Note that some conversations are only one or two lines.)

Lessons

Users are surprisingly revealing of things like their HIV status and sexual behaviors. This could be because IM mobile chat is a completely private medium. It's also clear that people still need basic information on HIV (like whether it is transmitted by kissing, or the fact that with medication you can live a long life).

Anecdotal evidence from the counselors indicates that they can provide as much meaningful counseling in one two-hour session as they can in a week of telephone counseling. One reason for this is that they can have multiple conversations at the same time. Also, up to 86 percent of NAHL telephone counseling calls are hoax calls (including abusive callers, wrong numbers, children playing, etc.) (Katz, 2004); by contrast, the IM chat counseling service does not suffer from this problem. (This could be because users have to spend even a tiny amount on airtime to text-chat whereas the NAHL is free from a landline; there could also be something about text-chat that makes it less "satisfying" for hoax calls.)

Counselors have indicated that the fact that previous conversations can be viewed means that counseling can have a degree of continuity that is not possible with telephone counseling (where the caller is allocated to the first available counselor and thus has to repeat ground covered in previous conversations). They have also indicated that mobile-chat counseling affords the client a degree of privacy not possible with telephone counseling: with the latter the counselors often hear background traffic noise (from public telephones) and clients using "bland" language (not mentioning HIV), whereas on mobile clients can text-chat from anywhere.

Cost is a major factor in the popularity of the service and its potential for scale-up and rollout in other countries. A counseling conversation using mobile-voice costs the user in the region of US$1 (for a four-minute call); a similar conversation on MXit costs less than US$0.01. This provides a means for organizations to provide low-cost call centre services via text counseling.

Provision of HIV-related content via MXit

The problem

With South Africa's high HIV prevalence rates comes a need for information to be disseminated. There are a range of HIV information services like loveLife and Khomanani, which largely rely on mass media. The country has low Internet penetration rates at around nine percent in 2008 (ITU, 2008). Despite the fact that many have mobiles that could be used to browse the Internet, relatively few do (60 percent of urban users could browse, but only 21 percent do) (World Wide Worx, 2010).

The intervention

While MXit is a mobile IM application, it can be used to serve content. Cell-Life set up an HIV information service called Red in August 2009. Red covers HIV basics including transmission, testing, prevention and living with HIV.

Outputs/outcomes

Since Red went live, over 500,000 "pages" of content have been viewed. While a mobile page contains nothing like the amount of information of a web page, this is still a significant amount of information viewed.

Lessons

Serving content via an IM chat application like MXit is not the same as using the Internet as users have to have the service (in this case Red) as a contact/buddy in the application. So users cannot find the content via a search function; the service thus has to be marketed so that the contact is added. Experience thus far has shown that advertising on MXit is very effective and that people, especially youth (MXit's main user base), do want to read about HIV.

Project Masiluleke

The problem

The project aimed to address low rates of HIV testing, delayed initiation of HIV treatment, and high rates of defaulting on that treatment (Pop!Tech, n.d.).

The intervention

South Africans make extensive use of "please-call-me" (PCM) text messages, which are a free way to get someone to call you back, particularly if you have no airtime or are loath to use it. PCMs have 120 characters of empty space in them, which is either left blank or sold as advertising (for instance to banks and other corporations). For the period October 1, 2008 to July 4, 2010, over 818 million PCMs contained Project Masiluleke messages; this was around 1.2 million messages per day (personal communications with Marcha Neethling of Praekelt Foundation, August 2010). Messages were written in local languages, and directed people to call South Africa's National AIDS Helpline (Vital Wave, 2009). Here are two examples of messages included in PCMs:

> HIV + and scared to tell your partner? For help with disclosure, call the AIDS Helpline 0800012322.

> Feeling sick and worried that you might be HIV positive? Call AIDS Helpline 0800012322 and find out where to test.

Outputs/outcomes

The project was simple in design, and had a simple, significant impact: it resulted in nearly a tripling of call volume to the National HIV/AIDS Helpline (Vital Wave, 2009).

Lessons

A key strength of this project was its use of a strong local partner, the MTN network, which is the second-biggest network in South Africa. MTN donated the PCM advertising space in PCMs sent over their network; this allowed for the leveraging of MTN's subscriber base. Also, local partners with expertise in content development were used (Vital Wave, 2009).

Prenatal SMS support, Thailand

The problem

All women worry, to varying degrees, about the safety of themselves and their unborn baby. Antenatal visits are often short, which does not always allow for sufficient time for expectant mothers' questions to be answered, thus leading to higher anxiety levels and potentially negative health outcomes for the mother an unborn baby (Jareethum *et al.*, 2008).

The intervention

A randomized, controlled study was done at a hospital in Bangkok, Thailand in May to October 2007 (Mechael *et al.*, 2010), in which healthy, pregnant women received two prenatal support SMSs per week from 28 weeks' gestation until birth.

Outputs/outcomes

The study found that women who received SMSs benefited in a range of ways:

- They had higher levels of satisfaction, both before birth and during labor.
- They had higher confidence levels.
- Their levels of anxiety were lower.

However, there were no significant differences in pregnancy outcomes (Jareethum *et al.*, 2008).

Projects to watch

This section describes some projects that at time of publication were in their early stages, and evaluations had not yet been done.

M4RH (Mobiles for Reproductive Health)

M4RH is an interactive menu-based SMS system that gives people access to information to help them chose and better manage their contraception (personal communication with Kelly L'Engle, Family Health International, 2010). The service was launched in Kenya in May 2010, and is free to users on the Zain network. Negotiations were underway in July 2010 to extend this to all Kenyan networks. It was due to launch in Tanzania in August 2010. Formative research was done to shape the project: it was found that users would welcome and trust messages on family planning options via text, and that they would share such messages with their partners and friends. The project is an initiative of Family Health International, with technical programming and hosting provided by Text to Change.

mDhil

mDhil is a for-profit initiative in India that provides people with health-related SMSs on a range of topics. Users can subscribe to messaging on topics including general health, sexual health, TB, weight, diet, stress, skin and beauty, and diabetes (mDhil.com, n.d.;

Mechael *et al*, 2010). The company started in March 2009 and in February 2010 boasted 150,000 users (MobileHealth, 2010).

Beba Dolazi

Beba Dolazi means "the baby is coming" and is a Serbian project. Automated weekly health-promotion SMSs are sent to pregnant women, and beyond birth for the baby's first three years. Three to six messages are sent per week on topics like the stages of development of the fetus, and when gynecological visits are needed. The information has been verified by professional medical associations and approved by the Ministry of Health of the Republic of Serbia. Subscribing cost US$1 (naslovi.net, 2008; Beba dolazi, n.d). In 2007 there were 3,200 women using the service (Mechael and Dodowa Health Research Service, 2009).

Text4baby

Text4baby is an American service very similar to Beba Dolazi that provides thrice-weekly SMSs to women during pregnancy and for the first year of the baby's life. Registration for the service is online or via SMS. The SMSs are timed to the due date or baby's date of birth and cover topics like birth defects prevention, nutrition, immunization, and referrals to relevant services (babycentre.com, 2010). The service is free and run in English and Spanish. The project has a broad range of sponsors and partners that includes government agencies, private companies, mobile networks and academic institutions (text4baby.org, n.d.). In early May 2010, over one million messages had been delivered (whitehouse.gov, 2010) and the service had over 60,000 subscribers in late July 2010 (personal communications with Arlene Remick, July 2010).

VidaNET, CardioNET

VidaNET was launched in Mexico in 2008, and provides users with free SMSs and email tips on living with HIV and AIDS, information on medications, and support to adhere to medications and keeping appointments (Royal Tropical Institute, 2009; voxiva.com, n.d.). CardioNET was also launched in 2008, and has around 5,000 subscribers (just-means.com, 2010). These projects are a partnership between the Carso Health Institute and Telcel, Mexico's largest mobile network.

Discussion

While these case studies show many interesting examples, there are still remarkably few widespread uses of mobile technology for health communications – a situation that is likely to change rapidly. The case studies above and a scan of the literature both indicate that examples of mhealth communication being done at scale do not exist, other than Project Masiluleke. This is likely to be due to three main challenges:

- *Cost*: especially in developing countries, mhealth communication shows particular promise (due to high mobile penetration rates and the lack of access to other ways of getting and distributing information, e.g., the Internet). But running projects at scale is unaffordable to most, given commercial charging for SMS and other mobile channels (e.g.,USSD). Only when projects make use of public–private partnerships or substantial donations by mobile networks, will projects be able to go to scale.

- *Mhealth communication is not mainstreamed*: the use of mobiles for large-scale health communication is relatively new, and is not yet a channel that is automatically considered along with others such as print, radio, etc.
- *Skills*: while the existence of commercial services such as downloadable ring tones would indicate that there are skills in the private sector, in the public and NGO sectors skills such as strategizing mobile campaigns, content writing and technical programming are thin on the ground.

The projects described above also rely almost exclusively on SMS, which is understandable given that all phones can get SMSs, and SMS coverage is ubiquitous (i.e., where there is mobile coverage, users can get SMS). The significant constraint with SMS is cost – it is an expensive form of data transmission.[3] For instance, in South Africa, it costs about eighty times more to send 1kb of data via SMS than it does via GPRS (i.e., via an Internet connection from the phone).

SMS is also mostly used for one-way or broadcast communications, which means that one of the benefits of mobile – its interactivity – is not being leveraged. Interactive SMS services such as M4RH have been piloted, but with interactivity (e.g.,where SMS is used to navigate through menus to drill down to content) costs escalate rapidly.

Interestingly, no case studies could be found that involved mobiles being integrated into a multi-channel communication program (for instance involving a combination of TV, radio, print and mobile). This is a potentially exciting application of mobiles, where messages from other media are extended via mobile, or where interactivity via mobile is added to traditionally "one-way" campaigns. This is one of the areas in which mobile phones can greatly strengthen health communications – allowing people to "talk back" to broadcast media. Behavior-change communication is most effective when there is a dialogue rather than simply a one-way flow of information. However, broadcast media are very poor at allowing interaction – radio phone-ins or letters to the editor do not provide a meaningful one-to-one conversation. Mobile phones can be used to allow people to interact with the TV or radio communications. For example, after a program on a given topic, viewers can be encouraged to SMS in their comments; vote in a poll; join a subscription list by sending an SMS (or Please Call Me) to a number; or find their local clinic or health facility by an SMS/PCM to another number. If they want to discuss the issue, they can go to an Instant Messaging chat room (e.g., through MXit); or if they have a serious issue they can seek counseling. This can allow the wide reach of the broadcast medium to be the first stage of an ongoing interaction.

IM chat applications present a potentially exciting way of reaching people and building communications services, especially as IM chat is so cheap to use, and allows for both one-way and interactive communications. The constraints with IM chat are that users usually have to download an application onto their phone; the phone needs to be Java-enabled (which means the most basic phones can't use IM chat); and the user needs GPRS coverage, which in many developing countries is still patchy.[4]

Conclusion

Mobiles clearly show immense promise in communication for health and development, and interesting projects highlight some of the dynamics around using mobiles in this way. But mobile as a channel for these kinds of communication is still in its infancy, as evidenced by the lack of projects that have gone to scale. Case studies show a dominance of one technology (SMS), which is understandable given the ubiquity of SMS.

In communications, mobiles should be though of as another medium (like print, the Internet, etc.). One that is potentially rich, given the potential for interaction (two-way communications) and the ability to carry voice, text, images, video and sound; but nevertheless, another medium. As such, the opportunities and constraints presented by mobile need to be carefully evaluated in projects, to ensure that the medium is used appropriately and in a way that strengthens communications and does not push technology for technology's sake. Principles of good communication design should be applied on mobile, as in any other medium. Mefalopulos (2008) puts this another way: "media are no longer the central element of communication, but one of the tools to be used according to the circumstances."

Hopefully a similar chapter written in a few years' time will see four major changes:

- The use of a wider range of technologies or channels on mobile (like IM chat and WAP).
- The use of mobiles having been "mainstreamed" and integrated with other media as a way of reaching the millions of people in need of health information and messaging.
- Greater interactivity being incorporated into health communications via mobile.
- More public-private partnerships that see mobile networks hosting free services for "social good" or development communications (for example free SMSs, free access to mobisites for users).

Notes

1 Based on a comparison of various translated texts at www.capegateway.gov.za
2 See www.jamiix.com for more on this application.
3 For a useful opinion piece on this subject, see Jonathan Gosier's "On Love and Hate for 160 characters" at http://appfrica.net/blog/2010/05/03/on-love-and-hate-for-160-characters/
4 For coverage maps see http://maps.mobileworldlive.com/#selectCountry

References

AIC and TTC (2009). Report: Text to Change/ AIDS Information Centre: HIV/AIDS SMS Program, Arua, Uganda. www.texttochange.com/AIC-TTC%20Arua.pdf

Atun, R. A. and Soalen R. S. (2006). *A Review of the Characteristics and Benefits of SMS in Delivering Healthcare. The Role of Mobile Phones in Increasing Accessibility and Efficiency in Healthcare.* Vodafone Policy Paper series no. 4.

BabyCenter.com (2010). BabyCenter® Partners in Promoting Safe and Healthy Pregnancies through Text4baby. Retrieved from http://www.babycenter.com/100_press-release-babycenter-174-partners-in-promoting-safe-and_10327479.bc

Beba dolazi (n.d.). Home page. Retrieved from http://bebadolazi.net (English version retrieved from http://translate.google.com/translate?sl=sr&tl=en&js=n&prev=_t&hl=en&ie=UTF-8&layout=2&eotf=1&u=http%3A%2F%2Fbebadolazi.net%2F&act=url).

Guthery, S. and Cronin, M. (2001). Mobile Application Development with SMS and the SIM Toolkit. New York: McGraw Hill.

ITU (International Telecommunication Union) (2008). ICT Statistics Database. Retrieved from http://www.itu.int/ITU-D/ICTEYE/Indicators/Indicators.aspx#

ITU (International Telecommunication Union) (2010). *Measuring the Information Society* (executive summary). Retrieved from http://www.itu.int/ITU-D/ict/publications/idi/2010/Material/MIS_2010_Summary_E.pdf

Jareethum, R., Titapant, V., Chantra, T. *et al.* (2008). Satisfaction of healthy pregnant women receiving short message service via mobile phone for prenatal support: A randomized controlled trial. *Journal of the Medical Association of Thailand*, 91(4). http://www.mat.or.th/journal/files/Vol91_No.4_458_1404.pdf

Justmeans.com (2010). *Healthy Tech: Mexico's Mobile Health Reminders*. Retrieved from http://www.justmeans.com/Healthy-tech-Mexico-s-mobile-health-reminders/9688.html

Kaplan, W. A. (2006). Can the ubiquitous power of mobile phones be used to improve health outcomes in developing countries? *Globalization and Health* 2(9). Retrieved from http://www.globalizationandhealth.com/content/2/1/9

Katz, I. (2004). *The South African National AIDS Helpline: Call Trends from 2000–2003*. CADRE research paper. Retrieved from http://www.cadre.org.za/node/170

Kinkade, S. and Verclas, K. (2008). *Wireless Technology for Social Change*. Washington, DC: UN Foundation–Vodafone Group Foundation Partnership.

Levine, D (2009). Using new media to promote adolescent sexual health: Examples from the field. *prACTice Matters*. Ithaca, NY: ACT for Youth Center of Excellence. Retrieved from http://www.actforyouth.net/documents/NewMedia_Oct09pdf.pdf

Levine, D., McCright, J., Dobkin, L. *et al.* (2008). SEXINFO: A sexual health text messaging service for San Francisco youth. *American Journal of Public Health* 98(3). Retrieved from http://www.ncbi.nlm.nih.gov/pmc/articles/PMC2253571/?tool=pubmed

Ling, R. (2004). *The Mobile Connection: The Cell Phone's Impact on Society*. San Francisco, CA: Elsevier.

mDhil.com (n.d.). *mDhil Better Health Care Information for Everyone*, home page. Retrieved from http://www.mdhil.com/

Mechael, P. (2009). The case for mHealth in developing countries. *Innovations: Technology, Governance, Globalization*, 4(1), 103–118. Retrieved from http://www.k4health.org/system/files/case%20for%20mHealth.pdf

Mechael, P., Batavia, H., Kaonga, N., *et al.* (2010). *Barriers and Gaps Affecting mHealth in Low and Middle Income Countries: Policy White Paper*. Center for Global Health and Economic development, Earth Institute, Columbia University. Retrieved from http://www.globalproblems-globalsolutions-files.org/pdfs/mHealth_Barriers_White_Paper.pdf

Mechael, P. and Dodowa Health Research Center (2009). *MoTECH: mHealth Ethnography Report*, for the Grameen Foundation. Retrieved from http://www.grameenfoundation.applab.org/uploads/Grameen_Foundation_FinalReport_3_.pdf

Mefalopulos, P (2008). *Development Communication Sourcebook: Broadening the Boundaries of Communication*. World Bank, Washington, DC. Retrieved from http://web.worldbank.org/WBSITE/EXTERNAL/TOPICS/EXTDEVCOMMENG/0,,contentMDK:21890561~pagePK:34000187~piPK:34000160~theSitePK:423815,00.html.

Mobile Marketing Association of South Africa (2009). Mobile Research Data SA: Useful extractions from AMPS. (presentation). Retrieved from http://mmaglobal.com/research/mobile-research-data-sa-useful-extractions-amps

MobileHealth (2010). @mHI Startup boasts 150K paying mHealth users. Retrieved from mobi-healthnews.com/6381/mhi-startup-boasts-150k-paying-mhealth-users/#more-6381

Naslovi.net (2008). SMS vodič kroz trudnocu – "Beba dolazi" [SMS guide to pregnancy – Baby is coming]. Retrieved from www.naslovi.net/2008-04-09/mondo/sms-vodic-kroz-trudnocu-beba-dolazi/634336

Pop!Tech (n.d.). *Project Masiluleke: A Breakthrough Initiative to Combat HIV/AIDS Utilizing Mobile Technology and HIV Self-Testing in South Africa.* Retrieved from http://poptech.org/system/uploaded_files/27/original/Project_Masiluleke_Brief.pdf

Republic of South Africa (2010). *South Africa Country Progress Report on the Declaration of Commitment on HIV/AIDS, 2010 Report.* Retrieved from http://www.unaids.org/en/dataanalysis/monitoringcountryprogress/2010progressreportssubmittedbycountries/southafrica_2010_country_progress_report_en.pdf Vital Wave Consulting (2009). *mHealth for Development: The Opportunity of Mobile Technology for Healthcare in the Developing World.* Washington, DC: UN Foundation-Vodafone Foundation Partnership

Royal Tropical Institute (2009). *mHealth in Low-Resource Settings.* Retrieved from http://www.kit.nl/smartsite.shtml?id=36966#vn Accessed 5 April 2010

text4baby.org (n.d.). Shjeis One Smart Mom, She's Got text4baby. Retrieved from http://www.text4baby.org.

voxiva.com (n.d.). *Cell-phone Medicine Brings Care to Patients in Developing Nations.* Retrieved from http://www.voxiva.com/company/news/voxiva_support_mexico.html.

whitehouse.gov (2010). *Free Text4baby service for Moms and Moms-to-Be is Growing Up Fast.* http://www.whitehouse.gov/blog/2010/05/07/free-text4baby-service-moms-and-moms-be-growing-fast.

Winchester, W. W., III (2009). Catalyzing a perfect storm: Mobile phone-based HIV-prevention behavioral interventions. *Social Interaction Design,* 16(6). Retrieved from http://dl.acm.org/citation.cfm?id=1620696&dl=ACM&coll=DL&CFID=51203542&CFTOKEN=12207323

World Wide Worx (2010). *Mobile Internet in South Africa 2010 Study.* For more on this study, see http://www.worldwideworx.com/2010/05/27/mobile-internet-booms-in-sa/

Further Reading

Cole-Lewis, H. and Kershaw, T. (2010). Text messaging as a tool for behavior change in disease prevention and management. Epidemiologic Reviews. Retrieved from http://extension.missouri.edu/hes/conference/txtmsgbehaviorchgYaleArticle.pdf

Earth Institute (2010). Barriers and Gaps Affecting mHealth in Low and Middle Income Countries: A Policy White Paper. Washington, DC: mHealth Alliance, 2010. Retrieved from http://www.mhealthalliance.org/content/barriers-and-gaps-affecting-mhealth-low-and-middle-income-countries

Fjeldsoe, B. S., Marshall, A. L., Miller, Y. D. (2009). Behavior change interventions delivered by mobile telephone short-message service. American Journal of Preventive Medicine, 36(2), 165–173.

Whittaker, R., Borland, R., Bullen, C., et al. (2009). Mobile Phone-Based Interventions for Smoking Cessation. Cochrane Database of Systematic Reviews 4. Retrieved from http://www.thecochranelibrary.com/userfiles/ccoch/file/World%20No%20Tobacco%20Day/CD006611.pdf

16

Social Marketing and Condom Promotion in Madagascar
A Case Study in Brand Equity Research

W. Douglas Evans, Kim Longfield,
Navendu Shekhar, Andry Rabemanatsoa,
Ietje Reerink, and Jeremy Snider

Introduction

"A brand is a set of differentiating promises that link a product to its customers."
Stuart Agres
"The three key rules of marketing are brand recognition, brand recognition, brand recognition." Anon.

As the preceding quotes suggest, brands are more than the products, logos, promotions, or other physical manifestations of marketing efforts. Brands are "promises," they are "recognized" – in short they live in the mind of the consumer. Brands have been defined as "a set of associations linked to a name, mark, or symbol associated with a product or service" (Calkins, 2005, p. 1). "Brand equity" is the overarching construct that characterizes brands and brand identification among target audiences (Evans and Hastings, 2008) and is defined as "a set of assets (and liabilities) linked to a brand's name and symbol that adds to (or subtracts from) the value provided by a product or service to a firm and/or that firm's customers" (Aaker, 1996). Thus, consumer perceptions – that a product has certain characteristics or provides value – define a brand. Recently, branding has been used as a social marketing strategy in public health to increase avoidance of health risks and adoption of healthy behaviors, including condom product purchase and consistent condom use (Evans and Hastings, 2008).

The purpose of brands and branding is to organize and frame choices – to buy a product, to use a service, or to live a physically active lifestyle or use condoms. Brands use symbols and imagery – colors, shapes, sounds – to organize our potential choices and frame the benefits a particular product, service, or behavior has to offer. Nike has the "swoosh" and Coca-Cola has the distinctive red color and shape of its iconic bottle. In recent years, public health social marketers have begun to use similar approaches, as in campaigns such as *truth* and *VERB* in the United States (Evans, Price, and Blahut, 2005; Huhman, Price, and Potter, 2008) and *loveLife* and *Trust* in Africa (Evans and Haider, 2008; Agha, 2003).

In public health we must always keep in mind that, for the most part, programs and the behaviors they promote are voluntary in nature. That is to say, our prospective customers are free to accept or reject the products or services that we offer them. Our success, therefore, typically hinges on our ability to design products and services that members of our intended target audience – i.e., our prospective customers – will see value in and embrace. That insight suggests that branding must be a central strategy in promoting value for public health customers. Brands and the role of brand research can be explained using the concept of the brand onion. Brand development can be largely explained in terms of 3 basic nested concepts: (1) Positioning, (2) Personality, and (3) Execution. Brand positioning is often summarized in a "positioning statement." Positioning statements have 3 basic components:

1   Statement of the target audience
2   Description of the frame of reference (of choices in which the brand exists)
3   Point of differentiation (PoD, or benefits) of the brand from competitors including both social (emotional) and functional benefits.

Brand personality is the expression of the emotional PoD of the brand, the social and emotional features that distinguish the brand and its identity from others. It can be expressed in adjectives like "fun," "sexy," or "serious," like describing a person. These features can shape the tone and sometimes the content of brand promotion and marketing. They can also be measured as brand personality traits in brand research, and represent predictors of brand choice.

Brand execution is how the brand is implemented in the real world. It is the images, colors, symbols, logo, tag lines, shapes, type fonts, language, touch/feel, sound/music, scent, and any other physical manifestations of the brand position and personality used to represent the brand and market it to consumers. It is what the consumer experiences when he or she comes in contact with the brand in the real world and what shapes brand associations. Thus, like personality, it can be measured – how did consumers experience the brand execution and what were their reactions?

This chapter focuses on brand research in social marketing using the principles just described, development of a brand research agenda at PSI (www.psi.org), and a case study of brand research in the PSI-Madagascar social marketing platform. The following discussion also seeks to position brand research in the toolkit of social marketing research methods. We argue that branding and brand equity research should be standard practice – part of the tool kit available to practitioners and researchers – in global social marketing programs.

Brand research serves two functions, and occupies two places on the social marketing research continuum. First, it is about measuring and evaluating *determinants of brand choice*. Consumers choose to use a category of branded product or behavior (e.g., condoms as a *category* of product) and individual branded *products* within a category (e.g., *Trust* socially marketed condoms in Kenya) due to market factors such as price, availability, and to the brand associations they form with the category or individual product. Brand research is concerned with identifying and analyzing those determinants of brand choice and informing brand managers to improve brand positioning and execution. Thus it represents a kind of formative research.

Second, brand research is concerned with *evaluating the outcomes of brand choice.* Consumers that use the category of condoms, or individual condom products, will have different health outcomes than those who do not. What effect do brand choices and utilization of brands (categories or individual products) have on individual health outcomes? Brand research, in its outcome evaluation function, is concerned with this question. In particular, it is concerned with the role of brand associations as *mediators* of health outcomes. This chapter explores brand research and a case example of how it served both of these functions for PSI's Madagascar social marketing efforts.

Brand Research Methods

First, formative research on what the audience values and how they think about a product, behavior, or category is crucial to establishing positioning. Social marketers need *audience insight* in order to build a solid brand positioning statement and develop subsequent brand promotion strategy. Audience insight can also identify what kinds of personality traits might best convey the brand positioning and establish the value of the brand in the minds of consumers. In this way, social marketers segment consumers and identify determinants of consumer brand choice.

Second, research on the effectiveness of a brand can identify whether its personality is perceived as intended. Brand personality is projected through imagery, logos, colors, shapes, and other features used in brand execution. It can be measured through brand associations – personality traits such as being fun, serious, sexy, or cool – and through social norms, attitudes, and behaviors the target audience associates with the brand. To the extent that these associations represent social or functional benefits for the target audiences, they will be more likely to engage in the target behavior (e.g., purchasing a particular brand of condoms or using condoms in general). Brand research can measure these associations and the extent to which they are associated with engaging in target behaviors.

Third, the effectiveness of brand executions (e.g., advertisements) in changing consumer knowledge, attitudes, beliefs, and behaviors can be evaluated. Executions are the promotional activities designed to project brand personality, establish the brand's position, and build equity with the audience. As noted earlier, the consumer only experiences the brand execution, not the strategy behind it. So to the extent consumers are (1) aware of brand executions (i.e., actually exposed and capable of recalling exposure to executions), and (2) react positively to those executions, we expect that they will form the desired associations and build brand equity.

Brand Equity and PSI Brand Research

Brand equity is what the brand stands for in the hearts and minds of consumers, and as a metric it captures their identification with and intentions to purchase, use, and engage with the brand (Keller, Aperia, and Georgson, 2008). It is a primary driver of product and behavioral choice, especially for health commodities with little functional attribute differentiation (e.g., what tangible functions they perform), such as condoms. Given that most purchase decisions are made within the market context of various brand choices (e.g., a luxury brand of condoms, inexpensive, or perhaps free), marketers need reliable measures of brand equity in order to understand consumers' purchase decisions (Evans, 2009).

PSI is a worldwide leader in the social marketing of disease prevention and health promotion products and services (PSI, 2010). Many PSI socially marketed brands, such as subsidized condoms and bed nets distributed in the developing world, have existed for years and thus may have established brand equity, the extent of which is unknown. However, as is common in social marketing settings in the developing world, that equity has often not been actively managed or measured. Once positioned and promotions initiated, little is typically done to understand changes in marketplace dynamics and consumer brand perceptions that may impact purchase and use decisions (Evans, 2009). Until recently, PSI did not have a research methodology to assess brand equity and its relevance and appeal to target audiences.

Previously, PSI relied on mostly formative research, monitoring and evaluation tools and methodologies that provided its marketers with evidence for use in designing messages, developing campaign strategy, tracking progress, evaluating outcomes, and allocating resources accordingly (PSI, 2010). These tools provide useful insight to marketers, but there remain unmet needs within PSI's approach for understanding target audiences' purchase decisions, or "choice" to buy a product, and their associated determinants, as well as the context in which those decisions are made. This understanding will enable marketers to develop more effective marketing strategies using all 4 Ps (place, price, product, and promotion) and more effectively segment target audiences. It will also aid in the development of source-of-volume projections and resource allocation based on purchase patterns (e.g., shifting brand switchers to increasing loyalty).

In addition to its role in the consumer purchase decision, the need to measure brand equity is magnified by the changing epidemiology of some diseases, in particular for HIV and the role condoms play in prevention efforts. This is not unlike the situation many commercial brands face in an evolving marketplace, with new competition and lifestyle preferences driving consumer decision making. Think of the declining market share and threat from Pepsi that led Coca-Cola to introduce the ill-fated New Coke (Schindler, 1992). Ultimately, the original "Classic Coke" proved to be the enduring branded product, and the corporate Coca-Cola brand was strengthened in the long-run through product extensions (e.g., flavored versions of Coke, new product extensions such as water and flavored waters).

When many PSI condom brands were launched in Africa, they were positioned to appeal to youth given that group's perceived high risk profile. However, the original audience members have now aged and recent evidence suggests that older cohorts are now most at risk for HIV and STI, especially those with concurrent sexual partners. In response, marketers may be tempted to reposition existing brands to this older audience (in many cases the same individuals in their original target segment). However, this should not be done without a clear understanding of existing brand equity and audience segmentation data.

Similarly, marketers may wish to alter a brand's equity based on a new benefit (e.g., shifting a condom brand's primary benefit from HIV prevention to contraception), or based on an increased price for cost recovery. However, these shifts may compromise a brand's existing equity. Brand equity is based in part on a price point, and the metric "price premium" (or "willingness to pay"). The marketer needs to understand a brand's equity among purchasers to effectively manage and promote the brand.

As a result of these insights, in 2009 PSI began a brand equity research initiative in collaboration with researchers at the George Washington University. The overall objectives of this initiative are to develop a conceptual model of brand equity for use in PSI social marketing platforms, design a research agenda and overarching methodologies, and initiate a series of pilot studies to validate the methodologies. Ultimately, when validated, these methods would become part of the overall PSI research, monitoring and evaluation toolkit.

Brand research agenda

The first objective of the PSI brand research agenda is to define what we mean by brand equity, how it applies to PSI marketing activities, and the framework for how we will measure it. Evans and colleagues (2008) define brand equity as a "mediator" of the relationship between consumer marketing exposure and behavior. Figure 16.1 captures this conceptual model of brand equity:

Objective 2 is to develop an immediate strategy to apply brand equity metrics, research methods, and analytics to new and existing PSI brands. Brand research methods apply to the full spectrum of social marketing research and evaluation – from formative to outcome. The PSI brand research agenda includes formative research using PSI's Framework for Qualitative research in Social Marketing, known within PSI as "FoQus" (PSI, 2010), to assist in planning for repositioning, rebranding, and marketing planning efforts. It includes audience segmentation and understanding determinants of brand choice following the two major functions of brand research discussed earlier.

The third objective is to develop and implement a long-term strategy for applying brand equity metrics, methods, and analytics across the lifecycle of PSI brands. This involves developing a process for integrating brand equity methods into the planning process for all new PSI brands. Evaluation planning will include a process for developing brand-specific outcome metrics based on standardized brand equity scales. The existing framework, known within PSI as "PERForM," is used in managing programs and will incorporate the new brand equity analytic methodologies (PSI, 2010).

As a first step in developing the long-term strategy, PSI and collaborators at the George Washington University designed a series of pilot brand equity scales and segmentation and evaluation studies. The PSI-Madagascar study described below is the first such pilot study with outcome data to report. Results of this and forthcoming studies will be used to implement and advance the long-term strategy.

One important dimension in piloting this effort is the diversity of marketing environments in which development organizations such as PSI work. It is important to recognize multiple market environment scenarios in a total market approach that includes free,

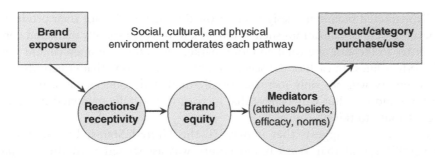

Figure 16.1 Brand equity conceptual model.
Source: With kind permission by PSI-Madagascar.

subsidized (socially marketed), and commercial brands (UNAIDS, 2010). In a total market approach, the need for and uses of brand management, brand measurement, and research efforts will differ depending on market environment. Generally speaking, for social marketers in developing countries, there are 3 types of scenarios (with variations within and between them). In addition to freely available, unbranded condoms distributed by governments, we have:

- Scenario 1: Total or near total market share of socially marketed product,
- Scenario 2: High-percentage market share of social marketed product, with some commercial market competition; and
- Scenario 3: Mature market in which socially marketed product is one among many competitors along with commercial offerings.

The marketer's need for brand equity data differs to some extent depending on which of these scenarios, or their variants, he or she faces. For example, in scenario 1, the social marketer needs regular brand equity data not to compete head-to-head, but to keep the brand fresh, relevant, and appealing to the market, and to expand the total number of category consumers. The goals are (1) maintenance, and (2) expanding the total market size over time. Also, market conditions may change and periodic monitoring of societal changes, behavioral epidemiology, introduction of new products, and other factors may be needed.

In scenario 2, the range of competition may be limited, but the issue arises whether socially marketed brands are hitting their intended target within the total market. In this case, active brand management to compete head-to-head on brand equity associations (e.g., creating and maintaining a more appealing brand personality or building popularity or loyalty) are essential. Segmentation analysis will be informative, as well as providing continuous monitoring for the position of socially marketed brands in the minds of consumers.

In scenario 3, social marketers may be trying to gain market share but still need to avoid encroaching on commercial brands. In this case, active brand management is more challenging, so more frequent head-to-head brand equity comparisons may be needed. Also, brand equity data can help to avoid encroachment on an audience intended for public or commercial brands by identifying equity and explaining purchase decisions in distinct audience segments.

Socially marketed brands are designed to grow the total market for their product line. Thus, development organizations such as PSI seek to increase socially marketed condom sales in order to increase the total condom market, including commercial and governmental product lines. In each of the scenarios above, we assume that effectively managing brand equity will not only increase socially marketed condom sales, but also the category of condoms. But why believe that increasing a socially marketed brand equity would contribute to this objective?

Previous research suggests that it may. In the United States, Evans, Price, and Blahut (2005) found that *truth* brand equity was associated with the *category* of reduced smoking initiation behavior, and Berkowitz, Huhman, and Nolan (2008) found that *VERB* brand equity was associated with the category of increased physical activity in both preadolescent boys and girls. In developing settings, Agha (2003) found brand equity in *Trust* was associated with increased condom use overall. Evans and colleagues (2008) review of branded social marketing, which examined both developed and developing world brands, suggests that category promotion may result from individual product brand promotion in developing country contexts. However, most of the studies examined lacked rigorous evaluation designs, and thus more research is needed to examine the question of how product brand equity and category promotion interact.

Brand equity pilots will ultimately be conducted in each of these environments to identify research and marketing planning needs and develop appropriate research methodologies. In the following, we report on the first such pilot, conducted in a scenario 1 environment in the PSI-Madagascar condom social marketing platform.

Madagascar Protector Plus Brand of Condoms

The Madagascar Protector Plus (P+) condom brand was developed by PSI in 2000 to grow the total market for condoms and as an HIV and STI prevention strategy. Following nearly a decade of SM efforts with little to no competition, either from the public sector or from commercial brands, the situation changed in late 2008 with the introduction of a free condom and an increase in commercial brands targeted at higher-end consumers. Marketers realized they had little to no information about consumer choices and the perception of P+ as a quality first-choice condom. A price change and new positioning were also considered, in line with a new packaging to refresh the product. In the following, we describe the repositioning effort, social marketing and brand strategies, evaluation of the rebranding effort, and possible implications for future condom brand social marketing.

P+ has had the same packaging and price for over 10 years and brand equity has not been actively managed. The PSI Madagascar team recognized that with the threat of a growing HIV epidemic and new condom brands entering the market, there was a need to reposition and reprice P+.

Previously, P+ did not have a clearly defined brand position and its old packaging highlighted an image of a loving couple silhouetted naked against a beach sunset. While this imagery was appealing, it did not clearly communicate what P+ stood for or represented to consumers. There were also concerns that the price was too low in the

Madagascar marketplace, and did not reflect a "high-quality" product. As a result, the team decided to increase the price by 100 percent (from 100 to 200 ariary, with 2100 ariary equaling about $1US) based on a review of available data on local spending for typical household goods. Additionally, the revised brand positioning clearly promises "peace of mind," and the new packaging pictures a leaf resting on calm water. This concept was tested among men who had sex with commercial sex workers (CSWs) who represented a key user category. This formative research suggested the audience is looking for peace of mind, and would value a high-quality condom that assured them they could live their lives free from fear of contracting HIV or an STI.

Social marketing benchmark criteria

The P+ brand utilizes the full set of social marketing benchmark criteria (French *et al.*, 2010). It thus represents a robust example of a social marketing brand and an illustrative example of the process and outcomes of brand research.

- *Methods mix*: P+ uses a "4P" strategy. Condoms are promoted based on the brand position and personality of providing peace of mind while offering excitement. Placements include "hot spots," like bars and clubs and widespread distribution to ensure access near the point of decision to have commercial sex. Pricing has been increased to raise the perception of brand quality and the product is designed to meet audience quality needs identified in formative research.
- *Customer orientation*: The lifestyles and social needs of young, sexually active men in their mid 20s to 30s (as these are the primary segment visiting CSWs) are central to the P+ brand strategy.
- *Insight*: Formative research on the brand was conducted as part of the repositioning effort, and has fed into the evaluation design reported below.
- *Behavioral goals*: To build the total market for condoms in the country and increase sales of P+ to serve public health objectives of reducing HIV and STI rates.
- *Segmentation*: P+ targets sexually active men aged 18–49, and has specific promotional strategies for young men who frequent CSWs, targeting their need for "sensation seeking" (Palmgreen *et al.*, 2002; Zuckerman, 1979).
- *Exchange*: The brand explicitly offers peace of mind while maintaining sensation value for the target audience in exchange for the monetary and non-monetary (loss of pleasure, potential social costs) price of using condoms.
- *Competition*: P+ recognized two forms of competition: (1) health risk due to unprotected sex with CSWs, and (2) increasing competition in the condom market from new entrants, and the competition from consumers choosing not to use condoms. This was explicitly reflected in the promotion and pricing strategies developed during the marketing planning process, highlighted by a five-day workshop that brought together marketers, researchers, and program staff that addressed HIV prevention and the role of condoms in reducing health risk behaviors among clients of CSWs.
- *Theory*: Social cognitive theory (Bandura, 2004), and recent work on public health branding (Evans and Hastings, 2008) was used in the brand repositioning.

Table 16.1   Sampling strategy for photo narrative.

Peri-urban areas of Tana	Young at-risk men Young (25–35)	Older at-risk men Old (36–44)	Non-at-risk men (no age distinction)	Total
Loyal users of P+	2	2	3	7
Nonusers of any condoms	2	2	3	7
Non-loyal users of P+	2	2	–	4
Total	6	6	6	18

Source: With kind permission by PSI-Madagascar.

Formative Research

We first integrated a line of brand equity questioning into formative research conducted by the PSI-Madagascar research team with input from researchers at GWU. A group of 18 Malagasy men aged 18–49 from Antananarivo (Tana), Madagascar were interviewed in-depth by six male researchers in the same age group about their condom use, attitudes, beliefs, preferences, brand awareness, and brand choice. Some of these men were condom users, and some weren't; some were considered "at risk" (defined as having had sex with a CSW in the past three months), some were considered "not at risk." They were also disaggregated by age, as shown in Table 16.1.

All 18 participants were provided with a pocket camera and asked to document a typical day in their life, paying specific attention to what brings them joy, what inspires them, what instills fears in them and where they get information about topics of interest to them (e.g., sports, music). Researchers collected the pictures and the stories behind them and presented these to the marketing team in a subsequent interpretation workshop. As a result, marketers were able to construct an archetype of a typical P+ user (at risk), gain insights into brand perceptions for P+, and promote beliefs to reinforce or to change. They also discussed strategies to behave (i.e., use of condom during high-risk sex) among users of condoms and P+.

The formative research helped the marketing team to: (1) rebrand P+ including positioning, personality, and execution strategy; (2) develop plans for active brand equity management; and (3) design a program of brand equity outcome evaluation research. Content analysis of interview transcripts showed that many audience members lacked positive perceptions of the condom product itself, social norms around product use, and often did not perceive it to be a product for them. Lack of active brand management may have contributed to these perceptions. This highlights the potential for brand equity research to explain impact of brand perceptions on condom use.

The P+ social marketing team used these results to rebrand and reposition the condom product. The P+ brand has been the predominant in-country condom brand, but new brands including those produced for-profit have recently entered the market. Figure 16.2 depicts the repackaged P+ brand.

To evaluate the repositioned brand and its effects over time on P+ brand choice and overall condom use behavior, we developed plans for long-term monitoring and evaluation of brand equity in Madagascar. The first step in this plan, the collection of baseline brand equity data prior to P+ repositioning, was implemented through a PSI TRaC (surveillance) study.

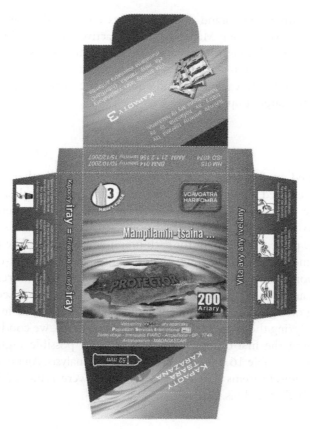

Figure 16.2 New Protector Plus package.
Source: With kind permission by PSI-Madagascar.

Evaluation and Results

In the following, we report on baseline results from the evaluation, including measures of perceptions of the brand positioning, personality, and product characteristics. Drawing from baseline findings from a cross-sectional, nationally representative survey of men aged 18–49 who reported having sex with CSWs, 87 percent of respondents reported they would use a P+ condom next time they used a condom. Over 82 percent said they would recommend their friends use P+. In terms of perceptions, 87 percent reported that the brand was "for them" and that P+ was "the leading brand of condoms," and 95 percent reported that it was a "good value for the money." However, product quality and other perceptions were more varied, with some measures of quality scoring low, such as feel, smell, durability (not breaking during sex), with each of these indicators under 50 percent. We additionally report on multivariable logistic regression results relating these brand equity indicators to condom use and attitudes and beliefs related to condom use. Results are being used in the brand repositioning effort, and the evaluation will be followed up over time to monitor changes in brand equity over time for future marketing efforts and to determine effectiveness in growing the total condom market in Madagascar.

The following summarizes brand equity analyses conducted using the 2009 PSI/ Madagascar TRaC survey among Malagasy sexually active men aged 18–49 who visited CSWs, noted earlier. Specifically, these analyses include factor analysis of the brand equity scale that was a module within the survey, and a series of descriptive and multivariable logistic regression models to examine brand equity in the Protector Plus (P+) brand of condoms among the target population.

Factor analysis

First, we conducted confirmatory factor analysis to identify whether, as hypothesized, brand equity represented a single factor for use in subsequent analysis. Results of the factor analysis are shown in Table 16.2, along with percent agreement for each item (dichotomized to agree/disagree from a 4-point strongly agree to strongly disagree scale) and average percent agreement for each brand equity factor. The results preceded by "[removed]" indicate measured items that did not load on the first-order factor (the factor resulting from factor analysis of measured items) and were thus removed from the factor for further analysis. We followed the widely used Comrey and Lee (1992) criteria (.5 factor loading or higher) to determine whether to include a variable in the factor.

After factor-analyzing the measured brand equity scale items, we conducted secondary factor analysis using the first-order factors to identify a possible higher-order, single "brand equity" factor. Table 16.3 presents results of this analysis. Again, results preceded by "[removed]" indicate items that did not load and were removed from the brand equity factor for further analysis.

Multivariable models

After completing the factor analysis, we used the higher-order brand equity factor and the second-order factors in all subsequent analyses. First we developed a logistic regression model using both the brand equity factor and each individual first-order factor as follows: Model 1 – Amongst those who have had sex (survey question), those who have vs. have not used a condom regularly when paying for sex. Tables 16.4 and 16.5 summarize these results. Thus higher odds ratios indicate a higher probability of using any condom brand (category of condoms) given brand equity.

In Table 16.4, the overall brand equity factor strongly predicts whether respondents used a condom when paying for sex, as they are 70 percent more likely to do so if they have expressed brand equity. In Table 16.5, we find the same result for the individual price-ever (87 percent more likely), satisfaction (more than twice as likely), and quality (75 percent more likely) factors. In other words, these individual first-order factors were significantly associated with regular condom use among men paying for sex, in addition to the overall result that the higher-order brand equity score has that significant association.

Next, we developed a second logistic regression model using the brand equity factor and first-order factors as follows: Model 2 – Amongst those who have had paid for sex recently, those who have vs. have not consistently used a condom. Thus higher odds ratios indicate a higher probability of using a condom given brand equity.

Table 16.2 Confirmatory factor analysis for brand equity scale items.

Question	First-order Factor	Factor Loadings	% Agree	Avg. % Agree
I will use Protector Plus brand the next time…	Satisfaction	0.6341	87.2%	75.8%
I would wear Protector Plus brand [gear].	Satisfaction	0.767	58.0%	
I would recommend my friends use P+ brand.	Satisfaction	0.7837	82.4%	
Protector Plus brand:				
• is better than other condom brands.	Quality	[removed] 0.0666	84.0%	
• has advertisements that are better than others for condoms.	Quality	[removed] 0.0530	92.3%	
• does not break during sex.	Quality	0.8069	47.3%	45.6%
• gives a pleasant sensation during sex.	Quality	0.6609	42.2%	
• does not smell like latex.	Quality	0.7705	42.7%	
• is not too thick.	Quality	0.7826	41.8%	
• is there when you need it.	Quality	0.8558	49.5%	
• is available at an outlet near you.	Quality	0.8703	47.3%	
• has sufficient lubricant.	Quality	0.8001	48.7%	
• is becoming more popular with people like you.	Leadership/Popularity	0.7662	90.7%	88.6%
• is for people like you.	Leadership/Popularity	0.7704	87.6%	
• is the leading brand of condoms.	Leadership/Popularity	0.6703	87.6%	
There are good reasons to buy P+ over other brands.	Value	0.773	68.0%	81.2%
Protector Plus brand is good value for the price.	Value	0.6148	94.5%	
Protector Plus brand is better value than other condoms.	Value	0.736	81.0%	
People who use Protector Plus brand:				
• Are strong	Personality	0.5149	54.2%	68.6%
• Are confident	Personality	[removed] 0.4754	74.9%	
• Have a lot of freedom	Personality	0.5085	70.6%	
• Have fun	Personality	0.6417	71.0%	

Table 16.2 (cont'd)

Question	First-order Factor	Factor Loadings	% Agree	Avg. % Agree
• Find it easy to have girlfriends	Personality	0.5526	53.4%	
• Are just like you	Personality	0.5472	79.6%	
• Are like the people that you hang out with	Personality	0.5325	83.2%	
At which of the following outlets have you purchased				
P+ in the past 30 days				
• Gas Stations	Price	[removed] 0.2973	5.7%	5.1%
• Pharmacy	Price	0.6296	8.3%	
• Grocery store	Price	[removed] 0.3118	66.7%	
• Sales representative	Price	[removed] 0.1426	3.4%	
• Doctor's office	Price	0.6759	4.4%	
• Community health clinic	Price	0.7102	2.6%	
• Friends or peers	Price	[removed] 0.2860	7.1%	
• Other (please specify)	Price	[removed] -0.2236	17.7%	
At which of the following outlets have you ever				
purchased P+				
• Gas stations	Price ever	0.5844	11.9%	11.5%
• Pharmacy	Price ever	0.5917	17.6%	
• Grocery store	Price ever	[removed] 0.2675	80.6%	
• Sales representative	Price ever	[removed] 0.4680	6.1%	
• Doctor's office	Price ever	0.7282	10.7%	
• Community health clinic	Price ever	0.7038	5.1%	
• Friends or peers	Price ever	0.5537	12.3%	
• Other (please specify)	Price ever	[removed] -0.1304	21.3%	

Table 16.3 Secondary factor analysis.

First-order factor	Factor loadings
Price	[removed] 0.1496
Satisfaction	0.7402
Quality	[removed] 0.0794
Leadership/Popularity	0.7917
Value	0.7839
Personality	0.7274

Table 16.4 Logistic regression of overall brand equity factor on regular condom use when paying for sex.

Variable	Odds Ratio	P-value
Brand Equity	1.689	0.001

Table 16.5 Logistic regression of first-order brand equity factors on regular condom use when paying for sex.

Variable	Odds Ratio	P-value
Price-ever	1.87	0.049
Satisfaction	2.03	0.016
Quality	1.75	0.013
Leadership	1.13	0.734
Value	0.98	0.951
Personality	0.75	0.404

In Table 16.6, the overall brand equity factor again strongly predicts whether respondents used a condom when paying for sex, as they are 63 percent more likely to do so if they have brand equity. In Table 16.7, we find the same result only for the individual price-ever (89 percent more likely) factor.

Then we developed a third logistic regression model using the brand equity factor and first-order factors as follows: Model 3 - Amongst those who have paid for sex recently, those who have vs. have not consistently used P+. Thus higher odds ratios indicate a higher probability of using P+ given brand equity.

In Table 16.8, the overall brand equity factor again strongly predicts whether respondents used a condom when paying for sex, as they are 84 percent more likely to do so if they have brand equity. In Table 16.9, we find that none of the individual first-order factors predicts P+ use.

Next, we examined the association between individual first-order brand equity factors and additional personality traits associated with the brand, but separately from the brand equity scales. We developed logistic regression models as follows: Among condom users when paying for sex, those who use vs. don't use P+ 100 percent of time. We were interested in identifying whether brand equity factors predicted consistent P+ choice.

Table 16.6 Logistic regression overall brand equity factor on consistent condom use among those who recently paid for sex.

Variable	Odds Ratio	P-value
Brand Equity	1.627836	0.000

Table 16.7 Logistic regression of first-order brand equity factors on consistent condom use among those who recently paid for sex.

Variable	Odds Ratio	P-value
Price-ever	1.888119	0.008
Satisfaction	1.237427	0.309
Quality	1.330381	0.103
Leadership	1.029702	0.89
Value	1.131603	0.533
Personality	0.9758534	0.912

Table 16.8 Logistic regression overall brand equity factor on consistent P+ use among those who recently paid for sex.

Variable	Odds Ratio	P-value
Brand Equity	1.84	0.012

Table 16.9 Logistic regression first-order brand equity factors on consistent P+ use among those who recently paid for sex.

Variable	Odds Ratio	P-value
Price-ever	1.85	0.167
Satisfaction	1.07	0.87
Quality	1.02	0.96
Leadership	1.66	0.146
Value	1.04	0.912
Personality	0.83	0.641

Table 16.10 Logistic regression of first-order brand equity factors on use of p+ 100% of time when paying for sex.

Variable	Odds Ratio	P-value
Price-ever	1.06	0.752
Satisfaction	1.47	0.146
Quality	1.09	0.692
Leadership	1.40	0.24
Value	1.09	0.734
Personality	0.59	0.113

Table 16.11 Logistic regression of first-order brand equity factors on use of p+ 100% of time when paying for sex.

Variable	Odds Ratio	P-value
Strong PP	0.87	0.417
Confident PP	0.93	0.722
Peace of Mind - FSW	0.75	0.582
Peace of Mind - outside	1.70	0.196
Avoid Blame STI	0.62	0.176

In Table 16.10, none of the first-order scales are associated with 100 percent P+ use. In Table 16.11, none of the personality traits associated with P+ are associated with 100 percent P+ Use. In other words, we find no significant association between brand equity factors and 100 percent consistent use of the P+ product when paying for sex.

Discussion

Overall, these findings indicate that the higher-order brand equity factor is a strong predictor of both condom category use and P+ brand use. This suggests that actively managing brand equity is important for the PSI/Madagascar marketing team.

Efforts should be made to increase brand equity to increase the total condom market, and P+ use in particular. There is evidence that individual brand equity factors such as price ever paid, satisfaction, and quality predict condom use and P+ use to varying degrees. These factors may represent targets for marketing efforts, such as increasing perceptions of product quality through a mass media campaign. Additionally, PSI/Madagascar is considering doing more with strength, confidence, and peace of mind when promoting P+ (these factors were measured separately in the survey and are not reported here). Separate analyses revealed that these factors are central to the brand personality of P+. The next phase of a media campaign targeting men with high-risk behaviors will seek to reinforce these personality traits associated with P+ use.

In terms of implications for further research, brand equity for P+ must be tracked and monitored going forward. The PSI/Madagascar program would also benefit from more in-depth research on how and why brand equity predicts category and P+ use, both alone and against market competitors, among the overall target population of sexually active men and among subgroups such as those who pay for sex. In other words, conjoint studies that compare P+ with other brands and brand attributes consumers hold for those brands should be conducted. Likewise, the strength, confidence, and peace of mind factors should be added to the brand equity scales so that they can be included in future factor analyses and multivariate modeling. Future research should examine how these variables are associated with brand equity as well as how respondents think about "strength," "confidence," or "peace of mind" as marketing constructs.

Conclusion

In conclusion, the P+ research process demonstrates the potential importance of brand equity research in global social marketing and public health programs. While P+ has been a successful brand in many respects, the changing marketplace for socially marketed and commercially available condoms suggests the need for active brand management. Brand equity research can be a valuable tool for management purposes and to evaluate the effects of the P+ repositioning efforts on P+ and overall condom category use. Brand equity research methods are currently being translated into public health practice and are poised to become an important source of social marketing evidence. Future research should utilize more rigorous designs, compare brand equity between commercial and socially marketed brands within markets, and shed light on the "Total Market Approach" to global social marketing of condoms and other products.

References

Aaker, D. (1996). *Building strong brands.* New York: Simon and Schuster Inc.

Agha, S. (2003). The impact of a mass media campaign on personal risk perception, perceived self-efficacy and on other behavioral predictors. *Aids Care, 15*(6), 749–762.

Bandura A. (2004). Health promotion by social cognitive means. *Health Education and Behavior, 31*(2), 143–164.

Berkowitz, J. M., Huhman, M., and Nolan, M. J. (2008). Did augmenting the VERB™ campaign advertising in select communities have an effect on awareness, attitudes, and physical activity? *American Journal of Preventive Medicine, 34*(6, supplement), S257–S266.

Calkins, T. (2005). The challenge of branding. In A. M. Tybout and T. Calkins (Eds.), *Kellogg on Branding* (pp. 1–10). New York: John Wiley and Sons..

Comrey, A. L., and Lee, H. B. (1992). *A First Course in Factor Analysis.* Hillsdale, NJ: Lawrence Erlbaum Associates.

Evans, W. D. (2009). BRAND-MAP (Strategic Brand Research for Management Action Planning). Population Services International Concept Paper. Retrieved from http://www.psi.org/sites/default/files/publication_files/Concept%20Brief%20Brand%20Equity%20-%20final%20 2-26-10.pdf

Evans, W. D., Blitstein, J. Hersey, J. *et al.* (2008). Systematic review of public health branding. *Journal of Health Communication, 13*(8), 351–360.

Evans, W. D., and Haider, M. (2008). Public health brands in the developing world. In W. D. Evans and G. Hastings (Eds.), *Public Health Branding: Applying Marketing for Social Change* (pp. 215–232). Oxford: Oxford University Press.

Evans, W. D., and Hastings, G. (2008). Public health branding: Recognition, promise, and delivery of healthy lifestyles. In W. D. Evans and G. Hastings (Eds.), *Public Health Branding: Applying Marketing for Social Change* (pp. 3–24). Oxford: Oxford University Press.

Evans, W. D., Price, S. and Blahut, S. (2005). Evaluating the truth® Brand. *Journal of Health Communication, 10*(2), 181–192.

French, J., Blair-Stevens, C., McVey, D., and Merritt, R. (2010). *Social Marketing and Public Health.* Oxford: Oxford University Press.

Huhman, M., Price, S., and Potter, L. (2008). Branding Play for Children: VERB™ It's What You Do. In W. D. Evans and G. Hastings (Eds.), *Public Health Branding: Applying Marketing for Social Change* (pp. 109–126). Oxford: Oxford University Press.

Keller, K. L., Aperia, T., and Georgson, M. (2008). *Strategic Brand Management: A European Perspective*. Harlow, UK: Prentice Hall.

Palmgreen, P., Donohew, L., Lorch, E. P. *et al.* (2002). Television campaigns and sensation seeking targeting of adolescent marijuana use: a controlled time-series approach. In R. Hornik (Ed.), *Public Health Communication: Evidence for Behavior Change* (pp. 80–101). Hillsdale, NJ: Lawrence Erlbaum Associates.

Population Services International. (2010). *Research Approaches*. Retrieved from: http://psi.org/resources/research-metrics/research-approaches

Schindler, R. M. (1992). The real lesson of New Coke: The value of focus groups for predicting the effects of social influence. *Marketing Research, 4*, 22–27.

UNAIDS (Joint United Nations Programme on HIV/AIDS) (2010). *Global Report: UNAIDS Report on the Global AIDS Epidemic 2010*. Retrieved from: http://www.unaids.org/globalreport/Global_report.htm

Zuckerman, M. (1979). *Sensation Seeking: Beyond the Optimal Level of Arousal*. Hillsdale, NJ: Lawrence Erlbaum Associates.

17

Participatory Health Communication Research
Four Tools to Complement the Interview

Karen Greiner

"You're not in the medical field, are you?" asked Glenn Buzzelli, a registered nurse (RN) at the Veterans' Hospital in Pittsburgh. His question came after showing me something I had never seen before and thus had no name for – some grey wires that looked to me like a short extension cord. The "grey wires" were, in fact, Electrocardiogram (EKG) lead wires used to help detect and monitor heart conditions. Glenn showed them to me during the guided visit he was giving me of the Veterans' Hospital. This "guided visit," in research terminology, can also be called an ethnographic "go-along," a term proposed by sociologist Margarethe Kusenbach (2003, p. 462) to describe a tool that complements two common ethnographic methods, participant observation and the "sit down" interview.

On Glenn's "go-along," he was in charge: he decided where we would go and, to a large extent, what would be discussed. He led me to different rooms, pointing out different items of equipment, especially hard-to-clean surfaces, and explaining at each destination how Intensive Care personnel were fighting hospital-acquired infections. My questions were mostly reactive: "What is the importance of these EKG lead wires?" "Can you explain how and why you began ordering these EKG lead wires instead of the ones you used before?" The utility of the go-along is the increase in visual information it offers. On a go-along, the researcher can be exposed to the unknown, to things one might not have thought to ask about for lack of awareness or vocabulary. Moving through different spaces while talking, the researcher and research participant come across a variety of sights and situations that would not normally occur in a fixed-place interview. A defining characteristic of the go-along, and of each tool I will discuss in this chapter, is that it is visual and participatory: it offers an increase in visual stimuli and it invites the research participant to take the lead in generating and interpreting information.

The Handbook of Global Health Communication, First Edition. Edited by Rafael Obregon and Silvio Waisbord.

Participatory Research Approaches

We can trace participatory approaches to health communication research to their roots in the fields of agriculture and rural development where practitioners first began developing participatory approaches for the collection, analysis, and dissemination of data (De Koning and Martin, 1996). Participatory research emerged as scholars and practitioners began recognizing that the use of nonparticipatory research methods resulted in a great power imbalance between researchers and respondents: researchers decided which issues to study, which questions to ask, and which analyses would be included in research reports and publications. Participatory research methods were developed to shift this imbalance in power by expanding the role of community members. Participatory research advocates De Koning and Martin (1996) write that participatory research emphasizes the generation of knowledge "from the perspective not only of the researchers but also of the researched" (p. 1). In agriculture and rural development researchers and practitioners employ a variety of participatory methodologies, including "participatory rural appraisal" (PRA), "rapid rural appraisal" (RRA), and "participatory action research" (PAR). Participatory methodology expert Robert Chambers (1992) describes the difference between Rapid Rural Appraisal (RRA) and Participatory Rural Appraisal (PRA) in this way:

> An RRA is intended for learning by outsiders. A PRA is intended to enable local people to conduct their own analysis, and often to plan and take action (p. 13).

While RRA, as described by Chambers, is "extractive" and designed to elicit information for the benefit of outsiders, PRA is meant to be empowering to local community members who conduct their own researcher with only the guidance of outsiders who serve as facilitators (See Chambers, 1992, p. 14; 1997, p. 206). Both RRA and PRA borrow from methodological tools used originally in the analysis of agro-ecosystems in including "transect walks" (systematic walks and observation), mapping, diagramming (seasonal calendars, flow and causal diagrams, bar charts, Venn diagrams, etc.).[1] While RRA and PRA are forms of inquiry, Participatory Action Research (PAR) can be described as both inquiry and intervention. Colombian sociologist Orlando Fals-Borda (1987) suggests that PAR is a combination of research, education and "political action" (p. 330). With PAR, inquiry is designed to lead to action, and inquiry, according to Fals-Borda (1987), should allow community members to "articulate and systematize knowledge ... in such a way that they can become protagonists in the advancement of their society" (p. 330). Placed on a continuum of community engagement, the three approaches described above could be illustrated as shown in Figure 17.1.

The idea of placing community engagement in participatory processes along a continuum is not a new one. Two scholars, writing 30 years apart, have offered a "typology" (or "ladder") of participation in acknowledgement that the word "participation" can mean everything from attending a meeting (a low level of engagement) to having decision-making power (a much higher level of engagement). Sherry Arnstein's (1969) classic "ladder of citizen participation" had eight "rungs," which ranged from "manipulative nonparticipation" whereby citizens are convoked and "informed" under the guise of

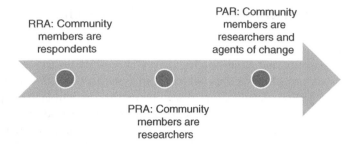

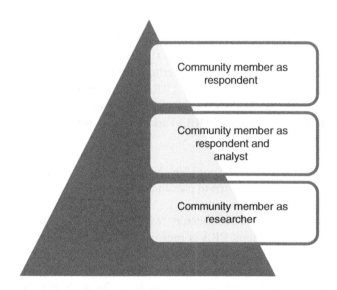

Figure 17.1   Increasing levels of community engagement along a continuum.

Figure 17.2   Role of community member in the interview process, from less to more control.

participation, to "citizen control" which involves citizens being involved as equals in the decision-making process (see p. 217, Figure 2).

Describing the challenges to women's engagement in participatory processes in India, Bina Argawal (2001, p. 1625) created a typology of participation that focused on the "extent of activeness." At the less active end of the continuum were group membership and passive acceptance of group decisions, and at the most active end was "interactive participation," defined as "having voice and influence in the group's decisions" (p. 1624). Inspired by these two typologies, I offer my typology of participation in the interview process. Figure 17.2 outlines the various roles community members can take, ranging from having less control to more control, in descending order.

In most research contexts involving interviews, the role of community members is limited to that of respondent: researchers ask questions and community members respond. Fixed-choice surveys or questionnaires that give the respondent a series of pre-determined answers to choose from give the respondent the least amount of control, for they can alter neither the question nor the response, they can only choose from available choices or not respond. Open-ended questions give the respondent more freedom in crafting their response. A life-history interview might include the question: "Tell me about your childhood," the response to which could last anywhere from minutes to hours. The tools I describe in this chapter place community members in the role of respondent and analyst. The answers provided by community members are analyzed first by community members themselves. This analysis can help the researcher gain a deeper understanding of the community members' responses and also help the researcher gauge which issues are deemed most important. Here the researcher need not engage in guesswork because respondents take the lead in explaining the answers to each question. The cases I describe in this chapter involved questions conceived by researchers who were external to the community and thus community members do not take full control as would be the case in the "community member as researcher" role described in Figure 17.2 above. I make this distinction because of the wide number of meanings attached to the word "participatory." I feel it is important to situate the research described in this chapter within this typology to illustrate that, in this instance, community members participate first as respondents to open-ended questions posed by external researchers and second as analysts of their own responses, which in these cases take the form of (1) drawings, (2) guided walks, (3) network maps, and (4) life maps.

Health communication researchers stand to gain from research methods that enable community members to participate in the interpretation and analysis of research findings. The meaning of "health" may vary between and even within communities; thus, inviting respondents to explain and interpret their own forms of expression ensures that the first layer of analysis is from the local community members' perspective. Health communication scholar Collins Airhihenbuwa (1995) argues that too often efforts to understand and promote health do not adequately respect local perspectives. He notes that public health practitioners and researchers alike only pay "lip service" to local community members' understanding of health and illness, an understanding rooted in a "cultural framework" that may be unknown to or misunderstood by the researcher (see pp. x–7). Designing research studies to include the perspectives and analyses of community members ensures that the values and interpretations of external researchers do not drown out local perspectives.

In this chapter I draw on four health communication case studies in community and health care settings to describe and discuss four different participatory research tools: (1) sketching, (2) the ethnographic go-along, (3) network mapping, and (4) life mapping. Each case includes a brief introduction to the research study, a discussion of the use of one research tool, a section on practical issues that may arise while using the tool, and finally the potential utility of each tool for health communication researchers.

Some of these tools have been described elsewhere. The ethnographic go-along, for example, has been amply and ably discussed by Kusenbach (2003), who coined the term. Scholars have also paid attention to participatory sketching as a research method, which has been used in a variety of international settings and contexts (Singhal and Rattine-Flaherty, 2006; Greiner, Singhal, and Hurlburt, 2007; Singhal and Dura, 2010). The other two tools I discuss in this chapter, life mapping and network mapping, are being introduced here.[2] I present the four tools together to illustrate, in very practical terms, how these visual, participatory methods can contribute to health communication research.

Each tool has its strength. Participatory sketching enables research participants to identify and depict the topics that are most salient for them. The detailed illustrations and the explanation that accompanies them can help the researcher understand a small slice of the world as seen by the participants themselves. The ethnographic go-along is an ideal tool for accessing information that is space-specific. If one wants to understand what happens in a hospital, for instance, it is useful to move *through* the hospital accompanied by individuals who can explain objects or phenomena that are unfamiliar to the researcher. Network mapping helps make relationships visible. It is a tool that provides structure during an interview: once relationships are made visible they can be more easily discussed. Asking research participants to create life maps is a way to access how they see their life and how they want their life to be seen. The life map, like the network map, can become a recurrent reference during an interview. Once relationships and life moments are charted, they can be returned to again and again. They can be elaborated upon, corrected, and used as a basis for a new, related topic. These tools share the same limitation, which is that they yield information that is specific to each participant and thus nonreplicable and nongeneralizable. The results of a sketching exercise in Khartoum, Sudan, for instance, are limited to that context. The symbols and colors used in participants' sketches are bound by culture and experience, and each sketch represents the unique perspective of its creator. The limitations of these tools can be tempered by making limited claims. When using tools that do not allow generalization, I advise making specific, context-specific claims. In my discussion of the life map tool, for instance, I gained understanding about the effect of a breast cancer diagnosis on the life of *one* woman. I tell Tammi's story, based on what I learned from her during our interview and our discussion of her map. The life map exercise gave Tammi the first opportunity to interpret her story. As with the other tools, the life map accesses subjective experience and perspectives and makes them visible. Once visible, subjective experience and perspectives can be easily referred to and discussed.

Radio Dramas and Female Genital Cutting (FGC) in Sudan: The Role of Participatory Sketching

Asking adults to draw is not easy. Asking through an interpreter adds another layer of difficulty. To overcome this difficulty in a hot, airless room in Khartoum, Sudan in the summer of 2006, my colleagues and I resorted to an American classic: Coca Cola. We encouraged our research participants with sugar. And when everyone had cooled down a bit and smiles began replacing the skeptical scowls that had appeared when we first mentioned sketching, we explained, again through the interpreter, that, indeed, what we wanted was an answer to the question we had just posed in the form of a *drawing*. We were conducting an evaluation of a radio soap opera called *Ashreat al Amal*, which had storylines that focused on health and, in particular, female reproductive health.[3] We had asked participants to give us a summary of what the soap opera was about. This question was somewhat of a "warm-up": it was meant to get the participants, all faithful listeners of the soap opera, thinking about the story lines and to help them become more comfortable expressing themselves visually, through sketching.

What happened next illustrates our first mistake. We had not sufficiently explained the methodology to the interpreters. Our one-minute English explanation became a six-minute explanation in Arabic as the interpreters added to our deliberately brief explanation with what they imagined to be helpful examples. If "do-overs" were possible, we would sit down with interpreters beforehand to explain that during a participatory sketching exercise, it is best to not provide examples because it can influence what participants choose to draw. Instead, the participants should fill the blank page with their own interpretations and preferences – images of their own choosing. Unlike a survey questionnaire, which asks respondents to select from among set of pre-established answers, participatory sketching enables research participants to craft an answer that is unanticipated by the researcher. Further, a participatory sketching exercise allows the research participant to provide the first layer of interpretation: when the drawings are finished and participants explain what they have drawn to the researchers they interpret their own drawings and reveal what different symbols and colors mean for them.

Our first round of questions with research participants in Sudan led to many drawings with scenes of hospitals and doctors, a result, I believe, of the interpreter having provided this example to participants. Our second question, however, led to very surprising responses. We asked participants: "As a listener, which scene from the radio soap opera was most meaningful to you?" We were familiar with the storylines of the soap opera, one involved drug use and many more related to female reproductive health, birth spacing, and so on. My colleagues and I were working in three teams, two female researchers, each with a female interpreter, with sets of 8–10 female listeners and one male researcher, with two male interpreters and 12 male listeners. Since we were working separately, it was not until the end of the day that we realized that the stories we had each heard separately had one major theme in common.

Figure 17.3 was created in one of the women's groups. The creator of the sketch, Ibtisam, explained her drawing to the group:

> I drew my two daughters. One of them was circumcised before the radio program. She is sad and depressed – also she bled a lot after the operation. But my other daughter was not circumcised. She's always happy and in good health. I drew our village, the nature, the fields and our houses.

Like many other participants, Ibtisam highlighted the female circumcision storyline as being most important to her. Also, like many other participants, she said that the radio soap opera was the reason her family ceased the practice. After Ibtisam explained the meaning of her drawing, many conversations broke out between group members, only some of which were translated by the interpreter: "They are sharing similar stories," I was told, without further details. This phenomenon of bursts of conversation after narrated drawings occurred several times during the day. Although I lamented the content I was missing because of having to work through an interpreter, I was glad that the women were sharing their stories as a group. We had deliberately worked in groups to create opportunities for exchange between participants. Our research design included ample time for participants' responses and ensuing discussion.

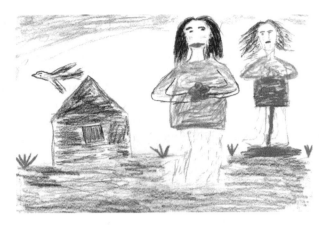

Figure 17.3   Two daughters.

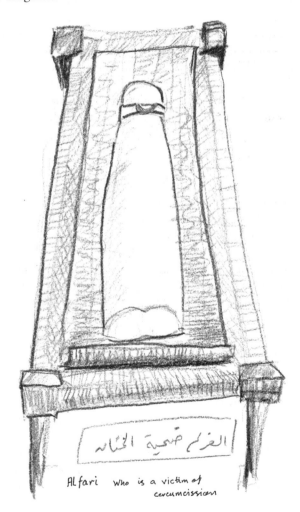

Figure 17.4   A funeral.

The drawing in Figure 17.4 was created in the men's group by a young man named Yaseen. He explained:

> This is a bed on which the dead are carried – the *Alangaraib*. The little girl was a victim of circumcision and died. She was a little girl and her mother insisted that she must be circumcised. I think this scene is representing the whole idea of the program. I added the crescent on the forehead of the girl which is a symbol of circumcision in Sudan.

When my colleagues and I discussed the preponderance of drawings related to "Khitan," as our participants called it, or female genital cutting (FGC) as it is commonly called in English, it came to light that the soap opera story line had coincided with a news item that many of our participants had mentioned, which involved a very young girl who had died from complications of FGC. The news story brought additional attention to an issue being discussed in the radio soap opera, and several research participants explained that when showing their sketches. As foreign researchers, we were not familiar with current events or local customs and thus would not have thought – or dared – to ask about an issue as sensitive as FGC. The sketching exercise, however, brought the issue to light and resulted in many group conversations. Our team of Sudanese interpreters shared with us that they were very surprised to hear the participants talking openly about the issue.

And the end of the day we made arrangements to continue the evaluation with 13 research participants who had volunteered for an additional exercise, this time using participatory photography.[4] As we were leaving the meeting room, I noticed that several research participants were in discussion, gathered around one woman. I asked Diana, one of the interpreters, to inquire about what the group was discussing. Diana explained that the research participant at the center of the group was a journalist: "They're talking with her about what they can do raise more awareness about female circumcision." Two days later, when listening to participants describe the content of the photographs they had taken, we would again witness how explaining a visual object in a group setting can lead to a lively group discussion. I do not know what, if any, follow-up action might have resulted from these group discussions. I do know, however, that the use of participatory sketching had yielded rich accounts on a variety of themes from the soap opera including the unexpected and taboo topic of FGC. Further, as a visual method, the approach resulted in colorful and powerful images to highlight participants' viewpoints in our final report.

Practical issues

Conducting participatory sketching in a group setting has advantages and disadvantages. One advantage is the inevitable outcome of group discussion following the presentation of each individual's sketch to the group. Group discussion can provide insights into other group members' experiences, how they are similar or how they differ, from the individual presenting the sketch. Group discussion can also provide support and reassurance to individuals: when their stories find resonance in others, individuals may feel validated and less alone. Some disadvantages of the group setting are (1) the time it takes to have each individual present each sketch and discuss each sketch within the group and (2) the possibility that the group setting will lead to "sidebar" discussions, separate conversations between pairs or subgroups, making it more difficult to hear the research participant explain the content of their sketch. To address these disadvantages I recommend (1) allowing ample time for the participatory sketching exercise, keeping in mind that discussion and interpretation will always add considerably to the time required and (2) if "sidebar" discussions pop up, moving away from the featured speaker and positioning yourself at the farthest end of the table thereby forcing the speaker to raise their voice to talk "over" others who may be having separate discussions.

I recommend digitally recording participants' narration of their sketches. If you require an interpreter, the digital recording serves to back up and complement the simultaneous translation. For the sake of time, it is possible to ask the interpreter to provide only the most salient details since you know you will have the digital recording for the full account. Be sure to ask the participant to state their name before they begin narrating their sketch and, once all the narrations are finished, it is important to also ask all the participants to write their name (and age, if desired) on the back of the sketch so that you can match each oral narration with its corresponding sketch. Given the group setting, if research participants have difficulty writing they will most likely ask a neighbor to assist them. It is a good idea to review the sketches to ensure that you have all the identifying information you need. At the end of our sketching exercise in Sudan, for instance, we required the assistant of our interpreters to convert all the names and some words on the drawings from Arabic to Latin script.

The utility of participatory sketching

My experience with participatory sketching in Sudan taught me that a blank page can be a powerful tool. Our research participants filled the pages with their ideas, preferences, and symbols. During their presentation of their sketches to the group, individuals had the opportunity to interpret their own representations and could explain symbols, color choices, and meanings that might not be obvious to all. In Sudan, many of our research participants depicted scenes related to female genital cutting, a theme of the radio soap opera that we had been told was a minor storyline. Our participants' sketches initiated frank discussions on a taboo topic that we would not have asked about in a traditional interview setting. A participatory sketching exercise conducted with listeners of a radio series in the Philippines[5] that had themes also included in the Sudan series including health, family planning, and HIV prevention yielded a different set of images; listeners signaled the domestic violence story line as one of the most relevant to them (Singhal, Rattine-Flaherty, and Mayer, 2010, p. 345). The fact that the same tool used in two contexts to evaluate similar radio series led to very different images is not surprising given the nature of the tool. In each case, research participants are free to depict the issues that matter most to them. Rather than a questionnaire with fixed questions, the radio series listeners were given a blank page, which they filled based on their own preferences, experiences, and worldviews. This tool is very useful for understanding what research participants understand and what they prefer when they have faithfully listened to (or watched) an entertainment-education series. Participatory sketching is also useful when the aim is to gain a better understanding of the everyday life of research participants. I once asked university students in Barranquilla, Colombia[6] to draw "a typical day in the life of a university student" and got very rich results. Here, when I write "very rich results" I mean that before the sketching exercise I knew nothing about the life of university students in Barranquilla and after the exercise I had images and accompanying narratives that explained, in great detail, what it meant to be a student, from the students' own perspectives.

The participatory sketching tool provides a great amount of freedom to the research participant. It invites the participant to share their ideas, understanding, and preferences through sketches they produce and then again, through the explanation of those sketches. An advantage of this tool is that it allows the researcher to report the participants' own interpretations and explanations when writing up the results of the exercise. The broad questions and blank pages initiating the participatory sketching exercise invite research participants to depict and describe their world, when their thought process is completely unknown to and unsuspected by the researcher.

Infection Control at the Pittsburgh VA Hospital: Learning by "Going Along"

The ethnographic go-along with Glenn Buzelli that I described in the opening paragraphs of this chapter took place during one of a series of visits to the Veterans' Hospital in Pittsburgh Pennsylvania (VAHPS) in 2006–2007. Invited by the VAHPS along with Dr. Arvind Singhal of the University of Texas El Paso, we conducted research on the VA Hospital's successful efforts to reduce hospital acquired infections (HAIs), with a particular focus the communication practices that led to a steep reduction in antibiotic-resistant staph infections (MRSA). The hospital had implemented two different strategies[7] over a four-year period that had resulted in a 64 percent hospital-wide reduction in the incidence of MRSA (Singhal and Greiner, 2007, p. 11). The VA Hospital had data to demonstrate the success of their infection control practices and they wanted further research to help document the "who and the how" behind those practices.

The ethnographic go-along was a key tool in our research design. We did conduct several "sit-down" interviews in offices and conference rooms in the VA Hospital, but the majority of our interviews were "on the go," moving through different spaces throughout the hospital. Each space we moved through generally corresponded with the work area of a staff member who was leading us while explaining their work. For instance, the physical therapists showed us the physical therapy room and explained how patients were transferred there from several different units. They discussed how, as a result of being included in the infection control effort, they were able to point out that patients that were in isolation rooms due to MRSA infection were often mixed with MRSA-free patients during physical therapy sessions. Orderlies took us to the areas where long-term-care MRSA-infected patients might interact with MRSA-free patients, such as the outdoor smoking area or the pottery workshop. Physicians showed us the

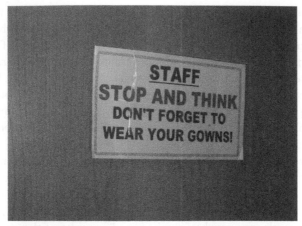

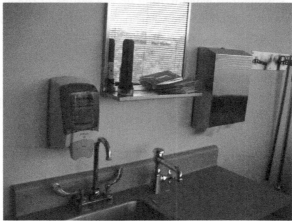

Figures 17.5   Items assisting infection control pointed out by staff during a hospital "go along."

red, "dedicated" stethoscopes in patient rooms. Rather than bringing the same stethoscope from room to room, which increased the possibility of germ transfer, the room of each MRSA-infected patient was equipped with its own stethoscope. Staff members decided that each stethoscope should be red to remind physicians to "stop" before removing the dedicated stethoscope from the room. Cleaning staff took us on a tour of patient rooms and pointed out staff-created signs on doors and the strategic placement of cleaning products in highly visible locations to encourage other hospital staff members to assist them in reducing germs on room surfaces (see Figure 17.5). A registered nurse showed us an innovation she came up with for reducing germs on her unit's emergency equipment cart – the "crash cart" as she called it. She explained how she noticed that the keyboards on the technical equipment quickly became worn-out due to repeated cleaning, which resulted in her designing a protective plastic cover for the cart, wisely reasoning that it was easier and more cost effective to clean and replace the plastic cover than to clean and replace the equipment.

Each go-along brought us into a new world. As nonmedical professionals, we had no previous experience with crash carts, dedicated stethoscopes, and the challenges of keeping patient room surfaces germ-free. As we moved through the hospital, we came across dozens of people, spaces, and objects that served as a catalyst for follow-up questions. Each new question led to detailed discussions about the "who and how" of infection control. We learned about the work and daily routines of staff members (the "who") and we learned the exact nature of their efforts to combat infections in the hospital (the "how"). Without the visual stimuli encountered on each go-along, it is doubtful that our conversations with staff members would have been so rich in details.

Practical issues

The ethnographic go-along is not ideal for digitally recording conversations with research participants. The presence of the digital recorder converts a casual stroll into a formal interview, which can lead to research participants being overly concerned with saying "the right thing." I found that writing notes in a small notebook during pauses in the go-along and taking photographs (when permitted) of key objects and spaces provided sufficient detail to document the salient information gleaned during the go-alongs. I was also able to ask staff members follow-up questions once we returned to a stationary position, making reference to things we had seen on the go-along. For example, I could ask cleaning staff: "Do you remember when you made reference to the lift in one of the empty patient rooms? Can you explain to me again what that piece of equipment does and why it is difficult to clean?" In the case of the ethnographic go-along, the ignorance of the researcher is not necessarily a disadvantage: a lack of understanding is fertile terrain for in-depth questioning. "What is this?" "What does this machine do?" "Why did you place the sign on *this* door?" "How do patients go from their room to physical therapy?" "Who orders the gowns and gloves?" "Where are they stored?" Each question can lead to an extension of the go-along, a trip to the storage room, a walk down the hallway to the physical therapy room, a visit to the pottery workshop. Each new destination is likely to lead to new questions and explanations.

As with any form of interview, it is always a good practice to verify your understanding and quoted statements with research participants. Our account of infection control practices at the VA Hospital in Pittsburgh, the people behind them and the details surrounding them was read by multiple staff members at the hospital, including administrators, prior to finalizing our report. We were able to correct the spelling of names, add precision to technical information we had included, and make corrections to terminology we had misunderstood or processes we had inaccurately described. Having recognized the importance of accuracy in research in general and of research in health care settings in particular, we were grateful for the thorough review of our work by VA Hospital staff members.[8]

The utility of the ethnographic go-along

The strength of the ethnographic go-along is the visual and spatial complement it provides to the traditional "sit down" interview. Led through different spaces by research participants, the researcher is consistently confronted with new objects, people, and situations, each of which can be a subject for further inquiry. A member of the cleaning staff who describes his duties while walking the route he normally takes on an average workday is more likely to speak of context-specific details than if sitting in a conference room. Why? Because he may not think of the details until he *sees* them. And, likewise, the researcher is more likely to ask context-specific questions when confronted with an unfamiliar sight. A researcher cannot ask "How do you clean *this* machine?" if they do not see the equipment found in patients' rooms. Like the participatory sketching exercise, the ethnographic go-along serves to make *visible* the unknown and unimaginable. Once information or issues are rendered visible, they make further inquiry possible. The photos taken during a go-along also provide visual evidence to complement research participants' observations and other data to be included in the final research report. Kusenbach (2003) signals two strengths of the ethnographic go-along that address the limitations of other ethnographic methods such as observation and the interview. It overcomes the static and stimulus-poor nature of the "sit down" interview (p. 462) and it allows research participants to express their perceptions and interpretations of spaces and events, something which is lacking in observation situations when the researcher is alone (p. 461). The go-along allows the researcher to encounter new objects and situations while moving through space, and it includes a local guide.

Learning about Collaborators in an HIV Prevention Intervention through Network Mapping

How does one make relationships *visible*? This was the challenge I sought to address as I prepared for five weeks of field research in Senegal in late 2007. On my desk sat a pile of books on social network analysis. I read about the sophisticated statistical analyses made possible through network analysis: I learned that I could measure frequency of contact, the centrality and prestige of members of a network – or "nodes" in technical language (Wasserman and Faust, 1994, p. 169). Flipping through the pages, I thought to myself: "This is much more than I need." I wanted to understand more about the members of a network of individuals and organizations implementing the biannual Scenarios from Africa scriptwriting contest, an HIV prevention and awareness-raising intervention that was entering its seventh edition in Senegal. The contest was a complex several-month-long process involving dozens of organizations and individuals. There were organizations that provided HIV-related information to would-be contestants, organizations that distributed and collected submission forms, individuals who served as script-writing mentors and jury members who read and evaluated contestant submissions. I wanted to understand the extent of this "Scenarios" network. I was interested in learning who worked with whom and in what capacity. I did not intend to make claims about the centrality, prestige, or degree of connectedness of network members. In essence, I wanted to map rather than measure. For this reason, I call this tool "network mapping" rather than "network analysis." June Holley[9], a colleague well versed in social network analysis, including the latest available software, proposed a solution:

> Why not map the members of the network manually – that is, ask participants to draw nodes and connections on a piece of paper, rather than having them answer the lengthy electronic questionnaire that would be required to perform more sophisticated analyses? … After creating maps manually, you can use software to create a visual depiction of the network. You can create an image that makes relationships visible without using measurement indicators and performing statistical analyses. Ask people to depict the group of people they work with when implementing the contest.

In my notebook, I drew a simple diagram that had the research participant (RP) at the center and additional circles representing relationships.

Thinking aloud, I shared with June my understanding of how I could use network maps in Senegal. "I can ask research participants to map their "Scenarios" network – to draw all the people that they work with when implementing the Scenarios scriptwriting contest – placing themselves or their organization at the center."

"Yes, it's that simple," June confirmed.

And it was simple: simple and incredibly rewarding. Sitting in June Holley's kitchen, learning about the manual mapping of networks, I did not know that this research tool would yield much more than I had hoped. With the network-mapping exercise, not only was I able to make relationships visible, which was my main aim, but I was also able to ask detailed questions about the nature and genesis of network member relationships. "So, you met this person here (pointing to a node on the network map) while serving as a jury member?" "And have you worked with the person since then in a different context?" With questions like these I discovered that individuals who met each other while implementing the contest in some cases continued collaborating long after the contest was over. I also learned the extent to which the contest served as a bridge between organizations that were working in the same city or village and often knew one another, but had not previously collaborated. The contest, I learned, often provided the occasion for individuals and organizations to get to know one another and eventually to even help one another professionally. The map below depicts a network featuring a relationship of this nature.

The network map shown in Figure 17.7 was created by Abdoulaye Konaty, a Program Associate with Africa Consultants International, a nongovernmental organization (NGO)

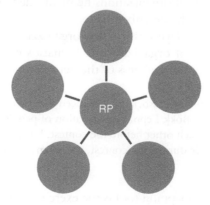

Figure 17.6 The research participant at the center of his or her "Scenarios" network.

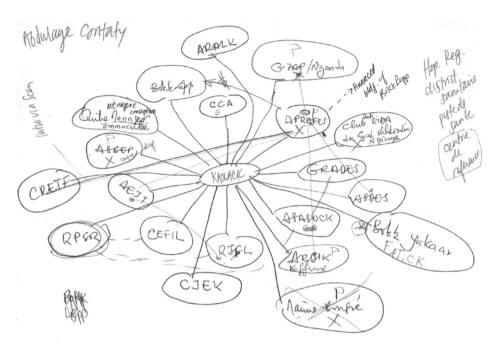

Figure 17.7   Hand-drawn network map.

based in Dakar, Senegal, which has helped to implement the Scenarios contest since its inception in 1997. As he drew his map, Abdoulaye described the relationships he had formed with organizations in Kaolack, the city he worked in most often when not in the capital. After he drew the nodes representing the organizations he worked with on the Scenarios contest, I asked him: "And were any of these organizations already in contact with one another prior to implementing the Scenarios contest?" On his map, he drew lines between several of the circles, each circle representing an organization, and each connecting line representing an existing relationship. As Abdoulaye discussed the organizations on his network map, I was glad to have the visual reference on the paper in front of us given the sheer number of organizations he mentioned and the complexity of the different types of relationships he described.

One question I asked Abdoulaye was whether organizations had begun collaborating with one another as a result of organizing the Scenarios contest. His response highlighted the strength and also the weakness of the network-mapping tool. He said:

> This organization here, a women's association, financed the construction of a new office for this other organization here, Bokk Lepp, an association of people living with HIV/AIDS. I do not know if they knew each other before the contest, but I do know that, as a result of getting to know one another during the contest, the women's association has invested in Bokk Lepp.

The strength of the network-mapping tool is the exercise of making relationships visible and then having a reference point for discussions and further comments about those relationships. The weakness of the tool is that a network map is only as complete and precise as the memory and awareness of its creator. For example, to know whether the women's association and Bokk Lepp knew one another prior to the Scenarios contest, I would need to ask follow-up questions with those organizations. Because I had chosen not to pursue or triangulate chronological details, I was limited in the claims I could make about causality or the precise sequence of events in many cases. As with other network-mapping exercises I conducted with research participants in Senegal, having a visual referent was a great asset during interview. Research participants often returned to the map to add or clarify information as our conversation continued. When the interviews were all completed, I used Smart Network Analyzer[10] software to create a "master" network map of organizations and individuals involved in implementing the Scenarios contest in Senegal (see Figure 17.8).

Practical issues

When I asked research participants to map their Scenarios-related networks, I began by demonstrating what a map might look like by drawing an example. I said:

> For example, if I was mapping my own personal network of the people I interact with in a given week, I would draw a circle in the center, like this (*I draw a circle and put my name in the middle of it*), and then I would add circles for each person or group of people I come into contact with on a weekly basis. So I might have a circle for my family, and then a circle for people at my office, etc. And each circle is connected to me with a line, like this (*I connect each circle to the circle with my name in it at the center*).

When research participants began drawing, they often began narrating details about each relationship. I digitally recorded the mapping exercise so that I could keep a good record of the details of each relationship discussed. The maps tended to be most complete when I did not ask questions while the research participants were drawing their initial maps. When the person stopped and seemed prepared to set the pen down, I often asked clarification questions or requested more detail. For example, Abdoulaye Konaty used many acronyms for organizations I was not familiar with. I asked him to say the full name of each organization so I could listen to the digital recording afterward and make note of each full name. I also asked questions about the nature of relationships. For example, "Were any of these organizations already in contact with one another prior to implementing the Scenarios contest?" as discussed earlier. In the early stages of my research, when I asked clarification or "nature of relationship" questions while the research participants were still mapping, I perceived that my questions were distracting. When I did not interrupt the initial mapping process, I felt that the conversations flowed more easily. Beyond not interrupting with questions, I was also careful to provide research participants with ample time to think before asking any questions. My silence was often rewarded when research participants added to their maps after long periods of reflection. On some occasions, I asked the research participants if they minded if I made notes directly on their maps. In the case of Abdoulaye Konaty's map, for example, I drew an arrow connecting the women's association with the association of people living with

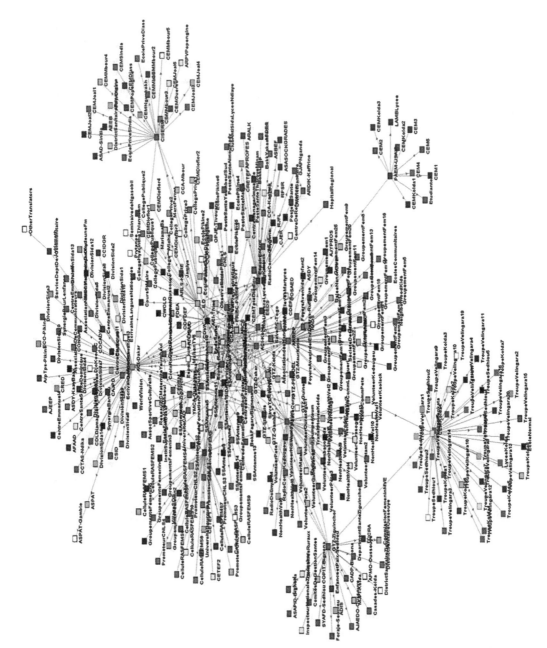

Figure 17.8 Network maps, compiled and entered in "Smart Network Analyzer" software.

HIV/AIDS, together with a dollar sign (a very North American symbol) to signal the relationship between the two organizations that had emerged as a result of collaborating on the Scenarios contest. If I had made note of this in a notebook rather than on the map directly, I would later have to match my separate notes with the network map and also the digital recording to recall the full story.

The utility of network mapping

Network mapping is useful both as a visual record and also as a tool to get more detailed information about relationships. In other words, network mapping is useful as both product and process. The map itself can be used as a visual display in a research report or article; it can also be combined with other maps to depict a larger network; and it can serve as an ongoing visual reference during an interview to access in-depth information about relationships among members of a network. Network mapping is appropriate when the object of research is to learn about the extent of a given network, but is not sufficient if the object is to measure and quantify relationships between network members. During the mapping exercise, the researcher can ask questions about the nature of a relationship but the responses will be qualitative and descriptive in nature. A standardized questionnaire would be required if the object of the study is to measure and perform statistical analyses on the relationships between members of a network. The network-mapping tool is ideal for learning about relationships or the size and nature of a network. In addition, the mapping exercise yields visual documentation that can supplement the written research report or article. Network mapping is ideal for understanding the extent and composition of relationship networks. The tool has great potential for understanding processes that involve multiple actors working in a decentralized fashion.

Life Mapping

I learned about the life-mapping tool in an informal meeting with Jerry and Monique Sternin, founders of the Positive Deviance Initiative, an organization that specializes in community inquiry for social change.[11] I had told Monique that I was beginning a study about health among women in Appalachia and was seeking a very open-ended interview protocol based on some study design advice I had received. I told Monique: "A colleague suggested to me that if I ask about health I will find out *only* about health.[12] I am thus seeking to broaden my approach, to 'cast a wider net' to see if health is a topic of interest and relevance to research participants themselves." Monique suggested life-history interviews.[13] She explained that by asking women broad questions about their life I would discover whether or not health issues were deemed central by participants. She added: "And you can begin each interview with a life map." I had never heard of a life map and so I asked Monique for more details. She began drawing an example on a napkin. As she drew, she explained:

> It's the "map" of a life charted on a very simple graph. You draw a happy face at the top of a vertical axis and sad face at the bottom of a vertical axis. You can also use positive and negative symbols if you prefer. Then you draw a horizontal axis with various points representing

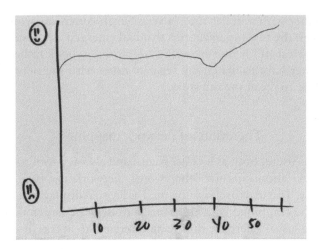

Figure 17.9   Tammi's life map.

decades or half decades, depending on the age of the interviewee. You ask the person to draw a line from left to write, starting with childhood and stopping at their current age. They can begin anywhere they like along the vertical "happiness" axis, and they should chart the high points and low points they have had over the years. The result is a visual rendering of the interviewee's own life as they choose to depict it.

After Monique's explanation I thanked her and carefully stored the napkin. I recall thinking: "This is really great but I have no formal reference for this tool. How will I cite this napkin?" When my study on women and health in Appalachia began I decided to put citation concerns aside and give the tool a try. I used it at the end of my interview with Tammi,[14] a woman in her late forties. Tammi had been telling me about various aspects of her life but the topic of health had yet to emerge. What follows is an excerpt of the transcript of one of my first experiences using the life-mapping tool.

> ME: It's called a life map...here's an example...This represents the good times up here (*pointing to a happy face*) and *this* is the represents the bad times...you sort of chart the highs and lows across the years, which run along this axis down here (*pointing to the line marked with decades along the bottom of the page*).

I passed Tammi the paper with the blank graph. She picked up a pen and began to draw. As she drew, Tammi narrated her map.

> TAMMI: I would say that up until here (*pointing to a dip at the 40-year mark*) I had just a little down, and then I'm up. I'm always up. Am I not? (*This last comment was directed to her son, who was sitting nearby*)
>
> ME: And what does this represent? (*pointing to the dip*)
>
> TAMMI: When I had cancer...when I found out.
>
> ME: It's not a very big dip...
>
> TAMMI: Because I never let it take me down. Did I? (*to her son*) I never let it take me down.

The life-mapping exercise with Tammi taught me that, although I had not asked directly about health, the issue of health, in this case breast cancer, was a major event in her life. The mapping exercise also taught me that Tammi was determined to fight her cancer and maintain a positive attitude. The life map is as much about Tammi's life as it is about the version of her life story that Tammi *wanted* to tell. When she discussed her cancer diagnosis she did so very briefly, and she hastened to stress her optimism. Would Tammi's map have been different if her son had not been in the room? It is hard to tell. The mapping exercise is not designed to access objective, verifiable information: it is designed to allow research participants to share their preferred life story in a visual way. The map is a starting point. Follow-up questions invite further explanation: "What happened here?" "What can you say about this high point here?" The questions are designed to elicit additional details from research participants. They are not designed to challenge or verify the participant's preferred rendering of their life.

I found that the life-mapping exercise richly complemented life-history interviews. Often, the maps contained information that had not already been discussed in the interview. I believe that asking participants to portray their life visually, and only afterwards with words, added texture and depth to their stories. The maps themselves provided a visual record of each participant's preferred life story that complemented their oral accounts. Given the broad, open-ended questions I had asked my research participants I was not surprised that health was only one of many topics they discussed. In that sense, the life-history interview and the life-mapping exercise were not the most direct way to inquire about health. The end result, however, was that when research participants did talk about health, it was because it was a topic that mattered to *them* – a topic they chose to discuss, on their own terms. The life-mapping tool, used in conjunction with any kind of interview, adds a biographical and visual chronology from the perspective of the research participant. This tool, like the network map, is both process and product. Conducting the exercise can lead to rich accounts from research participants and it yields a visual illustration of those accounts.

Practical issues

As with the network-mapping exercise, I found that research participants were more at ease when I did not ask questions while they created their maps. On most occasions, participants finished their maps in less than one minute. I learned to wait, without speaking. I waited until the research participant looked up from their map and I gave them the first opportunity to speak. Many simply asked: "Now what?" Upon which I asked various questions about the points on the map. Others began narrating as soon as they began to draw. Still others finished their maps and explained the highs and lows without prompting from me. All of the maps created by research participants in my study either depicted new information or provided greater detail about previously discussed topics. I was once asked by an acquaintance who knew of my study whether I had done the mapping exercise myself. "You mean, have I done my *own* life map?" I asked. "Yes," they responded. "And if you have not done one, I think it would be a good idea if you did." I agreed and immediately realized how difficult an exercise it actually is. The deceptively simple "happiness" axis caused me deep pause. When have I been most happy? What about least happy? As my acquaintance waited for me to finish and begin narrating my map I began to feel anxious. Did I know this person well enough to discuss the death of my mother? Should I deliberately ignore that "valley" and stick to a straight line? I recount my own experience with the life-mapping exercise as a cautionary tale. Life maps can get personal. It is therefore important to establish some level of rapport with research participants before beginning and it is equally important to tell them that the exercise is optional. In the case of my own study, none of the participants refused to draw a life map. Without exception, they charted the version of their life they were ready and willing to share.

The utility of life mapping

The life map is a tool that goes nicely with life-history interviews. It can also be used to provide biographical information to complement more specific studies. The map can be tailored to access information about a fixed period in a given life. One can ask about "adolescence," "student years," "life since motherhood," or "life since diagnosis," in the case of a health study. The important thing to remember is that the life map is a tool put in the hands of the research participant: the map they create is their unique and subjective perspective. It is a visual rendering of their own perspective that they have *chosen* to share. Including life map images along with transcriptions of interviews is one way to ensure that research participants get to interpret and illustrate their *own* stories, and that they have the opportunity to convey what events matter most to them. The researcher is then free to add analysis or a different interpretation of what the participant has chosen to share. In the case of my interview with Tammi, it was her narration of her life map that kept me from focusing exclusively on the breast cancer aspect of her story. She chose to minimize its important in her life. What right did I have to make it my focus? Life maps are visual complements to an interview. Including them in research reports ensures that participants' stories, as they themselves tell them, remain present and visible.

In Summary

During my own research experiences, the four tools presented here have performed a "double duty." Each tool led to useful visual evidence, sketches depicting preferred themes in the case of radio listeners, photos of important objects or spaces in the case of the go-along, and charted relationships and life events in the case of the network and life maps. For the studies I describe in this chapter, these tools were at the center of my research design, and each tool complemented traditional "sit down" interviews. On each occasion, I found that both the process of using the tool and the product generated from the tool were extremely useful. Each tool generates a visual reference that can serve as a catalyst for discussion and that visual reference becomes a record that can be included in the research report or article. The question of which tool, or which combination of tools, should be used depends on the objective of the study and the willingness of research participants to respond to questions in new ways.

For research exploring the subjective experience and preferences of research participants, sketching can be useful. Augusto Boal once asked residents of Lima Peru to respond in photos to the question: "What is exploitation?" (Boal, 1979, p. 125). The photograph-responses demonstrated that each participant, as a result of their own personal experience, had a different vision of exploitation to offer. The question "What is exploitation?" would also work well with sketching. The results would likely be as diverse as the photograph-responses submitted during Boal's exercise. Any question about personal experience or perspective can be fruitfully answered with a sketch. For example: "What is your life like as a University student?" "What was the most important theme, for you, of the radio (or television) soap opera?" "What does happiness look like to you?" "How would you depict a healthy life?" The answers to these questions enable the researcher to learn about the world as seen through the eyes of the research participant. The explanation of the sketch by the research participant ensures that all the elements of a sketch are made clear, such as the use of color or symbols. Further, the narrative accompanying the sketch provides insight into the participant's own interpretation of their image.

The ethnographic go-along is essentially a mobile interview. If a researcher wants to understand the daily activities of someone, and those activities involve movement, a go-along is a perfect tool. For example, to understand what is involved in the work of a letter-carrier, the best way to learn this would be to "go-along" on a mail route. Not only would the letter-carrier explain the ins and outs of delivering mail, but the researcher would experience things for herself: she would feel the rain, walk the distance, see threatening dogs, and listen to the conversations with residents. The objects and places seen by the researcher and participants together become subjects of discussion and further inquiry. In a "sit down" interview, the postal worker may not remember or may not think to comment upon the smaller details of their day to day experience. The go-along allows the researcher and participants to experience and see things together. If the researcher sees something unfamiliar to them, they only need to ask: "What is that?" and they have a local guide on hand to answer.

The network map is useful for documenting and exploring relationships. The initial mapping exercise documents the relationships and the follow-up questions allow the exploration. For example, if I wanted to understand the relationships between workers in an office, I could ask an office worker to draw a map depicting everyone they work with during a typical week. The drawn network can serve as a reference point for a series of follow-up questions, such as: "Who on this map do you work with most often?" "Who is the first person on this map that you would go to if you needed advice?" "Is there anyone that is *not* on your map but you would like them to be?" The answers to these questions will give insight into the working relationships that exist in an office. After doing a series of individual maps one might learn that the accountant is the one person in the office that everyone sees reliably each week or that no one in the office sees the vice-president of the company but several would like to. In any study where relationships and interaction are of interest, the network map can be useful.

The life map is a tool that helps the researcher explore biographical details and events over a given period of time ranging from an entire life to one slice of life. I found that, when used at the end of a life-history interview, the life-mapping tool can provide an additional layer of information that may or may not have emerged during conversation. When participants chart the "highs and lows" of a given period, these points on the map, as well as the participants' perspectives on them, become the subject of further inquiry. For example, when Tammi charted a low point on her map at the age when she was diagnosed with cancer, I remarked to her: "This is not a very big dip." Her response illustrated her optimism in the face of her diagnosis. The life map tool helped me learn about a major event in Tammi's life and also about her desire to portray it as *not* major. Before using the life map tool with others, it is a good idea for researchers to chart their own life. The self-life-mapping experience will help underscore that the tool gives insight into how participants' see and want to portray their life. As philosopher Alfred Korzybski (1995[1941]) once famously said: "The map *is not* the territory it represents" (p. 58). A life map is not a life; it is the research participant's preferred representation of that life.

The best way to learn about the potential of each of these tools is to try them. An easy way for a researcher to begin is to start with their own experience. Think about what you would draw if someone asked you to depict "health." Walk through your workplace or another place you frequent and think about how you would explain it to another person. Which spaces would you point out and which would not merit your attention? Map your relationships. Map your life. Then think about how you would narrate your maps. Next, try the tools out on a friend or colleague. Practice remaining silent as respondents discuss their drawing or map: let the respondent fill the empty space you have created as a silent listener. When designing your next research study consider how the tools discussed in this chapter can complement the standard qualitative interview in the ways shown in Figure 17.1.

Each of these tools allows researchers to gain insight into the subjective experience and perspective of the research participant. Whether moving through space, as with the ethnographic go-along, or using participant sketches and maps as a visual reference and catalyst for discussion, these participatory research tools can be a valuable complement to other qualitative research methods. Their greatest strengths, beyond those listed above, are the freedom they accord respondents in the crafting of their responses and the invitation they extend to respondents to be the first to interpret and analyze what they choose to share with the researcher. When using these tools, the role of the researcher is to listen, and follow, as participants take the lead.

Table 17.1 Four participatory research tools, each with a different strength.

Tool	Strength
Ethnographic go-along	Adds dimensions of space and interaction to interview.
Sketching	Allows respondent to depict and narrate their own perspectives.
Network map	Makes relationships of respondent visible and available for comment and analysis.
Life map	Allows respondent to identify and narrate important moments of their life, both good and bad.

Acknowledgments

The author gratefully acknowledges the contributions of research team members Dr. Arvind Singhal of the University of Texas, El Paso, and Sarah Hurlburt, formerly of Population Media Center, currently a Program Manager at Boston University's Center for Global Health and Development. I would also like to acknowledge the guidance of my "methods mentor," Dr. Devika Chawla, and the financial support provided by the Department of Communication Studies, the African Studies Program and the Office of the Vice President for Research at Ohio University.

Notes

1 This list is adapted from Chambers (1994, p. 965).
2 I describe the life map tool, albeit very briefly, in Greiner (2010).
3 The radio soap opera, *Ashreat Al Amal* (Sails of hope), was implemented by the Population Media Center (PMC) with financial support from the David and Lucille Packard Foundation. Our research team included PMC staff member Sarah Hurlburt and Dr. Arvind Singhal, an expert in the field of Entertainment Education. Our research would not have been possible without the skills and patience of our team of interpreters, Diana William, Walaa Ali Mohamed, Hamid, Abd Alraheim Abusibah, Ibrahim Abd Ulghani Mohammed, Bassam Abubakr, and Amna Ahmed.
4 The use of participatory photography in research has received extensive academic attention and for this reason I do not discuss it in this chapter. For information on this visual method, see: Wang and Burris, 1994; Wang, Burris, and Xiang, 1996; Moss, 1999; Wang, 1999, 2003; Singhal and Devi, 2003.
5 This series, *Sa Pagsikat Ng Araw* (Hope after the dawn), was implemented by Population Media Center with financial support from the United Nations Population Fund (UNFPA). This evaluation was conducted by Dr. Arvind Singhal, Dr. Elizabeth Rattine-Flaherty, and Molly A. Mayer. See http://www.populationmedia.org/where/philippines/
6 Thank you to Professor Jesus Arroyave and his Communication for Social Change masters students at the Universidad del Norte in Barranquilla, Colombia who participated in this exercise. And a special thanks to Professor Jair Vega who showed me that when research participants are asked to draw they can rebel and make a collage/sculpture instead.
7 The VAHPS implemented organizational principles and error reduction measures with a Toyota Production Systems (TPS) intervention, inspired by innovations in manufacturing, complemented subsequently with the Positive Deviance (PD) approach, a process that begins with identifying community members (in this case, hospital staff members) that are already practicing the desired behavior (in this case, effective infection control measures). See http://www.positivedeviance.org/
8 Special thanks VAPHS staff members Dr. Rajiv Jain, Dr. Bob Muder, Dr. Jon Lloyd, Cheryl Creen, Candice Cunningham, Jennifer Scott, Edward Yates, Glen Buzelli, Donna Luck, Kathleen Risa, Dora Gentile, Kathy Hill, Joyce Ewing and Tanice Smith and to Monique Sternin of the Positive Deviance Initiative.
9 June Holley is the founder of the Appalachian Center for Economic Networks (ACEnet), a committed "network weaver," and a generous mentor. I am grateful to June for her assistance and encouragement.

10   Smart Network Analyzer software was developed by June Holley and Valdis Krebs. For more information, see http://www.networkweaver.com/networkservices/index.html

11   See: http://www.positivedeviance.org/

12   I thank Dr. Devika Chawla for this perceptive observation.

13   The life-history (sometimes called "life-story") interview is a biographical approach to inquiry in which the research participant responds to very open-ended questions about their life. For example: "What do you remember about your early childhood years?" Research participants select and recount the moments of their life that are most salient to them. In his book *The Life Story Interview*, Robert Atkinson (1998) describes the life-story interview as a way to learn about how people see themselves and how they want to be seen. For more information on the life-history method in health-related setting, see Goldman *et al.* (2003).

14   "Tammi" is a pseudonym.

References

Airhihenbuwa, C. (1995). *Health and Culture: Beyond the Western Paradigm*. Thousand Oaks, CA: Sage.

Argawal, B. (2001). Participatory exclusions, community forestry and gender: An analysis for South Asia and a conceptual framework. *World Development, 29*(10): 1623–1648.

Arnstein, S. (1969). A ladder of citizen participation. *AIP Journal*, July, 216–224.

Atkinson, R. (1998). *The Life Story Interview*. Thousand Oaks, CA: Sage.

Boal, A. (1979). *Theater of the Oppressed* London: Pluto Press.

Chambers, R. (1992). Rural appraisal: Rapid, relaxed and participatory. *IDS Working Paper* 311, Brighton: IDS.

Chambers, R. (1994). The origins and practice of participatory rural appraisal. *World Development, 22*(7), 953–969.

Chambers, R. (1997). *Whose Reality Counts? Putting the First Last*. London, UK: Intermediate Technology Publications.

De Koning, K., and Martin, M. (1996). *Participatory Research in Health: Issues and Experiences*. London: Zed Books.

Fals-Borda, O. (1987). The application of participatory action-research in Latin America, *International Sociology, 2*(4): 329–347.

Goldman, R., Hunt, M. K., Allen, J. D. *et al.* (2003). The life history interview method: Applications to intervention development. *Health Education and Behavior, 30*(5), 564–581.

Greiner, K. (2010). Coming in from the margin: Research practices, representation and the ordinary. *The Qualitative Report, 15*(5), 1191–1208.

Greiner, K., Singhal, A., and Hurlburt, S. (2007). With an antenna we can stop the practice of female genital cutting: A participatory assessment of *Ashreat al Amal*, an entertainment-education radio soap opera in Sudan, *Investigacion y Desarollo, 15*(2), 226–259.

Korzybski A. (1995[1941]). *Science and Sanity: An Introduction to non-Aristotelian Systems and General Semantics*. Lakeville, CN: International Non-Aristotelian Library Publishing.

Kusenbach, M. (2003). Street phenomenology: The go-along as ethnographic research tool. *Ethnography 4*, 455–485.

Moss, T. (1999). 'Photovoice', *Children First, 3*(26), 28–29.

Singhal, A., and Devi, K. (2003). Visual voices in participatory communication, *Communicator 37*, 1–15.

Singhal, A., and Durá, L. (2010). *Protecting Children from Exploitation and Trafficking: Using the Positive Deviance Approach in Uganda and Indonesia.* Westport, CT: Save the Children Federation.

Singhal, A. and Greiner, K. (2007). Do what you can, with what you have, where you are: A quest to eliminate MRSA at the VA Pittsburgh Healthcare System, *Plexus Institute Deeper Learning Series, 1*(4), 1–12.

Singhal, A. and Rattine-Flaherty, E, (2006). Pencils and photos as tools of communicative research and praxis: Analyzing Minga Perú's quest for social justice in the Amazon. *Gazette, 68*(4), 313–330.

Singhal, A., Rattine-Flaherty, E., and Mayer, M. A. (2010). Can communication be socially responsible and commercially viable? An assessment of *Sa Pagsikat Ng Araw*, an entertainment education radio series in the Phillipines. In M. B. Hinner (Ed.). *The Interrelationship of Business and Communication* (pp. 331–347). Berlin, Germany: Peter Lang.

Wang, C. (1999). Photovoice: A participatory action research strategy applied to women's health. *Journal of Women's Health, 8*(2), 185–92.

Wang, C. (2003). Using Photovoice as a participatory assessment and issue selection tool: A case study with homeless in Ann Arbor. In M. Minkler and N. Wallerstein (Eds.), *Community-Based Participatory Health Research* (pp. 179–195). San Francisco, CA: Jossey-Bass.

Wang, C. and Burris, M. (1994). Empowerment through photo novella: Portraits of participation. *Health Education Quarterly, 21*(2), 171–186.

Wang, C., Burris, M., and Xiang, Y. P. (1996). Chinese village women as visual anthropologists: A participatory approach to reaching policy-makers, *Social Science and Medicine, 42*(10), 1391–1400.

Wasserman, S. and Faust, K. (1994). *Social Network Analysis: Methods and Applications,* Cambridge: Cambridge University Press.

18

Egypt's *Mabrouk!* Initiative
A Communication Strategy for Maternal/Child Health and Family Planning Integration

Ron Hess, Dominique Meekers, and J. Douglas Storey

Q: Are you using the *Mabrouk* book?
A: Using it? We're living by it!

(One of the original 2004 Minya newlywed wives, one year later)

Introduction

One of the most successful domains of health communication globally over the past 30 years has been in the area of fertility management. Many low-income countries have initiated family planning programs since the 1970s that have resulted in smaller family sizes, longer intervals between births, and slower population growth rates. With fewer births and more time between them, maternal and child health have also improved, aided by improved access to affordable health services. However, in many low-income countries that saw initial gains, the pace of the fertility decline has slowed, leveling off above replacement level. At the same time, maternal and neonatal morbidity and mortality levels in many of those countries remain unacceptably high, underscoring the challenge of sustainable change in public health.

This chapter describes the *Communication for Healthy Living* (CHL) project in Egypt.[1] CHL was part of the larger Health Communication Partnership (HCP), which was the flagship global communication project supported by the United States Agency for International Development (USAID). The CHL project in Egypt was a national effort that used a strategic, life-stage approach to design an integrated maternal and child health (MCH) and family planning (FP) communication program, resulting in improved health outcomes among young couples. The project implemented a full-scale national

The Handbook of Global Health Communication, First Edition. Edited by Rafael Obregon and Silvio Waisbord.
© 2012 John Wiley & Sons, Inc. Published 2012 by John Wiley & Sons, Inc.

and community-based communication campaign – supported by advocacy, capacity building, and coordination with service delivery – to address the health needs of family members in various life stages, with a special emphasis on newlywed and young couples. This emphasis was named the *Mabrouk!* Initiative using the Arabic word for "congratulations" to reflect the celebratory spirit of the key life events, marriage, childbirth, successful birth spacing, and child raising, while emphasizing the promise of a lifetime of family health. Given the complexity of the project, we will first describe its demographic context, as well as the conceptual and systematic approaches used in its design, implementation and evaluation, before turning to the specifics of the interventions and evidence of their impact.

The Egyptian Context

Although Egypt has been described as a low health-care spender (WHO, Regional Office for the Eastern Mediterranean, 2006), it has worked closely with international agencies and donors over many years to curb its population growth rate and to improve the health of its population. The main international donor is the United States Agency for International Development (USAID), which has provided assistance to Egypt in the areas of population and health since 1977. By 2010, USAID had obligated an estimated $1.5 billion (2010 Presentation by James Bever, USAID-Egypt Mission Director) to help achieve Egypt's strategic objectives in population and health. During the past three decades, Egypt has expanded the number of available health facilities, and most of the population now has access to affordable basic health services. The country has achieved substantial reductions in mortality rates, and has improved control of infectious diseases. It has also made major progress in reducing fertility and population growth rates (USAID, Office of Inspector General, 2006; WHO Regional Office for the Eastern Mediterranean, 2006).

Recognizing the strains that a burgeoning population creates on clean water, educational systems, and other resources, Egypt has long prioritized the management of population growth. It has had a family planning program since the 1960s. An extensive network of public, semi-public, and private outlets provide family planning services. In the public sector alone, over 4,470 public sector family planning clinics provide services at nominal fees (Adbel-Tawab and Roter, 2002; Ministry of Health and Population, Egypt, El-Zanaty and Associates, and ORC Macro, 2003, p. 94). Additionally, since the early 1980s the government of Egypt, in partnership with USAID, has consistently supported national-scale family planning information, education, and communication programs (Robinson and El-Zanaty, 2006) with the aim of achieving replacement level fertility by the year 2015 (USAID, Office of Inspector General, 2006).

Survey data show that the total fertility rate declined from 5.3 children per woman in 1980 to 3.5 in 2000 and to 3.0 in 2008, the most recent year for which national data are available (El-Zanaty and Way, 2009; Robinson and El-Zanaty, 2006; USAID, 2009; Vignoli, 2006). The same 2008 data show that 67 percent of currently married women were recently exposed to family planning messages (mostly from television) and that 60 percent are currently using a method of family planning. The 2008 data also show that 82 percent of eligible women have used family planning at some point, and that 87 percent of demand for contraceptive services has been satisfied (El-Zanaty and Way, 2009).

Demand for any service such as family planning can be represented as a primary demand curve (Rothschild, 1999), and progress toward satisfaction of that demand can be conceptualized in stages, as illustrated by Rogers' (1983) S-shaped diffusion curve. According to Rogers' stages of adoption, Egypt's demand for contraception has reached an advanced stage. With 87 percent of demand satisfied, family planning has become a well-established norm. The remaining population of nonusers of contraception includes both the pool of potential new users and those who have discontinued family planning use but still wish to delay or limit childbearing. Potential new users include the large group entering their reproductive life stage as well as potential "late adopters" from among challenged, hard-to-reach populations – often from rural or poor urban communities. Discontinuers are distributed throughout the population.

As with any enterprise, Egypt's family planning program must attract new clients and retain old ones. Attracting new clients from among the very late adopters is especially challenging, but Egypt's family planning program must overcome this challenge to achieve its goals of reaching replacement-level fertility and sustaining FP adoption and use. Robinson and El-Zanaty (2006, p. 123) identify a threefold approach to closing the remaining demand gaps in this mature market: (1) encouraging young, low-parity couples to delay childbirth and increase birth-spacing (emerging prospects); (2) encouraging existing users who have achieved their desired family size to maintain contraceptive use and reduce discontinuation (retaining customers); and (3) encouraging adoption among rural or poor urban nonusers (challenged, or underserved groups).

The *Mabrouk!* Initiative seeks, in some measure, to address all three of these goals, but prioritizes a focus on young couples entering the childbearing stage – an audience segment that we refer to as the *young family cohort* (YFC).

Conceptual Approach

The *Mabrouk!* Initiative was designed carefully and systematically according to the principles of the P-Process (Health Communication Partnership, 2003; Piotrow *et al.*, 1997), an iterative approach that progresses in stages from Situation and Audience Analysis to Strategic Design and Development to Implementation and Evaluation. The tools of analysis were drawn from the fields of public health as well as marketing communication.

Role of theory

Health competence. It is increasingly recognized that to achieve enduring, sustained demand for good health, the population must be *health-competent*. The health competence approach derives from the call by WHO, as early as the 1950s, for a shift in thinking toward health as "a state of complete mental, physical and social well-being and not merely the absence of disease" (WHO, 2006, p. 1). Building on the concepts of social capital and health literacy, Storey, Kaggwa, and Harbour (2008, p. 2) define health competence as "having the knowledge, attitudes, skills, and resources to act consistently and appropriately across multiple health behaviors."

In their analysis of data from Egypt and South Africa, Storey, Kaggwa, and Harbour (2008) found that individuals with basic health knowledge about causes of disease and wellness, positive attitudes toward preventive health, and access to health information and social support were more likely than individuals without those assets to display not just single disease-specific behaviors but to perform better across a spectrum of family health actions (in the case of Egypt) or of HIV/AIDS prevention actions (in the case of South Africa). But it is not enough for health programs to create health-competent *individuals;* they need to help create health-competent *households* and *communities* within which individuals live. This, in turn, requires a fundamental shift toward the view that households, not health care systems, are the primary producers of health. Households become health-competent when they are enabled to mobilize the resources they need – including information, social support, and greater control – in order to make health decisions consistently and gain greater ownership over positive household health outcomes.

While building health-competent societies is a challenging task, especially in contexts with limited resources and relatively low levels of education, strategic health communication programs are ideally positioned to help accelerate the process. Strategic health communication programs, designed in accord with communication theory, are based on evidence, oriented toward results, and implemented, monitored, and evaluated using the best practices from communication, epidemiology, demography, and other subfields of public health.

Communication theory. Health-competence communication builds on elements of various social science theories commonly used to predict health behavior (Edberg, 2007; Glanz, Rimer, and Viswanath, 2008). It also draws on theories at levels of aggregation above the individual level, including newer versions of health literacy (e.g., Kickbusch and Nutbeam, 1998) and social capital (e.g., Kawachi, Kennedy, and Lochner, 1997) that describe elements of capacity to respond to health challenges and characteristics of social organizations that "combine to facilitate cooperation among people for their mutual benefit" (Putnam, 1993, p. 36).

Putnam (1993, 2001), for example, identifying these facilitating traits, focuses on trust and reciprocity among group members (cognitive dimensions), but also on patterns and levels of participation in groups (a structural dimension). Health competence also draws on the model of Participatory Communication for Development and Social Change (Kincaid and Figueroa, 2009), which is built around the process of community dialogue leading to collective action and draws from a broad literature on development communication, particularly the work of Latin American theorists (Beltrán, 1974; Díaz-Bordenave, 1994), as well as theories of group dynamics, conflict resolution, networks/convergence, leadership and equity (see, e.g., Chemers, 2000; Gumucio-Dagrón, 2001; Lord and Brown, 2004; Moser, 1993; Senge, 1994; Stogdill, 1974; Tirmizi, 2002; White, 1994).

While different theories emphasize different aspects of social interaction, there is broad consensus that behavior is influenced by a combination of factors, such as the intent to perform the behavior, perceived and actual barriers and constraints, skills, attitudes, perceived social norms, self-efficacy and the influence of social networks (Salem *et al.*, 2008). Together, these conceptual elements helped inform analysis of the evidence base and the design of strategies, activities, and materials for the *Mabrouk!* Initiative from the beginning.

The marketing perspective. While public health tools and concepts help planners to analyze health issues at a population level, the marketing perspective emphasizes a view of the customer or client as an active partner in any health transaction, making decisions based on perceived value or benefit. Additionally, the marketing perspective focuses on return on investment, seeking to answer the question of where change can be achieved most cost-effectively, as well as on market readiness, to identify the margins of change where growth is most likely. The field of social marketing, which applies marketing principles to social goals is well elaborated elsewhere (Kotler, 1999; Kotler and Lee, 2008). Storey and colleagues (2008) describe the application of these principles to health behavior and health promotion.

Analysis

The audience

Data from the 2008 Egypt Demographic and Health Survey (EDHS) indicate that it is common for households to have members in several different life stages. Egyptian households are larger on average and somewhat more complex generationally than those in most Western countries. In rural Upper Egypt, 88 percent of households (n=4806) have a male head of household and an average of 5.8 residents (El-Zanaty and Way, 2009). Breaking down household members into five life stages,[2] we find that 91.6 percent of households include one or more ever-married older adults aged 30 or older; 39.9 percent include one or more married young adults aged 29 or younger; 53.1 percent include at least one never married person (most likely unmarried youth) over 15 years of age; 60.2 percent include one or more children aged 5–14; and 52.8 percent include one or more children below five years of age. Overall, 90 percent of the households in rural Upper Egypt have members in two or more different life stages. Over one-third of all households, 37 percent, have household members representing three different life stages; 25 percent have members presenting four different life stages; and 7 percent have members representing all five life stages.

Life-stage approaches to health communication are somewhat rare because funding streams tend to be vertical – aimed to achieve disease-specific objectives – rather than to cut across health areas. USAID, under its flagship global project – the Health Communication Partnership, of which CHL was a part – adopted an innovative cross-cutting communication design to see if such an approach could add value in terms of health outcomes across different health sectors as well as enhance the sustainability of health communication efforts. Another reason is the logistical challenges of an ambitious cross-cutting health program that not only addresses multiple health areas, but also simultaneously targets different life stages.

As a strategic entry point into the life stages of Egyptian households, the *Mabrouk!* Initiative selected the young family cohort (married couples under 30 years of age) as the primary audience segment, based on a variety of demographic and behavioral factors. Thirty-seven percent of married women fall into this category. Selection of this segment was guided by health need, as well as by considerations of market size, the long-term dividend on an investment in the health of young families, and readiness. The concept of "readiness" is vital to strategic communication for two main reasons: (1) because "change happens at the margins," a phenomenon well known in political communication circles, and widely observed in both the physical and social sciences (Kincaid, 2004); and (2) because communication empowers people to act rather than impels them. Communication-enabled change is voluntary, not coercive; if people find value in the offering and are ready, willing, and able, they are more likely to act.

The health issues

A complex and interrelated set of health issues confront new families. It has been widely recognized for some time that babies are more likely to survive if their mother gives birth less often and less frequently. Evidence is growing that the reverse may be true as well, that as more children in society survive, fertility rates go down (Udjo, 1997), underscoring how maternal and child health may be interconnected in ways we do not fully understand yet. Contraceptive use can reduce maternal and child morbidity and mortality and, conversely, successful outcomes in postpartum maternal and child health can influence family planning preferences and practices. The move toward lower fertility, or reduction in *quantity* of children may be driven in part by an increase in the *quality* of reproductive outcomes (increased child health and survival resulting in increased investment per child) (Becker, 1993; Robinson and El-Zanaty, 2006, p. 131). This complex interaction underlies, in our view, the integrated health competence approach adopted by the *Mabrouk!* Initiative.

Members of the YFC, if they have at least one child, in some ways represent more than one life stage. The couple itself faces the challenges of Young Marrieds around fertility planning, prenatal care, safe delivery, and postpartum care, while simultaneously facing the challenges of all adults, including smoking, nutrition, and other aspects of lifestyle health. Their children, of course, face the challenges of Early Childhood, particularly nutrition and immunization.

Family planning. Egypt's largest group of new FP users is young couples entering the childbearing stage. This demographic segment of young families is of vital importance to Egypt's future, due to its sheer magnitude and its great potential to affect Egypt's health status through the trends it sets in motion. More than 50 percent of Egypt's estimated 80 million people are under 25 years of age. It is at the stage of early adulthood and marriage when major reproductive health events begin, such as the onset of sexual activity and childbirth. Even in developed countries, the first pregnancy may be the very first time a young woman interacts with health services. Therefore, prenatal care provides an important opportunity to provide young adults with health education, including how to use contraceptives.

In Egypt, childbearing, as a rule, begins after marriage (Kashan, Baker, and Kenny, 2010; Population Council, 2010), and there are an estimated 1.2 million marriages per year (Minister of State for Family and Population, Mushira Khattab, personal communication, 2010). Nine out of ten married couples with no children say they want to have a child soon, so there is very little demand for delaying the first birth. However, six out of ten women with no children say they intend to use family planning *in the future* (El-Zanaty and Way, 2009), so the socially acceptable entry point for family planning is *after* the first birth, with 76 percent approving of the use of contraceptives at this stage. By contrast, only 1.2 percent consider it appropriate to use contraception before the first birth and less than half a percent of couples without children use contraception. However, after the first child is born, most Egyptian couples are ready, willing, and able to use contraception. This is the key point of market entry for family planning. Contraceptive use after the first birth, or at parity 1, has risen from 29 percent in 1995 to 35 percent in 2000, to 58 percent in 2008. El-Zanaty and Way (2009, p. 51) confirm that fertility has declined most rapidly among the 15–19 and 20–24 age groups. For example, between 1995 and 2008 (EDHS), the age-specific fertility rate for 15–24 year olds declined by 16 percent, but only by 12 percent among 25-34 year olds.

The second source of new contraceptive users comes from among the hard-to-reach populations that have lagged behind the national norm in contraceptive adoption, such as those in the economically disadvantaged or socially marginalized areas of urban slums or rural Upper Egypt. Though these areas still trail the national average on most indicators, in the last decade significant advances have helped to narrow the gap between the underserved areas, such as rural Upper Egypt, and the nation as a whole (El-Zanaty and Way, 2009). While the national contraceptive prevalence rate (the percentage of married women of reproductive age currently practicing family planning) has increased by 12.4 percent from 1995 to 2008, the rate in rural Upper Egypt has increased by 24.4 percent during the same period (El-Zanaty and Way, 2009).

Maternal and child health. In addition to advances in family planning, Egypt has achieved significant gains in maternal and child health (El-Ghazaly and Meekers, 2007; El-Zanaty and Way, 2009; Khalil and Roudi-Fahimi, 2004). The percentage of pregnancies for which regular antenatal care (four or more antenatal visits) was obtained increased from 28 percent in 1995 to 66 percent in 2008, and the percentage of medically assisted deliveries increased from 46 percent to 79 percent during the same period (El-Zanaty and Way, 2009). The coverage rates for child vaccinations are also very high (USAID, 2009). These changes have contributed to important declines in infant and child mortality. In 2008, the infant mortality rate was estimated at 24.5 deaths per 1,000 live births, and the under-five mortality rate at 28.3 per 1,000 live births (USAID, 2009). Although maternal mortality has decreased, it remains relatively high at 84 per 100,000 live births. The large majority of these maternal deaths are avoidable with sufficient prenatal care (Khalil and Roudi-Fahimi, 2004; USAID, 2009).

While recommended child vaccinations are nearly universal and full antenatal care coverage is increasing, not all aspects of family health receive the same degree of programmatic attention or are as widely addressed within households. Lifestyle diseases related to unhealthy diet, lack of exercise, and smoking make up an increasing proportion of the disease burden in Egypt (WHO Regional Office for the Eastern Mediterranean,

2006). Hence, there is an increasing need to integrate healthy lifestyle initiatives into larger efforts to improve family health and help move Egypt toward full health competence.

Health competence. Addressing the YFC for maternal and child health is vital to establishing positive health practices and health competence early, laying the foundation for a lifetime of family health. Hillary Clinton, in a 2010 United Nations Summit on the Millennium Development Goals (MDGs) endorsed a worldwide donor initiative aimed at improving MIYCN (Maternal, Infant and Young Child Nutrition) for the "First 1,000 Days" – the critical window for infant and child development, from conception to two years of age (–9 to +24 months) (Clinton, 2010). Programs that prepare young women for their first birth by promoting prenatal care, medically assisted delivery, and postnatal care, help to build the health competence of the young family cohort at a critical life stage and increase the likelihood of a pattern of healthy behaviors (Bandura, 2004) that will be sustained as the cohort ages and moves on to subsequent life stages. More health-competent parents, in turn, are more likely to consciously or unconsciously model health behaviors (e.g., handwashing, avoiding secondhand smoke, family planning, birth spacing), which has an educational effect on their children and results in more sustainable changes in family health patterns.

Integration across health issues. Integration across health issues is not a novel idea. For example, it has been fairly common practice for some programs to link family planning programs with post-abortion services (Youssef *et al.*, 2007) or with HIV prevention activities. The basic premise of many of these integrated programs is that a visit to a health care worker or facility for one specific health problem creates a unique opportunity for trained health professionals to also provide the client with information about other health issues. Such integrated approaches take advantage of existing face-to-face contact with trained health professionals. This is particularly important in developing country contexts where people do not always have good access to health information and services and where contacts with health care workers may be infrequent.[3] But many of these programs tend to focus almost exclusively on health services, or the supply side of health care. Few programs have tried to promote integration on the demand side of health, among the public.[4]

Typically, programs that focus on the demand side by promoting preventive and health-seeking behaviors among the public, have tended to focus on vertical health areas. For example, HIV prevention programs often focus on discouraging risky sexual behavior, increasing condom use, and promoting HIV testing. But very few programs are designed to address these issues in combination with other non-HIV-related health issues that individuals may face during their life course, and that families may have to deal with simultaneously, or in a relatively short time span.

One notable exception is the *Mabrouk!* Initiative, which was purposely designed to provide crosscutting communication support to increase positive behaviors and demand for services across a range of family health areas. The key maternal and child health goals addressed by the program were to increase prenatal care visits (including maternal nutrition), medically assisted delivery, neonatal birth weight, postpartum care (including immediate initiation of breastfeeding, use of contraception within two months of delivery), increased birth intervals, and infant health and nutrition. However, the health-competence platform on which the program was based allowed it to respond to other health issues as they emerged over time, including new activities related to second-hand smoke and smoking cessation, hepatitis-C, and avian influenza, among others. The next sections of the chapter describe the program strategy derived from this analysis, followed by a description of the program itself.

Strategic Design and Development

Based on this analysis of the situation and audiences in Egypt, the *Communication for Healthy Living* project selected the following two crosscutting goals:

1   To improve health outcomes in the areas of family planning and reproductive health, maternal and child health, and other public health threats, including infectious disease (avian and pandemic influenza, viral hepatitis, safe injection practices, and hygiene) and noncommunicable diseases or /healthy lifestyles (tobacco, breast cancer, cardiovascular disease, and diabetes).
2   To improve the capacity and sustainability of health communication programs in the public, NGO, and commercial sectors, as well as to establish enduring public demand for good health (Center for Communication Programs, Johns Hopkins University, 2010; Communication Initiative, 2005; Johns Hopkins University, 2005a).

The conceptual framework that was used to design the CHL project is based on three main guiding principles:

Households are primary producers of health. Families use their knowledge and information about health, and their access to services in the communities where they live, to avert risk, prevent illness, and stay healthy, thus "producing" their own health on a daily basis. Because such health decisions are made at the household level, it is essential to give ownership of "good health" to the families themselves.

Program activities and messages must be crosscutting and integrated. Because health information and messages from vertically funded service delivery programs converge at the household level, it is important to develop crosscutting messages and integrated programs that address fundamental household health needs. A unified health approach that promotes positive behaviors across the health domain can produce both synergistic outcomes across health areas and longitudinal gains in positive health effects. Integration of this type requires a multisectoral program that draws on the respective strengths of the public sector, the NGO sector, and the private sector. It also requires a multifaceted media campaign that uses a wide range of communication channels (including forms of mass media and forms of interpersonal communication).

Sustainability should be built into the system. The capacity of the health communication system as a whole must be strengthened. This includes building up: the essential capacity of households to access information, seek services, and practice healthy behaviors, thus creating an enduring demand for good health; the capacity of community networks to share information and offer access to basic quality health services; and the capacity of institutions and organizations in the public, private, and NGO sectors to play complementary, decentralized roles in providing credible health information and service-seeking opportunities for the public.

In line with the strategic objectives of the project donor, the United States Agency for International Development (USAID), the focal point of the CHL strategic framework is the "Healthy Families, Healthy Communities" concept. From the top down, national health policies and service delivery systems provide households and families with messages that promote healthy families, particularly with respect to family planning and reproductive health, maternal and child health, and infectious diseases, while, from the bottom up, households and communities are empowered through communication to demand the information and services that allow them to produce and take ownership of better health (Johns Hopkins University, 2005a). Specific behavior-change communication activities were designed using a detailed conceptual framework that outlines the underlying conditions that may affect the outcomes, and the pathways through which communication activities can help achieve improved family planning and reproductive health (Johns Hopkins University, 2005a; Salem *et al.*, 2008; Storey, Kaggwa, and Harbour, 2008).

Consistent with the analysis of the structure of Egyptian households above, the *Mabrouk!* Initiative segmented the family according to the age- or stage-appropriate needs of each member, addressing the household as a decision-making unit. At the same time, this approach addressed the needs of entire age cohorts in society (for example, "Children under 6 years" or "Unmarried Youth"), allowing for messaging that was relevant to the population as a whole. While each life stage has specific behavioral objectives, the Life Stage conceptual framework acknowledges that every stage is transitional and operates within the context of the family and community as a whole. Good health behavior adopted at an early stage, or collectively, represents a positive health investment and will have a cumulative, sustainable impact on future health behavior. Figure 18.1 shows how these life stages are depicted by CHL.

In early childhood, the main health needs include immunization, proper nutrition, and prevention and treatment of acute respiratory infections and childhood diarrhea. In its community program, CHL gives special focus to the critical window of maternal health and child development, from conception and pregnancy to the child's age of 2 years (–9 to +24 months), in line with the MDG "First 1,000 days" initiative. By the time these children reach school age, the needs shift toward nutrition, female genital mutilation, and healthy lifestyles, such as smoking prevention (Population Council, 2010; Suzuki and Meekers, 2008). Unmarried youth and adolescents continue to face a need for proper nutrition and healthy lifestyles. Moreover, since many Egyptian males start smoking at an early age, unmarried males also have a need for smoking cessation programs (Meekers and El-Ghazaly, 2005; Population Council, 2010). Young married couples also face the risk of HIV infection and other sexually transmitted diseases. Because this life stage is associated with the onset of childbearing, there is also a need for safe motherhood and birth spacing. Older men and women face exceeding their desired family size, and therefore may have a need for family limitation. Proper nutrition and healthy lifestyles are also key concerns for this life stage (El-Zanaty and Way, 2001, 2006, 2009).

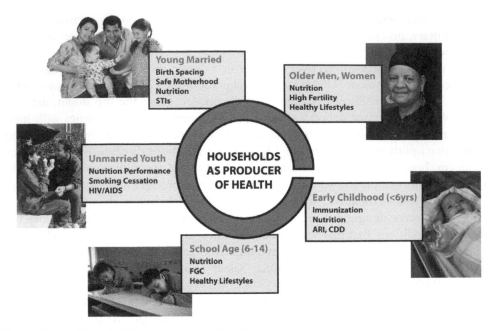

Figure 18.1   Households as producers of health.
Source: Developed for the CHL/Mabrouk initiative, created under the auspices of Johns Hopkins University.

The fact that health needs vary by age suggests that health competence is also life-stage-specific to a certain extent, as well as crosscutting. While some behaviors, such as hand washing, basic hygiene practices, and nutrition are relevant at all stages, other different sets of knowledge, attitudes, skills, and resources become necessary as one progresses to a new life stage and faces new health challenges (e.g., reproductive health in adolescence and young adulthood). Furthermore, people who practice health-competent behaviors at an earlier point in time are more likely to practice other healthy behaviors later. For example, analysis of survey data collected for the CHL project in 2004, 2005, and 2008 following a panel of 1,661 married women aged 15 to 49 showed that those who reported in 2004 that they had adopted family planning after the birth of their first child were significantly more likely in 2008 to report breastfeeding their most recent child, to have received regular antenatal care during that pregnancy, to have a smoke-free area in their home, and to practice handwashing before preparing food and after defecation. Consistent with social learning theory (Bandura, 1997, 2004), success in one aspect of health behavior results in self-efficacy perceptions that increase confidence in one's ability to achieve other health goals, so health competence is cumulative.

Program Implementation: The *Mabrouk!* Initiative

The *Mabrouk!* Initiative was implemented using an Integrated Marketing Communication (IMC) approach (Arens, 1999; Kotler, 1999) that has been widely applied and validated globally for social and behavioral change. Not to be confused with integration across focal areas of health (e.g., integrated approaches to FP/MCH/Nutrition), IMC seeks to unify and coordinate as many communication forms and approaches as possible (e.g. advertising, public relations, Internet communication, community mobilization, counseling) to reinforce and complement each other. At a deeper level, IMC means that all client contacts and messages are designed to communicate the same fundamental value associated with proposed actions and desired outcomes. The strength of this approach lies in the trust established between the client and the provider of the product or service. By focusing on the client–provider relationship, or trust, this approach recognizes that the client or customer is the main actor and decision maker with regard to the exchange.

The *Mabrouk!* Initiative used a full spectrum of communication approaches (ranging from mass media and publicity events, to community mobilization and empowerment, to client–provider counseling support) to promote the value of birth spacing and to help couples achieve their desired family planning outcomes (Center for Communication Programs, Johns Hopkins University, 2010; Communication Initiative, 2005; Salem *et al.*, 2008; Soul Beat Africa, 2010).

In line with Integrated Marketing Communication principles, the *Mabrouk!* Initiative (and, in fact, the entire CHL project) maintained a consistent, unifying focus on the value of good health, based on the deeply held cultural belief in Egypt that health is a gift that should be cherished and protected. This core value and unifying idea was embodied in the campaign's signature message, "*Sahetak Sarwetak*," or "Your Health is Your Wealth," which was featured and reinforced in virtually all program materials and activities over a span of more than six years.

Campaign highlights

Enabling environment

The national crosscutting communication program was made possible through the leadership of Egypt's Ministry of Health (MOH) and its long-term institutional partners, principally the Ministry of Information/State Information Services (Piotrow *et al.*, 1997). Crucially, MOH policy created the enabling environment for the crosscutting communication program, supporting the integration of the various health sectors (including Population, Maternal/Child Health, and Infectious Disease), and a platform for interministerial coordination as well as partnership with the nongovernmental and commercial sectors.

As a first step, the MOH and national partners in the USAID-supported Communication for Healthy Living project identified the country's strategic health priorities, forming a technical strategy whose implementation was overseen by an MOH-chaired Executive Steering Committee. The Executive Steering Committee coordinated sectoral workplans and joint activities. After a series of activities designed to strengthen the governmental officials' leadership capacity to conduct integrated programs, and to develop an agreed set of family health messages, the program was launched.

The national media campaign

The reach of communication programs is an essential precondition for impact. As with any program seeking to have population-level effects, the CHL program sought to achieve the greatest reach at the lowest cost per person. Since the Egyptian public's access to and viewership of television is almost universal – even among rural populations – television played an important role in the communication mix.

Because over 95 percent of Egyptian households own a television, the program launched *Sahetak Sarwetak* and other specific family health messages in a series of television spots. The signature TV spot featured a marriage party on a boat, with parents and friends wishing the couple, *Mabrouk!* (Congratulations), Happiness and Good Health! The message positioned health as both a desired goal and a responsibility, and modeled parental and social support to young couples making family health decisions, including family planning.

Other TV messages addressed the specific health needs of young couples, including antenatal care, medically assisted delivery, breastfeeding, and postpartum care, as well as family planning initiation after the first child, (re)initiation of FP use within two months after delivery, and three- to five-year birth spacing. The spots also modeled husband–wife communication (a strong predictor of family planning use globally; see Lozare *et al.*, 1993), parental– and client–provider communication, women's education, as well as timely information- and service-seeking.

The TV messages, in various combinations, were broadcast periodically throughout the life of the project from 2004–2010. Overall, the TV campaigns reached an average of between 52–65 percent of the adult population, or roughly 20–30 million adults every year (El-Zanaty and Way, 2009; PARC, n.d.).

Mabrouk! *wedding celebrations*

In Egypt, marriage is the foundation of family life, and wedding festivities are an important part of the local culture. Group wedding receptions are a customary way for families and friends of several newlywed couples to stage a major festivity jointly and to share in the costs. CHL launched the *Mabrouk!* Initiative locally in conjunction with the national *Sahatek, Sarwetek* media campaign by cohosting such a group wedding celebration in Minya Governorate in September 2004 (see Figure 18.2).

The celebration involved 150 newlywed couples and 9,000 guests, and was held in the Minya community sports stadium under the auspices of Minya Governor Hassan Hemeida and the Ministry of Health (Center for Communication Programs, Johns Hopkins University, 2010; Hammond, 2005; Johns Hopkins University, 2005b; Soul Beat Africa, 2010). The event was hosted by the popular Egyptian television personality Tarek El-Allam, included performances by several other major national celebrities, and attracted a broad range of private sector sponsorship. Major media coverage, including a feature on the global Arabic-language *Al Jazeera* network, and national and regional media, amplified the *Sahatek, Sarwetek* message, contributing to its success as a publicity event.

Edutainment: Mabrouk! *newlywed game show*

Similar but smaller wedding events were subsequently staged in several governorates of Egypt, in collaboration with event host Tareq El-Allam and his popular national television variety show, *Al Afdal.* As part of the collaboration, the *Al Afdal* TV program incorporated a *Sahetak Sarwetak* game show in the newlyweds segment. The segment was produced on location in the governorates. Each one featured a small-scale newlywed

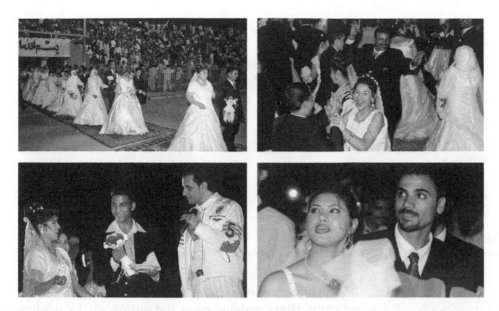

Figure 18.2 Group wedding celebration in Minya Governorate in September 2004.
Source: Developed for the CHL/Mabrouk initiative, created under the auspices of Johns Hopkins University.

event open to the public, with the governor, celebrity Tarek El-Allam, and musicians on stage, joined by up to a dozen local newlywed couples. The segment took the form of a loosely structured contest in which the celebrity would quiz the new couples on their plans for a healthy family, addressing a variety of health themes, as well as husband–wife communication and gender roles. Stage props included crying baby dolls and cooking utensils, among other objects. The host would end the newlywed game by reminding participants and viewers, "Your health is your wealth." The segment was then aired nationally as a segment within *Al Afdal* broadcasts and viewers were encouraged to call in for a chance to win prizes. In 2004 and 2005, the show aired during the 30 days of the Islamic holy month, Ramadan, when viewership was at its peak. In 2004, the show attracted an estimated 15 million viewers, and received almost 8.5 million calls over the Ramadan period. In 2005, the show was named by one of the national newspapers as the most popular television program during Ramadan (Communication Initiative, 2005; Johns Hopkins University, 2005b; Salem *et al.*, 2008; Soul Beat Africa, 2010).

Additional edutainment media programs included magazine-format TV and radio shows for young couples with children, featuring popular pediatrician, Dr. Mohamed Refaat. Dr. Refaat's 30-episode program *Youm Wara Youm* [Day after Day] was coproduced by CHL, Procter and Gamble, and the Showtime channel in Dubai. It aired on satellite television during Ramadan in 2007 and was rebroadcast the next year on the national Egyptian terrestrial broadcast channel, Channel One. A complementary radio program of daily health tips and a weekly call-in show were also aired on the popular *Nogoom* FM radio station. In his programs, Dr. Refaat gave health tips for young couples on infant and young child care, including support for breastfeeding, nutrition at weaning, birth spacing and a wide range of other child care issues.

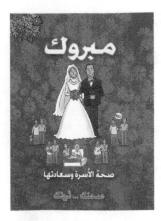 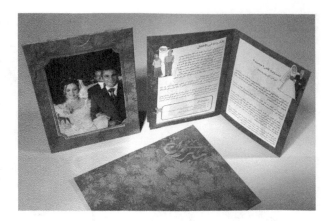

Figure 18.3 *Mabrouk!* family health booklet.
Source: Developed for the CHL/Mabrouk initiative, created under the auspices of Johns Hopkins University.

Mabrouk! *family health booklet*

All couples who participated in the Minya wedding event and subsequent TV newlywed shows, as well as hundreds of thousands of other couples over the life of the project were provided with a specially designed *Mabrouk!* family health booklet (see Figure 18.3). The *Mabrouk!* booklet guides the couple through the main health issues that they are likely to face during the first few years of their marriage, and that may have a lifelong effect on their family health (including family planning, safe pregnancy and delivery, pre- and post-natal care, breastfeeding, and child immunization). It is packaged in a standing picture frame that can be used to display the couple's wedding or other family photo with the booklet stored behind it to encourage keeping the book and having it accessible for easy reference (Salem *et al.*, 2008; Soul Beat Africa, 2010).

The booklet opens by wishing the couple happiness and good health, and then proceeds to give essential health information on the key health events (see Figure 18.4), with a double page for each reproductive life cycle event. For example, the section "You're pregnant" emphasizes the importance of visiting a doctor to monitor the pregnancy and the growth of the baby and to receive vaccinations and nutritional supplements that may be needed. Each section of the booklet also lists the warning signs that would require visiting a doctor and more serious danger signs that would require immediate emergency medical consultation. The booklet also contains a schedule of recommended vaccinations for children and space to record important information such as doctors' contact information, appointments, the mother's weight gain, and the child's weight gain.

The project distributed the booklet and related health communication materials wherever it made contact with young couples. In addition to the wedding event, over 100,000 booklets were distributed by MOH outreach workers and facility-based health workers to newlywed couples throughout the country (Salem *et al.*, 2008; Soul Beat Africa, 2010). The *Mabrouk!* booklet was inserted in special wedding issues of popular women's magazines on nine occasions, reaching an estimated 1.36 million purchasers directly, with additional pass-along readers assumed for each issue.

CHL also partnered with the *Maazoun* Association, or association of Islamic Marriage Registrars, and with priests of the same specialty, to deliver the *Mabrouk!* booklet to

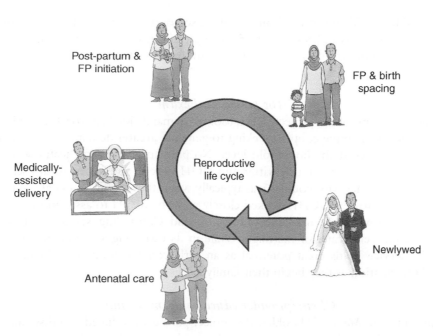

Figure 18.4 Reproductive life cycle from the *Mabrouk!* family health booklet.
Source: Developed for the CHL/Mabrouk initiative, created under the auspices of Johns Hopkins University.

newlywed couples applying to register their marriages (Center for Communication Programs, Johns Hopkins University, 2006). And in 2007, CHL entered an agreement with Procter and Gamble under which the company includes the *Mabrouk!* booklet in gift bags distributed to 130,000 new mothers annually. Through the variety of channels mentioned above, the project has distributed an estimated two million *Mabrouk!* booklets to couples throughout the country.

Interpersonal communication and counseling at the service-delivery level

The project also had goals to improve interpersonal communication linking MCH and FP within the service-delivery system. The enabling environment created by the MOH for an integrated, family health approach played an important role in supporting linkages between antenatal care, safe delivery, postpartum care, and family planning within the service-delivery system. After launching the integrated technical strategy, the training of providers, and the development of a set of integrated, family health messages, CHL continued to work with the MOH leadership to include family planning information in the antenatal care package, as well as to develop an integrated postpartum protocol. The protocol pioneered links between the hospital (curative sector) where most couples deliver, and the primary health care unit (preventive sector) that initiates the postpartum home visit. Additionally, the protocol linked the postpartum home-visiting service provided by an MCH nurse (who conducts a basic exam and checks for any signs of distress or complications) and that of the female health visitor, or *Raida Refaya*, who provides family planning, breastfeeding and MCH counseling and support. This integrated protocol was adopted and applied by the MOH throughout its public sector program, reaching an estimated 80,000 postpartum couples from 2005 through 2010. CHL and Save the Children through the Community Health Program conducted another 50,000 postpartum home visits.

The premarital exam

From the beginning of the project, CHL took a "demand side" approach to addressing the health needs of young couples, seeking to generate greater demand for health information and services at the household level. No premarital exam or health service for newlyweds had existed previously within the MOH system, so the first health service or "supply side" contact with couples was typically when they sought antenatal care for a first pregnancy. However, CHL worked closely with the MOH to assist in the development of a nationwide Premarital Examination and Counseling service that issues a required health certificate for marriage. While in its early stages of implementation in 2010, the service holds great potential as an early contact point to offer newlyweds essential information as they begin their family lives.

Client/provider educational materials

In addition to the *Mabrouk!* booklet, the project partners produced and disseminated a wide range of client education materials and provider counseling aids to improve interpersonal communication linking MCH and FP. Simple flyers for low-literacy clients address subjects such as danger signs and proper prenatal care during pregnancy, safe delivery, postpartum care and danger signs, proper breastfeeding, as well as family planning methods, including the lactational amenorrhea method (LAM). These, and posters covering the project's other main health areas, have been disseminated widely throughout the MOH health system with its estimated 5,000 service sites (Ministry of Health and Population, Egypt, El-Zanaty and Associates, and ORC Macro, 2003), as well as by NGOs and through a private sector pharmacy network, which has been developed and supported by the project and now consists of an estimated 30,000 neighborhood pharmacies nationally.

In addition, a client-provider counseling flipchart with a section for each MCH and FP health issue was developed for use in MOH primary health care centers. CHL and MOH together printed nearly 150,000 flipcharts on MCH, FP, and breastfeeding.

Production and distribution of such media and materials were strategically planned to reach and support, in as many ways and places as possible, the millions of young couples nationwide who were beginning family life: managing pregnancy, safe delivery, postpartum care, breastfeeding, and birth spacing.

The Community Health Program

To complement the national approach, the CHL project designed an intensive community health program to serve vulnerable groups in hard-to-reach, economically disadvantaged areas. What distinguished these subgroups from the majority was less their access to media than the psychosocial patterns of influence that created barriers to good health practices. The CHL program used community programs to "go the extra mile" and engage the social networks to affect change in rural Upper Egypt. This component was implemented in cooperation with one of JHUCCP's Health Communication Partnership partners, Save the Children, in a select number of villages. As noted in the early sections of this chapter, areas of Upper Egypt (in more isolated south central parts of the country) have traditionally lagged behind the rest of the nation on major health indicators. CHL's Community Health Program under the *Mabrouk!* Initiative, therefore, focused initially on these governorates.

The Community Health Program initially started in seven focal villages in Minya governorate in 2004, and expanded to villages in Qena and Fayoum governorates in 2005.[5] By September 2009, the program had expanded to 206 villages and hamlets with an estimated population of two million in five governorates (three in Upper Egypt and two in Lower Egypt). In these areas, CHL worked closely with community development associations (CDAs), which are local nongovernmental organizations, to assess the health needs of the village, to form village health committees where influential locals and the clinic doctor were represented, to build groups of women and men leaders, and, finally, to implement an easily managed family health program (Center for Communication Programs, Johns Hopkins University, 2010; Salem *et al.*, 2008; Soul Beat Africa, 2010). The core of the community health program is the *Mabrouk!* package on a village scale, with newlywed visits, pregnancy classes, safe delivery referrals, postpartum home visits, and infant nutrition classes, as well as special activities for avian influenza and school health and hygiene.

The Community Health Package: newlywed visits, antenatal care, postpartum home visits, and child nutrition sessions

As part of this community mobilization program, CDAs train outreach volunteers to help extend the reach of the *Mabrouk!* Initiative through the local social network. These CDA volunteers – who come from the community and know the members of their neighborhoods – make home visits to the newlywed couples to wish them "Happiness and Good Health," hand out the *Mabrouk!* booklet, introduce them to the health facilities that are available in the community, provide basic counseling on family health issues, distribute health-related information materials, and invite the couple to participate in various community activities.

CDAs also assist in organizing pregnancy classes in the local health facility. The CHL project has conducted community-based sessions with over 12,000 women who needed antenatal care especially those identified as being "at risk" because they were pregnant for the first time, had a pregnancy with low weight gain, or had previously delivered infants with low birth weight below the WHO standard of 2.5 kg (Center for Communication Programs, Johns Hopkins University, 2010). The safe pregnancy program conducted home visits to identify all pregnant women in the village and track their antenatal care and weight gain on a monthly basis. Women who were pregnant for the first time and those with low weight gain were recruited into health awareness classes. Volunteers facilitated regular antenatal classes in the local clinic and also assisted couples to make arrangements for medically assisted delivery at the local hospital, usually in a district center at a distance from the village.

During the first week after the delivery, CDA volunteers worked with nurses at the local primary health care unit to conduct postpartum home visits. Because most women conceive within the first few years of marriage, many women involved in the community health program have received a newlywed visit, antenatal classes, and a postpartum visit. Postpartum home visits by birth attendants are common in Egypt (Darmstadt *et al.*, 2008), so familiarity with and acceptance of this practice provides an opportunity to meet women in the privacy of their own home and to use interpersonal communication to reinforce and expand on the national messages seen in the media or in the government service delivery setting. During postpartum home visits, nurses and CDA volunteers discuss infant health and postpartum care for the mother, support them in breastfeeding the newborn, and encourage women to start using family planning within 40 days of the delivery, as well as to space their children three years apart.

In addition to this antenatal/postpartum care component, the CHL community health program sought to reduce malnutrition among children 6 to 24 months of age – a critical transition period in child development. Children that were underweight for their age were identified by weighing all the community babies in this age cohort – with findings showing malnutrition rates of typically 25–30 percent. CDA volunteers then led nutritional rehabilitation sessions in which the mothers with underweight children joined other village mothers in similar social circumstances with well-nurtured children to cook, eat, and learn together, using commonly available foodstuffs and sharing personal experience. After a series of such sessions, usually lasting less than six months, community malnutrition rates were reduced significantly, typically to levels of 5 percent or less.

Arab Women Speak Out (AWSO) Training Program

In conjunction with the *Mabrouk!* Initiative, CHL's Community Health Program also organizes Arab Women Speak Out (AWSO) sessions for young female leaders. AWSO is a long-standing female empowerment training program for women in the Near East (Underwood and Jabre, 2008). The program was designed and implemented by the Johns Hopkins University Center for Communication Programs in collaboration with the Center of Arab Women for Training and Research in Tunis, beginning in late 1999. It was later implemented in several countries in the Middle East, including Egypt (Center for Communication Programs, Johns Hopkins University, 2001; Soul Beat Africa, 2009). It has also been adapted for use in sub-Saharan Africa under the new label of African Transformations.

Consisting of video case studies, discussion guides, and other supporting materials, the program is specifically designed to be incorporated into existing community-based programs that are being implemented by organizations working in the area. CHL draws on the AWSO training program to prepare female leaders to serve as active agents to promote health and gender equity in their communities. This program helped identify, train, and recruit women volunteers (outreach workers) who implement Mabrouk Initiative as described above in all CHL focal villages.

CHL has trained over 430 female community leaders in its identified focal villages to implement this process and the discussion groups they organize reach an estimated

10,000 women annually (Center for Communication Programs, Johns Hopkins University, 2010). During fiscal year 2009 (October 2008–September 2009), nearly 13,000 women attended AWSO meetings through the CHL Community Health Program. Female leaders who have completed the AWSO training also conduct home visits with women, thereby increasing the outreach of the AWSO programs. One of the crucial roles of the AWSO program in CHL's community program has been to build social support among elder women in the community for delaying marriage, supporting female education, and supporting positive health practices among young couples.

Evaluation: CHL Program Results

Campaign exposure

A number of studies have shown that recall of CHL campaign activities is high (Hutchinson, 2010; Meekers and Nauman, 2006b). Figure 18.5 shows that in late 2007, almost half of all adult Egyptians could recall seeing safe motherhood messages on television within the past six months, while two thirds recalled seeing family planning messages. Recall of handwashing and passive smoking messages were 73 percent and 78 percent, respectively, while recall of safe injection and HIV/AIDS messages were 81 percent and 88 percent. Ninety-six percent recalled seeing avian influenza messages on television. Overall exposure to FP messages nationally has been high by communication campaign standards: 83 percent in 1995, 96 percent in 2000, 91 percent in 2005 and 67 percent in 2008 (El-Zanaty *et al.*, 1996; El-Zanaty and Way, 2001, 2006, 2009). The decline from 2005 to 2008 is partly explained by the Egyptian MOH's enthusiastic embrace of mass media as a public health tool and its use to address an expanding portfolio of health issues, such as avian influenza (as opposed to using mass media only promote FP and MCH, as was the case in the past).

Program Outcomes

There is strong evidence over time, as well as cross-sectionally, that exposure to the CHL health communication campaign activities had a positive effect on health competence, attitudes toward healthy behaviors, and several family planning outcomes. (Hutchinson, 2010; Meekers and Nauman, 2006a, 2006b; Storey *et al.*, 2008). We draw on two data sources to illustrate the effects of the CHL project at the national and community levels. Nationally, mass media, advocacy, and service quality improvement efforts are assessed using national Egypt Demographic and Health Survey (EDHS) data at four points in time: 1995, 2000, 2005, and 2008 (El-Zanaty *et al.*, 1996, El-Zanaty and Way, 2001, 2006, 2009). These surveys drew nationally representative samples of married women aged 15–49 years that can be disaggregated to the regional and governorate level. For the purposes of the *Mabrouk!* evaluation, we focus on a subset of these national samples,

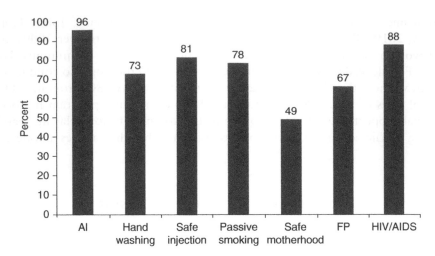

Figure 18.5   Television exposure by health topic, 2008.
Source: Egyptian Health Communication Survey, January 2008 (n=3770, 15–49 adults in 21 governorates).

namely the YFC of women under the age of 30 who reported at least one birth in the five years preceding the survey.

Respondents in the Demographic and Health Surveys are asked a wide variety of questions about pregnancy, childbirth, prenatal and postnatal care, and family planning, corresponding to all of the key indicators targeted by the *Mabrouk!* Initiative. In addition, respondents are asked an extensive battery of questions about their demographic and household conditions, including ownership of television, radio, computers, and mobile phones. They are also asked questions about their media use and interpersonal communication habits and about whether or not they have been exposed to family planning and safe pregnancy messages through television, radio, print or interpersonal channels (including at service facilities or through personal networks).

At the community level, we rely on monitoring data collected systematically by project partners in the focal villages of Minya, Fayoum, and Qena in Upper Egypt to assess impact of the intensive home visiting, counseling, nutrition, and empowerment activities conducted under the *Mabrouk!* Initiative by CDAs and local health-service providers. Standardized forms developed by Save the Children in the 1990s for monitoring prenatal progress, postpartum care, infant growth, and malnutrition, are used to record prenatal care visits, birth statistics (e.g., birthweight and birth intervals), postpartum care, and timing of contraceptive use.

National broadcast and print media reach families in the focal villages and countrywide alike. But focal village families also benefit from the community-based program, while the rest of Egypt does not. For some analyses, in order to compare the impact of the combined national and local *Mabrouk!* activities in the focal villages with the impact of the national program alone, we compare the subset of DHS cases in Upper Egypt – the larger sociopolitical region within which the CHL community-based program was implemented – with cases from the focal village monitoring data. Focusing on the *Mabrouk!* Initiative, we further restrict most of our analyses to women in the YFC. These restrictions help ensure that the respondents in the monitoring data and DHS data are roughly comparable in terms of the region, rural–urban residence, demographics, and other sociocultural characteristics.

Our analysis focuses mostly on seven key family planning and maternal health variables that are described below:

Maternal/child health variables

- Percentage of women in the YFC who report that they had four or more antenatal care (ANC) visits – the WHO recommended minimum – for their last birth;
- Percentage of women in the YFC whose last delivery was medically assisted (assisted by a medical doctor, as opposed to a midwife, traditional birth attendant, neighbor/ relative, or no one);
- Percentage of women in the YFC for whom the birth to birth interval for the two most recent births was more than 33 months (the lower end of the WHO standard range for optimum birth interval), and
- Percentage of women in the YFC whose most recent baby had a birth weight of over 2.5 kilograms (the WHO standard for acceptable birth weight).

Family Planning variables

- Percentage of women in the YFC who report that they ever used family planning;
- Percentage of women in the YFC who report using family planning within 8 weeks after their last delivery (among those women who adopted family planning).
- Percentage of women in the YFC who report using family planning after the birth of their first child (parity 1 use).

National trend results

Figures 18.6–18.8 show national trends in prenatal care, medically assisted delivery, and birth interval for the young family cohort across the four waves of DHS data. The launch of the *Mabrouk!* Initiative is indicated between the 2000 and 2005 data points. The percentage of YFC women who report having at least four ANC visits for their most recent birth has increased steadily from 30 percent in 1995, to 41 percent in 2000, 63 percent in 2005 and 69 percent in 2008, with a jump of over 21 percentage points between 2000 and 2005 when the *Mabrouk!* Initiative started.

Figure 18.7 shows that the percentage of YFC women nationally whose most recent delivery was medically assisted has increased from 40 percent in 1995 to 57 percent in 2000, 70 percent in 2005, and 75 percent in 2008. Although the increases are somewhat less dramatic for birth interval, Figure 18.8 also shows an upward trend over time in the percentage of YFC women nationally whose two most recent births were spaced at least 33 months apart, from 39 percent in 1995 to 51 percent in 2008. That gains in birth

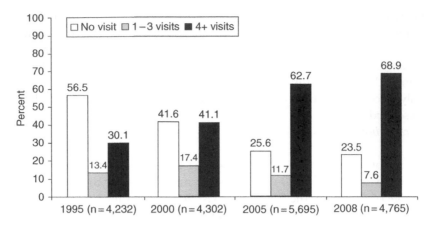

Figure 18.6   Four+ antenatal visits. YFC = Currently married women, < 30 years old, birth in past 5 years.
Sources: EDHS, 1995, 2000, 2005, 2008.

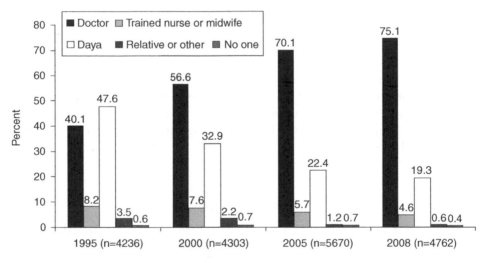

Figure 18.7   Medically assisted deliveries. YFC = Currently married women, < 30 years old, birth in past 5 years.
Sources: EDHS, 1995, 2000, 2005, 2008.

interval within this cohort are modest compared to some of the other indicators is probably explained by the fact that in Egypt newlywed couples face social pressure to demonstrate their fertility after marriage and particularly to produce a son. That much change over time was observed at all may speak well to the successful promotion of post partum and low parity family planning use.

Figure 18.9 shows trends in family planning use (either new use or reinitiation of prior use) within two months after the delivery of one's most recent child. Over time,

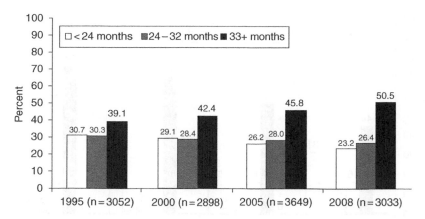

Figure 18.8 Birth interval of 33 months or longer. YFC = Currently married women, < 30 years old, birth in past 5 years.
Sources: EDHS, 1995, 2000, 2005, 2008.

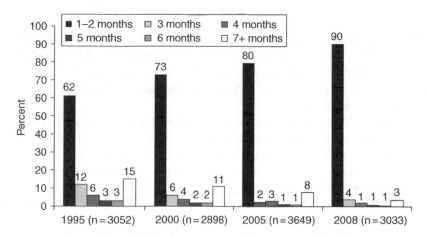

Figure 18.9 FP use within two months of delivery. YFC = Currently married women, < 30 years old, birth in past 5 years.
Sources: EDHS, 1995, 2000, 2005, 2008.

this has increased strongly from 62 percent in 1995 to 73 percent in 2000, 80 percent in 2005 and 90 percent in 2008. That 9 out of 10 women who use contraception report initiating use within two months of delivery provides strong evidence that women are proactively trying to manage their fertility by taking the precaution of starting contraception within the period before postpartum fertility returns in order to avoid unwanted pregnancy.

Finally, at the national level, the percentage of YFC women who say they first started to use FP after the birth of their first child has also climbed steadily. Figure 18.10 shows

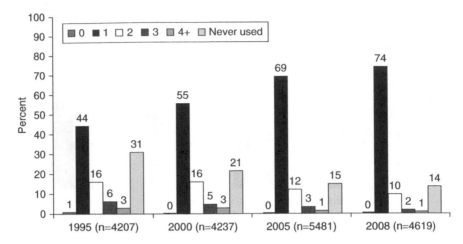

Figure 18.10 Number of children at first use of contraception. YFC = Currently married women, < 30 years old, birth in past 5 years.
Sources: EDHS, 1995, 2000, 2005, 2008.

that in 1995 only 44 percent of YFC women said they started using contraception when they had one child. That percentage climbed to 55 percent in 2000, to 69 percent in 2005, and to 74 percent by 2008. This figure also shows that the percentage of women who report never having used contraception has steadily declined from 31 percent in 1995 to 14 percent in 2008.

Taken together, these figures show consistent progress over time across the range of maternal and child health and family planning outcomes that were the focus of the *Mabrouk!* Initiative. At least two of these five indicators (prenatal care and parity 1 FP use) show particularly strong increases between 2000 and 2005 when the *Mabrouk!* Initiative was launched.

Focal village compared to national YFC outcomes

To further examine the question of program impact, we compare the outcomes on major MCH and FP indicators between YFC women in Upper Egypt and their counterparts in the CHL focal villages of Upper Egypt. Because YFC women everywhere could have been exposed to the national *Mabrouk!* Components, but only the focal village YFC women had access to the community-based program, outcomes in focal villages should be better – other things being equal – if outreach activities somehow complement or reinforce national program components.

The table in Figure 18.11 compares outcomes for YFC women in all of Upper Egypt with those for YFC women in the focal villages on seven MCH and FP indicators. The percentage of women who received the intensive focal village interventions (postpartum home visits, pregnancy classes, family planning counseling, and infant care classes) was statistically higher on six of seven indicators, compared to the larger population of women

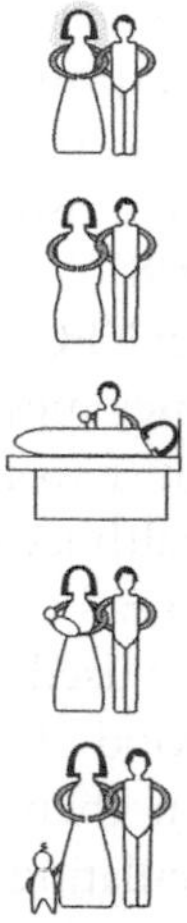

Indicator	All Upper Egypt		Focal villages Upper Egypt		P-value
	n	%	n	%	
4+ ANC visits	2,051	60.8	6,893	82.4	0.001
Delivery assisted by doctor	2,050	67.9	6,890	84.6	0.001
Birth weight > 2.5Kg	778	85.9	6,886	98.6	0.001
Ever use of FP	2,051	80.2	6,893	83.0	0.002
FP use within < 8wks after delivery	1,068	69.9	5,654	77.9	0.001
FP after birth of first child	2,051	61.4	6,893	82.5	0.001
Birth interval > 33 months	1,335	45.8	436	33.1	ns

Figure 18.11   Focal village compared to population outcomes (YFC in Upper Egypt). Members of young family cohort = married women aged 30 or less with a birth in the past 5 years.
Sources: EDHS, 2008, 9 governorates; CHL M&E data 2005–2009. 32 focal villages in 3 governorates.

in Upper Egypt. Only birth interval was not statistically different, probably due to the low number of women in the focal village monitoring data who had the two births within a five-year period needed to calculate the birth interval.

Because the women who participated in the community-based sessions and were captured in the monitoring database were by definition "high-risk" cases due to having low weight gain during pregnancy, delivering infants with low birth weight, or having malnourished children, the fact that these challenged women could in the end outperform their regional counterparts speaks to the power of the CDA-led activities.

Impact of communication at the national level

A critical question all communication programs should try to answer is whether change can be attributed to the program or if it is related to other factors, such as wealth, literacy, or access to media. Exposure to family planning messages was measured in the EDHS 2008 survey as recall of up to 12 different sources of information, including mass media, community outreach, and facility-based contacts. This scale was dichotomized at the median to create a low (0–1 sources) versus high (2+ sources) exposure variable. Exposure to safe pregnancy messages was measured in the EDHS 2008 survey as recall of up to nine sources of information including mass media, community outreach, and facility-based sources. This scale, too, was dichotomized at the median to create a zero (no sources) versus any (1+ sources) exposure variable.

Randomized assignment to treatment or nontreatment is not an appropriate design for evaluating national programs like *Mabrouk!* that aim to reach everyone, so the issue becomes how to create a comparison group that permits measurement of exposure effects. Also, disadvantaged individuals tend to have reduced opportunity or motivation to be exposed to a program, so a comparison of outcomes based on raw exposure can be biased. To address these issues, we use a technique known as propensity score matching (PSM) to control for exposure bias and to create valid treatment and comparison groups (Do and Kincaid, 2006; Rosenbaum and Rubin, 1983; D'Agostino, 1998).

From the EDHS 2008 data, we identified a set of variables that predict YFC women's reported exposure to FP messages, on the one hand, and to safe pregnancy messages on the other hand. We found 10 variables that predicted whether or not a woman was exposed to any FP messages in the broadcast or print media, through health facility contacts or through outreach and nine variables that predicted exposure to safe pregnancy messages.[6] Using STATA (v11) algorithms for PSM, these variables were used to calculate propensity scores for each person representing the predicted likelihood of exposure to FP messages and to safe pregnancy messages. The PSM algorithm then matches exposed and unexposed cases at the same level of propensity before calculating an average matched difference in outcome percentages between exposed and unexposed cases, controlling for the likelihood of exposure. The result is an estimated percentage point difference between exposed and unexposed (matched control) cases adjusted for exposure bias.

Figures 18.12 and 18.13 show the results of this analysis. Exposure to FP messages accounted for a 12.0 percentage point difference in current use of a modern contraceptive method and an 11.5 percentage point difference in use of FP after the birth of the

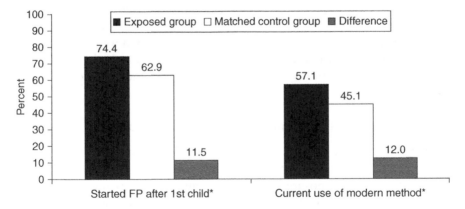

Figure 18.12 Impact of FP message exposure on FP behaviors among YFC, adjusted for exposure bias (EDHS 2008). Recall of up to 12 sources of FP information including mass media, outreach, and facility contacts (range 0–9); median split; matched control group = 0–1 sources, exposed group = 2+ sources. Controlling for 10 predictors of exposure to family planning messages. * p < .001.

Sources: EDHS 2008 (the YFC is n = 2774 exposed and 1837 unexposed CMW, < 30 years old, birth in past 5 years).

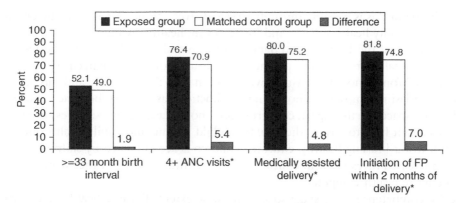

Figure 18.13 Impact of safe pregnancy message exposure on antenatal and postnatal behaviors among YFC, adjusted for exposure bias (EDHS 2008). Recall of safe pregnancy messages from any of 9 sources including mass media, outreach and facility contacts. Controlling for 9 predictors of exposure to safe pregnancy messages. *p<.05 or better.
Sources: EDHS 2008 (the YFC is n=1146 exposed and 3659 unexposed currently married women aged 30 or less with a birth in past 5 years).

first child. Exposure to safe pregnancy messages accounted for a 5.4 percentage point difference in having 4+ prenatal care visits, a 4.8 percentage point difference in medically assisted delivery and a 7.0 percentage point difference in FP use within 2 months of one's most recent delivery. Only the effect of safe pregnancy message exposure on birth interval was not statistically significant.

Discussion

The *Communication for Healthy Living* (CHL) project in Egypt implemented an unusually sophisticated full-scale national and community-based communication campaign – supported by policy change and service delivery quality improvement – to address the health needs of family members in various life stages, with the special *Mabrouk!* Initiative focused on newlywed and young couples. The achievements documented in national and community-based data could not have been realized without the political will and commitment over time of the Government of Egypt, particularly the Ministry of Health, and of one particular donor agency, USAID, to not only mitigate specific health deficits but to achieve sustainable healthy practices.

In a mature "market" like Egypt where 87 percent of the demand for family planning services is already satisfied – but where continued population growth threatens already stressed health and environmental resources – strategies must be developed to help new families become producers of health, help sustain healthy behaviors where they already exist, and help extend access to those who still face social and material barriers to good health. None of this is possible through service delivery alone. There must be enduring demand for quality health services and for achieving healthy living.

We believe that the EDHS trend data indicate an enduring demand for better health and generational shifts in health practices that could not have occurred without communication. Women now are having fewer children than their parents, and this has enormous, long-lasting impact on how families function: as families become smaller and children are spaced farther apart, concerns about how a large family survives turn toward concerns about how to ensure the quality of child rearing and family health outcomes. The shift toward raising healthy, educated children is accompanied by shifting priorities such as increased investment in education and healthful foods. In other words, families become more health-competent.

Health competence is life-stage-specific to some extent. Because health needs vary by age, individuals at each life-stage require a different set of knowledge, attitudes, skills, and resources to achieve healthy behaviors. But in the longer term, *households* become health-competent when they are enabled to mobilize the resources they need – including information, social support, and greater control – in order to make health decisions consistently and gain greater ownership over positive household health outcomes. CHL aimed to facilitate this and the *Mabrouk!* Initiative found an appropriate entry point in newlywed couples.

Space prohibits us from describing in any detail other documented outcomes associated with the CHL program, but the partnerships established with ministries, universities, the private sector, and CDAs helped the government and communities to respond rapidly and effectively to a number of emerging health issues. We mention only a few brief examples here. CHL's work with medical students to organize university campaigns on viral hepatitis vaccination and prevention resulted in an increase in vaccinations and in a new university policy requiring all college students to be vaccinated for viral hepatitis before graduation. Getting young people actively involved in health promotion helps establish interest in good health before marriage. When a series of studies drew attention to the high breast cancer mortality rate in Egypt due to delayed detection and treatment, CHL worked with partners to help organize a Komen Foundation "Race for the Cure" event, media coverage, and other breast cancer awareness activities.

One of the most striking achievements of the CHL program was its timely response to the avian influenza (AI) outbreak in February 2006 and continued efforts to fight seasonal AI and pandemic influenza outbreaks. In 2005, anticipating an AI outbreak, CHL partners produced television spots, print materials, and outreach activities and were able to launch a national campaign on the day the first AI case was reported. Within hours of the confirmation of cases, all the major state-owned television channels were broadcasting the news to the public as well as airing an informative TV spot showing families how to protect themselves from the deadly virus. PARC Media Monitoring Services reported that the TV message reached 82 percent of Egyptian adults, or 34 million people, within a day of its launch. A battery of AI-related questions developed by CHL for its 2007 national health communication survey was adopted and included in the 2008 EDHS survey (El-Zanaty *et al.*, 2008; El-Zanaty and Way, 2009). Data from the survey revealed that recall of program messages predicted higher levels of protective knowledge among poultry owners. Knowledge, in turn, predicted higher levels of self-efficacy and together, program recall and self-efficacy were the strongest predictors of household risk reduction behaviors in families that raised poultry (Center for Communication Programs, Johns Hopkins University, 2007).

In short, the innovative part of the CHL program – illustrated in the *Mabrouk!* Initiative we have focused on here – lies in its approach for simultaneously developing health competence at different levels: at the organizational level for timely, effective, high-quality health communication, at the community level for mobilization of health resources and outreach by civil society groups, and at the household level where newly-wed couples begin to develop health-competence from the earliest days of their family life together. Although unique in its local configuration, CHL's program focus on households as producers of health, supported by their community and by public and private health service providers, including the media may be an approach that holds promise for other and could potentially change the way we think about the implementation of family planning and family health programs.

Acknowledgments

The Egypt Communication for Healthy Living Project was funded by the United States Agency for International Development (USAID) through Cooperative Agreement No. 263-A-00-03-00053-00 ("Associate Award") and the Leader with Associate Award, Cooperative Agreement GPH-A-00-02-00008-00 ("Leader Award"). The authors are grateful to Dr. Catherine Harbour and Mr. Mahmoud Mahmoud Al Said for their assistance with the data analysis, and to Dr. Paul Hutchinson and Dr. Tawhida Khalil for their input and suggestions.

Notes

1   CHL was a seven-year project (2003–2011) funded by the United States Agency for International Development with technical assistance from the Johns Hopkins University Center for Communication Programs (JHUCCP). The program is part of the larger USAID-funded *Health Communication Partnership*, a global communication initiative also led by JHUCCP in partnership with the Academy for Educational Development, Save the Children, the International HIV/AIDS Alliance, and Tulane University's School of Public Health and Tropical Medicine.

2   These categories are *rough* proxies for the life stages identified by the CHL project. However, because of the way the household datasets are set up, creating the exact same categories was not feasible. Note also that, due to the age differences between spouses, it is possible for a husband and wife to be classified in different life stages.

3   A similar logic is used by programs that integrate health information and/or services in other sectors, such as agriculture or education. In Egypt, Pathfinder International's *Takamol* project trained agriculture and irrigation workers to provide reproductive health information (Salem *et al.* 2008) and the CHL project mobilized existing networks of local NGOs and neighborhood pharmacies that had previously supported family health initiatives to rapidly scale up avian influenza prevention efforts when the first cases appeared in Egypt in February 2006.

4   A notable exception is a recent eye care program in Menya Governorate that used female health
    visitors to talk to the entire family about the importance of seeking eye care for women in the
    household and to explain that saving or restoring women's eye sight would benefit the whole
    family (Mousa, Ezz El Arab, and Rashad, 2009).
5   The selected governorates are among the seven governorates that have been targeted for special
    USAID-sponsored family planning and health initiatives (El-Zanaty and Way, 2006, p. 6).
6   Statistically significant predictors of FP message exposure were: visited a health facility in the
    past year, had autonomy to make household decisions about money, had ever discussed female
    circumcision with spouse, had any barriers to health care access, region of residence, had con-
    versations with anyone about health, watched TV daily, listened to radio daily, ever read a
    newspaper, spouse had at least primary education. Predictors of safe pregnancy message expo-
    sure were: literacy, wealth quintile, age, had visited a health facility in past year, had ever dis-
    cussed female circumcision with spouse, had conversations with anyone about health, listened
    to the radio daily, ever read a newspaper, owned a TV.

References

Abdel-Tawab, N. and Roter, D. (2002). The relevance of client-centered communication to family
    planning setting in developing countries: Lessons from the Egyptian experience. *Social Science
    and Medicine, 54*(9), 1357–1368.
Arens, W. (1999). *Contemporary Advertising*, 7th edn. New York: Irwin/McGraw Hill.
Bandura, A. (1997). *Self-Efficacy: The Exercise of Control.* New York: Freeman Press.
Bandura, A. (2004). Health promotion by social cognitive means. *Health Education and Behavior,
    31*(2), 143–164.
Becker, G. (1993). *A Treatise on the Family: Enlarged Edition.* Cambridge, MA: Harvard University
    Press.
Beltrán, S. L. R. (1974). *Rural Development and Social Communication: Relationships and
    Strategies.* Proceedings of the Corner-CIAT International Symposium on Communication
    Strategies for Rural Development, Cali, Columbia, 17–22 March, 1974. (pp.11–27). Ithaca,
    NY: Cornell University.
Center for Communication Programs, Johns Hopkins University. (2001). AWSO program helps
    Arab women redirect their lives. *Communication Impact*, 13. Retrieved from http://www.
    jhuccp.org/sites/all/files/13.pdf
Center for Communication Programs, Johns Hopkins University. (2006). *CHL's Mabrouk
    Initiative Scales Up in Partnership with the Maazoun Association.* Retrieved from http://www.
    comminit.com/global/node
Center for Communication Programs, Johns Hopkins University. (2007). Communication for
    Healthy Living's campaign improves responses to avian influenza in Egypt. *Communication
    Impact*, 22. Retrieved from http://www.jhuccp.org/sites/all/files/22.pdf
Center for Communication Programs, Johns Hopkins University. (2010). Communication for
    Healthy Living. Retrieved from http://www.jhuccp.org/node/680
Chemers, M. (2000). Leadership research and theory: A functional integration. *Group Dynamics:
    Theory, Research, and Practice, 4*(1), 27–43.
Clinton, H. (2010). *1,000 Days: Change a Life, Change the Future.* Remarks by Secretary of State
    Hillary Rodham Clinton, InterContinental Hotel, New York, September 21, 2010. Retrieved
    from http://www.state.gov/secretary/rm/2010/09/147512.htm
Communication Initiative (2005). Programme Experiences: Communication for Healthy Living
    (CHL) – Egypt. Retrieved from http://www.comminit.com/global/node/128040

D'Agostino, R. B., Jr. (1998). Propensity score methods for bias reduction in the comparison of a treatment to a non-randomized control group. *Statistics in Medicine, 17*(19), 2265–2281.

Darmstadt, G., Hussein, M. H., Winch, P. *et al.* (2008). Practices of rural Egyptian birth attendants during the antenatal, intrapartum and early neonatal periods. *Journal of Health, Population, and Nutrition, 26*(1), 36–45.

Díaz Bordenave, J. (1994). Participative communication as a part of building the participative society. In S.White and N. Sadanandan (Eds.), *Participatory Communication: Working for Change and Development* (pp. 35–49). Thousand Oaks, CA: Sage Publications.

Do, M. and Kincaid, D. L. (2006). Impact of an entertainment-education television drama on health knowledge and behavior in Bangladesh: An application of propensity score matching. *Journal of Health Communication, 11*(3), 301–325.

Edberg, M. (2007). *Essentials of Health Behavior. Social and Behavioral Theory in Public Health.* Boston: Jones and Bartlett.

El-Ghazaly, N. and Meekers. D. (2007). Trends and determinants of maternal health indicators in Menya Governorate, Egypt. Poster presented at the Annual Meeting of the Population Association of America, New York, March 29–31, 2007.

El-Zanaty, F., Hussein, E., Shawsky, G. *et al.* (1996). *Egypt Demographic and Health Survey 1995.* Cairo and Calverton, MD: National Population Council and Macro International, Inc.

El-Zanaty, F., Storey, D., El-Saied, M. *et al.* (2008). *Egypt Health Communication Survey Report,*unpublished report. Cairo: Communication for Healthy Living Project.

El-Zanaty, F. and Way, A. (2001). *Egypt Demographic and Health Survey, 2000.* Calverton, MD: Ministry of Health and Population [Egypt], National Population Council and ORC Macro.

El-Zanaty, F. and Way, A. (2006). *Egypt Demographic and Health Survey, 2005.* Cairo: Ministry of Health and Population, National Population Council, El-Zanaty and Associates, and ORC Macro.

El-Zanaty, F. and Way, A. (2009). *Egypt Demographic and Health Survey, 2008.* Cairo: Ministry of Health and Population, National Population Council, El-Zanaty and Associates, and Macro International.

Glanz, K., Rimer, B., and Viswanath, K. (2008). *Health Behavior and Health Education. Theory, Research, and Practice,* (4th edn. San Francisco: Jossey-Bass.

Gumucio Dagrón, A. (2001). *Making Waves: Stories of Participatory Communication for Social Change.* New York: Rockefeller Foundation Report.

Hammond, S.-E. (2005). Nice day for a mass wedding. *Egypt Today, 26*(11). Retrieved from www.egypttoday.com

Health Communication Partnership. (2003). *The New P-Process. Steps in Strategic Communication.* Retrieved from http://www.jhuccp.org/sites/all/files/The percent20New percent20P-Process.pdf

Hutchinson, P. (2010). Estimating causal effects from family planning health communication campaigns: An analysis of the "Your Health, Your Wealth" communication campaign in Menya Villages, Egypt. Paper presented at the Annual Meeting of the American Public Health Association, Denver, CO, November 7–10, 2010.

Johns Hopkins University. (2005a). *Health Communication Partnership 2004–2005 Annual Report.* Baltimore: Johns Hopkins University.

Johns Hopkins University. (2005b). Egyptian health program generates 8.5 million calls from TV viewers. Press Release. Baltimore: Johns Hopkins University.

Kashan, A, Baker, P., and Kenny, L. (2010). Preterm birth and reduced birthweight in first and second teenage pregnancies: A register-based cohort study. *BMC Pregnancy and Childbirth, 10*(36) DOI: 10.1186/1471-2393-10-36.

Kawachi, I., Kennedy, B. P., and Lochner, K. (1997). Long live community: Social capital as public health. *The American Prospect, 8*(35), 56–59.

Khalil, K. and Roudi-Fahimi, F. (2004). *Making Motherhood Safer in Egypt*. MENA Policy Briefs. Washington, DC: Population Reference Bureau.

Kickbusch, I. and Nutbeam, D. (1998). *Health Promotion Glossary*. Geneva: World Health Organisation.

Kincaid, D. L. (2004). From innovation to social norm: Bounded normative influence. *Journal of Health Communication, 9* (Supplement 1), 37–57.

Kincaid, D. L., and Figueroa, M. E. (2009). Communication for participatory development: Dialogue, collective action, and change. In L. Frey and K. Cissna (Eds.), *Handbook of Applied Communication* (pp. 506–532). Mahwah, NJ: Lawrence Erlbaum Associates.

Kotler, P. (1999). *Kotler on Marketing. How to Create, Win, and Dominate Markets*. New York: The Free Press.

Kotler, P. and Lee, N. (2008). *Social Marketing. Influencing Behaviors for Good*, 3rd edn. Thousand Oaks, CA: Sage Publications.

Lord, R. G. and Brown, D. J. (2004). *Leadership Processes and Follower Identity*. Mahwah, NJ: Lawrence Erlbaum Associates.

Lozare, B. and Hess, R. (1993). *Improving Husband–Wife Communication on Family Planning through TV Drama – Pakistan*, Paper presented at the Annual Meeting of the Association for Public Health, San Francisco, CA, November, 1993.

Meekers, D. and El-Ghazaly, N. (2005). Smoking and attitudes toward smoking cessation in Menya Governorate, Egypt. Poster presented at the Annual Meeting of the American Public Health Association, Philadelphia, PA. Retrieved from http://apha.confex.com/apha/133am/techprogram/paper_118010.htm

Meekers, D. and Nauman, E. (2006a). Effect of exposure to health communication activities on awareness of healthy behaviors in Menya, Egypt. Paper presented at the Annual Meeting of the American Public Health Association, Boston, MA. Retrieved from http://apha.confex.com/apha/134am/techprogram/paper_141200.htm

Meekers, D. and Nauman, E. (2006b). Reach and impact of the Communication for Healthy Living (CHL) project in Menya, Egypt. Poster presented at the Annual Meeting of the American Public Health Association, Boston, MA. Retrieved from http://apha.confex.com/apha/134am/techprogram/paper_140235.htm

Ministry of Health and Population Egypt, El-Zanaty and Associates, and ORC Macro. (2003). *Egypt Service Provision Assessment Survey 2002*. Calverton, MD: Ministry of Health and Population, El-Zanaty and Associates and ORC Macro.

Moser, C. O. (1993). *Gender Planning and Development: Theory, Practice, and Training*. London and New York: Routledge.

Mousa, A., Ezz El Arab, G., and Rashed, E. (2009). Reaching women in Egypt: A success story. *Community Eye Health Journal, 22*(70), 22–23.

PARC (Pan Arab Research Center) (n.d.). *Media Monitoring Reports*. Cairo: Pan Arab Research Center.

Piotrow, P. T., Kincaid, D. L, Rimon, J. G., and Rinehart, W. E. (1997). *Health Communication: Lessons from Family Planning and Reproductive Health*. Westport, CT: Praeger.

Population Council. (2010). *Survey of Young People in Egypt. Preliminary Report*. Cairo, Egypt: The Population Council.

Putnam, R. D. (1993). The prospective community: Social capital and public life. *The American Prospect, 13*, 1–8.

Putnam, R. D. (2001). *Bowling Alone. The Collapse and Revival of American Community*. New York: Simon and Schuster.

Robinson, W. and El-Zanaty, F. (2006). *The Demographic Revolution in Modern Egypt*. Oxford: Lexington Books.

Rogers, E. (1983). *Diffusion of Innovations*, 3rd edn. New York: The Free Press.

Rosenbaum, P. and Rubin, D. B. (1983). The central role of the propensity score in observational studies for causal effects. *Biometrika, 70*(1), 41–55.

Rothschild, M. (1999). Carrots, sticks, and promises: A conceptual framework for the management of public health and social issue behaviors. *Journal of Marketing, 63*(4), 24–37.

Salem, R., Bernstein, J., Sullivan, T., and Landa, R. (2008). *Communication for Better Health*. Population Reports, Series J, No. 56. Baltimore, MD: INFO Project, Johns Hopkins Bloomberg School of Public Health.

Senge, P.M. (1994). *The Fifth Discipline: The Art and Practice of the Learning Organization*. New York: Doubleday.

Soul Beat Africa. (2009). *Arab Women Speak Out (AWSO) – Middle East/North Africa*. Retrieved from http://www.comminit.com/es/node/119815/38

Soul Beat Africa. (2010). *Mabrouk! Initiative*. Retrieved from www.commitinit.com/en/node/276306/38

Stogdill, R. M. (1974). *Handbook of Leadership: A Survey of the Literature*. New York: Free Press.

Storey, J. D., Kaggwa, E., and Harbour, C. (2008). *Communication Pathways to Health Competence: Testing a Model in Egypt and South Africa*. Paper presented at the Annual Meeting of the International Communication Association, Montreal, Canada, May 22–26, 2008.

Suzuki, C. and Meekers, D. (2008). Determinants of support for female genital circumcision among ever-married women in Egypt. *Global Public Health, 3*(4), 383–408.

Tirmizi, S. A. (2002). The 6-L framework: A model for leadership research and development. *Leadership and Organizational Development Journal 23*, 269–279.

Udjo, E. O. (1997). The effect of child survival on fertility in Zimbabwe: A micro-macro level analysis. *Journal of Tropical Pediatrics, 43*(5), 255–266.

Underwood, C. R. and Jabre, B. (2008). Enabling women's agency: Arab women speak out. *Journal of Communication for Development and Social Change, 2*(2), 13–32.

USAID. (2009). *USAID Country Health Statistical Report: Egypt*. Washington, D.C.: USAID and Analysis, Information Management and Communication Activity (AIM) Project.

USAID, Office of Inspector General. (2006). *Audit of USAID/Egypt's family planning activities*. Audit Report No. 6-263-06-001-P (September 28, 2006). Cairo, Egypt: USAID/Egypt.

Vignoli, D. (2006). Fertility change in Egypt. From second to third birth. *Demographic Research, 5*(18), 499–516.

White, S. A. (1994). *The Concept of Participation: Transforming Rhetoric to Reality*. Participatory communication: Working for change and development. Newbury Park, CA: Sage.

WHO (World Health Organisation) (2006). *Constitution of the World Health Organisation*. Retrieved from http://www.who.int/governance/eb/who_constitution_en.pdf

WHO Regional Office for the Eastern Mediterranean (2006). *Egypt: Country Cooperation Strategy for WHO and Egypt, 2005–2009*. Cairo: World Health Organisation, Regional Office for the Eastern Mediterranean.

Youssef, H., Abdel-Tawab, N., Bratt, J. *et al.* (2007). *Linking Family Planning with Postabortion Services in Egypt: Testing the Feasibility, Acceptability and Effectiveness of Two Models of Integration*. Washington, DC: Population Council, FRONTIERS in Reproductive Health.

19

Risk Communication and Emerging Infectious Diseases

Lessons and Implications for Theory–Praxis from Avian Influenza Control

Ketan Chitnis

Background and Scope

The year 2006 witnessed an international public health emergency unfold as the highly pathogenic avian influenza virus (H5N1 HPAI/Type A virus, hereafter referred to as AI) emerged in Southeast Asia. AI was detected in 2003 among wild and domestic poultry. However, when large numbers of human cases of avian influenza were reported in 2006, the global community was on high alert, given the experience of SARS in 2003. The concern was well placed, given the case fatality ratio among adults and children infected was close to 70% in the years 2006, 2007, and 2008, fearing an emergence of a novel influenza virus (UNSIC and World Bank, 2006, 2007, 2008).

The fact that the disease was quickly spreading across countries in Southeast Asia and to other regions including South and Central Asia, Europe, and parts of Africa, indicated an imminent risk of a potentially fatal pandemic. It was feared that, once the AI virus became entrenched among humans, the new virus would cause a serious influenza pandemic, such as the 1918 pandemic that killed millions (UNSIC and World Bank, 2006). Figure 19.1 provides a snapshot of the numbers of AI cases reported globally from 2003 to 2011. While the outbreak was concentrated in parts of East Asia, clearly the disease was spreading fast and manifesting in regions far and wide such as Africa and Central Asia, with 130 cases reported in Egypt and several cases in Turkey and Azerbaijan.

The international community was quick to mount a rapid response to prevent, control, and mitigate the impact of AI, beginning late 2005. The response plan initiated by the United Nations to assist national governments identified public information and supporting behavior change as one of the seven core objectives.[1] While informing the

The Handbook of Global Health Communication, First Edition. Edited by Rafael Obregon and Silvio Waisbord.

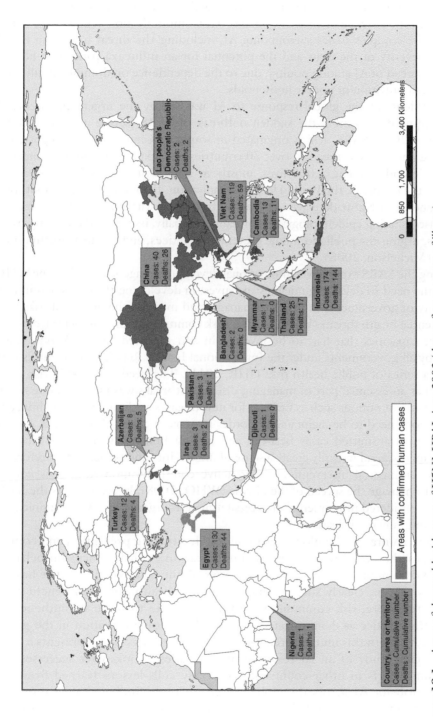

Figure 19.1 Areas of the world with cases of H5N1 HPAI since 2003 (date refers to onset of illness).

Source: (c) World Health Organisation, Global Health Observatory Map Gallery. Retrieved from http://gamapserver.who.int/mapLibrary/app/searchResults.aspx

public through the media to manage public perceptions was crucial, so was the need to protect communities by promoting preventive practices and behaviors, the best option at hand given the absence of a vaccine against AI. Communication actions were aimed to address the complex issues surrounding AI, including the threat to human health due to the severity of the virus and the potential for an influenza pandemic, how to control the spread of AI among poultry, due to the dependence on domestic poultry for livelihood and nutrition of poorer households.

The precedent for the global response to AI was set by the urgent public health response required to combat the sudden outbreak of SARS (severe acute respiratory syndrome) in 2003. SARS, which originated in southern China, was first reported in Hong Kong and quickly spread to over 30 countries in a span of six months, infecting 8,500 people and claiming 1,000 lives, mostly in Southeast Asia (WHO, 2003). In response to the outbreak, the World Health Organisation, through the Global Outbreak Response and Alert Network, played a proactive role along with governments in reporting new cases, sharing epidemiological information globally, issuing and enforcing travel restrictions, urging the public to follow preventive practices, and, in turn, averting new infections (Michelson, 2005).

Following the SARS experience, international development agencies such as the WHO identified the need to develop guidelines and invest in developing the core communication capacity of governments to plan for, manage, and mitigate the impact of risks with real or potential health threats (WHO, 2008). Risk communication was identified as one of the core capacities that had to be invested in and reported to the World Health Assembly by all governments under the International Health Regulation that deals with managing a series of public health risks (IHR, 2011). The need to invest in risk communication as an essential part of managing disease outbreaks was identified due to the fact that treatment options such as vaccines for new diseases are limited or take time, and public reactions need to be maintained in order to avoid a crisis. Also, diseases such as SARS that are transmitted easily between and among humans, within countries and across continents, tend to easily create a sense of uncertainty and panic, and therefore, in addition to biomedical interventions, a proactive communication strategy is equally important to manage the spread of the disease (WHO, 2008). In recent years the SARS outbreak is considered monumental in necessitating a resurgence in risk communication efforts around infectious diseases.

This chapter unravels the global response to AI, situating prevention and control efforts within the broad realm of risk communication, with the focus on behavior change and communication among communities. While much of the practice has not been theory-driven, clearly such an eminent public health crisis can benefit from theory. Furthermore, risk communication theory can, in turn, be strengthened by public health practice as demonstrated by the role of communication in the global response to AI. With this mutually reinforcing objective, this chapter presents a comprehensive case study of an AI response in Bangladesh, looks over successes and failures from efforts in other countries, and finally culls lessons learned from risk communication for AI across the globe. Based on these findings, implications for theory–praxis and recommendations to strengthen risk communication efforts are presented.

Risk Communication Approaches and Theories to Inform Action

The field of risk communication has its roots in the United States, dating back to the 1980s with environmental risks dominating public discourse and policy-making efforts (Covello and Sandman, 2001). Risk communication can be defined as the "interactive process of exchange of information and opinion among individuals, groups, and institutions concerning a risk or potential risk to human health or the environment" (National Research Council, 1989, p. 21). Some approaches to risk communication continue to build on the traditional one-way communication process where a source sends a message using a certain channel to a receiver. Others view the process as two-way and less linear. Among the various approaches to communicating risk, some are particularly relevant to AI efforts. For instance, the social constructionist approach puts forward the idea that the flow of information travels both ways between the scientific community and the stakeholders, as the scientific community has inherent values, beliefs, and emotions and the stakeholders have a store of technical knowledge, both of which affect the communication process. This approach recognizes that social context and culture affect beliefs and actions and emphasizes that giving due attention to the context can aid in the exchange and flow of information, attitudes, values, beliefs, and perceptions between the stakeholder and the source of the information, leading to better "risk decisions" (Lundgren and McMakin, 2009).

Another approach suggests that risk should be viewed as both a potential hazard and an outrage. This approach recognizes the danger or the hazard in the actions as well as the emotions people attach to their actions. So, while the hazard is the technical or scientific aspect of the risk assessment, the outrage is the emotional and nonscientific aspect of the information or assessment as experienced by the average person. The value addition of this approach is that it goes beyond the technicalities of the information and stresses that audiences require their feelings and concerns to be addressed through the communication response in addition to a presentation of the facts about a health threat (Covello and Sandman, 2001).

Applying some of the above principles, crisis and risk communication has been classified by some scholars as understanding how to prepare and help the public to manage events ranging from natural disasters, public health emergencies, and bioterrorism (Aakko, 2004; Abraham, 2009; Reynolds and Seeger, 2005). While each of these events involves a role for communication, behavioral actions and public education goals are different depending on the threat posed to the public and the country context in which the emergency unfolds. Communication components in the form of warnings, risk messages, evacuation notifications, messages regarding self-efficacy, and information regarding symptoms and medical treatment, are just some of the examples of the role of communication following an event. Simply put, crisis communication is usually communication after an event such as a disease outbreak, an earthquake, or a nuclear leak. Risk communication is linked to the identification of a risk to the public and the provision of information and use of communication to alleviate that risk through the adoption of protective practices.

A nuanced understanding of risk communication by several scholars has advanced the concept of dealing with how the public senses an impending threat based on people's own assessment of it. Communication deals with controlling the risk either pre- or post-event, based on a mix of technical information being exchanged by experts, the public, and other interested entities such as governments. Particularly with regard to behavior change, Witte (1998) elaborates that risk communication uses fear appeal to communicate possible threats, but also offers solutions by promoting preventive practices to alleviate the threat by underscoring self-efficacy, that is, the ability to adopt positive health behaviors. This approach extends risk communication to include a dialogue between the authorities and the public.

CDC has combined crisis and emergency risk communication approaches by putting forward a process model of dealing with a crisis or emergency situation before, during, and after the event. The five-stage model is based on the assumption that crises will unfold over a period of time requiring preparedness, control, and mitigation strategies. While the value of this model is to reduce uncertainty by investing in preparedness activities for risk communication, the model does acknowledge that not all crises can be planned for and communication may be required to deal with situations and audience needs that are uncertain (Reynolds and Seeger, 2005).

A further analysis of risk communication is the role of behavioral theory in understanding and identifying how beliefs influence risky behaviors (Fishbein and Cappella, 2006). While it has been established that behaviors are determined by individuals' beliefs, identifying people's beliefs is not enough to make communication efforts effective, as the communication process still needs to involve people and build a certain level of trust to change negative beliefs into positive behaviors. Fishbein and Cappella (2006) in their work on the role of theory in health communication interventions have proposed an integrated model that blends behavioral theory and communication theory to promote healthy behaviors or alter unhealthy practices. The integrated model for successful health communication builds upon extensive research into the subject and uses concepts such as existing behavioral beliefs and attitudes, normative belief systems, perceived self-efficacy to change, and prevailing power structures as determinants of whether or not people will adopt new behaviors. It also charts the environmental factors, skills and abilities of individuals, and people's intention to change. A combination of these behavioral factors, supported by trustworthy, credible, and appropriate communication, including involving communities in the process, will result in positive behavioral changes, it proposes.

The integrated model for health communication was applied to people's intention to quit smoking (Fishbein and Cappella, 2006). It was found that people's intention to quit smoking significantly predicted quitting behavior – in other words, if people had made up their mind to quit smoking then they were more likely to quit after being exposed to communication than were those people who had not decided to quit smoking. The study found that communication would be most effective in achieving the desired outcome – reducing the number of smokers – when it was aimed at persuading those people who did not intend to quit. A combination of factors including attitude, social norms, and self-efficacy together made up people's intention to quit or not to quit smoking. However, in this study the authors argued that good communication-theory-driven messages are required to ultimately change attitudes. Therefore, the study pointed out that successful health communication is a combination of understanding behavioral determinants and designing messages that people will act upon; it is not enough to have just one of the elements covered when designing campaigns.

The range of risk communication approaches provides us with several insights that apply differently to different situations, depending on contexts, audiences, and the types of risk being communicated. While there is no best approach for all contexts and risks, Lundgren and McMakin (2009) reiterate that "understanding the various approaches and their implications can provide us with a repertoire of ways to develop our risk communication efforts, giving us a greater chance of success than if we were communicating without this knowledge" (p. 20).

In recent years a spate of life-threatening public health emergencies such as the rapid spread of infectious diseases like AI and West Nile Virus, together with bioterrorism threats like anthrax and natural disasters, has reinforced the need to deepen the study of health and risk communication efforts to counter serious health crises (Kreps, 2009). The health- and life- threatening aspects of these emergencies are further exacerbated by the fact that most of them either involve large numbers of people or are highly transmittable, having epidemic and pandemic potential and therefore requiring both an immediate and an effective response. The subsequent sections of the chapter look at communication efforts for AI control and present a detailed case from Bangladesh, while also presenting the successes and challenges of current efforts and recommendations for future action.

Communication for Avian Influenza Control

The comprehensive AI strategy necessitated two types of broad-based communication responses (1) outbreak/risk communication focused on how the authorities responsible for animal and human health can assist in mobilizing the media and other channels to provide timely, trustworthy, and accurate information that reflects the needs of communities, and (2) behavior change communication focused on how individuals, communities, and institutions can reduce risks through changed or modified behaviors and, in turn, protect themselves from the disease. Advocacy with national and subnational government counterparts underpins the success of behavior change and outbreak communication, as both strategies remain the responsibility of government authorities (Strickland and Nabarro, 2006; UNSIC, 2006).

Standard and simplified behavioral actions were formulated by epidemiologists, veterinary scientists, and communication professionals, which were to be adapted to local conditions and promoted widely to urgently halt the spread of AI (WHO/FAO/UNICEF, 2006). The key actions promoted were grouped under four categories – report sickness or death among poultry or fever in humans after contact with poultry; separate poultry by species and separate from children and living areas; wash hands, clothes, cages, etc. after contact with poultry; and cook fully. These actions were deemed sufficient to control the rapid transmission of AI, provided there was an enabling environment to support them, which included public trust, awareness and recognition of risks and symptoms, and an understanding of cultural practices related to food handling, preparation, and consumption.

The overall response aimed to promote standardized behaviors to avert the rapid spread of AI. To this effect, actions were promoted to capture a range of behaviors that would limit transmission of AI from poultry to other domestic animals, as well as to protect humans from becoming infected. At the community level, the services that complemented uptake of protective behaviors were culling, if poultry was found to be infected, compensation to farmers/households who lost their livestock, vaccination, and, in some cases, alternative livelihood options. In principle, the strategy being promoted and implemented was sound, since what was expected from communities as a result of adopting new behaviors was complemented by adequate services to ensure households did not fall further into poverty. The integrated communication approach used in Kurigram district in Bangladesh, provides a good example of how outbreak and long-term behavior change communication interventions can be promoted simultaneously. The case study, described below, situates the background and outcomes of the Kurigram communication experience with a broader national risk communication response to AI.

Community-based Risk Communication for AI Control: The Kurigram Case

In response to the AI outbreak in Bangladesh in 2007, the government of Bangladesh, with support from agencies, spearheaded a program to reduce the risk of transmission of AI (UNICEF, 2010)[2]. UNICEF supported a national communication strategy aimed at creating awareness and promoting preventive practices to reduce the spread of the disease based on a knowledge, attitudes, and practices (KAP) survey among the urban and rural general public and backyard poultry farmers. In addition, UNICEF supported a five-month-long pilot communication project closely linked with the national strategy in Kurigram district, which accounted for over 15 percent of AI cases in the country, all of which were in backyard farms. Kurigram is one of the most inaccessible districts in the country, with no electricity and an almost complete absence of media reach in about one third of the district.

The Kurigram pilot aimed to provide a rapid response to the expanding pandemic situation in the country and create high-impact contact with the general population, while setting a national standard for interpersonal communication in response to AI. Given the challenging geographical context, the project provides experiential insights on conducting community mobilization and behavior change interventions in hard-to-reach terrains. The pilot project raised awareness on AI. However, at the later stage, when the H1N1 virus broke out in 2009, relevant messages were included in the communication activities to link up with the national efforts undertaken in response to pandemic flu.

Project implementation

The pilot was carried out using an integrated communication strategy, combining components of behavior change, community mobilization, and advocacy, drawing upon entertainment education as well as participatory communication methods. The approach extended beyond individuals and households to include service providers, traditional and religious leaders (i.e., Imams), key decision makers, and influential people in the community in order to ensure systematic social change with measurable impact. The multipronged activities included:

- *Screening videos:* Miking was used in crowded areas to announce the screening of videos as well as when 30 key messages developed by technical and communication agencies were disseminated. The video was shown in schools followed by a facilitated discussion.
- *Teacher training:* A ToT (training of trainers) of 30 master trainers was held at the Primary Training Institute (PTI) on effective utilization of the interactive games kit on AI prevention for school children. One teacher from each of the 563 government primary schools in Kurigram was trained and a Students' Day was organized in each of the 563 schools where teachers talked about AI prevention and showed the children how to play the interactive games, reaching out to a total of 20,000 school children.
- *Training and advocacy with religious leaders:* A pool of master trainers was developed to train imams in their respective *upazilas*. The imams delivered sermons from a booklet developed using teachings from the Holy Quran and creating a link with flu prevention behaviors, they promoted the use of soap during ablution and other preventive behaviors among the local population. A total of 2,898 imams were trained.
- *Mobilization of herbal medicine vendors:* Three hundred herbal medicine vendors were mobilized as partners, they put up posters with key messages, wore tee shirts that identified themselves as participants and handed out flyers containing AI messages to their customers.
- *Interactive popular theatre (IPT) performances with participatory scripts:* In collaboration with the Gram Theatre, a popular theatre organization in Bangladesh, 72 shows were performed, each show watched by around 650 people. Prior to the performance, the actors went from house to house generating interest and awareness about the show and AI issues. The scripts were developed by local boys and girls over a five-day workshop. Some 46,800 people were reached, 45 percent women and 35 percent adolescents.
- *Ongoing monitoring:* Both internal and external monitoring activities were carried out. The internal monitoring included tracking of IPT performances (village details, attendance, etc.) by the local government chair and the external study covering about half the 72 unions of the district included implementation, process, and outcome monitoring.

Outcome analysis

The KAP survey of 2010 assessed the differences in knowledge, attitude, and practice between the respondents in Kurigram and those from other areas of the country as well as from the national-level 2007 KAP survey. The assessment shows the impact of communication activities in Kurigram and its effectiveness in raising awareness and promoting behavior change among participants.

A significant proportion (77 percent) of survey respondents in rural and 16 percent in urban areas of Kurigram claimed to have heard of AI. Those who had heard of it were aware that it spread through contact with infected birds (67 percent) as well as a contaminated environment (29 percent). Over half of the respondents believed that humans were susceptible to the disease and knew about the means of human contamination (56 percent cited consumption of infected meat/eggs from poultry and 25 percent cited contact with infected poultry).

The practice of proper disposal of waste showed a positive trend as 35 percent of the general public and 24 percent of backyard farmers in the district mentioned burying waste in compost pits, which is an improvement from the previous practices found by the 2007 KAP survey. Poultry manure compost pits were found in about 22 percent of households with separate pits for burial of dead birds – both positive indicators compared to the national estimates of 2007 and 2010. All wet market vendors were well aware of AI. In fact, 100 percent of them reported awareness. They were found to be significantly aware of the importance of washing hands, which they demonstrated to the survey teams.

As a pilot project, the Kurigram experience may be considered to have fulfilled all expectations. Significant levels of community participation ensued involving different stakeholders and ownership of the project was demonstrated by the District Information Officer, whose cooperation was crucial to the project's effectiveness and was cited as a key source of information on AI in the pilot district. The Imams, scriptwriters and performers of the IPT shows, and medicine vendors all felt ownership towards the project. The detailed planning, the course corrections made based on feedback, the adjustments made to the activities to suit the audience, all contributed to making a difference in the AI-related KAP level of the people of Kurigram. The pilot, in fact, has demonstrated that a communication program has the potential to be really effective if all possible communication methods and channels are employed together.

Successes and challenges of risk communication for AI control

The urgency of communicating risks and preparing communities to manage the threat of avian influenza led to remarkable successes early in the response. Globally, between 2006 and 2007 several achievements were noted with regard to successful communication to control AI. With increasing global commitment and investments to contain the spread of the disease, most countries created intersectoral partnerships including a national interagency communication taskforce and advocated with relevant ministries and departments in health, agriculture, veterinary science, and livestock to develop and implement communication plans. This was achieved even in regions where AI outbreaks had not occurred, such as in Latin America and the Caribbean and Eastern and Southern Africa (UNICEF, 2008).

Rapid development and implementation of national communication strategies and plans, resulted in increased awareness of the risks and knowledge of how to mitigate these risks in at least 70 percent of the people in affected countries and over 90 percent in some countries like Indonesia, Cambodia, and Thailand. In over 20 countries where knowledge, attitude, and practice surveys were conducted in 2006 and 2007, it was found that knowledge and awareness of AI was high in the general population and in high-risk groups. However, people continued to practice high-risk behaviors when handling poultry as their risk perception of AI was quite low.

Hickler (2007), through a series of participatory action researches with farmers and rural communities, found out that a primary challenge to behavior change was rooted in the conflicting perception of AI among the local taxonomy and the technical experts. Farmers in Cambodia often refer to seasonal illness and death among chickens as *dan kor kach*. In order to communicate the severity of AI, experts coined the term *pdash sai back sey*. However, because the symptoms of AI are similar to the common seasonal illness among poultry caused by Newcastle disease, which is endemic, the new term did not really increase the risk perception among communities. The research also revealed that "the degree to which groups reported changes in community behavior was not correlated with higher levels of awareness or fear, but was rather positively proportional to the degree to which people saw their poultry and families at risk" (Hickler, 2007, p. 2).

In addition, in other countries it was found that people did not practice preventive behaviors due to lack of resources, difficult living conditions, and deep-rooted cultural practices. Surveys revealed that communication promoting desired behaviors to control AI is dependent on factors such as compensation policies, functioning surveillance systems, and veterinary and animal health infrastructure. On the ground, operational challenges revealed that communication dealing with the intersection of animal and health requires a specialized approach and increased communication capacity, especially within the animal health sector where communication capacity was weak.

Despite the well-intentioned global communication guidance and its adaption in countries that were most severely affected by AI, professionals and governments were concerned that AI communication efforts were resulting in increased levels of awareness and limited knowledge gained about the new virus, but that communities were unable to practice the recommended behaviors (UNICEF, 2008). The prospective assessment funded by the European Union, reported that communication systems that were put in place did result in "(strengthened) capacities for outbreak and risk communications among, in particular, Ministries of Agriculture, which can be objectively verified in those countries where the UNICEF coordination has been successful" (HTSPE, 2010, p. 53). The report goes on to illustrate that "the social mobilization with technically accurate messaging has resulted in an objectively verifiable impact as many KAP studies clearly demonstrated the high levels of knowledge and awareness of the contents of the messages. However, the anticipated behavior change stemming from those messages has not been achieved; thus the massive financial inputs have not contributed to a possible limitation in virus dissemination" (HTSPE, 2010, p. 53). Finally, the report concludes that "to achieve behavior change multidisciplinary intervention programs must combine risk perception communication with local values and priorities, feasible and practical recommendations including economic considerations for resource-poor settings, and must offer farmers that have limited materials for personal protection alternative methods to safely work with livestock on a daily basis" (HTSPE, 2010, p. 53).

These findings point to the challenges that were faced by professionals engaged in controlling the risk of the spread of AI at a time when a novel virus was spreading fast across countries and claiming several lives. However, in the long run the communication response had to be weighed against the programmatic response and the broader issue surrounding the economic situation of households with small numbers of backyard poultry with little access to protective gear and alternative livelihood options. Communication failed in ensuring sustainable changes in behaviors needed to limit the transmission of vectors within poultry and between poultry and humans, primarily because local adaptation of technically sound actions could not be carried out in many countries as one was dealing with an emergency.

Behavior change, however, does go beyond aspects of localizing technical information, addressing risk perceptions and ensuring communities are part of the communication process. While all these aspects are pivotal for good communication strategies, following a surge of human cases of AI in 2009 the European Commission study proposed that:

> human cases arise from direct and possibly indirect contact with infected birds and, therefore, humans can act as sentinels for disease in the poultry population. These figures [human cases of AI in 2009] may indicate that the incidence of AI in birds may, in fact, not have been falling, but that levels and standards of surveillance and diagnosis in poultry are falling because of low risk perception and major disincentives such as the economic and social consequences of reporting. Absence of, or insufficient indemnification/compensation is also a cause for under-reporting of outbreaks. Worldwide there is a large variety in compensation schemes, policies and payment mechanisms but little compensation is actually paid. Compensation for culled poultry has proved to be a contentious subject (HTSPE, 2010, p. 3).

Lessons Learned from Global Experiences in AI Control

Among the varying opinions and evidence on the efficacy of behavior change communication for AI control, several good practices emerged particularly from countries that were severely impacted by outbreaks of the disease among poultry and those with relatively higher numbers of human cases. A mix of communication interventions that resulted in positive communication outcomes have been recorded from Cambodia, Egypt, Indonesia, Thailand, Turkey, and Lao PDR (UNICEF, 2008). Several reviews and assessments from a global and regional level point to a number of lessons that could be gleaned from the communication experience of AI (Chitnis and Mansoor, 2007; Coker *et al.*, 2011; UNICEF, 2008). These lessons can be broadly categorized as (1) Supporting national AI responses and (2) implementing integrated BCC campaigns.

Supporting national AI responses

Coordination mechanisms for communication were established in most countries, which helped ensure that communication plans for AI in view of a potential pandemic influenza threat were in place by 2008 as part of the national response to AI. Investments in strengthening communication capacity to deal with AI and other zoonotic diseases led to positive outcomes among agriculture ministries, which otherwise tended to relegate communication to mere information dissemination. Over time the national media coverage of AI improved, as governments applied risk communication principles to build trust, reduce panic, and provide timely and correct information on outbreaks and actions to be taken to protect especially the vulnerable, children and the elderly, from AI. While the imminent threat was global, with the disease reported in 40 countries in 2006, it was hard to convince governments and the public to be vigilant about a health threat that had not been reported in their own country. Communicators had to walk a fine line between preparing communities to manage AI on the one hand and not raising panic and undue alarm on the other hand.

An interagency communication response for AI with buy-in from across sectors (agriculture, health, trade, livestock) and involving technical experts to deal with an emerging and evolving health issue requires time and can be challenging. Lack of clarity of roles and a need to have a lead ministry to manage communication is essential for accountability. Furthermore, investments in strengthening the capacity of national counterparts to plan and implement communication strategies to prepare for and respond to new public health crises requires ongoing actions as outlined in the IHR, with close coordination between animal and human health sectors to manage new and emerging zoonotic diseases.

Implementing integrated risk communication campaigns

Where AI was entrenched, positive changes were seen in adopting risk reduction practices when existing health and outreach worker networks, with additional training and investment in interpersonal communication skills, were mobilized early on (e.g., in Bangladesh, Egypt, Indonesia, Thailand, and Turkey). Standardized guidelines and several communication planning and training toolkits have been developed and used with different stakeholders ranging from government officials at various administrative levels to outreach workers to civil society and faith-based organizations (www.influenzaresources.org, http://avianflu.aed.org, www.createforchildren.org). While media and other channels were used extensively to sensitize the public about the threats of AI and how to protect oneself, groups who handle poultry on a daily basis (such as the women and children who care for backyard poultry, or transporters or wet market workers, who tend to be men), were not always reached with realistic preventive behaviors. Furthermore, for such high-risk groups, the simplified, technically sound messages relating to hygiene and separating poultry from other domestic animals were not practical even when these groups were reached with extensive communication networks. Rapid research in Burkina Faso and Nigeria revealed that there is a need to identify specific AI communication strategies that reach the hard-to-reach and those potentially at risk of AI, with credible information on an ongoing basis and to promote realistic behaviors grounded in the local context. Behavioral actions such as "keeping children away from chicken" or "separating birds from humans" were not feasible in many countries (UNICEF, 2008).

The general public had to be made aware of the risks posed by AI to ensure that informed choices were made regarding protecting oneself as well as decisions regarding consumption of poultry. Undue panic was expected to severely impact the demand for poultry, which would, in turn, negatively affect producers and distributors along the food chain. Thus socioeconomic ramifications as a result of communication activities needed to be accounted for. Successful communication efforts to stop the transmission at source, i.e., among birds, to ensure humans are protected from AI need functioning surveillance systems, limited culling and adequate compensation for affected farmers. These programming imperatives were critical to motivate communities to report cases. Community-based surveillance systems policies were enforced and were successful in countries ranging from Bangladesh to Egypt to Lao PDR to Turkey. In a short period of time, the role of communication was to inform, empower, and motivate people to engage in protective behaviors for themselves and their families as well as to ensure that the disease was not spread widely. This was achieved with a varying degree of success. However, for new emerging infectious diseases in the future, a proactive strategy that halts the transmission at source needs to be planned for rather than an outbreak response.

Implications for Future Theory and Praxis

This review of the experience of behavior change communication to control AI as a facet of the broader risk communication response to the disease outbreak has pointed out several areas where theory could inform practice. Commonly applied theories in behavior change communication are a mix of psychological, sociological, and interpersonal communication. In addition, risk communication seeks to build trust by being transparent, open, and credible while dealing with the public. Key theoretical constructs to design future risk communication efforts, particularly around emerging infectious diseases, could include systematically understanding and assessing risk perceptions and thereafter engaging in a communication process that reinforces self-efficacy, addresses social and cultural norms, uses change agents, and continues to build trust and ownership of communication efforts. Therefore, what is proposed is the application of theory to guide interventions, lessons that would strengthen the conceptual underpinning of risk communication.

Focusing on risk perception

The first principle that could improve future communication efforts would be understanding how individuals and communities perceive risk. Building on the extensive work of Slovic (1987), where risk perception is considered as a subjective notion of the level of threat posed due to various events, and it is argued that perceptions can lead to an amplification of a risk well beyond the actual threat posed by the event, further evidence has demonstrated that risk perceptions are a result of complex interplay of the actual impact of the risk, sociocultural factors, and emotional reactions (Slovic and Weber, 2002). In other words, the cognitive and emotional elements of the different stakeholders involved in the communication process need to be deconstructed. The lessons from AI regarding the behavior change communication processes and activities rolled out in most countries clearly point out that the level of risk of AI perceived and understood by technical experts was not the same as that perceived by the general population. In particular, the risk perception of AI among the communities at the front line of the disease – communities with household/backyard poultry, transporters of poultry, wet market workers – was very low due to the newness of the disease, similarity of symptoms with other common illnesses that kill poultry routinely, and the lack of association between illness and death in birds with flu-like symptoms among humans. The risk of a health threat was very low among the at-risk communities, whereas the risk of loss of livelihood in case of culling or a sudden onset of AI among birds was high.

Intensive communication efforts around potential and perceived risks as opposed to communicating about protective actions alone, when risk perceptions were low or disproportionate to the level of exposure to AI, would have resulted in desired behavioral changes. Linked to the issue of risk perception, communication efforts would have done better had the communication actions and messages also focused on the ability of individuals and communities to prevent the spread of the virus. If self-efficacy, which includes the actions that people can take, was underscored in the communication for different audience groups (primarily, those at immediate risk such as those handling poultry; secondarily, those who are at a distant risk but need to be aware such as the general population; and, tertiarily, those who make decisions and can influence policies) rather than generic actions for all groups, then changes in behavior might have been more feasible.

Promoting self-efficacy and collective action

By providing options to communities as to what they can do (either new practices or adapting existing practices) to be self-efficacious would have improved their confidence in the actions being recommended. Involving at-risk communities from the start would have ensured that local practices around biosecurity or hygiene practices when dealing with poultry and other animals would be feasible. While the rapid outbreaks of AI in several countries in 2006 required urgent risk communication efforts, to ensure sustainable behavior change a more long-term perspective was needed that allowed community participation and ownership. Drawing upon the principles of the communication for social change model – initiating a community dialogue and promoting collective action – would have balanced the expectation of technical recommendations with locally appropriate actions. The Kurigram case study reveals that active and widespread community participation is feasible even in a short period of time, provided the right stakeholders are identified and direction is given through which behavior change communication can become locally owned.

Localizing the content through addressing social norms and individual behaviors could have spurred community dialogue and ultimately ownership. Emphasis was too much on the psychometric model of communication where the technical experts decided what to would be best to inform the public about the potential risk of AI (Abraham, 2009). Furthermore, communication around AI control relied heavily on local and media channels, which was effective in rapidly informing communities of risks but did not allow a chance for a two-way dialogue. Change agents and social mobilization efforts were also sporadic and not systematically integrated into the communication interventions. Blending principles of diffusion theory, particularly the role of change agents, along with promoting communication actions based on technical accuracy would have provided more room for dialogue and interactive communication. Change agents could also have been effective in alerting existing risk perception in communities that did not see AI as a threat or those that felt they had little control over the disease, as seen in the Cambodia experience (Heckler, 2007). Countries where positive changes in behaviors were reported, such as in Egypt and Indonesia (UNICEF, 2008) local leaders and community health workers played a significant role, underscoring the importance of change agents to mobilize collective action.

Outreach and interpersonal communication

Harnessing the expertise of change agents in mobilizing action to control and mitigate the risk posed by emerging infectious diseases could have furthered the success of AI communication efforts. To complement the media outreach activities, further investments in developing the interpersonal skills of outreach workers to facilitate adaptation of standardized preventive behaviors to local realities and enable action would have strengthened the integrated communication approach. Future behavior change communication interventions would benefit from the enhanced skills of outreach workers particularly to manage and tackle relevant and logical questions pertaining to new and emerging infectious diseases. Enhanced skills of outreach workers would allow for greater dialogue and transparency and for the establishment of trust between communities and health workers, who act as intermediaries for the local adaptation of technical information. While several studies on AI communication have documented empirically the knowledge–practice gap, a way to narrow the gap would be to encourage dialogue. Trained health and outreach workers with up-to-date knowledge about the health threat, as well as effective interpersonal skills, would provide communities with the means to raise questions, challenge prescriptive messages, propose local solutions, and, over time, establish rapport with the outreach worker. These principles that have resulted in positive outcomes in the field of community-based primary health care could be replicated and adapted to the behavior change component of risk communication.

Conclusion

The review of communication to control AI demonstrates that risk communication theory can inform future practice. While immediate and emergency responses are needed as a first line of response, sustainable behavior change requires community engagement. The role of interpersonal communication and promotion of dialogue among communities and between communities and decision makers cannot be undermined. Evidence reviewed here points to failures in translating information and knowledge into behaviors, and one reason for this is the lack of attention paid to communities' risk perceptions and to the favorable norms and environmental factors needed for individuals and communities to adopt preventive practices.

Second, the complexity of behavior change communication needs to be unpacked before interventions are designed even in an emergency context. As elaborated by the various risk communication concepts and models, people's intentions to change or not to change are determined by a combination of individual factors and social practices as well as the efficacy of communication efforts. Reliance on knowledge, attitude, and practice surveys needs to be limited to track trends; such instruments cannot explain why high levels of knowledge do not result in behavior change. Successful communication efforts, therefore, need to be put into the broader context within which communities live and interact, including their livelihood options. This is particularly important when dealing with new emerging diseases at the animal–human interface.

Finally, the emphasis on community preparedness to manage potential disasters as advanced by disaster risk reduction provides a natural entry point to mainstream risk communication as part of day-to-day communication efforts to empower communities, rather than a strategy that is used to manage risks alone. Risk communication in the future could focus more on: involving communities, including children, to identify risks faced; designing community early-warning systems to manage risks; and empowering communities to become involved in preparedness and response measures as part of development work rather than after an emergency unfolds.

Notes

1   The other objectives dealt with animal health and bio-security, sustaining livelihoods, human health, coordination of national, regional and international stakeholders, continuity under pandemic conditions, humanitarian common services support.
2   Information and data extracted from UNICEF (2010).

References

Aakko, E. (2004). Risk communication, risk perceptions and public. *Wisconsin Medical Journal, 103*(1). Retrieved from http://www.wisconsinmedicalsociety.org/_WMS/publications/wmj/issues/wmj_v103n1/aako.pdf

Abraham, T. (2009). Risk and outbreak communication: lessons from alternative paradigms. *Bulletin of the World Health Organisation, 87*, 604–607.

Chitnis, K. and Mansoor, O. (2007). Role of communication in avian/pandemic influenza programme. Paper presented at the Technical Meeting on Highly Pathogenic Avian Influenza and Human H5N1 Infection, June 2007, FAO, Rome.

Coker, R. J., Hunter, B. M., Rudge, J. W. *et al.* (2011). Emerging infectious diseases in Southeast Asia: Regional challenges to control. *The Lancet 377*, 9765: 599–609.

Covello., V. and Sandman, P. M. (2001). Risk communication: Evolution and revolution. In A. Wolbarst (Ed.), *Solutions to an Environment in Peril* (pp.164–178). Baltimore: Johns Hopkins University Press.

Fishbein, M. and Cappella, J. N. (2006). The role of theory in developing effective health communications *Journal of Communication, 56*, S1–S17.

Hickler, B. (2007). *Bridging the Gap between HPAI "Awareness" and Practice in Cambodia: Recommendations from an Anthropological Participatory Assessment.* FAO: Cambodia. Retrieved from http://www.fao.org/docs/eims/upload//241483/ai301e00.pdf

HTSPE (2010). Outcome and impact assessment of the global response to the avian influenza crisis. European Commission / Regional Programme Asia Cross-border Co-operation in Animal and Human Health. EuropeAid Cooperation Office. Retrieved from http://www.eeas.europa.eu/health/docs/health_grai_en.pdf

IHR (2011). *IHR Core Capacity Monitoring Framework: Checklist and Indicators for Monitoring Progress in the Development of IHR Core Capacities in States Parties.* WHO, Geneva.

Kreps, G. L. (2009). Health communication theories. In S. W. Littlejohn and K. A. Foss (Eds.), *Encyclopedia of Communication Theory.* Thousand Oaks, CA: Sage Publications.

Lundgren, R. E., and McMakin, A. H. (2009). *Risk Communication: A Handbook for Communicating Environmenal, Safety and Health Risks,* 4th edn. Placataway, NJ: IEEE Press.

Michelson, E. S. (2005). Dodging a bullet: WHO, SARS, and the successful management of infectious disease. *Bulletin of Science, Technology and Society, 25*(5), 379–386.

National Research Council (1989). *Improving Risk Communication.* Washington, DC: National Academy Press.

Reynolds, B. and Seeger. M. W. (2005).Crisis and emergency risk communication as an integrative model. *Journal of Health Communication,* 10, 43–55.

Slovic, P. (1987). Perception of risk. *Science, 236,* 280–285.

Slovic, P. and Weber, E.U. (2002). Perception of risk posed by extreme events. Paper presented at the conference on Risk management strategies in an uncertain world, Palisades, New York, April 12–13, 2002.

Strickland, S. and Nabarro, D. (2006). Avian and pandemic influenza: communicating the risks through deliberative dialogue. *The Commonwealth Health Ministers Reference Book.* Retrieved from http://docs.google.com/viewer?a=v&pid=sites&srcid=c3RyaWNrbGFuZC5hc2lhfHd3Hd3d3xneDozOWY5Y2Y5MzIzNTlhYTgy

UNICEF (2008). *Assessment of Communication Initiatives for Prevention and Control of Avian Influenza.* Draft report prepared by Silvio Waisbord. UNICEF New York. Retrieved from http://avianflu.aed.org/docs/pb_bcc.pdf.

UNICEF (2010). *Integrated Communication Response Project for Avian and Pandemic Influenza in Bangladesh: The Kurigram Case Study.* UNICEF: Bangladesh.

UNSIC (2006). *Avian and Human Influenza (AHI): Consolidated Action Plan for the Contributions of the UN System and Partner.* Retrieved from http://www.un.org/influenza/review06_07.pdf

UNSIC and World Bank (2006). *Responses to Avian and Human Influenza Threats: Progress, Analysis and Recommendations.* New York and Washington DC. Retrieved from http://www-wds.worldbank.org/external/default/main?pagePK=64193027&piPK=64187937&theSitePK=523679&menuPK=64187510&searchMenuPK=64187283&siteName=WDS&entityID=000090341_20060802111646

UNSIC and World Bank (2007). *Responses to Avian Influenza and State of Pandemic Readiness Third Global Progress Report.* New York, NY and Washington DC: UNSIC and World Bank.

UNSIC and World Bank (2008). *Responses to Avian Influenza and State of Pandemic Readiness. Fourth Global Progress Report.* New York and Washington, DC. Retrieved from http://un-influenza.org/files/12-18-07UN-WBAHIProgressReportfinal.pdf

WHO (2003). SARS: Lessons from a new disease. In *The World Health Report 2003* (pp. 71–82). Geneva, Switzerland: WHO.

WHO (2008). *Outbreak Communication Planning Guide.* Geneva: WHO.

WHO/FAO/UNICEF (2006). Adhoc meeting on behavioral interventions for avian influenza risk reduction. 14–16 March 2006, WHO Geneva. Retrieved from http://www.who.int/influenza/preparedness/measures/adhocsummaryreport.pdf

Witte, K. (1998). Fear as motivator, fear as inhibitor: Using the extended parallel process model to explain fear appeal successes and failures. In P. A. Andersen and L. K. Guerrero (Eds.), *Handbook of Communication and Emotion: Research, Theory, Applications, and Contexts* (pp. 423–450). San Diego, CA: Academic Press.

20

Journalism and HIV
Lessons from the Frontline of Behavior Change Communication in Mozambique

Gregory Alonso Pirio

Introduction

The southern African country of Mozambique confronts a serious HIV/AIDS epidemic, and public health experts believe that motivating Mozambicans to abandon risky heterosexual behaviors is central to reversing it. This chapter presents lessons learned from designing and implementing a public health intervention in Mozambique intended to inspire the media to become stronger allies in the country's effort to reverse the epidemic. It advocates a change in the way that much journalism in Mozambique (and possibly elsewhere) has covered the HIV/AIDS story, that is, a move away from the more traditional role of the journalist as the mere disseminator of information from experts and political elites to the public and toward an approach centered on journalists as promoters of community dialogue. This chapter suggests that journalists covering HIV/AIDS topics can potentially influence a shift in the public discourse about the epidemic in ways that encourage people to take greater personal and community responsibility in the areas of prevention and treatment and contribute to promoting the behavioral and attitudinal changes needed to reverse the epidemic. The impact of journalists on the public mind will likely increase if they embrace a more inclusive and pluralistic set of journalistic techniques in areas such as sourcing, selecting topics and formats, framing issues, and defining target audiences. Many of the lessons learned from this public health media intervention have applicability beyond Mozambique, especially in other African countries.

The Handbook of Global Health Communication, First Edition. Edited by Rafael Obregon and Silvio Waisbord.
© 2012 John Wiley & Sons, Inc. Published 2012 by John Wiley & Sons, Inc.

Media's Role in the HIV/AIDS Response

People worldwide obtain their knowledge of HIV/AIDS overwhelmingly from the traditional mass media, especially radio and TV. This phenomenon was strikingly borne out, for instance, by an extensive study of the topic by the UN in 2002 conducted in 39 African, Asian, and Latin American countries. It found that radio was by far the most cited source of knowledge about HIV/AIDS. About half of the female respondents and more than seven in ten male respondents had heard about AIDS on the radio. Second only to radio, friends and relatives proved to be the most important sources of AIDS information in many countries, and the mass media may very well have often been the original source of the information passed on by these friends and relatives. Television was an important source in countries such as Brazil, Colombia, the Dominican Republic, Jordan, Turkey, and Viet Nam. Newspapers came in fourth. Noticeably, few respondents mentioned channels that are often thought to be sources of information, such as clinics and health workers, community meetings, pamphlets and posters, churches or mosques, and the workplace (United Nations Department of Economic and Social Affairs, Population Division, 2002). Even in countries with high Internet accessibility, the traditional mass media remain a strikingly important source of information on HIV/AIDS. In a study of youth in Korea, for instance, respondents identified TV (52.5%) and school classes (32.1%) as the two major sources of information on HIV/AIDS. Only a few pointed to their parents (1.3%) as a source of information (Yoo, *et al.* 2005).

When health communications specialists are involved in the development of the behavior change media products on HIV/AIDS, it is possible to know with some certainty the quality and impact of the information transmitted through the mass media, often because of the guidance given and the impact assessments that are conducted (Bertrand and Anhang, 2006). One of the advantages of the direct placement of supervised messaging is that public health planners can be assured that the formats and content of the messages are consistent with best behavior change communication (BCC) practices and with the public health strategic objectives. In Mozambique, this traditional public health campaign model is an important part of the national BCC strategy to address HIV/AIDS. (Conselho Nacional de Combate ao HIV/SIDA (CNCS), 2004).

In the case of HIV/AIDS, such public health communications campaigns typically focus on designing messages that seek to motivate change in sexual behavior and practices that place individuals at risk of contracting HIV. They also seek to modify the target audience's ways of thinking that contribute to the stigmatization of, and discrimination against, people living with HIV/AIDS (PLHAs). The fear of becoming a victim of stigmatization and discrimination often deters an individual from seeking testing, counseling, treatment, and/or care and thus interferes with attempts to fight the HIV/AIDS epidemic as a whole (Rankin *et al.*, 2005). A PLHA may also internalize stigmatization, resulting in self-exclusion from health services and other social opportunities (POLICY Project, South Africa, n.d.).

There is less certainty, however, about the quality of media messages produced as part of the more routine output of programs and articles. Strengthening the media's capacity to produce its own quality articles and programs on HIV/AIDS on a routine basis is unlike the traditional public health communications campaign in that planners have much less control over content. Nonetheless, media institutions can be an important vehicle for BCC; they play a crucial role in health behavior because traditionally they act as key gatekeepers for disseminating information; and as they act as socializing agents – they have a powerful impact in legitimizing behavior norms. Messages conveyed through the mass media can have an effect on motivations, cognitions, involvement, attitudes and behaviors of the consumer (Finnegan and Viswanath, 2008). Within the journalism profession, this capacity to affect the public mind is called journalism's "agenda-setting" role, and it comes about by focusing the public's attention on a specific issue. It has the potential either to place issues at the centre of debate or to ignore issues that could steer debate in particular directions (de Wit, 2004).

Because of their capacity to focus the public's attention on HIV/AIDS issues, journalists are potentially powerful allies in the global public health effort both to curb the HIV epidemic and to mitigate its impact on individuals, families, and communities. In Uganda, for instance, the news and information media reportedly played a significant role in informing people of risk factors, in helping them adopt preventive behaviors, and in encouraging the public to leave behind the paradigm of fear and to assume one of responsibility before the HIV/AIDS epidemic (Batto and Mugenyi, 2002). However, research indicates that journalists can often be deficient in their knowledge of the HIV/AIDS issues and are often in need of training if they are to play a positive agenda-setting role (Isibor and Ajuwon, 2004).

This agenda-setting role is widely accepted in the profession, but the nature of the debate promoted likely has a determinant role in the media's effectiveness in enabling the community and the individual to embrace social and behavioral change. The intervention under study here challenged journalists to embrace a process that positioned journalists as promoters of community dialogue as opposed to mere disseminators of information, which has been the traditional approach for journalists working in health. Within such a framework, moreover, the journalist's power to set the stage for behavior change rests in choosing how to steer the public's perception of the debate at hand, that is, determining what sources, formats, etc. to employ in telling a story and in influencing the narrative framework of the story that gets told.

The often valid concerns that public health planners may have about the appropriateness, quality, and accuracy of messages and information conveyed by journalists may be offset by the advantages to be achieved by empowering these media professionals to be better purveyors of news and information on HIV/AIDS topics (Martinez-Cajas *et al.*, 2008). Local journalists with profound knowledge of the cultural, religious, and political complex in which they are operating can be real communications assets to campaigns. Knowledge of local conditions is certainly valuable in Mozambique – a country that enjoys rich cultural, linguistic, and religious diversity. The country has 13 main languages; Portuguese, the official language, and three main African language groups – Tsonga, Sena-Nyanja, and Makua-Lomwe. Its cultural diversity can be seen in various patrilineal and matrilineal kinship systems, in various systems of traditional political leadership, in strong traditions of African traditional religious and medicinal practices including initiation rites and, in some areas, ritual sexual customs, often existing side by side with Muslim and Christian belief systems. This complex of cultural, religious and linguistic diversity operates within the superstructure of a nascent secular multi-party democracy and a public health system grounded in Western scientific notions of medicine.

Taking advantage of local knowledge and expertise in the development of media messaging, especially within the more than 50 community, religious, private commercial, and government-owned radio stations that broadcast in local languages, is one of the ways of responding to the criticism that Mozambique's National Strategic Plan for Combating HIV/AIDS leveled at past HIV/AIDS communication campaigns. The Plan noted that "Communication, Information and Education activities are undertaken predominately in Portuguese and with less frequency in local languages. The content of the messages, moreover, does not take into consideration the socioeconomic and specific cultural contexts of the local community, with the result that individuals are not motivated to change attitudes or behaviors" (Conselho Nacional de Combate ao HIV/SIDA (CNCS), 2004). It suggested, for instance, that the involvement of community elders in communication, information, and education activities would likely help assure success of behavior change. The official document also criticized in certain instances the use of pamphlets and other printed materials when theatrical and dramatic production would be more appropriate.

Mozambique's Media Response to the National Health Emergency

Despite their potential, the Mozambican media have historically not fulfilled their potential role as allies of the public health effort to turn back the tide of the HIV epidemic. A study on the media's coverage of HIV/AIDS topics, which monitored a large cross-section of Mozambican media outlets (press, TV, and radio), described the media's coverage of HIV/AIDS topics as low, at about 5 percent of all topics covered by the media (The Southern African Media Action Plan (MAP) on HIV and Aids & Gender, 2004). A study of Mozambique's leading newspapers published in 2010 indicated that only around 1.2 percent of all coverage dealt with HIV/AIDS, and 40 percent of this small coverage was published at the end of November and beginning of December in association with World Aids Day, commemorated on December 1 (Nobre, 2010).

This level of coverage of HIV/AIDS issues appears strikingly low in a country such as Mozambique with an HIV/AIDS prevalence rate among the highest in the world; it hovers around 16 percent – a situation in which approximately one in every six adult Mozambicans is living with HIV/AIDS (International HIV/AIDS Alliance, 2008). In an epidemic of these dimensions, which was declared a national emergency by the national government in 2004 (UNICEF, n.d.), it would not be unreasonable to assume that most Mozambicans have been directly impacted by the epidemic. This is especially true in the southern region where there has been a troubling increase in infection from 19 percent in 2004 to 21 percent in 2007 (Mozambique Data Triangulation Project, 2009).

The scale of the epidemic offers journalists with a potentially interested audience as well as the opportunity to report on a large array of topics of individual, community, and national concerns in areas such as prevention, the treatment and care of PLHA, stigmatization and discrimination toward PLHA, the social impact of the epidemic such as the situation of orphans and other vulnerable children, and the economic developmental implications of an epidemic of this magnitude. Mozambique is a low-income country where the spread of HIV is affecting the economy and heightening poverty. (Agence France Presse, 2008) And even if these concerns may not be on the popular mind, the media can play its agenda-setting role by focusing on an urgent issue and compelling the public to pay attention to it.

Available evidence suggest that the Mozambican media have not met the public's information needs regarding HIV/AIDS, even though there appears to be a latent demand for such information. According to the above-cited 2004 study of the Mozambique's media coverage of HIV/AIDS, 54 percent of all topics covered by the media focused on prevention, but, quite alarmingly for those concerned about promoting behavior change, many of the behaviors and practices driving the epidemic, such as intergenerational sex, transactional sex, gender violence, and cultural practices, received scant or no attention. In coverage of treatment, the prevention of mother-to-child transmission of HIV received only 5 percent of the total coverage. Mother-to-child transmission (MTCT) is when an HIV-positive woman passes the virus to her baby. This can occur during pregnancy, labor and delivery, or breastfeeding. The administration of a drug therapy regimen and other measures can be highly effective in protecting the child from infection. Without treatment, around 15–30 percent of babies born to HIV-positive women will become infected with HIV during pregnancy and delivery. A further 5–20 percent will become infected through breastfeeding (De Cock, 2000) Another area in which the media was found wanting was the near total absence of the voices of PLHAs in HIV/AIDS coverage. (The Southern African Media Action Plan (MAP) on HIV and Aids and Gender, 2004). Much to its credit, the country's national AIDS control program, CNCS, had put in place an ambitious plan designed to engage and provide support to media institutions to enhance their coverage of HIV/AIDS-related issues as way of riveting the public's attention on the epidemic and of strengthening the country's response to the HIV crisis.

Evidence from parts of southern Africa suggests a public fatigue or weariness with public health messaging that focuses on HIV/AIDS prevention (C-Change Lesotho, 2008). While these research findings do not make it altogether clear why individuals may be developing resistance to HIV/AIDS messaging, it may be that they have grown tired of prevention messages that they perceive as focusing largely on sexual prohibitions. The move toward a communication paradigm of dialogue rather than unidirectional messaging may be capable of reinvigorating efforts at prevention awareness. Journalists may have something to learn from such a paradigm shift, in which the audience is no longer merely spoken to or at, but rather "feels" that he or she is part of a conversation, and indeed may end up a part of that conversation in the case of radio or TV. This shift represents a movement from objectification toward subjectification of the audience. To encourage journalists to experiment with techniques that would produce such a paradigm shift, the Johns Hopkins University Center for Communication Programs organized a series of journalism workshops in Sofala and Zambezia provinces, with support from both the United States Agency for International Development and from CNCS, Mozambique's national HIV/AIDS control program.

The Journalist's Role in HIV/AIDS Problem Solving

These workshops aimed to strengthen the capacity of journalists to produce programs and articles more likely to stimulate radio listeners, television viewers, and readers to abandon behaviors that put them and others at risk of contracting HIV and to adopt healthy sexual behaviors. The workshops focused on improving the journalists' understanding of several related heterosexual behaviors: the practice of having multiple concurrent sexual partners, intergenerational sex, and the frequency of commercial or transactional sex, all of which are fueling the transmission of HIV in Mozambique according to recent studies (Whitson, Horth, and Goncalves, n.d.; Magaia, 2008). The journalism workshops also sought to encourage journalists to produce stories and programs that would contribute toward eliminating the lingering and widespread stigma toward and discrimination against PLHAs. The workshops were also designed to urge journalists to help create a supportive environment for PLHA adherence to treatment and for pregnant women to be tested for HIV infection and to adhere to the treatment preventing mother-to-child transmission of HIV.

Asking journalists to affect the public mind in these ways amounts to a form of BCC, and this bumps into a classic tenet of journalism that calls for objectivity and neutrality, which dominated much of Western-inspired journalism in the twentieth Century (Mindich, 2000). In the journalistic profession, advocating a cause or expressing a viewpoint is known as advocacy journalism (Careless, 2000). In the context of so-called developing countries, "development journalism" is often used to describe the type of journalism that advocates. According to the objectivity and neutrality school of thought, high-quality journalism should be dispassionate, so that professionals do their jobs without advocating. For more than two decades there has been a raging debate within the journalist community internationally about whether it is professionally desirable or even ethical to engage in advocacy journalism (Shafer, 1998; Ogan, 1982).

This, however, is an essentially false dichotomy in the sense that either perspective taken to its extreme runs the risk of motivating the production of reports and programs that would likely be largely irrelevant to the public's interests. The objectivity and neutrality purist runs the risk of producing reporting that seeks universal truth and thus ignores the cultural and socio-demographic dimension of communication. The journalists who engage in the extreme end of this approach are much more likely to unwittingly transmit news narratives and messages that are reflective of their own cultural and socioeconomic perspectives in the name of objectivity and neutrality. Media critics such as Edward Herman and Noam Chomsky have described a propaganda model that they use to show how in practice such a notion of objectivity ends up heavily favoring the viewpoint of government and the powerful (Herman and Chomsky, 1988). On the other hand, a journalist who advocates a specific agenda is apt to ignore both dissonant voices and the ambiguities that may surround a given issue, however relevant that issue may be. In either extreme case, a journalist runs the risk of having his work enveloped in his own perspective, and the informational needs of the individual person and community to which he is communicating and serving may likely to be poorly addressed (Ricchiardi, 2000).

The didactic approach employed in the JHUCCP journalism workshops sought to sidestep the controversy by asking participants to assume the role of mediator in a public conversation about what actions to take to solve the HIV/AIDS crisis. In such an approach, a journalist can assume an appearance of impartiality at the same time as driving an agenda of promoting community discussion and debate. This requires the journalist not so much to be an advocate of a particular solution, but rather to provide the person and community with the information that they need to help solve what is a national health emergency and to do it in ways that communicate the human dimension of the problem, thus opening up the media consumer to the prospect of change. As the facilitator of a community or societal discussion of a problem and the range of possible actions that may be taken to solve it, the journalist frames the issues in ways such that it can be solved at personal and social levels, and, of course, the journalist may include expert opinion in this conversation. Such an approach is consistent with those in the public health field who advocate community empowerment interventions as a way of effecting community-wide change in health-related behaviors by organizing communities to define their health problems, to identify the determinants of those problems, and to engage in effective individual and collective action to change those determinants (Beeker, Guenther-Grey, and Raj, 1998). In journalism, the objectivity/neutrality model is arguably rooted in the cultural framework of Western individualism (Kasoma, 1996) and, as in the field of health communication, there are severe limits to the effectiveness of culturally bound individualism in more communal and socially participatory societies such as that of Mozambique (Airhihenbuwa and Obregon, 2000).

In addition, the approach advocated in the workshops diverged from another journalistic school of thought historically associated with the American intellectual, writer, reporter, and political commentator, Walter Lippman (1889–1973) who promoted a basic transmission model in which journalists took information given them by experts and elites, including policymakers, repackaged that information in simple terms, and transmitted it to the public, whose role was to react emotionally to the news. In his model, Lippmann supposed that the public was incapable of serious thought or sustained constructive action, and that all thought and action should be left to the experts and elites. Within this role, journalists are a link between policymakers and the public. A journalist seeks facts from policymakers that he or she then transmits to citizens who form a public opinion (Campbell, 2007).

An approach that was community-oriented necessitated challenging the journalists attending the HIV/AIDS journalism workshops to shift the ways in which they exercised certain aspects of their profession, particularly some of the common components of journalism production. These key components of the journalistic process include sourcing, the use of formats, audience targeting, and the framing of issues in story leads, in headlines, and in the posing of questions in interviews and during live broadcasts. The curriculum required participants to examine and conceivably reinvent how they went about producing their journalistic outputs so as to invite the public to be part of the solution to the HIV/AIDS crisis, in essence, to promote a sense of personal and community ownership of the HIV/AIDS problem. The curriculum also encouraged an examination of potential barriers to enhanced HIV/AIDS coverage that a journalist might encounter from editors and other gatekeepers within a media establishment and to devise ways to navigate around such obstacles in the workplace. Journalists shared with each other ideas on how to improve their pitch to editors, who might be looking at their bottom lines, for instance, by citing evidence from other countries that health stories help to build readership and audiences and as such can be a money maker for a media company.

The curriculum developed for these journalism workshops paid ample attention to both what to do and how to do it. The curriculum maximized practice in journalism skills such as interviewing, hosting of call-in shows, and moderating of round tables, and it provided an opportunity for self-criticism and feedback by the group. The curriculum required the journalists to work together in teams to devise a series of programs or stories on suggested HIV/AIDS topics. By the end of the workshop, each team of journalists had planned a series of reports or programs that they could use to enhance their coverage of HIV/AIDS topics when they returned to their places of work.

Narratives and Sources: Implications for the Public's HIV/AIDS Response

The workshop curriculum encouraged the journalists to use a wider array of sources in the production of their stories and programs on HIV/AIDS themes than is standard in the Mozambican media, and during the workshop journalists had ample opportunity to interact with diverse sources of information, including PLHAs, pastoral figures, traditional healers, public health officials, HIV/AIDS community activists, social workers, health care workers, and others, to give them the raw material to design a series of stories or programs. Encouraging participants to utilize a greater diversity in sourcing sought to move beyond an overreliance on official and established sources that may be undermining the capacity of media institutions to better play their part in helping to reverse the HIV/AIDS epidemic and its impact upon the country.

The use of sources is central to the production of news and information by media institutions (Sigal, 1973). Journalists typically consult with individuals who are credible and available and who must be able to supply reliable information. Often journalists seek out established or official sources routinely to gather information that they use to create news. Reliance on these types of sources also means that individuals or groups who have the resources and organization to hold press conferences, issue press releases, and who possess other means of communicating with and influencing journalists, can frequently dominate news production and affect the media. Reliance on a regular supply of information from established and official sources also channels the narratives and content of stories in certain directions, and it means that groups without social power are less likely to gain access to news making and therefore have less influence in society. This tendency may become more pronounced in resource-constrained settings, where the moneyed and politically powerful can more easily dominate in setting the news agenda and determining what gets the public's attention. The routine reliance on established and official sources is often a practical solution for journalists, who usually work under the pressure of meeting deadlines – a professional condition that deprives them of the time needed to cultivate and use a greater diversity of sources.

In Mozambique this journalistic inclination has, historically, had a number of implications for determining what the public focuses its attention upon in matters of HIV/AIDS, and an examination of sources used by the Mozambican media in HIV/AIDS coverage is revealing in this regard. The previously cited 2004 study of the Mozambican media's coverage of HIV/AIDS topics indicated that 56 percent of the sources consisted of government officials and representatives of United Nations agencies. Thirty-three percent came from Mozambican and international nongovernmental organizations. Only 4 percent of the sources cited were identified as PLHAs and a mere 2 percent of the sources were identified as individuals affected by HIV. Two percent of the sources were described as experts (The Southern African Media Action Plan (MAP) on HIV and Aids & Gender 2004).

The author's review of articles on HIV/AIDS that were published during 2006 in the country's most widely circulated newspaper, the government-owned *Notícias de Moçambique,* largely echoed the findings cited above – with government officials and representatives of UN agencies and international nongovernment organizations dominating the sources used by journalists. Virtually completely absent from the newspaper's coverage were the voices of PLHAs or other people affected personally by the epidemic. This sourcing pattern seen in the *Notícias de Moçambique*'s coverage appears to be a fairly consistent phenomenon in the print media regardless of whether the media institution is publicly or privately owned.

The preponderance of high-ranking government officials and representatives from multilateral organizations gives an authoritarian "feel" to the coverage of HIV/AIDS, even though this may not be the intent. This type of communication through the media may be described as "authoritarian" in the sense of creating a one-way communication from those in positions of authority to the public. It is worth considering to what extent this mode of one-way, authoritarian communication itself becomes part of the message relayed. To a large extent, it appears that the sources that a journalist chooses drive the story narrative conveyed to the media-consuming public.

The information conveyed through official sources tends to relate to the government's role in providing health care services to the public, for example, highlighting the dedication of new public hospitals and clinics. In summary, reports typically highlight what the government is doing for the public. In the area of prevention, high-ranking officials were often cited as exhorting the public, especially youth, to be responsible in sexual matters because of the risks of HIV infection.

Governments and international organizations have the right and, indeed, duty to reach the public with information about their activities through the media. However, from a journalistic point of view, it is worthwhile considering the possibility that the predominance of these sources in the coverage of HIV/AIDS topics may skew coverage in ways that have an inadvertent disempowering affect upon the public, by creating the impression that the responsibility for a response to the public health crisis rests solely with government. Moreover, though this chapter focuses on the coverage of HIV/AIDS topics in Mozambique, the patterns of coverage established for HIV/AIDS topics appear part and parcel of a journalistic archetype practiced widely in the country. Indeed, the implications of authoritarian messaging and top-down narratives discussed here for a Mozambican context hold significance for the practice of journalism more globally.

Unidirectional – what we have called here authoritarian – messaging is more likely to drive a narrative in which government and international agencies are those responsible for solving the HIV/AIDS crisis. This contrasts with a possible coverage of the HIV/AIDS topic using a diversity of voices from various segments of society that would create a more interactive, democratic "feel" to the country's approach. Arguably, deploying a more inclusive and diversified set of sources would contribute to creating a narrative and more powerful messaging that would validate the possibility of community involvement in finding and applying solutions to the HIV/AIDS epidemic and its worth; these types of sources might also carry with them a social valorization of personal initiative in face of the HIV/AIDS crisis and, by extension, underscore the importance of personal responsibility. Such news coverage is potentially more in concert with the objectives of BCC in the sense of creating messages that contribute to empowering individuals and communities. Indeed, problem-solving journalism of this type that employs a diversity of sources and narratives of empowerment can condition the public mind on issues that reinforce and articulate with the objectives of BCCs campaigns, whose messages are directly supervised by public health experts.

The practice of reliance on authority figures for sourcing often appears to be the result of habit and convenience. An editor of a leading Mozambican media institution explained to me in an interview that it is easy and inexpensive to cover high-ranking government officials due to the simple fact that they provide reporters with the transport to cover their activities; with this type of assistance, media institutions are able to cover influential and newsworthy public figures such as government ministers without incurring additional costs.

A senior editor for the government-owned *Noticias* explained that the newspaper's reporters became aware of this bias toward relying on official sources for coverage of HIV/AIDS during a meeting organized by the CNCS. At the suggestion of a CNCS representative, its reporters began to give a more human dimension to their stories on HIV/AIDS precisely to promote greater identification with the issue at a personal level. The CNCS suggestion came as part of a program that it launched to provide the country's media institutions with special funding to enable them to improve and expand their coverage of HIV/AIDS topics. Awareness of the implication of reliance on established and official sources combined with the availability of additional resources seemed to allow journalists to get off the deadline treadmill and away from the tendency to cover those who can provide transport, arrange events to cover, hold a workshop, and issue press releases.

Our review of the media's coverage of HIV/AIDS-related topics raised additional questions as to the possible influence of past coverage on the public mind. Through the mediation of news outlets, UN agencies and other international organizations appear to be attempting to accomplish a series of self-promotional objectives that have little to do with HIV/AIDS prevention and destigmatization. The stories that relayed information from these sources tended to make sweeping, often negative statements about the disastrous consequences of the epidemic on Mozambique in particular and sub-Saharan Africa in general. In response to what seemed like excessive "doom and gloom" reporting on health in Africa, our intervention with journalists asked them to think about the possibility that such reporting may contribute to a sense of hopelessness among the public, which may contribute to promoting a sense of apathy toward the HIV/AIDS crisis, and to consider the wisdom of also developing stories focusing on success, that is, highlighting instances where constructive behavior change has occurred. Focusing on success stories may also be an antidote to possible public fatigue at hearing unidirectional, prohibitive messages about HIV/AIDS prevention.

The authors' review of the print media also detected the proclivity to use statistics to illustrate the severity of the epidemic. In the context of the near total blackout of the voices of those affected by HIV/AIDS from the media, the public has little recourse to anything other than numerical abstractions for understanding the impact of the epidemic. Statistics possess significant meaning in scientific and technocratic settings but, when used in the popular media, arguably may not inspire the public to take a desired action and may even have a negative influence. Media coverage that combines public health statistics with concrete examples of the implications of the epidemic at a human level is likely to promote a feeling of identity with those affected by HIV/AIDS and arguably act to undermine the twin scourge of stigmatization and discrimination as well as making the media consumer more receptive to the information conveyed by the media coverage.

In workshops, journalists were encouraged to give coverage to "success stories," that is, to highlight instances where individuals and communities have made positive change, as a way of creating more empowering narratives. One example of a public health success story was relayed during one of our JHUCCP journalism workshops. It involved changing a risky sexual practice in areas of central Mozambique. There it had been common to practice one variant of traditional ritual known as *kupita kufa*, which requires a widow, after the death of her husband, to have sexual relations with a traditional healer as part of ritual purification (in some areas purification requires sexual intercourse between the widow and the dead husband's brother – levirate). In the era of HIV/AIDS, many traditional healers are put at risk of contracting HIV by this practice, and indeed, as the leader of the traditional healers association in Sofala Province noted at one of the workshops, healers were dying in increasing numbers from the complications of AIDS. In response, the healers association advocated that its members modify *kupita kufa*, so that the purification goals of the ritual could be achieved through the use of herbal remedies rather than risky sexual intercourse.

Formats and Targeting Audiences

Story formats are also likely to influence the receptivity of readers, viewers, and listeners to the messages and information on HIV/AIDS. In the case of radio, for instance, a call-in show featuring a couple living with HIV/AIDS may more likely create an emotional connection between the audience and the PLHA than a feature story read by a broadcaster. This is particularly true in what is fundamentally an oral culture as in Mozambique, where interactivity in communication is culturally compelling (Mutere, n.d.), and it is worthwhile considering the possibility that the authentic sharing of an emotion or a first-person description of human vulnerability may create identification with the PLHA and open the listener to a series of messages that may be conveyed in the program (Oscher and Barrett, 2001). This certainly appeared to be the case in the interviews with PLHAs conducted by workshop participants. Radio, moreover, has a unique capacity to convey to listeners the feelings expressed by those featured on programs. Attentive listeners can perceive nuances in interpersonal communications such as tone, hesitation, and the quivering of the voice, and the absence of visual images stirs the listener's imagination. In the print media, techniques that journalists can adopt to humanize their stories can include human interest stories, published interviews, first-person accounts, and emotive photography and drawings.

Workshop participants were also encouraged to consider using with more frequency interactive formats such as interviews, round tables, call-in shows, and *vox populi* (a Latin phrase that literally means *voice of the people* and is often used in broadcasting for interviews with members of the "general public") to help humanize their coverage of HIV/AIDS issues and to create a sense of identification with the subjects of the programs and articles. In the design of their series of programs on HIV/AIDS themes, the teams of radio broadcasters in the workshop frequently planned to broadcast interviews with PLHAs to launch community discussions about issues of stigma and discrimination.

During the course of the workshop, journalists were also asked to consider how they might target the information that they were conveying to a specific audience. For instance, on the topic of intergenerational sex among teachers and students, the teams of journalists had to reveal how they would write or program for a youth audience as opposed to an audience of parents. In this way, they had to suggest what sources would be appropriate for each audience, in the case of radio what type of music might be used as bridges between segments, what types of questions would be posed that would resonate with each audience, etc. – some examples of the final products/stories might make these references more illustrative or powerful.

Creating an Enabling Environment

Arming journalists with the knowledge and skills required to produce more effective reports and programs on the issues that are driving the HIV/AIDS epidemic in Mozambique does not necessarily guarantee that the desired changes in journalistic practices and approaches take place and that the public receives the information that it needs to create better solutions to the challenges of the epidemic. No journalist works in isolation; when a workshop is over, he or she returns to a workplace reality with its supervisorial and gatekeeper structure, a journalistic culture, competing demands on time and energy, resource constraints, and other factors that affect a journalist's desire to achieve performance goals and to expand his or her thematic scope of work.

Journalists require an enabling environment to exercise more effectively their craft; this is true for journalists whether they are working on HIV/AIDS or, for that matter, any other topic including what in the profession is called hard (usually political) news.

In their work environments, journalists report to superiors who give out assignments with deadlines, who establish for their operations coverage priorities from a universe of possible topics, and who have their own, often fixed, ideas about priorities that may not necessarily coincide with proposals that come from individual journalists. It is important to motivate these gatekeepers to approve of and support the enhanced coverage of HIV/AIDS on which the individual journalist may wish to embark. Our journalism and HIV/AIDS workshops provided opportunities for participating journalists to share ideas on how they would pitch or sell enhanced HIV/AIDS coverage to their editors. To achieve the goal of improved and increased HIV/AIDS coverage, it is thus critical to engage editors, media managers, and media owners in direct outreach advocacy to secure their buy-ins and to create opportunities for journalists to practice the skills that they learned in the workshop.

In addition, media institutions, especially commercial enterprises, need to be reassured that their readers, listeners, and viewers will welcome increased coverage of health topics such as HIV/AIDS. In the United States, for instance, decision makers in many traditional media institutions have come to the conclusion that there is a consumer demand for health reporting. (Judd, 1998) In developing countries, there is anecdotal evidence of consumer demand for health reporting, but few evidence-based findings on the matter. Though editors and media managers often express an interest in enhancing HIV/AIDS coverage out of a sense of public service, evidence-based findings demonstrating that health reporting "sells" would send a more convincing message that there is little bottom-line risk in increasing the output of good health coverage and it may indeed make a media institution more competitive. It is recommended that donors and governments support this type of research to help motivate the mass media to embrace the goal of enhanced HIV/AIDS coverage as vital part of a country's HIV/AIDS response.

Transforming the Journalistic Culture

It is critical to work with media professionals to assure that the journalistic culture is open to innovation in health reporting. Mozambican journalists and editors explained that there is really no such thing as a health beat, that is, journalists are not assigned exclusively to health reporting. This lack of specialization means that journalists do not have the opportunity to accumulate the expertise in the health arena that would optimize coverage of HIV/AIDS topics. Moreover, within the profession, a "hard" news assignment such as a national political controversy is more highly valued than assignments on "soft" topics such as health, and the road to professional advancement often lies in making a reputation in political reporting.

The establishment of health journalism courses in the country's three schools of journalism would likely help valorize health reporting within the profession and contribute to the creation of professional standards and expectations around health reporting. At the time of writing, Mozambique's journalism schools do not have such courses, and several editors indicated that the lack of professional preparation in health journalism prevented their institutions from improving their coverage of health topics including HIV/AIDS. In addition, support for more research on health journalism, including its ability to affect behavior and attitudes, would help the profession hone journalistic best practices in tune with the country's linguistic, cultural, and religious diversity.

Resource constraints

Resource constraints are among the greatest obstacles that journalists confront in enhancing their coverage of HIV/AIDS themes, according to a survey that JHUCCP conducted with more than 40 print and broadcast journalists participating in the journalism-HIV/AIDS workshops. The cost of transportation and the lack of professional equipment led the list of their concerns. Mozambique's national HIV/AIDS control program – CNCS – launched a program of support for media institutions that apply for funds to enhance their coverage of HIV/AIDS-related issues. As part of its plan of support, CNCS organized journalism workshops based on the JHUCCP workshop curriculum in a bid to strengthen the competency of individual journalists to report on HIV/AIDS topics, so that the funds invested in media institutions are effectively utilized. At the time of writing, CNCS was exploring ways of linking support for media institutions to specific desired outcomes to ensure that the funding is invested in effective journalistic products.

Training impact

The workshop curriculum, with its focus on shifting the journalistic paradigm to one that aims to create a greater sense of personal and community ownership of the challenges of the HIV/AIDS crisis, seems to have resonated with many of the journalists participating in the workshops. The workshop experience led many of them to experiment with the way that they approached coverage of HIV/AIDS topics. Both pre- and post-workshop knowledge assessments and follow-up group discussions approximately three months after the initial workshops provided the evidence for the observation that journalists intended to, and indeed had begun to, shift their approaches to HIV/AIDS coverage. The knowledge assessments indicated that journalists had acquired a more nuanced understanding of the themes that could be covered as part of HIV/AIDS coverage, and this increased awareness indicated that they had assimilated the themes stressed in the workshop curriculum.

In conversations with journalists three months after the workshops, journalists demonstrated how they were incorporating in their outputs features of the journalistic paradigm advocated in the workshop curriculum – with radio journalists seemingly particularly responsive to the suggestions made in the workshops. Journalists from community radio stations, for instance, noted that prior to the workshops they relied much more on brochures furnished by national AIDS authorities and on governmental health experts for background information. After the workshops, they devised programs much more centered on the experience of people from the local community and that they made efforts to broadcast interviews and programs originating from within local communities (*entrevistas e reportagens no terreno*) as distinguished from those conducted in studio. They described an increased use of radio dramas to address risky behaviors commonly practiced in their communities, reports about and interviews with individuals who were using local health services, and in-studio discussions with persons affected by and living with HIV/AIDS.

Journalists said that they were deploying formats that permitted a greater identification of the audience with the covered topics. A representative from the Community Radio Station of *Maganja da Costa* in Zambezia Province explained that "the better accepted programs are those in which each listener feels as if it is his personal problem that is being discussed or as if one is speaking personally with him" (at the Center for Communication Programs, Johns Hopkins University in 2008).

Some journalists also indicated that they had begun to produce their programs with an eye to avoiding further stigmatization of PLHAs and to encourage positive change in behaviors. This represented a shift from using a prevention message with "fear" as its basis to one that stressed assuming responsibility for one's actions. Such a shift is critical since fear-based motivation seems to contribute to the stigmatization of PLHAs. During workshop discussions, a few journalists spontaneously made the link between stigma and earlier anti-HIV/AIDS campaigns conducted in Mozambique. According to these journalists, these campaigns early on in the AIDS control effort were responsible for instilling fear that subsequently led to popular fear of PLHAs.

Some journalists proudly acknowledged that, as a result of their programming innovations, PLHAs were more willing to admit their HIV-positive status on the air (*quebrar o silencio* "break the silence"), and they also noted that young people were more likely to talk about their HIV status than married adults. Overall, they felt that married adults would only come forward more readily to discuss their experiences when HIV infection became less stigmatized, and the challenge to help destigmatize PLHAs seemed to energize the journalists to do more in this area.

Journalists also discussed limitations that they faced in enhancing their coverage of HIV/AIDS topics. Journalists indicated that

- they needed more training in gender issues and reproductive health (gender issues being particularly important to a discussion of multiple concurrent partners),
- radio personnel needed more training in the production of radio dramas,
- stations needed equipment to record and store programs so that they could be repeated at different times, and
- they would welcome additional training in how to better approach complex issues such as mulitiple concurrent partners and stigma.

The following items further highlight some of the achievements and constraints that journalists said that they had experienced following their workshop participation.

- "One of my programs helped an HIV-positive youth reunite with his family."
- "We were able to air a series of programs both with patients who had abandoned their antiretroviral treatment (ART) and with health providers to discuss barriers to adherence to ART."

- Some journalists said that they had problems at their own radio stations in covering the HIV/AIDS topics, because of the stigmatizing attitude of some of their colleagues at the station toward PLHAs. These attitudes discouraged PLHAs and others affected by HIV/AIDS from going to the studio to participate in programs.
- "Before my participation in the workshop, our programs were repetitive and did not add any new information to people. Today, our programs bring different perspectives about the same issues as seen by different segments of the community."
- Reporters noted that public health officials often do not cooperate with them and so they cannot access the information that they need; they said that this was especially true when they raised questions about the quality of health services provided to communities.
- One journalist introduced as a regular feature in his interview program the asking of the question "*Já fez o teste?*" (Have you been tested yet?) as a way of promoting testing for everyone in the community. In the words of the journalist, "This is something that will make people feel that it is just normal to be tested for HIV."
- Before the training, one radio station covered HIV/AIDS issues only in the town where the station was located, but, after the training, the station worked out an arrangement with a local NGO to provide support so that the station could develop radio programs on HIV/AIDS issues that confronted more remote communities in their listening area.
- Some journalists said that listeners had begun approaching them for advice on HIV/AIDS, saying that they couldn't trust the information that they were receiving from health care workers or that the attitude of health care workers discouraged them from asking questions about HIV/AIDS.

References

Agence France Presse (2008). High HIV rate heightens Mozambique poverty: UN envoy. June 13, 2008. Retrieved from http://povertynewsblog.blogspot.com/2008/06/high-hiv-rate-heightens-mozambique.html

Airhihenbuwa, C. O. and Obregon, R. (2000). A critical assessment of theories/modes used in communication for HIV/AIDS. *Journal of Health Communication, 5* (supplement), 5–15.

Batto, A. B., and Mugenyi, P. M. (2002). The role of the media in HIV prevention in Uganda. *International Conference on AIDS.* Retrieved from http://gateway.nlm.nih.gov/MeetingAbstracts/ma?f=102251494.html

Beeker, C., Guenther-Grey, C., and Raj, A. (1998). Community empowerment paradigm drift and the primary prevention of HIV/AIDS. *Social Science and Medicine, 46*(7), 831–842.

Bertrand, J. T. and Anhang, R. (2006). The effectiveness of mass media in changing HIV/AIDS-related behaviour among young people in developing countries. In D. Ross, B. Dick, and J. Ferguson (Eds.), *Preventing HIV/AIDS in Young People: A Systematic Review of Preventing HIV/AIDS in Young People* (pp. 205–241). Geneva: UNICEF.

Campbell, C. C. (2007). Journalism and public knowledge. *Kettering Review*, 39–49. Retrieved from http://www.kettering.org/File%20Library/ArticlePDFs/Campbell_JournalismandPublic%20KnowledgeReview.pdf

Careless, S. (2000). Advocacy journalism. *The Interim*. May 2000. Retrieved from http://www.theinterim.com/2000/may/10advocacy.html

C-Change Lesotho (2008). *The Language of Multiple Concurrent Partners, Sex and HIV/AIDS in Lesotho: Opportunities for Dialogue Promotion*. Research report in draft, 2008. Retrieved from http://c-changeprogram.org/resources/language-multiple-concurrent-partners-sex-and-hiv-and-aids-lesotho-opportunities-dialogue-

Conselho Nacional de Combate ao HIV/SIDA (CNCS) (2004). Plano Estratégico Nacional de Combate Ao HIV/SIDA [National strategic plan to combat HIV/AIDS]. Official Report, Maputo. Retrieved from http://www.misau.gov.mz/pt/content/download/469/2005/file/PENII.pdf

De Cock, K. M., Fowler, M. G., Mercier E. *et al.* (2000). Prevention of mother-to-child HIV transmission in resource-poor countries: Translating research into policy and practice. *Journal of the American Medical Association 283*(9), 1175–1182.

de Wit, G. (2004). Agenda setting and HIV/Aids news sources, implications for journalism education: An exploratory study. *Ecquid Novi, 25*(1), 94–114.

Finnegan, J. R. and Viswananth, K. (2008). Communication theory and health behavior change: The media studies framework. In K. Glanz, B. K. Rimer, and F. M. Lewis (Eds.), *Health Behavior and Health Education: Theory, Research and Practice* (pp. 361–388). San Francisco: Jossey-Bass.

Herman, E., and Chomsky, N. (1988). *Manufacturing Consent: The Political Economy of the Mass Media*. New York: Pantheon.

International HIV/AIDS Alliance (2008). International HIV/AIDS Alliance in Mozambique. . Retrieved from http://www.aidsalliance.org/linkingorganisationdetails.aspx?id=17

Isibor, M. D. and Ajuwon, A. J. (2004). Journalists' knowledge of AIDS and attitude to persons living with HIV in Ibadan, Nigeria. *African Journal of Reproductive Health, 8*(2), 101–110.

Kasoma, F. (1996). The foundations of African ethics (Afriethics) and the professional practice of journalism: The case for society-centered media morality. *Africa Media Review, 10*, 93–116.

Levander, M. and Judd, J. (1998). RX for Good Journalism & Good Ratings: A Strong Dose of Good Health Reporting. Retrieved from http://www.kff.org/about/upload/mediafellows_011005_goodhealthjournalism.pdf

Magaia, D. (2008).Audience Report – Multiple Concurrent Partners – Mozambique. Retrieved from http://www.comminit.com/?q=africa/node/286762

Martinez-Cajas, J. L., Invernizzi, C. F., Ntemgwa, M. *et al.* (2008) Benefits of an educational program for journalists on media coverage of HIV/AIDS in developing countries. *Journal of the International Aids Society 11*(2). Retrieved from http://www.ncbi.nlm.nih.gov/pmc/articles/PMC2580037/

Mindich, D. (2000). *Just the Facts: How Objectivity Came to Define American Journalism*. New York: New York University Press.

Mozambique Data Triangulation Project (2009). Mozambique. http://globalhealthsciences.ucsf.edu/PPHG/triangulation/data-synthesis-profiles/Mozambique.pdf (accessed April 14, 2010).

Mutere, M. An Introduction to African History and Culture. *John F. Kennedy Center*. Retrieved July 6, 2009, http://artsedge.kennedy-center.org/aoi/history/ao-guide.html

Nobre, J. (2010). *Estudo de Base acerca de Notícias sobre HIV/SIDA na Imprensa Moçambicana: Relatório Final* {Baseline study of papers on HIV/AIDS published in Mozambique: Final report]. Maputo: UNICEF and Agência de Notícias de Resposta ao SIDA/MISA.

Ogan, C. L. (1982). Development journalism/communication: The status of the concept. *International Communication Gazette 29*, 3–13.

Oscher, K. N. and Feldman Barrett, L. (2001). A multiprocess perspective on the neuroscience of emotion. In T. Mayne and G. Bonnano, *Emotion: Current Issues and Future Directions* (pp. 38–81). New York: Guilford Press.

POLICY Project, South Africa (n.d.). Siyam'Kela: Measuring HIV/AIDS-related stigma. Research Findings. Retrieved from http://www.policyproject.com/siyamkela.cfm

Rankin, W. W., Brennan, S., Schell, E. *et al.* (2005). The stigma of being HIV-positive in Africa. Essay, PLoS Med 2(8): e247 DOI:10.1371/journal.pmed.0020247.

Ricchiardi, S. (2000). Highway to the danger zone. *American Journalism Review*. Retrieved from http://www.ajr.org/article.asp?id=746

Shafer, R. (1998). Comparing development journalism and public journalism as interventionist press models. *Asian Journal of Communication, 8*(1), 31–52.

Sigal, L. V. (1973). *Reporters and Officials*. Lexington, MA: D. C. Heath and Company.

The Southern African Media Action Plan (MAP) on HIV and Aids and Gender (2004). *Moçambique: Estudo Básico do Género e HIV e SIDA* [Mozambique: Baseline study of gender and HIV/AIDS]. Summary of Key Findings. Retrieved from www.genderlinks.org.za/attachment.php?aa_id=12977

UNICEF (n.d.). Mozambique: HIV/AIDS Picture. http://www.unicef.org/mozambique/hiv_aids_2045.html (accessed March 13, 2010).

United Nations Department of Economic and Social Affairs, Population Division (2002). HIV/AIDS: Awareness and Behavior. Retrieved from http://www.un.org/esa/population/publications/AIDS_awareness/AIDS_es_English.pdf

Whitson, D., Horth, R., and Goncalves, S. (n.d.). Mozambique: Analysis of HIV Prevention Response and Modes of HIV Transmission: Mozambique Country Synthesis. Retrieved March 2010 from http://www.unaidsrstesa.org/files/MoT_0.pdf

Yoo, H., Lee, S. H., Kwon, B. E. *et al.* (2005). HIV/AIDS knowledge, attitudes, related behaviors, and sources of information among Korean adolescents. *The Journal of School Health 75*(10), 393–399.

jovenHABLAjoven
Lessons Learned about Interpellation, Peer Communication, and Second-Generation Edutainment in Sexuality and Gender Projects among Young People[1]

Jair Vega Casanova and Carmen R. Mendivil Calderón

jovenHABLAjoven Group, Third Phase: The Commitment to Methodological Learning

The text *jovenHABLAjoven: Una Experiencia de Comunicación y Salud en el Municipio de Malambo. Los y las Jóvenes Urbano/Rurales, su Cultura y sus Identidades alrededor de la Sexualidad* [jovenHABLAjoven: a communication and health experience in the municipality of Malambo.[2] The culture and identities of urban/rural young people regarding sexuality] (Suarez, Mendivil, and Vega, 2004) describes the process of creation and consolidation of the *jovenHABLAjoven Communication Group*,[3] as the result of a joint exercise between final-year students from the Universidad del Norte's Social Communication and Journalism program[4] and young people from the municipality of Malambo, who, since the beginning of 2003, had worked together on three objectives related to the sexuality of the young people from that locality: (1) characterizing the socialization spaces for the construction of their identities, (2) exploring the situational contexts generated by the culture in which their linguistic potential is built, and (3) identifying their collective imaginaries.

That first phase made it possible to create the following scenarios: (1) The *jovenHABLAjoven Group* as a "permanent production space in which the base group and the co-researchers could strengthen team work and develop the other scenarios through training sessions, discussions, and production of thought"; (2) *La Parla Directa* [Talking face to face], "a radio program aired Mondays and Wednesdays, that sought to appropriate new spaces where young people could publicly express their interests regarding sexual and reproductive health"; (3) *The jovenHABLAjoven Discussion Groups*, as "two-hour spaces for dialogue held on Wednesdays in zones frequently

The Handbook of Global Health Communication, First Edition. Edited by Rafael Obregon and Silvio Waisbord.

visited by young people, where recreational and participative approaches were used to formulate trigger-questions fostering open conversation regarding young people's sexuality" (Suarez, Mendivil, and Vega, 2004, p. 73).

Subsequently, in 2004 and 2005, the conceptual strengthening process of the base group continued with the support of the United Nations Population Fund and the Universidad del Norte through "a process of reflection among young people aimed at questioning those conceptions and practices rooted in their culture that affected gender equality and constituted risk factors for their sexual health". The radio program *La Parla Directa* was also continued, with its sections improved and enriched by the creation of a radio drama called *It Won't Be the First Time* (Vega and Mendivil, 2005).

Thus, by the beginning of the third phase, which lasted from March 2005 to March 2006, there were 10 members in the base group and approximately 30 young people from the community in the support group. Upon completion of the first two phases, the following facts were evident: the scarceness of autonomy and willingness on the part of parents, teachers, and young people to address topics related to sexuality; the marked patriarchal legacy; the presence of instrumental and utilitarian relations between men and women; and the existence of practices that foster risks such as sexually transmitted diseases, HIV/AIDS, teen pregnancies, and other situations related to the construction of identities (Suárez, Mendivil, and Vega, 2004).

The spectrum of research was expanded for the third phase. Beyond inquiring about the transformations that the process could generate in the population of young people, and beyond the interpellation of their sexual imaginaries from a gender perspective, the objective was to establish the scope of the communication strategy itself. The question that served as starting point for the study was then how to create spaces for dialogue among the community of young people in Malambo, which made possible the interpellation of their sexual imaginaries from a gender perspective. In this sense, the theoretical and methodological efforts focused on how to structure a strategy aimed at the interpellation of young people's sexual and gender imaginaries, on the basis of peer communication and within the framework of second-generation edutainment. For this purpose, a plan was designed that would make it possible to: (1) observe the evolution of the groups at two moments and account for the interpellations that could be made to the sexual imaginaries of young men and women studying in private or public schools of different zones of the municipality, who were listeners of the radio program *La Parla Directa* and participants in the discussion groups, as well as of the participants in the base and support sections of the jovenHABLAjoven Group; and (2) establish some of the lessons learned regarding the scope of the implementation of a communication strategy among peers within the framework of second-generation edutainment and of communication for social change.

This chapter presents some basic conceptual considerations on the project's communication approach, that is, on interpellation, imaginaries, communication for social change, and second-generation edutainment, and then goes on to describe the methodological process. Finally, on the basis of the conceptualizations regarding sexuality, gender, and body, it presents the results and includes a discussion on the implications and range of the project and its methodology.

Interpellation of Imaginaries, Second-Generation Edutainment, and Communication for Social Change

On the basis of the above-mentioned question, the project was committed from the start to interaction[5] (Franco, 2000) in its work with the young people, on the basis of what is known as Communication for Social Change. As opposed to other conceptualizations that address the relationship of communication, development, and social change, this perspective emphasizes: (1) the critique of a single conception of development, and, in this case, of a predetermined conception of sexuality or of adequate behaviors, conceived as an "ought"; (2) the conception of individuals and communities as agents of their own change, as opposed to considering them objects of intervention; (3) public debate instead of information transmission; and (4) an understanding of changes in social conventions, the cultural field, and policies, which goes beyond mere behaviors.

Communication for Social Change (CFSC) has been defined as "a process of public and private dialogue through which people define who they are, what they want and how they can get it," where social change is understood as "change in people's lives as they themselves define change" (Fundación Rockefeller, 1999).

For this reason, the approach to the young population of Malambo was not carried out through campaigns promoting knowledge, attitudes, or behavioral changes, but rather through a process of conversation and consensus building with respect to the young people themselves and to a reflection that would lead to the interpellation of their sexual imaginaries. The processes to be developed were agreed on and, although it had been initially considered that television might be a more attractive communication alternative, the group decided on radio, thus giving rise to the program *La Parla Directa*, which became their scenario for communication and for their own discussions.

In this sense, the change perspective was addressed on the basis of an edutainment strategy, which has been defined as a process aimed at proposing, designing, and implementing a media message that entertains and educates with the purpose of generating social change on the basis of behavioral changes in the members of the audience (Singhal and Rogers, 1999, 2002).

Edutainment has been recognized as an important vehicle for the dissemination of behaviors:

> The creation and dissemination of knowledge are key factors in the development process where the media have been instrumental as a means of storing and sharing knowledge. For example, the UK Department for International Development (DFID) cites the effectiveness of radio in promoting development in a wide range of disparate countries, including Afghanistan, Moldova, and Kiribati (DFID, 2006). The well-recognized functions of the media are to educate, inform, and entertain where the social and economic contributions of the media to development depend on the nature of the content delivered (Locksley, 2009, p. 2).

However, the idea of using Edutainment to position behaviors did not seem to be the ideal perspective. Thomas Tufte's considerations on the topic led to the idea that, rather than molding and proposing behaviors, the drama should generate situations that fostered debate among young people with respect to sexuality, gender, and rights, in such a way as to interpellate social conventions or pre-established truths that, if unquestioned, end up legitimating behaviors that do not give this population the opportunity to enjoy their sexuality fully.

Thomas Tufte (2004) speaks of the coexistence of three generations of edutainment. The first, developed in the 1960s and associated with social marketing, focuses on individual behavior changes and on fiction genres through the mass media. The second generation is associated with a revival of Freire's pedagogy (1986), which includes everything from theater for development on the basis of Boal's perspective to more strategic thinking such as that set forth by the Population Communication Services at Johns Hopkins University. In this case, the strategy focuses more on dialogic pedagogies aimed at creating awareness and connecting problems to issues of power, inequality, and human rights, pedagogies that we adopted in this project in the context of the discussion groups. Finally, the third generation integrates the two preceding ones, but also generates social mobilization and political advocacy processes aimed at generating more structural changes.

Given the possibilities of action and its scope, our project is framed in the context of second-generation Edutainment, insofar as it takes up Paulo Freire's (1970) dialogic pedagogy, based mainly on face-to-face communication and small-scale group interaction. Freire clearly understood the need to deal with social power structures and to include marginal sectors of society in order to recover spaces for their critical and dialogical reflections (Tufte, 2005).

This generation of edutainment seemed more compatible with the project's commitment to *interpellation*, since rather than proposing new knowledge or new practices, the goal was to "require, compel, or simply ask someone to give explanations or declarations regarding any fact whatsoever" (*Dictionary of the Spanish Language* – 22nd ed.). In this case, the young people asked one another questions and sought to account for their perceptions of sexuality. This concept has already been used in educational practice and assumes that

> on the basis of the practice of interpellation, agents are constituted as active subjects of education, who adopt new evaluative, behavioral, or conceptual contents from the interpellation, thus modifying their daily practices in terms of either a radical transformation or better justified reaffirmation" (Buenfil, 1998; cited by Álvarez and Errico, 2007).

Álvarez and Errico (2007), drawing on Da Porta (2005), state that, for an educational practice to take place, interpellation must be successful, on the basis of a communication process which puts different meanings into play so that they can bring about transformations in the participants. In this sense, interpellation is grounded in the discussion of assumptions, the formulation of a question, or an affirmation that makes visible what is hidden behind what is taken to be true. This concept was initially set forth by Althusser (1972) as a process that transforms individuals into subjects. Martín Barbero (1993) uses the term "interpellation" in a different sense, to characterize the process of appropriation of mass media messages by the low-income population and the use they make of them from their class perspective.

With respect to the object of interpellation, that is, social imaginaries, Taylor (2006) states that there are significant differences between a social imaginary and a social theory. The importance of working from the perspective of imaginaries is threefold. First of all, they refer to " "the way ordinary people "imagine" their social surroundings, and this is often not expressed in theoretical terms, it is carried in images, stories, legends" (p. 23). Secondly, Taylor states that theories are generally shared by a minority, while "what is interesting in the social imaginary is that it is shared by large groups of people, if not the whole society" (p. 23). Finally, in conformity with the above, "the social imaginary is that common understanding which that makes possible common practices and a widely shared sense of legitimacy" (p. 23).

The Third Phase: Interpellation of Social Imaginaries Regarding Sexuality Methodological Approaches

In the context of second-generation edutainment, the third phase focused on combining three scenarios: (1) support for the base group in its internal reflection regarding production of the radio programs and the implementation of discussion groups; (2) the radio program designed by the group in order to disseminate the work carried out on the suggested topics, including the radio drama[6]; and (3) traveling discussion groups aimed at peer dialogue, carried out by the members of the base group with students from the participating schools. The topics for each one of the scenarios were defined and adjusted on the basis of the focus groups that served as referents for the evaluation of the process.

The research project was thus conceived as a way of taking up the strategy formulated in the first phase of the project, but this time in relation to the work carried out by the base group in the school environment.

The idea was to identify how empowerment was being achieved among the members of the base group of the *jovenHABLAjoven* Communication Group, as protagonists and drivers of individual and community change processes, and to establish whether the interpersonal scenarios for communication with the young people of Malambo were, in fact, creating spaces for dialogue and discussion about the collective imaginaries regarding sexuality, gender equality, and sexual and reproductive rights.

First of all, with respect to the process of empowerment of the group members, follow-up was carried out through field logs of the different meetings with the base group. Also, upon completion of the project, a Memory Workshop was held, in which a patchwork quilt exercise made it possible to identify the progress made by the group, the main changes that had occurred, and the participants' point of view regarding the scope of the strategy. Riaño (2000), cited by Pérez and Vega (2010), points out that the use of unorthodox methodologies such as the Memory Workshop are the result of specific epistemological and pragmatic concerns, of a search for alternatives that make it possible to explore the diverse ways in which human groups and individuals construct meanings. This exercise is framed in what Parks and colleagues (2005) call MSCT (Most Significant

Change Technique), a technique used to inquire into the changes generated within projects, not from an external perspective, but on the basis of the most significant changes brought about in the participating population, on the understanding that the participating population or stakeholders can become evaluating subjects (Byrne, Gray-Felder, and Hunt, 2005; Parks *et al.*, 2005).

Secondly, given the impossibility of developing a complex exercise in the form of a longitudinal group evolution design or cohort study, in order to evaluate the process carried out with the population with whom the base group was interacting, a sub-population of students from three schools[7] who participated systematically in the discussion groups was selected. Three months into the study, and before starting the discussion groups and broadcasting of the radio drama, three focal sessions were held with one group from each school in order to talk about the strategy topics, which made it possible to establish a baseline for subsequent comparisons.[8] A second focal session was held six months into implementation of the project, and a third one at nine months, in order to follow up on the evolution of the imaginaries and discourses expressed by the young people.

The focal sessions were carried out on the basis of a guide with open-ended questions covering the categories of sexuality, gender equality, and sexual rights, which made it possible for the participants to express their social imaginaries regarding these categories during the conversations. Those same conversations made it possible to establish certain images that were immediately validated or confirmed with each group. Subsequently, an analysis was carried out on the basis of the interpretation of the discourses, and similarities among the groups were established.

The categories taken into account for the study were: sexuality, focusing on body and identity; gender equality, focusing on male and female social roles; and sexual rights, as a cross-cutting support for the discussion of each topic.

Table 21.1 Categories of the study.

CATEGORIES	CORRESPONDING TOPICS*	OBJECTIVE
SEXUALITY	1. The body as one's own	Get to know the body and the condition of sexual beings
	2. The importance of looking and touching oneself	
	3. Myths surrounding the body	
GENDER EQUALITY	4. Expressions of sexuality form a gender perspective	Make the meaning of gender equality evident
	5. Spaces	
	6. Roles	
SEXUAL RIGHTS	7. Expressions of male and female sexuality	Critically analyze sexual rights and the violation of these rights
	8. New masculinities, new femininities, new families	

*Topics related to the radio dramas.

Early Findings Regarding the Interpellation
of Sexual Imaginaries

Elvia Vargas (2007) considers that, although the definition provided by the World Health Organisation (WHO, 2004) sets forth the elements that constitute sexuality as a complex phenomenon that puts multiple aspects of the human being into play, it does not really define sexuality. Despite that fact, the WHO formulation was a fundamental starting point for the project, insofar as it involves sex, identity, and gender roles, sexual orientation, eroticism, pleasure, intimacy, and reproduction, while recognizing that biological, psychological, social, economic, political, cultural, ethical, legal, historical, and religious factors interact in sexuality.

The notion of sexuality was explored in order to get to know the imaginaries that are common regarding this concept. The first and most dominant perception of sexuality was that associated with "sexual relations between men and women," excluding other expressions and dimensions, as well as other relational options based on sexual diversity. Sexuality also appeared as a topic nobody talks about and which tends to disfigure the body as part of the human being.

> (Sexuality) Well, as people say, it means to make love.
> (Male, 9th–11th grade, Baseline)

Although by the end of the project, most of the participants continued to express more doubts than convictions regarding sexuality, the final personal conclusions the participants drew from the radio programs and the discussion groups did show that, at least at discourse level, their perception of sexuality had expanded and started to include other dimensions and perspectives, beyond genitality:

> My mentality has changed because before, when I heard someone talking about sexuality, I thought they were talking about sex; now I know that sexuality is part of human nature, for example your way of being, your way of living, etc. (Male, 9th–11th grade, Final Evaluation)

> It is fundamental for every young person to have a clear and precise idea of sexuality, since it gives us a model to follow in our reality, and teaches us to value our body with every right we have over it, thus sexuality covers everything. (Female, 9th–11th grade, Final Evaluation)

Perceptions of Interlocutors in the Dialogue
about Sexuality

Young participants in the discussion groups said that the reason they knew nothing about sexuality was that they had no interlocutors with whom to discuss their doubts and fears regarding the topic. They agreed that friends were their main source of information, followed by their teachers. Most of them know that their parents have a sexual life, but it is kept secret and does not come up in their conversations with them. In fact, parents are perceived to be the ones who most oppose and evade the subject at home, and, when they do refer to it, they limit themselves to information about the onset of menstruation in the case of women and to the risk of pregnancy, without talking about birth control methods, the risk of sexually transmitted diseases, or young people's autonomy to experience their own sexuality.

> Our parents have sex and, there they are, so quiet about it. (Female, 6th–8th grade, Baseline)

> My parents told me about menstruation, for example, but they did not tell me how to relate to men. (Female, 9th–11th grade, Baseline)

The conversations with students and the analysis of the radio dramas made it possible to reflect on the fear of talking about the subject and the importance of circulating information:

> "I thought it was very interesting especially because there are girls in my class who sometimes feel ashamed to abandon that taboo and ask questions; they gave us several examples, and told us that we had to do research, talk to our parents, or ask somebody who knows, but not strangers." (Female, 6th–8th grade, Final Evaluation)

With respect to the search for information about sexuality, reference was made to pornography, a topic that had also been dealt with in the radio dramas. The initial perception of the young people was that sexual relations and eroticism as portrayed in pornographic films represented the reality of adult couples.

In the final evaluation, the issue of pornography was discussed from two angles. On the one hand, some said that the sexual expressions of men and women could be similar to those portrayed in porn movies, although the latter tend to overemphasize arousal, the reactions of women, and sexual penetration. On the other hand, it was pointed out that pornographic movies offer no information regarding sexually transmitted diseases.

> With this we have learned that it is important to know one's body and to understand that sexual expressions are not limited to what is shown in the media, like pornography, and that there are many ways for men and women to have pleasure when it's time for sex. (Female, 9th–11th grade, Final Evaluation)

> I thought the radio program was very nice because it taught us that sex movies never teach us how to put on a condom. (Male, 6th–8th grade, Intermediate Evaluation)

> If we want to find out for sure, we don't need to watch porn movies; it's better to learn from things we are told about, and we can prevent diseases if we talk with our parents instead of believing our friends. (Female, 6th–8th grade, Final Evaluation)

Table 21.2 Comparative synthesis of the main findings regarding the sexual imaginaries of the young people from Malambo participating in the project.

	Baseline	Final Evaluation
SEXUALITY	• In the initial conversations, the young people – especially those in the rural groups – appear apathetic and reluctant to talk about sexuality. Their perception of sexuality is that it is something that must be hidden.	• The groups participated openly, especially those from rural institutions, telling stories about sexuality and drawing conclusions from each one of them. Although timidly, sexuality started to appear as something you can talk about, at least in order to learn about it.
	• In their imaginaries, sexuality is associated only with penetrative sex acts, and for this reason the exercise of sexuality at an early age is denied.	• Other perceptions of sexuality, related to caring for the body and appreciating it, appear, although sporadically, in the conversations of the focus groups.
	• Sexuality appears as a denial element, that is, an appropriation of the body through "don'ts": don't harm yourself; don't let people diminish you; don't sell your body, etc.	
	• Touching one's body is perceived as a "dirty" practice associated with prostitutes, gays, and lesbians, except for the case of male masturbation, which is considered normal.	• Some of the women accept the idea of touching their bodies as normal, especially when it is related to the importance of exploring the body to prevent diseases.
	• The status of authority figures granted to parents continues to determine behavior: dress styles, the couple paradigm, decision making, and repressive prevention.	• The young people stated the following as the main lessons learned from the experience: taking care of one's body, appreciating your body, trusting your parents, and questioning the information provided by friends.
	• Taking care of the body is an image associated with women: women are the ones who have to take care of their bodies and know how to dress; the possibility of men caring for themselves that way is ruled out.	• No changed perceptions were identified concerning this aspect. However, in the focus groups, the participants went back to the attitudes of the characters in the dramatization to compare them with situations that had taken place in their own environment.
	• Men assume body care more in terms of physical appearance and fitness than in terms of a healthy life.	• Also, they expressed interest in the contents, since they affirm that their families only comment on situations concerning body care but do not address decision-making situations as shown in the stories.
	• Occasionally, young women who have an active sexual life are associated with prostitutes.	

Source: Adapted and translated from Vega and Mendivil (2010), p. 78.

Perceptions of Gender and Sexuality

For this chapter, we decided to adopt a gender perspective, which was incorporated explicitly as one of the central topics of the radio dramas (sexuality, gender equality, and sexual rights), and which also cuts across the contents of all the stories produced for the dramatization *It Won't Be the First Time*, broadcast in the radio program *La Parla Directa*. For purposes of this analysis, gender is understood as "an ecosystemic concept, a constant learning, an individual and social construction that is experienced differently by each person; it refers to the way in which all societies, in a specific time, culture, and set of social relations, determine attitudes, values, and relations that affect men and women" (Proyecto Colombia, 2005).

> The sex–gender system introduced by G. Rubin (1975) is a formulation aimed at separating sex and gender from an anthropological perspective. In this proposal, sex refers to anatomy; it is sex in the biological sense. Gender, on the other hand, is considered to be a cultural construction that marks and gives meaning to anatomic sex. This conception implies a decentering of biological and naturalistic conceptions (Glocer, 2001, p. 144).

The starting point is the fact that "more than a biological reality, our male/female dichotomy is a symbolic or cultural reality" (Lamas, 1994, p. 10). Giddens (2001) states that both sex and gender are thus understood as socially and not biologically constructed products, which is essential in order to understand gender inequalities. The fact that people are socially induced to believe that inequalities between the sexes are based exclusively on an anatomic distinction makes these inequalities and even male dominance appear as completely natural differences or processes in thought systems (Bourdieu, 1998, 2000).

On the basis of these concepts, we started our analysis, understanding gender as a category that "makes it possible to understand that organizational patterns based on sexual differences (biological) are social and cultural constructions, established on the basis of those differences, which have led to unequal appreciations of men and women, resulting in discrimination against the latter", as we were able to confirm in our initial encounters (PESCC, 2008, p. 8).

In these results, we have also adopted the concept of gender roles, which refers to the gestures and behaviors associated with each sex. Although some gestures and behaviors tend to be attributed to one sex and some to the other, they are "nevertheless inter-changeable and flexible depending on adaptation and adjustment factors (Amezúa, 1999, cited in PESCC, 2008, p. 12).

The results included in the above table show that the evaluation group conversations reflected new perceptions of what it means to be a man or a woman, of the masculine and the feminine, or, at least, the understanding that their initial perceptions were not natural, or representative of the "normal," and that they could be changed. The participants brought up as objects of analysis situations of mockery or discrimination of people from their environment whose perceptions did not coincide with the stereotypes of masculinity and femininity they initially had. This mere fact demonstrates that that the established social imaginaries regarding what it meant to be a man or a woman had been

Table 21.3 Comparative synthesis of the main findings regarding the sexual imaginaries of the young people from Malambo participating in the project.

	Baseline	Final Evaluation
GENDER EQUALITY AND SEXUAL AND REPRODUCTIVE RIGHTS	• Although initially men and women agreed on the image of men and women as subjects of pleasure, what this image would be would depend on the type of relationship the couple has. • They also agreed on the perception that men get more sexually aroused than women, and, in the case of couples, on the image of women responding and consenting to their partner's requests. • The image they have of women includes restricted access to places such as bars, motels, and pool rooms because going to those places would compromise their reputation. On the other hand, there are no restricted places for men. • Men have few opportunities to worry about their image and self-care because they fear being classified as homosexuals. • Images of male activities that women cannot perform have to do mainly with sports, especially soccer and boxing. • Women who perform heavy duty work are classified as "machorras" (butches), that is, women with a male sexual orientation. • Women were described as weak, waiting for their men at home, and incapable of performing activities that require strength, although some men claimed that they shared cleaning chores at home. • The image of a house-proud, innocent, shy, delicate, and reserved woman is opposed to that of the man out in the street, the conqueror she must beware of.	• When debating the notions of equality of sexual rights, they at least accept the idea that women can be subjects of desire, independently of their partners. • Contrary to their response in the initial evaluation regarding access restrictions for men and women, many agreed that choosing the places where you want to be must depend only on the kind of entertainment activity each person chooses and, therefore, it is a right that must be respected. • Very few associated social concepts such as "delicate" and "weak" with women, or "strong" and "tough" with men. • They agreed that, although some of their male friends have sensitive behaviors, they cannot be classified as gay, and that those female friends whose behavior is frowned upon for being rough must be at least respected.

Source: Adapted and translated from Vega and Mendivil (2010), p. 81.

interpellated, and that the participants would now have to carry out a sort of collective construction of new perceptions.

Perceptions of the Body from a Gender Perspective

Fuller (2001) states that gender identities must be understood on the basis of the body, for which purpose it is necessary to understand the representations of the body, that is, those aspects usually considered to be natural and constitutive of masculine or feminine identities.

In the Introduction to the compilation "Body and sexuality," Vidal and Donoso (2002), in reference to a body language presentation by Josefina Hurtado, say that she addresses "the body as a cultural and historical construction in which bodily pleasure must be worked on by deconstructing the conceptions of sexuality imposed by both politics and religion. This deconstruction should facilitate the successive structuring, destructuring, and restructuring of corporal experience from the individual and collective perspectives" (p. 6).

During the discussions, the image of the body came up as an unknown territory that is sometimes abused and, in general, observed and criticized. The idea of identity was associated with that of the body, as one of the ways in which men and women show themselves to their peer groups. In the first conversation, the body was characterized as the starting point for the expression of desire and for initiating interpersonal relationships. The latter, in turn, are necessary for the approval or rejection of behaviors that reaffirm gender roles due to fear of being considered as a transgressor of hetero-normative relations, that is, acting in such a way as to leave no doubt about whether you are male or female. In the case of men, social attributions of masculinity include not being vain and not concentrating on looks, while in the case of women, they include being complaisant toward the male partner in order to guarantee a stable relationship.

> If they see that girls' breasts are too small, and this guy doesn't like small breasts, then they say they want to take flesh from their butt or their belly to put it in their breasts (Female, 9th–11th grade, Baseline)

> I say that the young people from Malambo, most of them, don't value their body; there are people who don't accept the way they are: most of the girls don't accept themselves because they are fat; they want to lose weight and perhaps they feel bad, and rejected, but it shouldn't be this way. They should love themselves the way God made them and they must have a high self-esteem so they can live better (Female, 9th–11th grade, Baseline)

According to these conceptions, women conceive their bodies as a temple that must be preserved and remain untouched by men. The idea that the body is immaculate and should not be exposed to males, unless a stable relationship is ensured, is common among young women, since the body is seen as a reward for the man who chooses them. This idea is reinforced not only by their peers, but also by adults.

To save yourself (the woman), meaning that if there is a man who wants to take advantage of you, you have to realize that a woman has to save herself for life and for the man that will be with her for the rest of her life. (Female, 9th–11th grade, Baseline)

If she did that (have sex), it should be with the person that's always going to be with her, instead of sleeping around for pleasure with someone that they allegedly love, but who will not value them all their life. Then, for me, the right thing is to resist the urge, as they say, and do it with your husband when you have a husband. (Female, 9th–11th grade, Baseline)

Exclusion is the social punishment for a woman who has decided to start her sexual life. In contrast, the sooner men initiate sexual activity, the greater the admiration they get from their peers.

INTERVIEWER:	What do young people think of a woman that has had sex while being single?
FEMALE 1, 6TH–8TH GRADE, BASELINE:	Her reputation is ruined because the other girls' parents forbid them to be with her, to hang out with her, because she will corrupt them."
MALE:	She is a person who doesn't respect herself.
FEMALE 1:	That no man will see her as a woman again, only as an object."
FEMALE 2, 6TH–8TH GRADE, BASELINE:	As a slut.
INTERVIEWER:	And what about the men who have already had sex for the first time?
MALE, 6TH–8TH GRADE, BASELINE:	Maybe as a 'chachito' because he has experience and the others don't, and they know he feels superior to them.

In this sense, a woman's body may only be touched by her male partner in order to preserve that purity (seen as kind of offering); therefore, a woman's self-exploration of her body is interpreted as a transgression. Likewise, genitals are conceived as that which is prohibited, untouchable, and unknown.

People who touch their bodies are sick, because if they already go as far as to touch what must not be touched, then, I think, if they do it to themselves, they might do it to another person. (Female, 9th–11th grade, Baseline)

Although the imaginary that considers a woman's body as untouchable prevailed until the end of the project, some young women began to relate self-exploration of the body to prevention of diseases and to understand it as part of their sexuality.

Touching your body is very important because if one touches one's breasts one can know, go to the doctor, and rule out a disease. (Female, 6th–8th grade, Intermediate Evaluation)

We, as young people, could know our bodies and not believe in rites that people talk about; if one knows one's body and sexuality, one can have a healthy sex life. (Female, 9th–11th grade, Final Evaluation)

I learned that to be able to know our body it is necessary to explore and be well aware of what having access to our body means. (Female, 9th–11th grade, Final Evaluation)

Just as in the case of the images of masculinity and femininity, here it was also possible to observe a process of interpellation of the perceptions they had regarding men's and women's bodies. Although this does not guarantee that their behavior in the future will be different from their current behavior, it is possible to affirm that, since these behaviors are grounded in perceptions that have been questioned, they will not have the same social support, at least not within the group.

Courting: Who Courts Whom?

When talking about sexuality, young people highlighted different ways of courting. The dialogue among peers made it possible to discuss the imaginaries in circulation regarding techniques to seduce members of the opposite sex. However, although peer pressure can be significant in this dialogue, we found that it was women who expressed some ideas that questioned the cultural conventions on gender, which tend to attribute to males the responsibility for courting and for taking the initiative in these situations.

We talk with our friends because sometimes one likes a girl and friends tell you how you can win her heart. Sometimes, one is shy and feels embarrassed. (Male, 9th–11th grade, Baseline)

The study of this context revealed that it was a male attribute to be able to express their interests freely, as well as the ways to seduce women, while restricting that freedom in the case of women.

The thing is that men speak more openly than women; even in the classroom, in front of the teacher, they say, 'Wow, teacher, that lady is hot", while girls express these things, but to a lesser extent. (Male, Baseline)

Women, on the other hand, use seduction techniques privately, resorting to superstitions in order to avoid expressing their attraction for someone openly. Expressing this desire publicly would harm their reputation and classify them as "easy."

(for seduction) My sister puts a piece of paper under her pillow every night; I have seen her. It works for her. (Female, 6th–8th grade, Baseline)

Before, it used to be said that the men from Malambo courted with pebbles; it was said that the guy threw a pebble at the girl, the girl turned, and that was it, they were boyfriend and girlfriend. (Male, 9th–11th grade, Baseline)

The application of the strategy opened up spaces to question those roles assigned according to gender, especially to young women, in whose case such initiatives would be considered inappropriate.

In the story, Andrés (a character in the radio drama) felt ashamed to tell Diana some things (that he was in love with her), and they were friends. I wish we didn't feel ashamed to talk to one another. (Female, 6th–8th grade, Final Evaluation)

If we are going to start a relationship with someone, we have to know their tastes, what they don't like, and not pretend but be just the way we are. (Female, 6th–8th grade, Final Evaluation)

Gender and Spaces to Be

Public and private spaces, as well as crowded or isolated rural places, are scenarios in which gender is constituted and reaffirmed. Parks, gardens, public squares, and schools serve to show how men and women are excluded or included just for being what they are.

The approach to the context through the Baseline made it possible to confirm the traditional spaces assigned to men and women: the private sphere as that reserved for women and represented by the home, closed spaces, daytime, company, care, and restricted access to certain activities, while the public sphere appeared as that reserved for men and represented by trips to the countryside, access to the river, and nighttime.

F1: Yes, I mean a beauty shop, a spa, where everything is delicate; women should be surrounded by everything that is typical of being feminine; and for men, what is typical here in Malambo is the pool room, bars, street corners.

F2: Well, if a boy is with a girl it should be at her house, and the boy should visit her and all that, but boys don't like that because they don't want to take it seriously; but those who take it seriously do want to be at the girl's house. (Females, 9th–11th grade, Baseline)

On the other hand, although some young women feel curiosity about some spaces that are exclusively for males, they refrain from going there for fear of being labeled as "easy," that is, as women who accept sexual activity easily, or to prevent their femininity to be questioned. However, after the reflections that arose from the strategy, the young people understood the use of spaces as a social construction that does not always correspond to the physical-biological possibilities of one sex or the other.

At the pool room, it looks terrible for a woman to come in when the men are there; I think women and men should be apart. Let them go to the pool room and we can go anywhere else, go out, or go dancing… whatever. (Female, 6th–8th grade, Baseline)

On the other hand, although the men have more freedom to circulate and access public spaces (pubs, motels, bars), they refrain from entering places classified as feminine, such as beauty parlors, for fear that their masculinity might be questioned.

In a beauty shop, because men have their nails done, but most have them done by girls that go to their place, but if a man goes in, ouch!, that man is a fag having his nails done. (Female, 9th–11th grade, Baseline)

In the final evaluation, when talking about restricted spaces, many of the young people agreed that the places where members of each sex choose to go, for fun or for whatever reason, is a right that should be respected.[9]

(of a man that walks into a gay bar) Maybe he doesn't go in for that but to look for his brother or his cousin... there are many reasons... I can't judge a person, and say that he walks into a bar and he is gay... I can't because I don't know what his position is. (Male, 6th–8th grade, Final Evaluation)

I think that is her business because if she wants to be in the pool room they should respect her right to be there. (Male, 6th–8th grade, Final Evaluation)

Gender Roles

Roles for each sex are also determined according to the public and private spheres. In this sense, the street, work, being the provider, and fun are associated more with masculine practices, while the home, care, and waiting are associated with femininity.

I think women belong in the house, in their homes; they don't have to go out to work; that's what men are there for. (Male, 6th–8th grade, Baseline)

Although the traditional images associated with gender persisted in the final evaluation, those roles were also questioned and some expressed the possibility of envisioning men and women in other scenarios.

I think the project expectations were fulfilled since I learned to know myself, my body, and for me sexuality isn't just talking about sex but also about rights; the fact that a woman fixes the lights or climbs a tree doesn't mean she is a lesbian but that this is what she feels like doing. (Female, 9th–11th grade, Final Evaluation)

The reflections also revolved around finding the meaning of what it is to be a man or a woman. After discussing the difference between the sexes, the young people arrived at the conclusion that most of these differences are marked by reproductive functions and that limitations are the result of cultural loads.

INTERVIEWER:	What do you think are the main differences between men and women?"
MALE, 9TH–11TH GRADE, FINAL EVALUATION:	That women can get pregnant and men can't."
FEMALE, 6TH–8TH GRADE, FINAL EVALUATION:	That women stay at home and men go out to work, but nowadays there are some women who go out to work.

Thus, the strategy implemented opened up spaces to analyze the reality of the young people's families and the execution of roles on the basis of daily activities, which do not necessarily correspond to the cultural loads assigned to the feminine and the masculine at home. It could be said that the discussion groups served as spaces for the young people to talk about the new masculinities and femininities that had begun to arise in their contexts.

> F1:   No, because all human beings are equal; also, men have to do those chores; there are women that want to be able to cope alone because sometimes they don't live with their husbands, then they have to do those things because otherwise, how are they going to support their children?
> F2:   But here in Malambo they take it as if she is a butch, and say she is doing things that are for men.
> (Females, 9th–11th grade)

> A man that helps at home isn't a bum, he is a househusband. Because not all men leave their house to help their families; some are out in the street doing what they must not do. (Female, 9th–11th grade)

> M1:   Women should not build walls, they should be housewives.
> M2:   No, because if she needs to help, she can do so.
> (Males, 6th–8th grade, Final Evaluation)

In conclusion, the issue of gender was understood more as a question of decision making, a process in which power has generally been assigned to the masculine role rather than to the feminine one.

> (Between men and women) I don't think there is any difference because both men and women are in equal conditions, not like some myths that say that men are the ones who give orders at home and that women have to do what they say. I don't think it's like that because men and women are equal and we all have rights and duties. (Male 6th–8th grade. Simón Bolívar, Final Evaluation)

Scope and Challenges Posed by the Reflection on the Strategy Implemented

The discussion groups made it possible to confirm changes in the discourse and imaginaries regarding sexuality, gender, and rights. In the above-mentioned comparisons of the conversations held with the young people about sexuality, gender, and rights on the basis of focus groups held at the beginning, middle, and end of the implementation of the project, it is possible to see how their imaginaries of rights and gender were gradually interpellated, understanding interpellation as the exercise of asking questions about the implications of those imaginaries, so that they could continue to use them as referents for their action or not, either individually or collectively.

This makes evident a type of interpellation that is different from that used in the analysis of interpellation (Butler, 1999; Amorós, 2005; Youdell, 2010), since it refers to the questioning carried out from the social norm to the behavior of the individual. Butler (1999), as cited by Amorós (2005), states that the performative constitution of a subject is defined on the basis of a reiterative summons or "interpellation" that permanently exhorts the subject to adhere to a gender norm. In the case of the implementation of this project, the social imaginaries that represent the social norm are interpellated by the process of peer communication, for example, the radio program *La Parla Directa*. This situation was evident in the discussions regarding the perceptions of what it means to be a man or a woman, and causes them to reconfigure, at least in discourse, the image they have built of people they know and against whom they hold stereotyped prejudices.

However, the idea of this final reflection is not only to focus on the changes achieved, but also on the subsequent discussions carried out by the research group and on the conversations with the jovenHABLAjoven base group regarding the scope and limitation s they considered significant (Parks *et al.*, 2005).

jovenHABLAjoven discussion groups: peer work

In general, conversation among peers on topics related to sexuality flowed easily, generating a climate of openness and trust and making it possible to express opinions without fear of being judged, something that required a lot of rigor and follow-up. This coincides with the ideas of Clark, MacGeorge, and Robinson (2008), who show how the processes that "should be taken into account" in the context of peer interaction processes such as "comradeship" and "optimism," fall into a moderate centrality range for people, for which reason they also include people's feelings, which is different from what occurs in counseling processes.

However, authors such as Paek (2009), citing Bearman (2002) and Paek and Gunther (2007), point out the multidimensional nature of the concept of peers, which depends on various factors such as proximity or distance within the social circle, and the limitations that can arise in communication processes focusing on peer work. Some of the limitations we found were that sometimes topics are not dealt with adequately, which generates confusion in the answers or requests not attended to. Although it is true that conversations are important spaces because they allow forbidden topics to be brought to the table, it is also true that when topics are not adequately dealt with, group consensuses begin to circulate as "truths" in their agendas.

jovenHABLAjoven: the group perspective

In the course of reflection on the project, the possibility of individual and collective transformation on the basis of communication was identified as the greatest potential of a process like this one. When the objective is to generate communication products and communication scenarios among others, the question of responsibility for the process arises. For this reason, the group studies, learns, reflects, and brings to the table its own imaginaries, using the same dynamics of proposing topics, writing scripts, and building questions and answers. Support and advice, reflection, and permanent questioning about each case set forth are very important here, as is the recognition of the diversity of organizational structures that these processes give rise to.

> Youth development organizations have begun to strengthen their organizational capacity to sustain themselves by focusing on their core goal: to improve the capacity of young people to be effective problem-solvers, communicators and citizens. In the areas of management and organizational studies, a new paradigm of egalitarian, flexible structure has been emerging in the last few decades, replacing more traditional hierarchical structures (Hobbs and Yoon, 2008, p. 149).

In our case, the process also had to take into account sustainability mechanisms. Once the group was established as a legal person, the responsibilities deriving from this led to concern on the part of the group members regarding their income. That is, although the group was set up as a young people's enterprise, their needs at home and their jobs jeopardized the possibilities of economic stability for the group.

Another risk perceived in this peer work process was the distinction between "those who have been saved" and "those who have not been saved."[10] This is one of the complex situations that these types of processes have to face. Those who perceive themselves as having been saved tend to project an image of themselves as persons "who have changed their imaginaries," who "already know everything about the topics," "who think of themselves as different," and "who have solved all their issues," and for this reason, they feel they can respond to any situation they face. It is essential to have them understand that projects like this entail processes and reflections that will always have to be contrasted with everyday life situations and that they do not lead directly to "salvation," but rather have to be defined at each moment of their lives. However, the groups of young people who think this way play a key role in the process of interpellation of social norms.

It Won't be the First Time: From the field of discussion to the field of production

In general, the radio drama became a key mechanism to generate discussion among the young people. The characters and situations allowed each participant to express his or her points of view, fears, experiences, and reflections on them. What should be criticized and what should be emulated were always discussed. The radio program also contributed to enriching the discussion groups since they expanded points of view on topics and persons, leading to the questioning and transformation of the participants' ideas.

Nevertheless, the participants continued to attach greater value to the production process of the radio dramas, to the reflections that arose when proposing the topics, and creating the characters, situations, and stories. The group kept asking why, instead of discussing the dramas, we did not go on to restructure them or create new ones, in the form of theater forums. This evaluation exercise is very important because, as demonstrated above, it consists in making communication one of the scenarios where it is possible for norms to be interpellated by the subjects, instead of the other way around.

In this sense, it was possible to confirm the potential of the appropriation of the production by the young people, in a process that, contrary to traditional processes that originate in adults – for example, teachers – is generated by the young people themselves. This type of process has also been carried out in other countries:

> Most people might assume that getting a participatory youth radio project off the ground is primarily about providing tools and training young people—that adult professionals already have the skills and will help transfer them to the youth. But what we found was actually the reverse. The young people embraced new technology, were hip to the latest global sounds, and liked to experiment with form and content. The adults, not so much (Ross and Obdam, 2008, p. 260).

Second-generation edutainment: limits and risks

Working with young people, students, and, in some cases, with their teachers was a key element in the process of establishing the potential of the radio program *La Parla Directa*, of the radio drama *It Won't be the First Time*, of the *jovenHABLAjoven* discussion groups, of the imaginaries that could be interpellated, and of the pleasure with which the young people participated and remained in the project.

Nevertheless, it was possible to identify fear of the challenges posed through some of the questions the young people asked one another. How can we make these discussions reach our parents and get out teachers involved? How can we avoid being judged at health centers? How can we obtain spaces for our sexuality other than the cemetery at night, the nearby hills, or a bedroom when our parents are not at home? How can we ensure access to condoms so that young people don't have to resort to Boli bags[11] and run the risk of getting the opposite of what they seek? How can we compete with widely listened to or watched radio programs or soap operas that propose exactly the opposite of what we are proposing and push people toward it? This is the gap between second and third-generation Edutainment that Tufte (2004) points out: the need to aim at more structural changes, to generate processes that have an impact on local and national public policies, to involve different actors who can make decisions and who can support those demands that cannot be satisfied specifically from the field of communication.

Given the scope, duration, and budget of a project like *jovenHABLAjoven*, it would be unrealistic to expect it to generate that type of impact. It might be that the actual scope of micro-projects such as this one is limited to developing experiences that show how peer communication can generate interpellations and changes in imaginaries. However, it is important to understand that for social change to be possible, it is necessary to work together with other actors, in other scenarios, and with other communication models and strategies (socio-ecological models and third-generation edutainment, for example).

Notes

1   This chapter presents the final results of the project *jovenHABLAjoven* (youngpeopleTALK-young) Communication Group: Implementation and Evaluation of a Communication Strategy in an Urban-Rural Population of the Department of Atlántico, developed as a result

of a research internship carried out by Carmen Rosa Mendivil in the context of the Universidad del Norte's Young Researchers Program 2005–2006, in its fourth internal session and within the framework of the strategy aimed at strengthening the Universidad del Norte's Groups and Centers. The internship took place as part of the project "jovenHABLAjoven: Communication for Participation of Young People in the Municipality of Malambo," led by Jair Vega Casanova and carried out by the PBX Communications and Culture Research Group. A preliminary version of these results was published in Vega, J. and Mendivil C. (2010) jovenHABLAjoven: A second-generation edutainment experience in sexuality and gender work with young people. *Revista Folios, 23,* 69–92. Facultad de Comunicaciones, Universidad de Antioquia.

2   Malambo is a municipality located in the Metropolitan Area of Barranquilla, Colombia.

3   There are other texts documenting the experience, such as: Vega, Arroyave, and Mendivil (2006), Vega, Obregón, and Mendivil (2005), and Vega and Suárez (2003). Although this was a peer project carried out by undergraduate students in the Social Communication and Journalism program and young people from the Municipality of Malambo, the project was supervised by the researchers belonging to the PBX Communications and Culture Research Group.

4   The following undergraduate theses in Social Communication and Journalism resulted from the process: Cuartas and Romero (2005), Mendivil (2004), and Suárez (2004).

5   The concept of "interaction" was proposed as an alternative to that of "intervention," insofar as it goes beyond the idea of an action executed from the outside on a population, in such a way that the latter is not considered an agent of its own process, but rather as the object of a change of interest or an action on the part of an external agent. This reflection was also carried out in the context of the social programs sponsored by the Fundación Social in Colombia, and is explained in several documents, such as the one written by the author cited.

6   The radio program aired over three months on the Sensación Estéreo community radio station in Malambo. Then it was broadcast at recess time in schools, and, during the last four months it aired on the National Police radio station.

7   The schools selected were considered to be socially representative of the population at large, given that they are the public and private institutions with the greatest number of students from different zones of the municipality. Twenty young people from each institution were selected and divided into two main groups: 6th to 8th-graders and 9th to 11th-graders. Discussion groups were carried out independently with the young people at each stage of the study. This same group of students was used to evaluate the discussion group process, since it was decided, together with the teachers, that this process would be incorporated into a classroom dynamics that helped generate greater trust between the teacher and the participating student group.

8   The findings of this first exercise were taken as baseline for the evaluation of the project and will be presented as such in the results.

9   It will also be interesting to expand the reflection on gender roles of young people in public spaces and spheres, contrasting it with other approaches not necessarily based on sexuality. See Pérez (2007).

10 The concept of "saved" individuals is used as an interpretation of those young people who assume that, just because they now handle new discourses about sexuality, they are somehow "protected" from any risk of falling into negative behaviors or of having health problems. The term is used as an interpretation and must be understood as specifically focusing on risks.

11 "Bolis" are low-priced refreshments packed and frozen in small plastic bags, approximately the size of a condom.

References

Althusser, L. (1972). Ideology and ideological state apparatuses. Notes towards an investigation. In L. Althusser, *Lenin and Philosophy and Other Essays* (pp. 127–186). New York: Monthly Review Press.

Álvarez, O., and Pilar y Errico, F. (2007). Comunicación, producción de sentidos y formación de sujetos en la "Escuela Pedagógica" [Communication, production of meanings and training of subjects in the "Pedagogical School"]. In V Congreso Virtual "La tesis en comunicación. Centralidad de los antecedentes y el estado del arte en la elaboración del Plan de Tesis". Universidad Nacional de la Plata. Argentina. Retrieved from http://www.perio.unlp.edu.ar/seminario/V_congreso_virtual/nivel2/mesa3/23_Alvarez%20Olaizola_Pilar_Errico_francisco_ponencia.doc

Amezúa, E. (1999). Teoría de los sexos: La letra pequeña de la sexología [Theory of the sexes: the small print of sexology]. *Revista Española de Sexología, 95–96*, 17–265.

Amorós, C. (2005). *La Gran Diferencia y sus Pequeñas Consecuencias para las Luchas de las Mujeres* [The big difference and its little consequences for women's struggles]. Premio Nacional de Ensayo. Madrid: Cátedra.

Barbero, J. M. (1993). *Communication, Culture and Hegemony: From the Media to Mediations.* Thousand Oaks, CA: Sage Publications Ltd.

Bearman, P. S. (2002). Social network context and adolescent STD risk. New York: Institute for Social and Economic Research and Policy, Columbia University.

Bourdieu, P. (2000). *Poder, Derecho y Clases Sociales* [Power, law, and social classes]. Bilbao: Editorial Desclée de Brouwer.

Bourdieu, P. (2001). *Masculine Domination.* Stanford: Stanford University Press.

Butler, J., and Laclau, E. (1999). Los usos de la igualdad [The uses of equality]. *Debate Feminista, 19.* Retrieved from http://www.debatefeminista.com/PDF/Articulos/losuso384.pdf

Byrne, A., Gray-Felder, D. and Hunt, J. (Eds.) (2005). *Communities Measure Change: A Reference Guide to Monitoring Communication for Social Change.* Communication for Social Change Consortium, New Jersey. Retrieved from http://www.communicationforsocialchange.org/pdf/communities_measure_change.pdf

Clark, R., MacGeorge, E., and Robinson L. (2008). Evaluation of peer comforting strategies by children and adolescents. *Human Communication Research, 34*(2), 319–345.

Cuartas, M., and Romero, X. (2005). Jóvenes, comunicación y salud: imaginarios sexuales. Diseño participativo de una estrategia de comunicación en el Municipio de Malambo [Young people, communication and health: sexual imaginaries. Participatory design of a communication strategy in the municipality of Malambo]. Thesis for the Communication and Journalism Pregraduate Program, Universidad del Norte, Barranquilla.

Da Porta, E. (2005). El vínculo comunicación-educación: Transdisciplina y articulación. Senderos y recorridos. Apuntes para un mapa de investigación [The communication–education link: Transdisciplinarity and articulation. Trails and paths. Notes for a research map]. *Revista "Tram[p]as" de la Comunicación y la Cultura, 29* "Investigación en Comunicación y Educación". Facultad de Periodismo y Comunicación Social – Universidad Nacional de La Plata. Argentina.

Franco, G. (2000). Culturas juveniles urbanas y convivencia democrática: "El caso de muchachos a lo bien" [Urban youth culture and democratic coexistence: "The case of Muchachos a lo bien"]. In C. Valderrama (Ed.), *Comunicación – Educación. Coordenadas, Abordajes y Travesías.* Santafé de Bogotá: Siglo del Hombre Editores, Fundación Universidad Central, Departamento de Investigaciones, DIUC.

Freire, P. (1970). *Pedagogía del oprimido* [Pedagogy of the oppressed]. Montevideo: Tierra Nueva.

Freire, P. (1986). *Hacia una pedagogía de la pregunta. Conversaciones con Antonio Faundez* [Towards a pedagogy of the question. Conversations with Antonio Faundez]. Buenos Aires: Ediciones La Aurora.

Fuller, N. (2001). *Masculinidades. Cambios y Permanencias* [Masculinities: Changes and permanencies]. Lima: Fondo Editorial de la Pontificia Universidad Católica del Perú.

Fundación Rockefeller (1999, enero). *Comunicación para el Cambio Social: Documento Programático e Informe sobre una Conferencia* [Communication for social change: Programmatic document and conference report]. Retrieved from http://www.comminit.com/en/node/150284/348

Giddens, A. (2001). Género y sexualidad [Gender and sexuality]. Chapter 5 in A. Giddens, *Sociología*, 4 edn. Madrid: Alianza Editorial.

Glocer, L. (2001). *Lo Femenino y el Pensamiento Complejo* The feminine and complex thought]. Buenos Aires: Lugar Editorial.

Hobbs, R., and Yoon, J. (2008). Creating empowering environments in youth media organizations. *Youth Media Reporter*, August 2008. Retrieved from http://www.youthmediareporter.org/docs/HobbsYoon2.pdf

Lamas, M. (1994). Cuerpo, diferencia sexual y género [The body, sexual difference and gneder]. *Debate feminista. Cuerpo y política.* 5(10), 3–31.

Locksley, G. (2009). *Media and Development: What's the Story?* Washington, DC: World Bank Publications.

Mendivil, C. (2004). Joven, contexto y sexualidad: Exploración socio-semiótica de los contextos de situación en los que se desarrollan los jóvenes de Malambo y su incidencia en la sexualidad [Youth, context, and sexuality: Socio-semiotic exploration of situational contexts in which the young people of Malambo develop and its impact on sexuality]. Thesis of the Communication and Journalism Pregraduate Program, Universidad del Norte, Barranquilla.

Paek, H.-J. (2009). Differential effects of different peers: further evidence of the peer proximity thesis in perceived peer influence on college students' smoking. *Journal of Communication, 59*(3), 434–455.

Paek, H.-J., and Gunther, A. C. (2007). How peer proximity moderates indirect media influence on adolescent smoking. *Communication Research, 34,* 407–432.

Parks, W. with Gray-Felder, D., Hunt, J. and Byrne, A. (2005). Who measures change? An Introduction to Participatory Monitoring and Evaluation of Communication for Social Change. Communication for Social Change Consortium. Retrieved from http://www.communicationforsocialchange.org/pdf/who_measures_change.pdf

Pérez, M. (2007). Cartografías de lo público: una aproximación desde los estudios culturales. Esferas públicas juveniles en la Comuna 13 de Medellín (Colombia) [Cartographies of the public: An approach from cultural studies. Youth public spheres in Commune 13 in Medellin (Colombia)]. *Revista Investigación y Desarrollo,* Universidad del Norte, *15*(2), 344–365.

Pérez, M., and Vega, J. (2010). Memorias de organizaciones juveniles, comunicación e identidades políticas. Estudio de caso del Colectivo Pasolini en Medellín [Memories of youth organizations, media and political identities. Case study of Colectivo Pasolini in Medellin]. In A. Garcés (Ed.), *Pensar la Comunicación II.* Medellin: Universidad de Medellín.

PESCC (Proyecto de Educación Sexual y Construcción Sexual y Construcción de Ciudadanía) (2008). La dimensión de la sexualidad en la educación de nuestros niños, niñas, adolescentes y jóvenes [Sexual education project, sexual construction and building citizenship. The dimension of sexuality in the education of our children and young people]. Bogotá: Ministerio de Educación Nacional – Fondo de Población de Naciones Unidas.

Proyecto Colombia (2005). Jóvenes re-corridos, Cuerpos con paisaje. Construcción de una respuesta intersectorial en salud sexual y reproductiva, con énfasis en prevención y atención a las ITS-VIH-SIDA, con jóvenes y adolescentes residentes en comunidades receptoras de población desplazada de Colombia [Young *re-corridos*, bodies with landscape. Construction of an intersectoral sexual and reproductive health, with emphasis on prevention and care of STI-HIV-AIDS, with youth and adolescents residing in communities hosting displaced people in Colombia]. Bogotá: Proyecto Colombia.

Riaño, P. (2000), Recuerdos metodológicos: El taller y la investigación etnográfica [Methodological memories: The workshop and ethnographic research]. *Estudios sobre las Culturas Contemporáneas*, *V*(10). Retrieved from http://redalyc.uaemex.mx/redalyc/pdf/316/31601008.pdf

Ross, J., and Obdam, E. (2008). Like a bell that calls: Participatory youth radio in Ethiopia. *Youth Media Reporter*, 6. Retrieved from http://www.youthmediareporter.org/2008/12/like_a_bell_that_calls_partici.html

Rubin, G. (1975). The traffic of women; Notes on the "political economy" if sex. In R. Reiter (Ed.), *Toward an Anthropology of Women* (pp. 157–210). New York: Monthly Review Press.

Singhal, A., and Rogers, E. (1999). *Entertainment-Education. A Communication Strategy for Social Change*. Mahwah, NJ: Lawrence Erlbaum.

Singhal, A., and Rogers, E. (2002). A theoretical agenda for entertainment-education. *Communication Theory, 12*(2), 117–135.

Suarez, L. (2004). Jóvenes y Sexualidad: Los Espacios y la Configuración de Identidades: Diseño Participativo De Una Estrategia de comunicación en el municipio de Malambo [Youth and sexuality: The configuration spaces and identities: participatory design of a communication strategy in the town of Malambo]. Thesis for the Social Communication and Journalism Pregraduate Program, Universidad del Norte, Barranquilla.

Suarez, L., Mendivil, C., and Vega, M. (2004). *jovenHABLAjoven: Una experiencia de comunicación y salud en el municipio de Malambo. Los y las jóvenes urbano/rurales, su cultura y sus identidades alrededor de la sexualidad* [jovenHABLAjoven: A communication and health experience in the municipality of Malambo. The culture and identities of urban/rural young people regarding sexuality]. *Revista Investigación and Desarrollo*, No. 1 Vol. XII. Barranquilla: Ediciones Uninorte.

Taylor, C. (2006). *Modern Social Imaginaries*. Durham, NC: Duke University Press.

Tufte, T. (2004). Eduentretenimiento en la comunicación para el VIH/SIDA más allá del mercadeo, hacia el empoderamiento [Edutainment communication for HIV /AIDS beyond marketing to empowerment]. *Investigación and Desarrollo, 12*(1), 24–43.

Tufte, T. (2005). Entertainment education in development communications. between marketing behaviors and empowering people. In O. Helmer and T. Tufte (Eds.), *Media and Global Change, Rethinking, Communication for Development* (pp. 159–176). Buenos Aires: Ed. Norden.

Vargas, E. (2007). *Sexualidad... Mucho Más que Sexo* [Sexuality ... much more than sex]. Bogotá: Uniandes.

Vega, J., Arroyave, J., and Mendivil, C. (2006). Project: jovenHABLAjoven (Young People Speak) a communication intervention for social change to improve sexual responsibility. In *World Congress on Communication for Development. Lessons, Challenges, and the Way Forward, the Communication Initiative*. Rome: Food and Agriculture Organization of the United Nations.

Vega, J., and Mendivil, C. (2005).Colectivo de comunicación jovenHABLAjoven: estrategia de comunicación para la prevención y promoción de la salud sexual y reproductiva, equidad de género y derechos sexuales y reproductivos en la población joven de malambo. Informe Final [JovenHABLAjoven Collective communication: Communication strategy for the prevention and promotion of sexual and reproductive health, gender equity, and reproductive rights of young people in Malambo. Final report]. Unpublished document, Universidad del Norte – UNFPA. Barranquilla.

Vega, J., Obregón, R., and Mendivil, C. (2005). Sistematización de experiencias de comunicación y participación. Caso Joven Habla Joven. Informe final de proyecto de investigación [Systematization of experiences of communication and participation. The case of Joven Habla Joven. Final report of research project]. Unpublished document, Universidad del Norte – Exchange, Barranquilla.

Vega, J., and Suárez, L. (2003). Jóvenes, Identidades y Salud: Reflexiones a partir de una experiencia de comunicación [Youth, identity and health: Reflections on a communication experience]. In *Memorias del Primer Congreso Latinoamericano de Comunicación y Salud* (pp. 115–124). Cochabamba: Centro de Programas para la Comunicación.

Vidal, F., and Donoso, C. (Eds.) (2002). Cuerpo y Sexualidad [The body and sexuality]. Santiago: Universidad Arcis, Flacso, Vivo Positivo. Retrieved from http://www.pasa.cl/biblioteca/Cuerpo_y_Sexualidad_Vidal,_Francisco;_Donoso,_Carla.pdf

WHO (World Health Organisation).(2004).Progress in Reproductive Health Research. Retrieved from http://www.who.int/hrp/publications/progress67.pdf

Youdell, D. (2005). Sex-gender-sexuality: How sex, gender and sexuality constellations are constituted in secondary schools. *Gender and Education, 17*(3), 149–170.

22

Changing Gender Norms for HIV and Violence Risk Reduction
A Comparison of Male-Focused Programs in Brazil and India

Julie Pulerwitz, Gary Barker, and Ravi Verma

Introduction

Substantial evidence indicates that inequitable gender norms negatively influence sexual and reproductive health-related behaviors and disease prevention, as well as men's use of violence against women (e.g., Worth, 1989; Campbell, 1995). These norms include support for men to have multiple partners, or to maintain control over the behavior of their female partners. Thus, addressing gender norms – defined here as the roles, responsibilities, and rights of men as opposed to women, based on societal expectations – is increasingly recognized as an important HIV and violence risk reduction strategy.

Recently, a number of behavior-change communication (BCC) programs that specifically promote gender-equitable norms and related behaviors have been implemented in different cultural settings. These are mainly small in scale and pilot programs, and have rarely been evaluated, but many have seemed promising (WHO, 2007). Many additional programs have described gender equity as a program goal, but have rarely assessed how the program interventions contributed to achieving gender equity and gender-equitable attitudes or behaviors among men (White, Greene, and Murphy, 2005). At this point, few interventions to promote gender-equitable behavior have been systematically implemented and evaluated, and little has been published about their effects, including on HIV/STI risk and violence, or their cost.

This case study is intended to bridge theory and practice, and highlight the impact of including a gender-focus in actual programs. Findings provide an opportunity to:

- Compare results of two similar intervention and evaluation designs, on key outcomes and lessons learned, in very different cultural contexts: Brazil and India (Pulerwitz *et al.*, 2006; Verma *et al.*, 2008; Pulerwitz *et al.*, 2010).

The Handbook of Global Health Communication, First Edition. Edited by Rafael Obregon and Silvio Waisbord.

- Test the effect of different combinations of communication activities.
- Directly and quantitatively measure gender dynamics/support for (in)equitable gender norms.
- Investigate the dynamics of programs that focus on young men.
- Assess the cost of intervention activities.

Our findings suggest that behavior-change communication interventions that explicitly focus on gender within the context of HIV and violence prevention, can both renorm gender for the young men exposed to the intervention and demonstrate HIV and violence risk reduction. Findings were positive in both Brazil and in India. A key component was the intentional process to conceptualize and operationalize how to promote gender equity. The intervention used an ecological model for its behavior change approaches, which led to the combination of interpersonal communication via participatory group education, and community-based media and mobilization activities to reinforce the messages on the community level. This chapter highlights the lessons learned from the Operations Research (OR) around these interventions. The OR tested the effect of different combinations of BCC activities on views towards gender norms, and HIV and violence outcomes, as well as determined programmatic lessons. In addition, a cost analysis was conducted at the Brazil site.

We will be describing a project designed and implemented in a low-income, urban setting in Brazil, and then adapted to a comparable setting in India (after a formative research and revision process). In both countries, similar research questions, methodologies, and communication approaches were applied.

Key questions we answer in the chapter include:

- What is the role of gender dynamics in HIV and violence risk for young men?
- How do you measure support for (in)equitable gender norms, so you know where you are at baseline and what you change?
- What kinds of communication activities will be effective to change attitudes towards gender norms, and related behaviors?
- How useful are these measures and strategies across different cultural contexts?
- What is the cost per beneficiary reached?

Literature Review

Both boys/men and girls/women receive and internalize societal messages about appropriate behaviors, roles, responsibilities and rights for men versus women. This socialization process can promote inequity between men and women, and can encourage behaviors that place men and their sexual partners at risk of various negative health outcomes (Rivers and Aggleton, 1998).

Studies from various countries have found that young men often view sexual initiation as a way to demonstrate that they are "real" men; that is, to affirm their identity as men (e.g., Marsiglio, 1988). Boys often feel that they must repeatedly prove their manhood through sexual activity. Furthermore, social norms frequently hold that it is the male's responsibility to acquire condoms, since for a young woman to carry condoms would suggest that she intends to have sex, which may be seen as "promiscuous" (Childhope, 1997). At the same time, the prevailing norms in many settings dictate that since reproductive and sexual health are "female" concerns, women must be the ones to suggest contraceptive use (Greene *et al.*, 2004). Gender-based power dynamics exacerbate these issues, and women often cannot negotiate condom use when they wish to do so (Amaro, 1995; Pulerwitz *et al.*, 2002).

Another relevant example of men's behavior toward women related to inequitable norms is the use of violence against women. Findings from a seminal, multi-country study among population-based samples in 15 sites in 10 countries indicate that between 15 and 71 percent of women of reproductive age have been subject to physical or sexual violence by a male partner, with seven sites reporting a prevalence of 25 percent to 50 percent and six sites a prevalence of 50 percent to 75 percent (Garcia-Moreno *et al.*, 2006). A survey of 750 men across various social classes in Rio de Janeiro found that 25 percent reported using physical violence against a partner at least once (Instituto Promundo and Instituto Noos, 2003). In India, the nationally representative National Family Health Survey (FHS) found that 34 percent of all women aged 15 to 49 have experienced violence at some time since the age of 15 (IIPS and Macro International, 2007). The causes and factors associated with men's use of physical and sexual violence against women are complex, but among them are the social construction of masculinity (Kaufman, 1993). A study in India, for example, found that use of violent behaviors was an integral component of describing a "real man" and manliness (Verma *et al.*, 2005).

Boys are also socialized into a set of ideas about household roles and childrearing. Studies conducted in various countries find that fathers tend to contribute about one-third to one-fourth of the time that mothers do in direct child care (Population Council, 2001). While there are substantial individual and context-specific differences, research suggests that boys and young men commonly identify less involvement in domestic roles as part of their understanding of masculinity.

A helpful World Health Organisation (WHO)-led review assessed the effectiveness of programs seeking to engage men and boys in achieving gender equality and equity in health, including programs that focused on HIV/STI and violence, among other topics. The review analyzed data from 58 evaluation studies (identified via an Internet search, key informants, and colleague organizations) of interventions with men and boys, including the two programs described in this chapter. Programs were rated on overall effectiveness, which included evaluation design (giving more weight to quasi-experimental and randomized control trial designs) and level of impact (giving more weight to interventions that confirmed behavior change on the part of men or boys). Overall, 29 percent of the 58 programs were assessed as effective in leading to changes in attitudes or behavior, 38 percent as promising, and 33 percent as unclear. Integrated programs and programs with community outreach, mobilization, and mass-media campaigns showed more effectiveness in producing behavior change than individual-only interventions. This highlights the importance of reaching beyond the individual level to the social context – including interpersonal relationships and community leaders. The authors conclude that the evidence is encouraging, although most of the programs were small in scale and short in duration (WHO, 2007).

Conceptual Framework

This work applied a social constructionist or interactive theory of gender socialization. In recent years many authors in the field of gender research, and specifically in the field of masculinities, have subscribed to this theoretical framework, which posits that any given cultural setting provides a version, or multiple versions, of masculinities (Connell, 1987, 1994). These gender "norms," which are passed on to young men by their family, peer group, and social institutions, among others, are interpreted and internalized by individual men. These individuals reinterpret and "reconstruct" the norms, and, as members of society, also influence the broader shared norms. This theoretical framework highlights that certain models of manhood or masculinity are promoted in specific cultural settings, but that individual men will vary in how closely they adhere to these norms. Furthermore, this framework indicates that norms can evolve over time as individuals and groups reconstruct them. The intervention activities were selected to address gender norms on a specific set of topic areas: sexuality, violence, reproductive health and HIV prevention, and daily/domestic life and decision making.

The study and intervention also drew upon the "ecological" model, and its guidance regarding the importance of addressing key issues from multiple levels, from the individual to the greater society. Hence, the intervention included the promotion of individual reflection, a peer and interpersonal group education component, and a broader community-based component. Finally, the interventions were guided by a participatory framework, where the young men helped design the intervention, such as key BCC messages.

Intervention: Development and Adaptation in Brazil and India

The intervention developed and implemented in Brazil was called Program H (for *homens*: "men" in Portuguese). Program H focuses on helping young men question traditional norms related to manhood and on promoting the abilities of young men to discuss and reflect on the "costs" of inequitable gender-related views and the advantages of more gender-equitable behaviors. One intervention component included interactive group education sessions for young men led by adult male facilitators. The other was a community-wide "lifestyle" behavior-change communication campaign to promote condom use, using a new condom brand and gender-equitable messages that reinforced those promoted in the group education sessions.

In India, the interactive group education sessions were adapted for the cultural setting, and then piloted and tested (Verma *et al.*, 2006), before being implemented in the evaluation describe in this chapter. The behavior-change communication campaign was also adapted. It focused on street theater, and small media (e.g., posters) to reinforce the gender equitable messages on the community level, but did not include a new condom brand. The intervention was named *Yaari-Dosti* (translated as "friendship" or "bonding" among men).

These projects were developed and implemented as a result of an ongoing partnership among a number of institutions. PATH and the Population Council (via the Horizons Program, which was funded by USAID/PEPFAR) led the evaluations, including measurement development, while Promundo in Brazil and CORO for Literacy (Committee of Resource Organization) in India led the implementation and adaptation of the interventions. The group education sessions, video, and "lifestyle" social marketing campaign were originally developed in Brazil by Promundo, Salud y Genero, Ecos, Instituto PAPAI, and JohnSnowBrazil.

Group education intervention

The curriculum includes an overview and framework for thinking about these issues, and a series of activities that were developed and pretested with groups of young men. As noted above, this group education component of the intervention was applied in both Brazil and India. In Brazil, 18 activities were selected from a larger manual of 70 activities, and 23 activities were adapted in India. The activities were organized under five themes: Sexuality and Reproductive Health, Fatherhood and Caregiving, From Violence to Peaceful Coexistence, Reasons and Emotions (including communication skills, substance abuse, and mental health), and Preventing and Living with HIV/AIDS. The activities in the manual were designed to be carried out in a same-sex group setting. They consisted of role plays, brainstorming exercises, discussion sessions, and individual reflection.

In Brazil, the 18 exercises (plus a video that was viewed and discussed at the onset of the activities) were conducted with the young men during once-a-week sessions for about two hours each over approximately a six-month period, for a total of about 28 hours. The study team considered the six-month period long enough to expect an effect from the intervention, yet short enough that it was not too much of a burden on the young men to complete, nor on future organizations that may be interested in implementing it. Eighteen activities deemed most relevant for the goals of the project were selected from the complete manuals by a Technical Advisory Group (TAG), comprised of project partners.

The video used during the sessions was a no-words cartoon called "Once upon a boy," which tells the story of a young man from early childhood, through adolescence, to early adulthood. The story highlights different experiences in the young man's life, including witnessing violence in his home, interactions with male peer groups, his first sexual experience, as well as his contracting a sexually transmitted infection (STI) and facing an unplanned pregnancy. Like the Program H group educational activities, the video was widely field-tested in Latin America and the Caribbean during its development and its content was based on previous qualitative research with young men in the region.

In India, youth working for CORO for Literacy – who were from the planned intervention communities – were engaged to work with Horizons and Promundo to adapt and implement the intervention. They underwent a two-week training program to strengthen their gender and HIV-related knowledge and facilitation skills and were trained in qualitative methods of data collection. Formative research, where information about the key gender-related themes in the community, and the appropriateness of the Program H activities, was conducted by the partners. Intervention activities for young men were then adapted and piloted. Based on the formative research, the key themes were quite similar in both contexts and interventions with a similar format could be used. When adapting the education sessions, some of the story lines were modified and the names in the stories were changed, but the general themes stayed the same. The participatory format, which focused on probes to prompt discussion, permitted applying these same exercises even in this very different cultural setting. In addition, instead of using a cartoon video, it was considered more appropriate in this setting to utilize written cartoons, which captured similar themes (e.g., gender, violence, and alcohol), and these were produced and distributed. Prior to piloting the activities, the same peer leaders were additionally trained to facilitate the adapted group education sessions.

In Brazil, the young men were recruited to participate in the intervention via a multistage process. Promundo held meetings with local community groups, resident associations, and local schools to discuss potential partnerships with the community and the availability of space for the educational workshops. A few of the community groups and schools offered space for the workshops and assisted in the recruitment of young men. In India, similarly, volunteers were sought from existing youth groups in the community, vocational training centers, and through word of mouth and the peer leaders' friends. Activities took place across the community, whether in established community centers or outside under a tree.

The facilitators of the education sessions were mainly young men from the same or similar communities as the intervention, who had some prior experience with health promotion activities. In Brazil, five adult men were selected to facilitate the group activities. Each of the facilitators had prior experience working with groups of youth from low-income communities on gender and health issues. Facilitators were additionally trained by program staff for a total of 24 hours (three days). In India, the nine peer leaders who participated in adapting the intervention originally took a leading role in implementation. Over time, additional peer leaders were engaged to implement the activities, and the original peer leaders and program staff were both involved in training them. The peer leaders in India had less prior, relevant experience than the facilitators in Brazil, and they were therefore initially teamed with adult "gender experts" when leading the activities.

Community-based BCC campaign

A behavior-change communication campaign to promote a more gender-equitable lifestyle and HIV/STI/violence prevention at the community level, and to reinforce the messages learned in the group education sessions, was also applied in both Brazil and India. Program staff worked with peer promoters – young men recruited from the community – to help develop and implement the campaign. The community-based BCC campaign encourages young men to reflect on how they act as men and enjoins them to respect their partners, to avoid using violence against women, and to practice safer sex. Related materials, such as posters and postcards, were developed and distributed.

In Brazil, as part of the campaign, the team produced and promoted a specific condom to be targeted for the intervention audience. Hence, the intervention also had a social marketing component, referred to here as "lifestyle" social marketing. The peer promoters who had helped design the campaign messages also engaged in the activities to promote the condoms and related messages in the community. For example, they would sit at booths to sell condoms and distribute related materials.

In India, after discussions with local groups, it was decided against focusing on promoting condoms or developing a specific condom, as this was perceived as more stigmatized than in Brazil and associated with a number of topics that would detract from the goals of the project. Instead, the main community-based intervention focused on street theater, and group discussions after the theater session ended. One of the themes of the performances was the use and appropriateness of condoms.

Measuring Gender Norms: the Gender Equitable Men Scale in Brazil and India

Before PATH/Horizons researchers began their work, few studies had attempted to quantitatively measure change in attitudes about gender norms related to violence and HIV/STI risk, and few scales were available to evaluate an intervention's effects on gender norms and sexual risk behaviors. In response to this important gap, PATH/Horizons researchers and partners (in particular, Promundo) developed and validated the Gender Equitable Men (GEM) Scale (Pulerwitz and Barker, 2008). This scale includes items on women and men's roles and responsibilities in daily life such as domestic work and child care, sexuality and sexual relationships, reproductive health and disease prevention, violence, and homophobia and relations between men. Items were based on previous qualitative work and a literature review.

The scale items were initially administered to a household sample of 742 men aged 15 to 59 years in Rio de Janeiro, Brazil. Factor analyses supported two subscales with 24 items in total, and the scale was internally consistent (alpha = 0.81). As hypothesized, more support for equitable norms (i.e., higher GEM Scale scores) was significantly associated with less self-reported partner violence, more contraceptive use, and a higher education level. The 17-item "inegalitarian" subscale was the one used in the evaluation of the young men described in this chapter, and the scale was again internally consistent (alpha = 0.78).

Table 22.1 displays examples of items from the original GEM Scale developed in Brazil and from its subsequent adaptation in India to a 15-item scale (alpha = 0.78), where certain items were removed (or added) for cultural specificity. Additional psychometric testing took place in India, and the adapted scale was found to be clear, internally consistent, and associated with key outcomes as expected. Further adaptations by PATH researchers, and the successful application of the scales, have since taken place in Ethiopia,

Table 22.1 Examples of GEM Scale items.

GEM Scale item	Examples*
Reproductive health and disease prevention	It is a woman's responsibility to avoid getting pregnant I would be outraged if my wife asked me to use a condom A real man produces a male child (I) Women who carry condoms on them are "easy" (B)
Sexuality	Men need more sex than women do You don't talk about sex, you just do it Men are always ready to have sex Men need other women even if things are fine with their wives A real man is one who can have sex with a woman for a long time (I)
Violence	It is okay for a man to hit his wife if she won't have sex with him A woman should tolerate violence in order to keep her family together There are times when a woman deserves to be beaten If someone insults me, I will defend my reputation, with force if I have to (B)
Domestic life and child care	A man should have the final word about decisions in his home Giving the kids a bath and feeding the kids are the mother's responsibility A man is happily married only if his wife brings a big dowry (I) A married woman should not need to ask her husband for permission to visit her parents/family (I)

* (I) Indicates India-specific items; (B) Indicates Brazil-specific items.

Kenya, China, and other countries. In addition to these studies, the GEM Scale is being used by other researchers in such countries as Mexico, Senegal, Tanzania, and Thailand to study different populations of males and females.

It is important to note that scale development in the field, especially related to a construct called "masculine ideologies," is not new. Since the 1970s, various researchers (e.g., Pleck, Sonenstein, and Ku, 1993) have sought to measure masculine ideologies or culturally defined standards for male behavior. While this previous scale development informed the development of the GEM Scale, the existing scales did not sufficiently meet the demands of the current project, and developing a new measure was deemed important. For example, few if any of the existing scales were developed for program evaluation – that is, to measure potential changes in attitudes towards gender norms as a result of a programmatic intervention. Additionally, the authors were especially interested in norms related to specific topics, addressed in the intervention, and other scales often focused on other topics. Thirdly, masculine ideology scales for the most part measure how men define themselves as men, while the focus of the GEM Scale is to compare how men "should" be compared to women, or relational issues related to gender equity.

Operations Research Design and Methods

These quasi-experimental intervention studies in Rio de Janeiro, Brazil, and Mumbai, India, compared the impact of different combinations of program activities. One arm of the study focused only on group education, while the second arm included a combination of group education and the community-wide behavior-change communication campaign. In a third community, a delayed intervention (to ensure that all participants benefited from some intervention activities) followed a control period.

In Brazil, three groups of young men aged 14 to 25 years, with a mean age of 17 (at baseline, n = 780), were followed over time. The sample included both in-school and out-of-school youth. The study population was based in three different but fairly homogeneous low-income communities or *favelas*. Surveys were administered to a cohort in each site prior to any intervention activities (n = 258 in Bangu, n = 250 in Maré, and n = 272 in Morro dos Macacos), after the intervention had been ongoing for six months (n = 230 in Bangu, n = 212 in Maré, and n = 180 in Morro dos Macacos), and again after one year (n = 217 in Bangu and n = 190 in Maré). The response rate overall was 80 percent at six months and 80 percent at one year. In addition, qualitative interviews were conducted with a subsample of young men in ongoing primary relationships, as well as with their female partners (n = 18). The costs of implementing the different components of the program were also tracked, and are discussed in the report.

In India, in each of the three sites, surveys were administered before any intervention activity (n = 886) and after the intervention had been ongoing for six months (n = 537). The sample included married and unmarried young men aged 16 to 28 years from low-income communities (i.e., "slums") in urban Mumbai. In addition, in-depth interviews with participants, and in some cases their partners, were collected to aid in the interpretation of the attitudinal and behavioral survey data.

In this report, matched cohort data from young men who were interviewed both during baseline and follow up are presented. In addition to responses on the GEM Scale, participants also provided information on HIV-related risk and prevention factors, including STI symptoms, condom use, number of sexual partners, and intimate partner violence, as well as sociodemographic characteristics.

Key Evaluation Findings

At baseline, young men reported substantial HIV/STI risk, and violence. In Brazil, at baseline, more than 70 percent of the young men across the three intervention groups were sexually experienced, with sexual initiation taking place at an average age of 13. Among the sexually experienced group, almost one-third (30 percent) reported having more than one sexual partner over the last month. Condom use was largely inconsistent with casual partners, where 49 percent reported that they used condoms with every casual partner during the last month. About two-thirds (63 percent) of the young men reported condom use at last sex with a primary partner. About 25 percent of the young men reported having STI symptoms during the three months prior to the survey. About ten percent of the young men indicated that they had been physically or sexually violent against their current or most recent regular partner.

In India, reports of at least one STI symptom or other factor indicative of poor sexual health in the three months prior to the survey was substantial in all groups. More than one-third of young men reported they had been physically or sexually violent against a partner in the three months prior to the survey. Across the three urban sites, 44 percent of respondents were sexually experienced, with an average age of 18 years at sexual initiation. At least one-fourth of young men who reported having sex in the last three months had reported having sex with two or more partners. Condom use at last sex with all partner types in the last three months varied from one-fourth to a little less than half, depending on the study site.

At baseline, views towards gender norms varied, and many supported inequitable gender norms. For ease of interpretation, GEM Scale scores were trichotomized into "high equity," "moderate equity," and "low equity." The categories were determined based on the range of possible responses, and distributed equally into the three categories (e.g., the top third of possible scores were categorized as "high equity"). At baseline in Brazil, about half of the young men were categorized as "highly" equitable, and the other half were distributed across the "moderate" and "low" categories. In India, at baseline, less than 10 percent of the young men in all the sites were categorized as "highly equitable." The majority of young men were distributed across the "moderate" and "low" equity categories.

Agreement with inequitable gender norms was associated with more risk. Support for inequitable gender norms was significantly associated with HIV risk at baseline. In Brazil, agreement with inequitable gender norms in the GEM Scale was significantly associated with reported STI symptoms ($p < 0.05$), lack of contraceptive use ($p = 0.05$), and both physical and sexual violence against a partner ($p < 0.001$). In India, combined data from the three urban sites indicate that young men reporting more support for inequitable norms were significantly ($p < 0.05$) less likely to use condoms and more likely to report symptoms of poor sexual health.

More equitable views towards gender norms can be successfully promoted. In Brazil, a comparison of baseline and six month post-intervention results revealed that a significantly smaller proportion of respondents supported inequitable gender norms over time ($p < 0.05$), while a similar change was not found at the control site. Specifically, 10 out of 17 items improved in the combined intervention site (Bangu) and 13 out of 17 items improved in the group education only site (Maré), while one item improved in the control site (Morro dos Macacos). These positive changes were maintained at the one-year follow-up in both intervention sites.

Similarly, in India, there was a significant ($p < 0.05$) positive shift of young men moving from the "low equity" category into the "moderate equity" and "high equity" categories in the intervention sites. Changes in the control site were not significant. Specifically, 9 out of 15 items shifted in the combined intervention group, 7 out of 15 shifted in the group education only group, and 2 shifted in the control group.

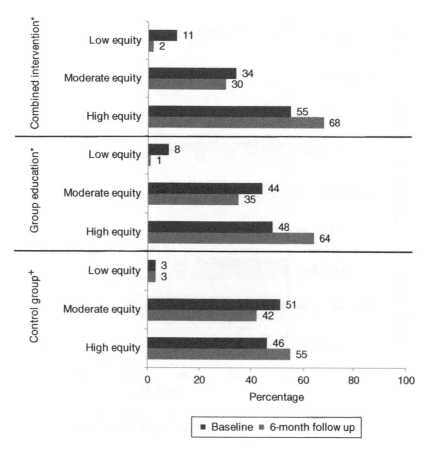

Figure 22.1 In Brazil, change in percentage toward greater support for gender equity in GEM Scale responses by evaluation arm. *p < 0.001; +no significant change.
Source: Adapted from Pulerwitz, Julie, Gary Barker, Márcio Segundo, and Marcos Nascimento, "Promoting more gender-equitable norms and behaviors among young men as an HIV/AIDS prevention strategy," Horizons Final Report, Washington, DC: Population Council (2006).

Logistic regression analysis at follow up found that a positive change in India in gender attitudes was correlated with exposure to the intervention. See Figures 22.1 and 22.2 below for a visual depiction of these shifts.

Significant improvements were found in HIV/STI and violence outcomes. Key HIV/STI-related outcomes improved. In Brazil, at both intervention sites, reported STI symptoms decreased, with the change in the combined intervention site being statistically significant (p < 0.05). In the control site, there was no significant decrease. Findings related to condom use were similar. In both sites, condom use at last sex with a primary partner increased, with a significant improvement seen in the combined site (p < 0.05) and no significant increase in the control site. Results at one-year follow-up indicate that the

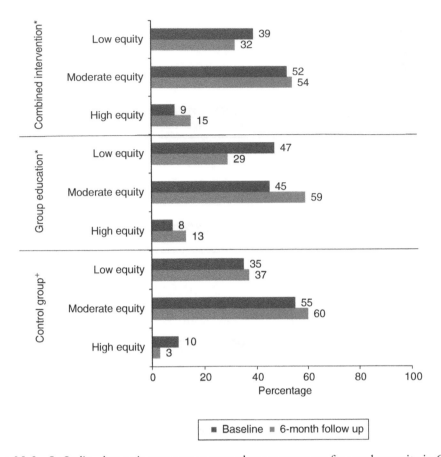

Figure 22.2   In India, change in percentage toward greater support for gender equity in GEM Scale responses by evaluation arm. *p < 0.05; +no significant change.
Source: Adapted from Verma, Ravi et al., "Promoting gender equity as a strategy to reduce HIV risk and gender-based violence among young men in India," Horizons Final Report, Washington, DC: Population Council (2008).

improvements in both condom use and reported STI symptoms were maintained. Qualitative data support this finding; for example, one young man indicated that he now was delaying sex with his girlfriend, saying:

> Used to be when I went out with a girl, if we didn't have sex within two weeks of going out, I would leave her. But now [after the workshops], I think differently. I want to construct something [a relationship] with her.

Another young man stated:

> Before [the workshops] I had sex with a girl…and then left her. If I saw her later, it was like I didn't even know her. If she got pregnant or something, I had nothing to do with it. But now, I think before I act or do something.

In all three Brazilian sites, reported condom use with casual partners and violence against a partner did not significantly change. At baseline, condom use with a casual partner was high, and reported violence low, so there was limited potential for movement.

Turning to India, among the young men who had sex in the last three months, reported condom use at last sex with all sexual partners increased significantly ($p < 0.05$) from baseline to follow up. In contrast, condom use stayed the same or decreased slightly in the control site. Logistic regression analysis at follow up showed that men in the intervention arms were 1.9 times more likely to have used condoms at last sex with all partners in Mumbai ($p < 0.001$) than those in the control arm. The proportion of men in the intervention sites who reported violence against a partner (both sexual and romantic but nonsexual) in the last three months declined significantly ($p < 0.05$) at endline. In contrast, reported partner violence increased significantly in the control group. Qualitative data suggest a positive change as well.

> As far as the sexual act is concerned, if my wife is uncomfortable I do not force her now, earlier I used to... Because of my participation in the YD program I have started respecting the feelings of my wife.

Another participant stated:

> After the session on gender and discussions with the peer leaders, I realized the importance of my wife. Slowly, slowly I started discussing with her, started helping with her work, and this has created more love and affection. I started respecting her and one day she asked me to keep away from my girlfriends... I have accepted it.

Communication between couples about HIV/AIDS remained relatively high or improved. In Brazil, survey responses indicate that a majority of participants communicated with their primary partners about key HIV/STI-related topics at baseline, and a similar pattern was found after the intervention period. In the qualitative interviews, some young men reported that they began to discuss new HIV-related topics with their partners, and their partners agreed that a change had taken place. For example, the female partner of one young man said:

> After the workshop ... He even talked about getting a blood test [HIV test] and he said: "You should get one too" and I said: "Okay, I'll do it, we'll do it together."

In India, in both intervention sites, the number of men discussing condoms, sex, STIs, and/or HIV with a partner increased almost one and a half times from baseline to follow up, while it decreased in the control site. Intervention participants spoke of the value of the information discussed during the program:

> After the program I can say that I got good information on gender roles and discrimination, sexual violence, sexuality, addiction, HIV/AIDS, etc. I have shared everything with my wife, which has resulted in us coming more close to each other.

Key Intervention Lessons

We also conducted "process" evaluations, to learn about successes and challenges of program implementation. Information from monitoring reports and attendance lists of the facilitators, interviews with the research and program staff, and statements from the young men themselves, and their female partners, are integrated below. Further, in Brazil, the team documented the costs of the intervention, and conducted a cost analysis.

Older or married youth difficult to engage
In general, it was more difficult to recruit and encourage attendance from older or married youth. In Brazil they were either working or searching for work, or they prioritized participation in professional training courses offered by other groups based in the community. In India, married men expressed the need to fulfill household responsibilities. However, those older and married youth that did attend often displayed more involvement and interest in the session topics, likely because they had more experience with intimate relationships.

Importance of male-only spaces to discuss these key topics
In both Brazil and India, young men and the facilitators said that it was quite important for these young men to participate in "male-only" groups, or safe spaces to openly address these potentially sensitive topics. In Brazil, the young men appreciated the opportunity "to be here among men and to be able to talk." The facilitators reported that, as the groups progressed, the participants became increasingly comfortable with contributing personal stories and opinions. In both India and Brazil, young men also reported that they appreciated the group sessions because they provided new information about sexuality or reproductive facts related to women that they hadn't understood previously. In India young men regularly reached out to the facilitators after sessions, to inquire about sexual and relationship concerns, and were then referred to counselors to discuss these issues.

Interest in reaching out to young women as well
While it was perceived to be important to have safe spaces for young men to discuss these issues amongst themselves, many young men (and their families) also expressed an interest in engaging young women in the discussions and program. This interest was found in both Brazil and India. In India, for example, there were regular queries from the family members of the boys and men about what this program was doing and soon there was a growing demand for a similar program for the girls and women.

Conflicts occurring during the sessions
Conflicts were periodically experienced during the sessions. In Brazil, the facilitators reported, many young men disputed over who spoke, interacted with each other using threats, and were generally disrespectful toward the facilitator. In such cases, it was important that facilitators felt trained and equipped to handle these conflicts and this

style of interaction, and that they consistently promoted a style of discussion that encouraged tolerance and respect toward one another. In both Brazil and India, there were periodic conflicts among the participants because of the themes they were discussing, such as homophobia. In such cases, the facilitators sought to use these moments of conflict, and the themes that provoked the conflict, to promote further discussions in subsequent sessions.

Cost analysis in Brazil

The goal of the costing analysis was to provide information on how expensive it was to reach a young man with the two different intervention components (i.e., a cost-per-output analysis). Providing information not only on the impact of interventions, but also on the cost of different types of interventions, can assist in decisions related to replication – and potentially the scaling-up – of these activities. As a special issue on cost-effectiveness analysis in the *Journal of Health Communication* highlighted, costing data contributes to "more rational decision making in the allocation of resources to communication programs" (Bertrand, 2006).

Several agencies and institutions provided funding for the two intervention components, including International Planned Parenthood Federation, Pan American Health Organization, US Agency for International Development, Summit Foundation, The MacArthur Foundation, The Moriah Fund, and SSL International, Inc. (the makers of Durex condoms). The Horizons Program paid for facilitator training costs, and "stipends" for participation to the young men.

Start-up and service delivery costs

The costs of the two project components were divided into two types: start-up and service delivery. Start-up costs largely encompassed training the facilitators for the group education sessions. Training costs included the value of the time of the trainers and trainees, as well as costs of travel to the training site and materials for the intervention. Project development costs (i.e., designing the interventions and materials), which are other potential start-up costs, are not included in the analysis. Many materials were already developed prior to this formal evaluation (e.g., the manual for group education), and the focus here is to cost the implementation of the activities. Further, adapting these materials to other settings – as was done in India – can be done without reincurring many of the costs.

The main cost of delivering the intervention was related to labor: i.e., the time spent by facilitators, program coordinators, and youth participating in condom distribution for the BCC campaign, and the stipend provided to the youth participants in the group education intervention. The value of the time spent by program coordinators was calculated based on their salary and benefits. Because most of the young men were unemployed, the value of the time they spent participating in program activities was estimated as the amount of the stipend (approximately seven dollars per month). Other costs included commodities such as posters (particularly printing the materials), transportation, and miscellaneous expenses (e.g., meetings costs). When potential costs were donated, such as meeting venues in the community for the group education sessions and condoms for the BCC campaign, they were not included in the costing analysis. An additional cost for the BCC campaign was the "launching" event in the community, for publicity purposes.

Results of cost study

The total costs of the two interventions (Bangu – combining group education and BCC campaign, and Maré – group education alone) were USD$35,856.87 and USD$21,060.28, respectively (USD$1 = R$2.93). The cost-per-output of the intervention, or the cost per youth reached, was USD$138.98 for Bangu and USD$84.24 for Maré. An additional analysis was done to determine the cost per participant, per hour of group education. There were approximately 28 hours of group education over six months, so the cost per participant per hour in Bangu was USD$4.96, and in Maré was USD$3.01.

If this intervention were to be adapted by other organizations, as was done in India, or scaled up, as Promundo was doing in the public education system in two states in Brazil, many of the costs would be removed. For example, facilitator training for the group education intervention included "experts" from other cities and countries, which added transportation and per diem costs. However, some costs would be added. For example, while condoms were donated by SSL International in Brazil, and were therefore not a significant expense, future applications of the intervention sometimes needed to take into account local costs for condoms.

Conclusion, Implications, and Recommendations

The findings indicate that the behavior-change communication strategies used in Brazil and India, which concentrated on promoting gender-equitable norms, successfully influenced young men's attitudes toward gender norms, reduced HIV/STI risk and violence, and led to healthier relationships. In both Brazil and India, disagreement with inequitable gender norms significantly increased for both intervention groups at endline, and a corresponding change was not seen in the group that was not exposed to any intervention, supporting the contention that the intervention had an impact on these views. In Brazil, we also conducted a follow-up study six months after the end of the activities, and these changes were maintained, indicating that they can be sustained over some time.

The positive changes in attitudes towards gender norms were equally great for young men exposed to the combination of interpersonal group education and the community-based behavior-change communication activities, and the group participating in group education activities alone. This finding underscores that the group education was key to address the gender-related attitudes, and an interactive and interpersonal process may be needed to influence often deep-seated and complex gender-related norms. As described above, this work applied a social constructionist or interactive theory of gender socialization. Findings from the evaluation suggest that this intervention can assist individuals to reinterpret and "reconstruct" the norms to be more gender equitable, and potentially, as members of society, also influence the broader shared norms.

Important HIV/STI and violence-related outcomes such as reported condom use, STI symptoms, and violence against a partner also improved for young men in the intervention groups, while the positive change was not found in the control groups that did not receive the interventions. In Brazil, the change was often greater for young men exposed to the combined intervention. In India, these changes were reported among both intervention groups. However, some young men in India also expressed concern during the qualitative interviews about their ability to maintain the changes without the support of a larger group. This highlights the importance of including both interpersonal and wider (e.g., community-based) strategies. The "ecological framework," which recommends including intervention activities at multiple levels that influence the audience in question, is helpful in this regard. Both small-group sessions (with their intensive impact on limited numbers of individuals) and broader communications strategies, such as widespread distribution of IEC materials (with their less intensive but broader reach) have a place in future efforts.

Qualitative evidence from both young men and their female partners indicates that many relationships, and sexual and reproductive health behavior within the relationships, have been substantially positively affected by the intervention. For example, some men in both Brazil and India reported having a new willingness to wait to engage in sexual activity with partners, to reduce sexual coercion of their partners, and to openly communicate with their partners about sexual risk reduction. They also reported paying more attention to other aspects of the relationship outside of the sexual component, such as, for example, assisting wives with household chores in India, and they showed more interest in the opinions of their girlfriends and wives in general.

The intervention activities were considered culturally appropriate for both urban settings in India and Brazil, based on qualitative findings. Other important lessons related to the process of implementing this type of intervention emerged as well. It was found to be more difficult to recruit and retain older or married youth, due to competing responsibilities. Young men greatly appreciated the "men-only" space as a place to openly address a number of sensitive issues, and at the same time, they expressed an interest in including young women in these discussions. Finally, there was sometimes conflict, even physical conflict, between participants, which meant that facilitators had to be trained and prepared to resolve a given conflict.

Directly measuring attitudes towards "gender-equitable" norms provides useful information about the prevailing norms in the community as well as the effectiveness of any program that hopes to influence or promote a modification of those norms. The study team developed and tested the GEM Scale with a representative sample of men in three communities in Rio de Janeiro. The resulting scale appeared to capture gender dynamics well, and be sensitive to locally relevant issues. In the subsequent intervention study with young men in Brazil, the 17 items of the inegalitarian subscale of the full GEM Scale were used as the gender norms measure. In India, after formative research to adapt the scale for this very different cultural context, a 15 item version of the scale was used. The GEM Scale has since been adapted and used with varied populations across multiple countries.

The cost analysis in Brazil provides additional information for those who may be interested in replicating this type of intervention. The cost per youth reached was USD$138.98 for Bangu and USD$84.24 for Maré, and the cost per hour of group education was USD$4.96 for Bangu and USD$3.01 for Maré. However, this analysis focused on the costs of reaching the young men who participated in the group education in both arms of the study (approximately 500). It does not take into account the many other young men and community members that were reached by the community-based BCC campaign, which included billboards, posters, and other materials.

There are limitations to the study that should be highlighted. The participants in both intervention groups were followed for six months in India, and up to one year in Brazil, so it is not clear if the positive changes were maintained longer-term. To maximize the chances of long-term sustainability of these positive outcomes, there is a need to further facilitate a supportive environment for these changes. It will be important to build alliances for large-scale and ongoing discourse on men and masculinities, and to include women in this dialogue as well. In fact, programs for young women were developed in both Brazil and India, and are currently being evaluated. Also, while various sources of data were triangulated within these evaluations (e.g., from participants, female partners, program facilitators), all data were self-reported. Future studies that include other measures, such as biological measures of STIs, would strengthen the findings. However, the nonsignificant change found among the control groups does support the validity of the findings.

Study findings demonstrate that confronting inequitable gender norms is an important element of HIV prevention strategies. Specifically, the findings provide empirical evidence that a behavior-change intervention focused on combating inequitable gender norms was associated with improvements in HIV/STI risk outcomes. The positive results suggest that it is in fact possible to question these inequitable views about manhood and in turn to change the attitudes and behaviors of young men in ways that are good for the health of themselves and their partners.

References

Amaro, H. (1995). Love, sex, and power: Considering women's realities in HIV prevention. *American Psychologist* 50(6): 437–447.

Bertrand, J.T. (2006). Introduction to the special issue on cost-effectiveness analysis. *Journal of Health Communication, 11*, 3–6.

Campbell, C.A. (1995). Male gender roles and sexuality: Implications for women's AIDS risk and prevention. *Social Science & Medicine 41*(2), 197–210.

Childhope (1997). Gender, sexuality and attitudes related to AIDS among low income youth and street youth in Rio de Janeiro, Brazil. *Childhope Working Paper No. 6*. New York.

Connell, R. W. (1987). *Gender and Power*. Berkeley, CA: University of California Press.

Connell, R. W. (1995). *Masculinities*. Berkeley, CA: University of California Press.

Garcia-Moreno, C., Jansen, H., Ellsberg, M. *et al.* (2006). Prevalence of intimate partner violence: Findings from the WHO multi-country study on women's health and domestic violence. *Lancet. 368*, 1260–1269.

Greene, M. E., Mehta, M., Pulerwitz, J. *et al.* (2004). Involving Men in Reproductive Health. Background paper to the report *Public Choices, Private Decisions: Sexual and Reproductive Health and the Millennium Development Goals*. New York. Retrieved from http://www. unmillenniumproject.org/documents/Greene_et_al-final.pdf

Instituto Promundo and Instituto Noos (2003). *Men, Gender-based Violence and Sexual and Reproductive Health: A Study with Men in Rio de Janeiro, Brazil*. Rio de Janeiro: Instituto Promundo and Instituto Noos.

IIPS (International Institute for Population Sciences) and Macro International (2007). *National Family Health Surveys (NFHS-3), 2005–6: Volume 1.* Mumbai.

Kaufman, M. (1993). *Cracking the Armour: Power, Pain and the Lives of Men.* Toronto: Viking.

Marsiglio, W. (1988). Adolescent male sexuality and heterosexual masculinity: A conceptual model and review. *Journal of Adolescent Research 3*(3–4), 285–303.

Pleck, J. H., Sonenstein, F., and Ku, L. (1993). Masculinity ideology: Its impact on adolescent males' heterosexual relationships. *Journal of Social Issues 49*(3), 11–29.

Population Council (2001). The unfinished transition: Gender equity: Sharing the responsibilities of parenthood. *Population Council Issues Paper.* New York: Population Coucil.

Pulerwitz, J., Amaro, H., DeJong, W. *et al.* (2002). Relationship power, condom use, and HIV risk among women in the US. *AIDS Care 14*(6), 789–800.

Pulerwitz, J., and Barker, G. (2008). Measuring attitudes toward gender norms among young men in Brazil: Development and psychometric evaluation of the GEM Scale. *Men and Masculinities 10,* 322–338.

Pulerwitz, J., Barker, G., Segundo, M., and Nascimento, M. (2006). *Promoting More Gender-Equitable Norms and Behaviors among Young Men as an HIV/AIDS Prevention Strategy: Horizons Final Report.* Retrieved from http://www.popcouncil.org/pdfs/horizons/brgendernorms.pdf

Pulerwitz, J., Michaelis, A., Verma, R., and Weiss, E. (2010). Addressing gender dynamics and engaging men in HIV programs: Lessons learned from Horizons research. *Public Health Reports 125,* 282–292.

Rivers, K., and Aggleton, P. (1998). *Men and the HIV Epidemic, Gender and the HIV Epidemic.* New York. Retrieved from http://content.undp.org/go/cms-service/download/asset/?asset_id=1703492

Verma, R., Mahendra, V.S., Pulerwitz, J. *et al.* (2005). From research to action: Addressing masculinity and gender norms to reduce HIV/AIDS related risky sexual behaviour among young men in India. *Indian Journal of Social Work 65*(4), 634–654.

Verma, R., Pulerwitz, J. Mahendra, V. S. *et al.* (2006). Challenging and changing gender attitudes among young men in Mumbai, India. *Reproductive Health Matters 14*(28), 1–10.

Verma R., Pulerwitz, J., Mahendra, V. S. *et al.* (2008). *Promoting Gender Equity as a Strategy to Reduce HIV Risk and Gender-Based Violence among Young Men in India. Horizons Final Report.* Washington. Retrieved from http://www.popcouncil.org/pdfs/horizons/India_GenderNorms.pdf

White, V., Greene, M., and Murphy, E. (2003). *Men and Reproductive Health Programs: Influencing Gender Norms.* The Synergy Project, Washington, DC. Retrieved from http://pdf.usaid.gov/pdf_docs/PNACU969.pdf

WHO (World Health Organisation) (2007). *Engaging Men and Boys in Changing Gender-Based Inequity in Health: Evidence from Programme Interventions.* Geneva: WHO.

Worth, D. (1989). Sexual decision-making and AIDS: Why condom promotion among vulnerable women is likely to fail. *Studies in Family Planning 20,* 297–307.

23

Women's Health and Healing in the Peruvian Amazon
Minga Perú's Participatory Communication Approach

Ami Sengupta and Eliana Elias

The rain had just stopped, leaving the community looking freshly washed. The foliage is a bright shiny green. The sun is out and a gentle wind blows. We sit outside talking to a group of women, all of whom are regular listeners of the radio program, *Bienvenida Salud* (Welcome to Health). The group comprises women of various age groups including a mother and her teenage daughter and a mother-in-law and her daughter-in-law, who is in her twenties. One of the women, Lucinda, is a 47-year-old from Gallito, she has been working as a health worker in her community for the past 30 years and is an avid listener of Minga Perú's radio program, *Bienvenida Salud*. She tells us with pride that she has been listening to the program since it was first aired in 1998. She thinks the program is helpful, as it teaches young couples to plan their families and provides useful information to pregnant women, thus promoting the health and nourishment of unborn children. Lucinda tells us that girls as young as 14 and 15 years of age are getting pregnant and they find the radio program particularly useful amidst all the frustration and despair that adolescents encounter in the Amazon. Our conversation with her reveals how health and human rights are inextricably connected in the worldview of Amazonian communities and how Minga Perú's entertainment-education-based radio program *Bienvenida Salud* reaches out to the needs, local realities, and belief-systems of these communities. Quoting Lucinda:

> About health I can say it is about having a good relationship in the family, like I have with my husband. It is about having a good understanding with people in the household – your husband, the children, and with your neighbors – with all the people in your community. Being united and together is health. Good relationships with the people you work with and your community is health. We listen to the program and it teaches us how to live better with your partner and teaches young people how to behave with their friends. Before there was so much fighting within the family and now we are learning that it is not good. We see

The Handbook of Global Health Communication, First Edition. Edited by Rafael Obregon and Silvio Waisbord.

among the adolescents that there are many problems in their daily lives. The program is very helpful for them. ... The Program also teaches us about our rights. If there is something we want to do, we have our rights just as men do. In the community we, the mothers, have the same rights as the men, we have a role to play in the community and [in local] organizations. It is very good for the community that we are able to practice our rights. Rights are very important, it means that as a woman I have the same rights as a man in my community and in different organizations within the community. I now know that I have the same rights as a man, and I have the right to live peacefully with my husband in my house. We listen [to the program] and absorb what we hear and put it into practice. It is very important because it teaches us, because without it people suffer from many ills.

In this chapter we present a case study of Minga Perú and its efforts to promote women's rights, health, and well-being in the Peruvian Amazon. We build on the Amazonian notion of health which is not just the absence of illness but a more inclusive understanding that encompasses overall well-being, marked by good relationships, self-esteem and a life free of negative or damaging forces, referred to as *cutipa*. Within the Amazonian worldview disease, domestic violence, discrimination, and disharmony are all forms of *cutipa* that damage the body and soul. By sharing and learning from participants' stories we highlight how Minga's efforts have improved women's "well-being" at three levels, (1) at an individual level by improving women's self-confidence; (2) at a spousal level by helping women ascertain their reproductive rights; and (3) at a family level by improving relationships and enabling women to live with reduced incidents of domestic violence and abuse.

This chapter describes the important elements of Minga Perú's efforts to facilitate sustainable and meaningful change in the Amazon. We provide a detailed description of the organization to provide a context and understanding of their vision, approach, and activities. We attempt to capture key processes employed by Minga in promoting health and human rights in the Amazon. In so doing we document how social issues such as health and gender equity can be communicated more effectively to communities and how communities can both envision and create healthier futures, by being active participants in the communication process.

Our Theoretical Standpoints

We found literature on participatory development as well as postcolonial feminist theorizing to be particularly enlightening as we tried to understand Minga's work, both its vision and its practices and the participants' response to the program. The participatory paradigm in development recognizes people as human beings and not as objects to be developed, treated, or cured and calls for a people-centered bottom-up approach as opposed to the previously prevalent top-down approaches. The participatory approach, also referred to as the alternative framework, moves away from blueprints to development work and encourages a localized and context-specific approach (Chambers, 1997; Gumucio-Dagron, 2001). This approach calls for an "endogenous" development, which stems from recognizing societal values and community's perception of their needs (Fraser and Restrapo-Estrada, 1998). The focus of development thus shifts from economic advancement to social change, focusing on bettering peoples' quality of life and overall well-being (Rist, 1997). This framework recognizes the value of going beyond economic and basic need indicators to include other aspects of human development, respectful of people and their lived realities.

The shifts in development theorizing were also reflected in communication for development theory–praxis, as scholars put forth the importance of "context evaluation," which encouraged the understanding of lifestyles and community needs (Wilkins and Mody, 2001). Communication for development scholars stressed that "understanding the context of implementation is critical if we are to gain a better understanding of community-responsive communication interventions" (Wilkins and Mody, 2001, p. 391). In similar vein, Sypher, McKinley, Ventsam, and Elías (2002) aptly state that "locally situated knowledge is an imperative for designing culturally sensitive, participatory campaigns; it provides the framework for understanding why and how a social system changes because of media interventions" (p. 193). This shift was concurrent with the shifts in international development that began, increasingly, to embrace multiple local voices and community participation, and were accompanied by the emergence of grassroots and community-based organizations. Such a framework leads us to privilege people's sociocultural realities and worldviews.

In line with the alternative approach, postcolonial feminist theorizing sensitizes scholar-practitioners to become "multicentered ... simultaneously self-critical of their own power/knowledge starting points, historically and contextually grounded, and yet unapologetically integrative" (Ferguson, 2000, p. 197). Ferguson calls for "situated ethics" (p. 198) over universal, North-centered ethics. Ferguson's suggestion to reorient and initiate development practice from the South, starting with the community's needs and participation, is timely and useful in (re-)envisioning feminist development practice and bears much in common with similar calls for "endogenous" development practices within communication for development (Singhal and Sthapitanonda, 1996).

Both feminist and development theory–praxis remain in the hands of "experts" most of whom belong to, or are trained in, the West. Similarly, the notion of what counts as knowledge continues to follow Western, scientific, and rational ideals, undervaluing indigenous knowledge (Chambers, 1997). For feminist theorizing to be truly (de)centered, the site of knowledge production necessitates a shift from ivory towers and academics to include the lived experiences and local knowledge systems of grassroots women (Harding, 2000).

Harding (2000) further elucidates the value and need for incorporating "local knowledge systems" within the development discourse. We seek to include indigenous health belief-systems into this discourse. She highlights how the Enlightenment paradigm that values scientific and universally valid knowledge claims, has shaped, and in turn limited, the efficacy of development practices. A development model that focuses solely on economic growth has several flaws, such as the devaluing and obscuring of other needs and interests. Following Harding's lead, we question the limitations of understanding health as only biomedical, viewed through a lens based on Western medicine, and attempt to include local understandings and conceptions of health into the health communication discourse. The Amazonian conception of health includes physical, emotional, and spiritual well-being, as elaborated in the research findings. Our findings reaffirm how such a broad understanding of health promotes a more holistic and grounded vision of health.

In the next section we elaborate upon Minga Perú's work and briefly describe the data collection process prior to detailing the key findings.

Description of the Project

Established in 1998, Minga Perú is a nonprofit community-based, communication for social change organization that addresses issues of social justice, human rights, reproductive health and gender equity (Minga Perú, n.d). The organization was cofounded by Ashoka Fellow[1] and social communicator Eliana Elías and Luis González, who had extensive experience in community development work in the Peruvian Amazon. Minga aims to provide culturally and regionally appropriate communication and training to community members to enable them to realize their basic human rights and attain a higher quality of life (Digital Pulse, 2003; Inter-American Development Bank, 2004).

Minga works to achieve women's rights and social justice in the Amazon. Minga recognizes health as an important aspect of women's rights and construes health broadly to include, but not be limited to, reproductive rights. It addresses women's health in particular, but situated and integrated within the larger realm of community health. Minga entered the arena of women's health by looking at reproductive health as a fundamental human right. Reproductive health was viewed as something that went beyond birth control and planning families and took into account women's concerns and sensitivities about reproductive health. The health training included learning about and respecting women's bodies, understanding how internal organs work, and building upon their existing and traditional knowledge base. Minga works primarily with women, but extends its work to include their families, thus it also looks into health issues concerning women's spouses and children. Minga has over the past few years begun to include a specific component on HIV/AIDS and domestic violence, both in its training courses for women and in the school curriculum in selected rural schools to target adolescents.

Minga's work is carried out in the Loreto province in the Peruvian Amazon. The population of Loreto province is spread over 146,000 square miles and there are about one million inhabitants, almost half of whom live in the communities. The region comprises rainforests and riverine areas traversed by the River Amazon and its tributaries which serve as the region's primary mode of transportation (Farrington, 2003; Minga Perú, n.d.). The inhabitants of this region are mostly peasants of mixed ethnic descent, referred to as *ribereños* or river people (Santos-Granero and Barclay, 2000). This area is ravaged by unemployment, malnourishment, low food security, and poor health exacerbated by very limited access to health facilities (Minga Perú, n.d.). Barring the main towns, the region has very limited access to power supply or telephone connections.

Though the Loreto province comprises almost a third of Peru's total area, the population accounts for less than five percent of the country's total population. Iquitos is the main city in the area and is home to almost half the population of Loreto. Over 500 communities spanning over 65 linguistic groups and representing over 13 main ethnic groups reside in the Loreto province (Farrington, 2003). Given the vastness of the area and its scattered settlements, radio serves as an effective means of communication between the riverine communities (McKinley and Jensen, 2003).

According to the United Nations Development Program (UNDP), Peru is categorized as a "medium developed nation," distinguishing its level of human development from either highly developed or least developed nations. Life expectancy at birth is almost 73 years, the literacy rate is almost 90 percent and the per capita GDP is US$7, 836 (UNDP, 2009).[2] However, the indicators for Loreto are well below national figures in all respects. The health indicators in Loreto reflect higher infant mortality and fertility rates than in urban areas of Peru. Life expectancy in Loreto is lower than the national averages (Sypher *et al.*, 2002). Regional reproductive health figures suggest that an indigenous woman in Loreto is likely to become sexually active by age 12, and bear 10 children in her lifetime (four times the national fertility rate of 2.5) and have a life expectancy below 50 years, which is 23 years less than the national average. In addition these women are very likely to lose at least one child and suffer from sexually transmitted infections and domestic violence (Farrington, 2003; UNICEF, 2009). Women begin having children early, and among the females between the ages of 15 and 19, 24 percent have had at least one child and 40 percent have had more than one child (Minga, n.d.).

In the early 1990s, when the second author, Elías, began working as a social communicator in the Amazon on a health, sanitation, and cholera prevention project, she realized the dearth of messages that were culturally appropriate and understandable to local communities. Realizing that most health material was produced by officials in Lima and used language and terminology inaccessible to indigenous communities, Elías recognized that in order to achieve the desired impact it was imperative that health messages were communicated in a manner that was appropriate to the intended audience (Farrington, 2003; personal communication, July 4, 2005).

Minga works primarily with the *Cocama* indigenous group living in the riverine communities in the El Tigré and Marañon basin. However, the radio program *Bienvenida Salud* includes a diverse audience spanning the *Bora, Witoto, Quichua, Urarina, Shawi, Iquito, Ticuna, Achuar, Aguahun,* and *Wambi* indigenous groups (E. Neira, personal communication, April 17, 2007). Minga recognizes health as an important aspect of women's rights and construes health broadly to include, but not be limited to, reproductive rights. Minga's primary purpose is to promote a healthy lifestyle by enabling local communities to be well informed through access to health materials and information that they can understand. All of Minga's health information including its radio program, videos, and training manuals are in local languages and use terms that are easily understood by local communities. Elías noticed that, in many cases, the Ministry of Health handed out materials full of technical jargon that were culturally inappropriate and could not be understood by anyone. For Minga Perú, producing culturally appropriate material goes beyond using local vocabulary and the right accent; it necessitates that the people you are trying to reach participate in forming the messages and that their sensitivities, values, attitudes, and emotions are integrated into them.

The core of Minga's initiatives is the radio program *Bienvenida Salud* (Welcome to Health) with over 120,000 listeners across Loreto, Ucayali, and Huánuco provinces. *Bienvenida Salud* is aired three times a week on Mondays, Wednesday, and Fridays, each episode lasting 30 minutes. The program is aired at 5.30 in the morning and repeated at 6 in the evening. The timing fits in well with the Amazonian routine where the days begin at the crack of dawn and end by early evening. Close to 1,300 episodes have been aired thus far. *Bienvenida Salud* has enabled a "mediated space in which population planning and gender-based development discourse can be contested, reworked, and negotiated" (McKinley and Jensen, 2003, p. 182). Women's concerns such as domestic violence and reproductive health, which were typically construed as private concerns, entered the public domain through *Bienvenida Salud* (McKinley and Jensen). The content of the radio program is collaboratively constructed by the audience and portrays local realities in local language and familiar accents. Radio listening and ownership in this area tend to be communal, thus the radio program encourages community listening, which is accompanied by group discussion and visits to neighbors and friends. The program is aired on the regional radio station *La voz de la Selva,* which has extensive reach in the Loreto province, as well as nine other local stations for areas where the regional station does not have reach. In over 10 communities, listeners have, with the support of Minga, set up loud speakers in central areas of the community to publicly broadcast the radio program (Dura, Singhal, and Elias, 2008).

The term "minga" refers to collaborative community work in the local dialect, Quechua. One of the ways in which Minga privileges collaboration is through valuing local knowledge and collective knowledge building. For instance, the story lines of the radio program are based on letters written by the community members to the producers. These letters help weave peoples' concerns and needs into *Bienvenida Salud's* storyline and consequently into Minga's programming. Minga pays boat companies for the delivery of these letters, which arrive by the dozen every week and average around 150 letters a month, with as many as 500 letters in some months.

According to Elías "asking for letters is not only a strategy to measure audience effects, it is a way to prepare the scripts of the program and a way to change the passive consumers of the program into active producers" (Singhal and Rogers, 2004, p. 17). As of July 2005, when this fieldwork was conducted, some 6,000 letters had been received, crossing the 14,000 mark by mid 2010. Similarly, health messages are designed incorporating ideas from local community members such as opinion leaders, traditional healers (shamans), and health workers (Farrington, 2003).

In addition, Minga has a network of 53 *promotoras* (peer facilitators) from around 35 riverine communities who provide outreach and leadership on health issues to community members. *Promotoras* provide ground-based support, reinforcing radio messages and training the community on issues they have learned at Minga workshops. They engage in peer education and training and are motivated women and girls from the communities, who have displayed commitment and leadership skills and are nominated by the community themselves. Each *promotora* works closely with about eight to twenty women from their community who are part of Minga's women's network. Presently, this network has more than 400 active women participants in the Peruvian Amazon. These women and others work with Minga to develop scripts and training materials. Minga's other activities include mobilizing around 40 youth correspondents who work with the adolescents and regularly write letters to Minga, serving as a link between the adolescents in the communities and Minga (Digital Pulse, 2003; L. González, personal communication, July 27, 2005; McKinley and Jensen, 2003; Sypher *et al.*, 2002).

The *promotoras comunitaria* are nominated by the community themselves. The listeners were asked to nominate women whom they consider to be leaders within the community, whom they thought capable of acting on behalf of the community, and whom they "considered a good neighbor with congenial relationships with the rest of the community." Minga representatives first discussed their idea with the local community leaders and, after explaining the proposed plan and gaining their consent and support, a community meeting was called where women were nominated and later elected as *promotoras*. Keeping local realities in mind and realizing the difficulty the women may face in leaving their families and communities to attend workshops and training sessions, two women were elected from each community, so that, if for some family- or health-related reason, one was unable to attend, at least the other could take her place. Further, the Amazonian people tend to move frequently and training two women served as a backup in case a family moved to another community.

As the title suggests, *promotoras* foster community well-being by promoting women's rights, reconciliation, and harmony. Luis González explained that "it was important to include the word community in their title as it conveyed both a sense of community and the organization's commitment to the community." *Promotoras* are "social entrepreneurs at the community level and they distinguish themselves by their sense of solidarity with and commitment for (*compromiso*) the women in their community and most importantly their eagerness to share what they learn [with the community]," emphasized Luis. He further explained that these women "do not have solutions for everything or everybody's problems but they are convinced about the power of sharing their personal knowledge with others and are determined to stand up with other women in their joint struggle against unjust practices of the establishment."

Minga's Regional Office in Iquitos serves as the center of their operations, the radio program is produced in-house, and all the outreach activities are managed from there. The entire team in Iquitos hail from communities in the Loreto province. The Lima office is a significantly smaller operation. At the Tambo training center, located near the town of Nauta about two hours by boat from Iquitos city, Minga conducts orientation and training programs for women on human rights, health, income-generation schemes such as handicrafts, carpentry, fish and poultry farming, and natural resource management. Special sessions are held for men too. Minga has also trained their *promotoras* to make handicrafts using local art forms and materials and are currently looking for markets to sell the products (personal conversations, Minga Team, July 2005).

Data Collection and Analysis

The present chapter draws upon a larger study and data set (see Sengupta, 2007). The findings are based on six weeks of fieldwork in Peru, where the first author (Sengupta) divided her time between Lima, Iquitos, and two riverine communities – Gallito (on the River Amazon) and Santa Cruz (on the River Marañon). The research drew upon a range of ethnographic methods including interviews, focus group discussions, participant observation, and qualitative content analysis of audience letters, involving a total of 124 participants (88 female and 36 male) and 160 hours of observation. Additionally, two participatory tools – sketching and skits – were included to add to the richness of data. We employ methodological triangulation to gain a holistic understanding of the multiple and complex processes that play out in social change efforts (Morgan, 1998; Papa, Auwal, and Singhal, 1995).

The interviews and the participatory research were conducted in Spanish and simultaneously translated into English by a bilingual translator. Both versions were audio-taped and the English version was transcribed. The data collection resulted in a total of 29 60-minute tapes and 359 pages of transcripts. The interviews could not be taped digitally as not all the research sites had electricity.

Data analysis consisted of manually coding and categorizing the transcripts of interviews, FGDs, and skits. After several readings of the transcripts the emergent themes were coded. We used a clustering technique whereby overarching and subthemes were grouped (Huberman and Miles, 1998). Research field notes were also referred to during the analysis. Analysis revealed that health and healing were manifested at three distinct levels, (1) at an individual level by improving women's self-esteem; (2) at a spousal level by helping women ascertain their reproductive rights; and (3) at a family level by improving relationships and enabling women to live with reduced incidents of domestic violence and abuse. In the proceeding section we elaborate upon these three themes as we share the narratives of the listener–producers of *Bienvenida Salud*.

Research Findings

The Amazonian conception of health

Being healthy is to be good. When I am healthy, I am without illness, without problems and nothing bad is going on. Sometimes when we are in poor health, we are sick or we have problems. Now I feel happy and healthy. Everything is good. I feel happy with my husband, my children, and my parents. (Mellita Chota Kachique, 46-year-old woman from Gallito Community)

Within the Amazonian worldview, health is construed very broadly and encompasses physical as well as emotional, relational, and spiritual well-being. Culturally, Amazonians consider all objects in the world, both animate and inanimate, as living beings, hence all elements of nature whether rivers, stones, plants, or animals have a soul and thus can be harmed or damaged by negative forces, referred to as *cutipa*. Within this worldview, all forms of disease, domestic violence, discrimination, and disharmony are different manifestations of *cutipa* that damage the body and soul. However, in the dynamic worldview of the Amazonians, this condition of ill-being can be reversed by positive forces that serve to protect from and cure disease and damage, referred to as *icara*.

Health is also construed as a relational construct and includes good relationships within the home and harmonious coexistence within communities. For instance, a community member from Gallito, Reynaldo Fasabi, emphasized: "The most important thing for our community is health. Health is when you have good health inside your house and outside in your community." Thus health was construed more broadly than as a physical state; being healthy entailed having good feelings, being motivated and inspired, having a positive attitude, and nurturing relationships with people.

Minga is cognizant of the local worldview and its understanding of health and frames health messages in a manner that respects the cultural ethos and belief-system. The radio program *Bienvenida Salud* means "Welcome to Health," but construes health broadly (beyond physical maladies) to include overall well-being. Our participants too understood health as beginning with individuals but extending beyond – to the family and community. As a community member from Gallito aptly explained to us: "health has various parts" and though "having a strong healthy body to walk and work," was an important aspect of health, the radio program had helped reinforce the notion that "there was more to being healthy."

Working towards healing or *icararse* is important in restoring balance and harmony to the universe and Amazonians give due attention to caring for the body to protect it from negative forces (ill-health as it is broadly construed) and restoring harmony, health, and overall well-being when the body or soul is *cutipado* (damaged or sick). In keeping with this cultural understanding of health, we seek to illustrate how the work of Minga Perú enables health and healing in three distinct ways.

Gaining self-confidence

> I was very shy and felt ashamed all the time. I was afraid to stand up and talk in front of people. I used to hide from the others. María [the regional coordinator and trainer] kept urging me to go in front and speak, I used to be so scared I felt the blood was draining out of my body. But that was in the past when I used to come for workshops, now I have the courage to speak in front of people. (Lourdes, a 36 year old *Promotora* from San Jose de Sarapanga)

The *promotoras* felt that overcoming shyness and the deep-rooted feeling of fear and shame that they associated with being indigenous and poor women was not easy. Emira, who was only fourteen years old when she became a *promotora*, shared that "It was not easy to participate and to talk with all the *Señoritas*. I was very afraid because I thought people would make fun of me and say that I was not talking well." Emira's father, like several men in the communities, didn't think she was capable of learning or teaching anything as she was "just a woman." However, Emira continued to attend training sessions as she gained encouragement and confidence. She recounted: "Slowly I grew up. After two years of receiving training as a *promotora* I told my father that I wanted to study [further]. I told him that if I did not study I would be nothing and would have no hope for the future." Emira joined a school and rowed her balsa boat two hours each way on a daily basis in her quest to seek education. Many women in the Amazon have gained a "voice" through their association with Minga's program. Marcelita a *promotora* from San Francisco community poignantly explained the changes these women had undergone:

> As we say, the air doesn't cost anything. We live because the air is free. Now we know so much more, we value ourselves as women and are so grateful to Minga. We have high self-esteem, we can talk with other people, we have opinions and we can talk at community

meetings. Before, we were not brave enough to talk or have any opinions, we stayed in our homes, thinking that we were just useful for serving other people and to make food and nothing else.

Promotoras agreed that, earlier on, they thought that only men "had a voice and a right to say things" but now they knew better. When asked to share how they had changed as individuals through their association with Minga, all their narratives traced a pattern of personal growth from their previous state of fear and shyness. Each one of them said they had lost their shame or fear using the word *vergüenza* (shame). In another conversation Lourdes, who is quoted above, stated: "because of María I have lost my shyness. Now I can talk with people, I am not afraid or scared of people. I have changed a lot and I continue to change every moment." Yet another *promotora* Leydis shared: "before I was shy and ashamed to participate in any event. I was afraid to talk, but after coming to the workshops I have changed. I have stopped being ashamed and now freely give my opinion." Enthused to share the story upon hearing her colleagues express themselves, Elsita stated:

> I have learned about self-esteem and I love myself as a person. I feel good about myself. I am so proud to know all the new things that I never thought I would learn. I am not shy, not ashamed, not afraid and I can travel alone.

Making reproductive choices

Consider this letter from a listener of *Bienvenida Salud*:

> December 17, 2000
> Minga Peru Nauta 446
> Miss Everli Egoavil Vasquez
> Program Bienvenida Salud
>
> I want to tell you that I have had malaria three times and that I have finally taken care of it at the health center in Morona Cocha.
>
> I also want to tell you that I have 4 children and I have decided along with my husband that I do not want to have any more children. I am taking care of myself with a family planning method from the nearest health center.
>
> Also, I have a group of citrus trees that are already producing fruit but all of the fruit is bad, it is black and falls to the ground. What can I do so that the fruit doesn't keep falling like this?
>
> Sincerely
>
> Mercedes Tuanama Lachuma
> Village of Nuevo Miraflores
> Itaya River

Women considered making informed reproductive choices as an important aspect of controlling and looking after their health and well-being. As the letter above suggests, illness could be something like malaria that affects the body physically, or it could be something affecting plants such as the condition afflicting the fruit trees. Similarly, better health or well-being could be brought about by preventing unwanted pregnancies. This view was reinforced by Ofelia, a listener from Gallito community, who shared with us that her grandmother had 19 children, while her mother had nine, and she had three "one is 11 years old and the other is 3, my third child died and I don't want any more," asserted Ofelia. Her friend Lucinda commended the radio program "for providing important information to these young mothers" on issues such as birth control and pre-natal care during pregnancy. Women's narratives suggested that, though the region is characterized by high fertility rates, the information and training made available to these women may have helped them to exercise more control over their bodies and themselves as reproductive beings.

However, in some cases, women decided to have more children after their association with Minga. A case in point – after learning about her reproductive rights, Adela Shapiama decided to make the choice of having another child. So, after a long gap, Adela had her fourth child. This was her way of asserting that she had control over her own reproductive decisions. On the contrary, the organization has also observed that, as women are gaining agency and leadership, the pregnancy rates are also increasing. The team believes this could be a way for men to control women's mobility and travel (as they will be less mobile when pregnant) or because men feel that women are less likely to leave them for another man if they have had several children together. Whatever the reason, the organization has had to take into account and accommodate the changing needs of these women.

Early childbearing was another challenge faced by several adolescents. Anyone with children and with a partner was considered an adult as they had to take on adult roles and responsibilities. Though still adolescents, many Amazonians slipped into adulthood as early as 13 or 14 years of age, as it was common for girls to get pregnant and start living together with their boyfriends. In a letter from Miraflores community, dated May 12, 2000, an adolescent girl wrote:

> I am a 14-year-old girl and I am in my first year of high school in the community of Miraflores. Also, since I am an adolescent, I am thinking about how I should plan my future and that I must take care of myself and protect myself from sexually transmitted diseases so that I do not get sick from one.

Judith, who has a teenage daughter, felt the program was well suited to the lived realities of the youth in the communities:

> The young people are helped too because they now know about family planning, before (the radio program) there was nothing to tell us about such things. Thanks to the program we have family planning now. I have a young daughter and I am teaching her to listen to the program so that she doesn't get pregnant.

Contextualizing the high fertility rates in the Amazon region, Luis González, cofounder and director of Minga explained the social pressures that lead to women having several children. According to González, high fertility rates exist in the region not merely because of the lack of birth control information and services but also because women tend to want more children as they feel this will make the men more "fulfilled" and happy. Similarly men feel the women are under their care if they have more children and aspire to be men whose "wives are full of children." Given the high fertility rates in the region and the physical risks involved in having too many children too soon with limited medical facilities, being proactive about reproductive choices becomes a key tool for improving maternal and child health and preventing maternal morbidity.

Improving Family Relationships

I will tell you about my life, before I was a victim of violence and abuse and I suffered a lot. I didn't know how to live, possibly because I was not educated. I had been living with my partner for two years when the violence began. He was a very jealous man and he didn't like me talking to anyone, he thought every man that talked to me wanted to seduce me, he also thought that I was having sexual relations with all the men I knew or talked with. In this manner, my abuse and physical violence continued. I was hit a lot. I was very afraid when he would drink. My children also felt very scared and would run out of the house. I have four children – all boys. I received no advice from anybody and I didn't know where to go or whom to turn to. [After receiving training from Minga] I began to explain to him what I had learned at the workshop. I talked to him about how we could continue to live in this manner. I told him that our children would grow up seeing this and when they grew up they would behave in the same way. We had many such conversations and he promised me that he would try to change and be less violent. However the problems continued and we would still fight and he even threatened to kill our children. I suggested that we separate and I took all my things and was ready to leave. Then he said where are you going to go you don't have family here (I come from another community)? He promised that he would change and he would no longer be violent like before. Now he looks like he had never been a bad man – or a violent or jealous man. He has changed a lot and so has my life changed a lot. (Rosa Mozambite, a 38-year-old *Promotora*, from Santa Cruz Community)

Narratives emerging from men, women, and children from these riverine communities, as well as members of the Minga team revealed that family-based violence was rampant in the Amazonian region. As one *promotora* stated "violence is the biggest problem in the communities." It is common for men to drink and be violent toward their spouses. Women would fight back, both physically and verbally, and often would vent their anger and frustration on their children. Most of the participants spoke about how their association with Minga, through training or listening to the radio program, or in some cases their interaction with the *promotora* had led to increased family harmony and had lessened the violence in the homes.

This theme emerged repeatedly in the data. For instance, Rosa told us that her husband had now become a new man; as if Minga had "cut his hands and stitched his lips because he didn't hit anymore and didn't say anything bad." However, violent behavior is not easy to stop overnight, and Rosa explained that, once in a while, her husband still gets angry and slips back into violent behavior. The *promotoras* explained that it had been both a difficult and a slow process, and their training and increased awareness of their rights had contributed to this noticeable change.

Promotoras played a vital role in improving their own and other community members' family relationships by stimulating dialogue on such topics. Several women negotiated with their partners by talking about the negative impacts of family-based violence on their children. As Martha noted:

> First I began to talk to my partner during mealtimes. Then when we were in bed I told him that we have kids and it is not good for him to talk to me like this. How can you say such things in front of them? We can't live like this in violence, because of the children. Someday they too will be parents, and do the same.

When possible, *promotoras* served as informal peer counselors in their communities, informing women about their rights and advising couples about the ills of living in violent relationships, particularly the detrimental impact on their children. Juana shared an incident in her community. A young woman was being beaten by her spouse and ran over to Juana's house to seek help. This woman was married to Juana's nephew, and her husband was in such a rage that Juana sought the help of local authorities at that time of the night. She asked that the man be punished for his irresponsible, violent behavior. The authorities put him in the community jail house (*calabozo*).[4] After serving his punishment (which required him to work on a large farm single-handedly), the man seemed to have realized his mistake. Juana noted that the couple are still together and "every time he sees me he says 'thank you *Tia* (Aunt) for helping my relationship and improving things with my wife.'" Clearly, the *promotoras* tread on delicate ground while playing the role of community mediators and counselors. In this case, the abused woman wanted to leave the man after she learned about her rights. Juana had to somehow explain to them that she "was not trying to separate them but instead wanted them to reconcile and live harmoniously." Further, to maintain harmony, she apologized to the couple if she had caused trouble and applauded the man for trying to change his behavior toward his wife. Fortunately, this couple worked things out, although Juana was not sure that everyone could.

Minga's efforts to increase family harmony include reducing domestic violence and promoting better communication and increased understanding among partners and between children and their parents. As Emira noted: "Minga's training has really helped me to develop as a person and has helped improve my relationship with my family." She added: "Now I see a lot more communication between couples. Before many did not talk and now through talking they have become closer to their spouse." Martha recounted her story to reinforce this point. She lived with her husband who was a jealous man and often violent toward her. She recalled that after a fight they would often not talk to each other for several days. When her community nominated her as a *promotora*, she told us that she "accepted without even asking my husband. I hadn't even talked to him and agreed without asking him. I used to do whatever I wanted." Martha shared that at the present time she and her husband talked about various things, and often settled their matters with words not blows. This began to happen particularly after her husband began to attend the workshops for men:

> I noticed that he began telling me what he had learned at the workshop – just the way I would tell him things when I returned from a Minga workshop. He changed a lot – for instance, he used to say he cared about me only when he wanted to have sex with me, but now he really cared about me. He was changing.

Many other participants also stated that the degree of physical and verbal violence had decreased in their homes. For instance, 46-year-old Nelida Macayuma said that previously she would argue a lot with her husband but now she didn't argue as much and didn't respond negatively when her husband was angry. She had learned from the radio program and from Minga's training that "families don't need to live in violence and parents need to show their children how to behave." Now she believed that she and her husband were setting a better example for their children to follow. Similarly Elsita confessed that previously she would hit or shout at her children whenever she was angry with her husband. She described herself as a "closed person" who didn't want to listen to her husband or to try to reason with him." Minga's workshops gave her a chance to reflect on her behavior and realize how badly it was affecting her children.

Our conversations with men from the community were suggestive of changes occurring in familial relationships. For example, Armando Arimuya, who lives with Milagros, a *promotora* from Santa Cruz community, felt that she has changed a lot and they now "live in a more solid home." He added that "her relationship with the children has changed totally," as she is no longer violent with them. Armando vouched for their relationship having evolved and improved over the six years that Milagros had been working as a *promotora*. Now both partners granted each other the freedom to travel away from the home and were no longer physically violent toward each other. However, Armando admitted that there were still moments when they would fight; but the confrontation was mostly verbal. Another man from Armando's community concurred that, though violence still exists in the community, it has decreased a lot compared to what it used to be. He added that one of the most important changes that had taken place in his community was the seemingly increased trust between couples, among parents and children, and within the community. He stated: "we never had conversations with them [children], but now there is more trust and we talk. There is also more solidarity within the family and in the community, and with other communities." Participants' accounts reveal how several women and families went through a process of "healing" as they resisted domestic violence and welcomed more harmonious and healthy family situations.

Conclusions and Future Directions

Our data speak to how gender roles were slowly but surely changing in the communities Minga Peru was working with. These changes led to an initial increase in domestic violence. Such conflict and resistance is common when long-standing social structures and hierarchies are challenged. As Chambers (1998) points out, "for gender equity, much that needs to change concerns the power and priority of males over females... [and] conflict can be an essential and creative factor in change for the better" (p. xviii). However, for women to gain equal power does not mean that men lose. Men gain by living less violent lives and enjoying more harmonious and productive relationships (Chambers, 1998). We see abundant examples of how women, men, children and communities in general have gained by living in more harmonious and thereby healthier relationships.

Development initiatives have always emphasized meeting peoples' physical and basic needs, undermining the need to meet emotional needs or privilege cultural realities and belief-systems. In similar vein, dominant discourses of health privilege the biomedical definition. Our work with the Amazonian people reflects how limited such discourses may be. Basic health and survival are crucial and necessary to achieve development goals, but these goals cannot be achieved without taking into account sociocultural aspects of health. Furthermore, when individuals and families are not healthy within, health in its complete sense cannot exist.

Minga works primarily with women but extends its work to include their families. It sees women as living situated lives where they are closely linked to their husbands and children. Therefore, it runs workshops for men too, so that they can also understand and help realize women's rights. By involving men, couples and families can have "healthier" relationships. The founders view communication for social change as a process that focuses on changing unequal power relationships into ones that are more just (personal conversation, July 7, 2005). The Minga team understands development as being communicative, that is, development and social change occur through communicative experiences and processes. Exclusion and discrimination are understood as occurring through communicative acts. Therefore, Minga chooses to work toward social justice and change using communication as a key resource. Communication is thus viewed as an essential and important part of every human being, family, community, and region and its role is emphasized to create possibilities for more equitable relationships. Minga endeavors to create "communicative spaces" where people are able to express themselves in multiple ways. For instance, Minga's radio program, *Bienvenida Salud* creates a space for voicing concerns and issues that affect indigenous communities whose points of view have otherwise been overlooked, silenced, or rejected.

Income generation is an important aspect of Minga's inclusive vision of social change which recognizes women's material and social needs. Minga's social change initiatives include training activities such as producing and marketing handicrafts, raising poultry and fish farming, and it teaches women to advocate for their rights through appeals to the local government. Developing women's income-generation skills enables them to earn a livelihood and support their families better. Women sell eggs, poultry, and fish in the community and with this money they are able to buy school supplies or medicines for their children. Similarly, the women make jewelry using Amazonian berries, beads, and wood for sale in local markets. Women also make embroidered handbags made out of the locally available *Chambira* fiber. They embroider patterns that reflect their dreams, as a way of telling their stories. These products are sold under the slogan of "buy a story, change a life," and are currently being marketed in Peru and the United

States as a part of fair trade practices, some of the buyers include The Rainforest Foundation, founded by the musician Sting, who bought 500 handbags. The money earned is distributed among the artisans and profits from the project are used to support workshops for *promotoras*. Minga's long-term goal is for *promotoras* to take on the responsibility of running local projects so that Minga can move its attention to other communities. Minga focuses on building capacities at all levels and, just as the radio production team have become proficient in producing the program without supervision from Lima, the organization expects the *promotoras* to independently lead community development and sustainable income-generation projects eventually. According to Luis González:

> Our institutional vision is that the power of knowledge is transferred to the technicians [i.e., *promotoras* trained in the technical aspects of poultry and fish farming] and to the women [in the community]. We know that Kiké [a Minga trainer and technical resource person] is important but we want that he and us can eventually be replaced by the people themselves. We wish that in the long run we are not needed and people can manage on their own....We don't want to be indispensable. If we want to grow, we will need to hire more and more people, but we don't want to do that, we don't want to be full of engineers and other staff, we want the women to grow and take charge.

In sum, this illustrates how Minga endeavors to put people and communities at the heart of their work in the Peruvian Amazon. Minga's vision is grounded in the belief that sustainable development privileges community ownership, and in doing so facilitators and technical experts need to provide space and opportunity for community members to own the program over a period of time.

Our review of literature speaks about the need for development efforts to focus on "the people." Minga takes this seriously, believing that people and their lived realities need to be privileged and that people should play an active role in planning their own projects. Minga's openness to learn from and with the people, and its willingness to work on an emergent agenda that is constantly whetted by the people, resonates with the dialogic and participatory tenets of the "alternative" (reversal) approach. Minga represents an instance of development practitioners valuing the voices, experiences, knowledge, desires, and needs of the community to collaboratively plan how to address them. As Huesca (2002) remarks "such a process result[s] in a 'cultural synthesis' between development collaborators to arrive at mutually identified problems, needs, and guidelines for action" (p. 502). The gaping divide between development agent and development client/beneficiary is thus bridged, leading to what Huesca refers to as "development collaborators." In addition we gain an understanding of how hard-to-reach populations can be reached and become engaged in health communication efforts that are culturally sensitive and contextually grounded.

Furthermore, alternative communication-for-social-change practices demand alternative ways of measuring their success. We draw upon traditional qualitative methods coupled with participatory tools to understand how Minga has affected the lives and well-being of community members. The narratives in this study point out clearly that Minga has made a qualitative difference to peoples' lives and that community members have been engaged meaningfully as program participants (see Dura, Singhal, and Elias, 2008; Sengupta, 2007; Singhal and Rattine-Flaherty, 2006; Sypher *et al.*, 2002 for additional assessments of Minga Perú's impact in the communities it works with). While advocating for the alternative approach, this study also makes a case for reassessing how we understand the success and impact of health communication efforts. As Ford and Yep (2003) put it:

> We must encourage the legitimacy of alternative outcomes as a measure of success for health communication [and other social change] interventions. For example, these emancipatory projects often do not conform to conventional time lines and frequently are met by surprises and setbacks. Further, hypothesis generation and testing as linked to communication effectiveness cannot be a goal. Success may be measured instead by the accomplishments, small and large, of individuals and communities and the type and quality of participation in the community dialogue. (p. 256)

We hope to have captured these "accomplishments, small and large" as we chart how the work of Minga Perú promotes health and healing in the Amazon, while endorsing a locally situated and inclusive conceptualization of health.

Notes

1 Ashoka is a global nonprofit organization that furthers international development goals by investing in social entrepreneurs around the world. Ashoka Fellows are extraordinary individuals who are leading social entrepreneurs, recognized for their commitment and innovative approaches to social change. Over the past 23 years, Ashoka has nominated over 1,500 Fellows from 53 countries (Ashoka, 2005).
2 To put this into context, developed countries such as Norway or the United States have a life expectancy of 80.5 and 79 years respectively and the per capita GDP for the United States is US$ 45,592.
3 Names of respondents have been changed in this section to protect the identities of women facing domestic violence and abuse.
4 Community authorities are called upon to negotiate domestic disputes when they either get very violent or when the couple cannot resolve the issue. In such cases the wrongdoer may be locked up in the *calabozo* (communal stockade). Receiving such punishment is considered very demeaning and shameful among Amazonian communities (Dean, 1995).

References

Ashoka. (2005). The Ashoka homepage. Retrieved May 24, 2005 from http://www.ashoka.org/home/index.cfm

Chambers, R. (1997). *Whose Reality Counts? Putting the First Last.* London: Intermediate Technology Publications.

Chambers, R. (1998). Foreword. In I. Guijt and M. K. Shah (Eds.), *The Myth of Community: Gender Issues in Participatory Development* (pp. xvii–xx). London: Intermediate Technology Publications.

Dean, B. (1995). Forbidden fruit: Infidelity, affinity and brideservice among the Urarina of Peruvian Amazonia. *The Journal of the Royal Anthropological Institute, 1,* 87–110.

Digital Pulse (2003). *The Current and Future Applications of Information and Communication Technologies for Developmental Health Priorities.* APRI – Minga Perú, Chapter 3, Section 3. Retrieved from http://change.comminit.com/en/node/1430

Dura, L., Singhal, A., and Elias, E. (2008). *Listener as Producer: Minga Peru's Intercultural Radio Educative Project in the Peruvian Amazon.* El Paso, TX: Sam Donaldson Centre for Communication Studies.

Farrington, A. (2003). "Family matters" in the Amazon. *Ford Foundation Report, 34,* 16–19.

Ferguson, A. (2000). Resisting the veil of privilege: Building bridge identities as an ethico-politics of global feminisms. In U. Narayan and S. Harding (Eds.), *Decentering the Center: Philosophy for a Multicultural, Postcolonial, and Feminist World* (pp. 189–207). Bloomington, IN: Indiana University Press.

Ford, L. A., and Yep, G. A. (2003). Working along the margins: Developing community-based strategies for communicating about health with marginalized groups. In T. Thompson, A. Dorsey, K. Miller, and R. Parrot (Eds.), *Handbook of Health Communication* (pp. 241–261). Hillsdale, NJ: Lawrence Erlbaum Associates.

Fraser, C., and Restrapo-Estrada, S. (1998). *Communicating for Development: Human Change for Survival.* London: IB Tauris Publishing.

Gumucio-Dagron, A. (2001). *Making Waves: Stories of Participatory Communication for Social Change.* New York: Rockefeller Foundation.

Harding, S. (2000). Gender, development, and post-enlightenment philosophies of science. In U. Narayan and S. Harding (Eds.), *Decentering the Center: Philosophy for a Multicultural, Postcolonial, and Feminist World* (pp. 240–261). Bloomington, IN: Indiana University Press.

Huberman, A. M., and Miles, M. B. (1998). Data management and analysis methods. In N. K. Denzin and Y. S. Lincoln (Eds.), *Collecting and Interpreting Qualitative Materials* (pp. 179–210). Thousand Oaks, CA: Sage.

Huesca, R. (2002). Participatory approaches to communication for development. In W. B. Gudykunst and B. Mody (Eds.), *Handbook of International and Intercultural Communication* (2nd edn., pp. 499–517). Thousand Oaks, CA: Sage.

Inter-American Development Bank. (2005). *Listeners from the Heart of the Amazon.* Retrieved from http://www.iadb.org/NEWS/DISPLAY/WSView.cfm?WS_Num=ws09204&Language=English

McKinley, M. A., and Jensen, L. O. (2003). In our own voices: Reproductive health radio programming in the Peruvian Amazon. *Critical Studies in Mass Communication, 20,* 80–203.

Minga Perú (n.d.). Minga Peru. Retrieved from link http://www.mingaperu.org

Morgan, D. L. (1998). Practical strategies for combining qualitative and quantitative methods: Applications to health research. *Qualitative Health Research, 8,* 362–376.

Papa, M. J., Auwal, M. A., and Singhal, A. (1997). Dialectic of control and emancipation in organizing for social change: A multitheoretic study of the Grameen Bank in Bangladesh. *Communication Theory, 5,* 189–223.

Rist, G. (1997). *The History of Development: From Western Origins to Global Faith.* (P. Camiller, trans.). New York: St. Martin's Press.

Santos-Granero, F., and Barclay, F. (2000). *Tamed Frontiers: Economy, Society, and Civil Rights in Upper Amazonia.* Boulder, CO: Westview Press.

Sengupta, A. (2007). Enacting an alternative vision of communication for social change in the Peruvian Amazon. Unpublished doctoral dissertation. Ohio University, Athens.

Singhal, A., and Rattine-Flaherty, E. (2006). Pencils and photos as tools of communicative research and praxis: Analyzing Minga Peru's quest for social justice in the Amazon. *The International Communication Gazette, 68,* 313–330.

Singhal, A., and Rogers, E. M. (2004). The status of entertainment-education worldwide. In A. Singhal, M. Cody, E.M. Rogers, and M. Sabido (Eds.), *Entertainment-Education and Social Change: History, Research, and Practice* (pp. 3–21). Mahwah, NJ: Lawrence Erlbaum Associates.

Singhal, A., and Sthapitanonda, P. (1996). The role of communication in development: Lessons learned from critique of the dominant, dependency, and alternative paradigms. *Journal of Development Communication, 1*, 10–25.

Sypher, B. D., McKinley, M., Ventsam, S., and Elías, E. (2002). Fostering reproductive health through entertainment-education in the Peruvian Amazon: The social construction of *Bienvenida Salud! Communication Theory 12*, 192–205.

UNICEF (United Nations Children's Fund) (2009). *The State of the World's Children 2009*. New York: UNICEF.

UNDP (United Nations Development Progam) (2009). *Human Development Report 2009*. New York: Oxford University Press.

Wilkins, K. G., and Mody, B. (2001). Reshaping development communication: Developing communication and communicating development. *Communication Theory, 11*, 385–396.

24

Positive Deviance, Good for Global Health

Arvind Singhal and Lucía Durá

In one of his many incarnations, Nasirudin, the mystical Sufi character, appears on earth as a smuggler. Each evening Nasirudin arrives at the customs checkpoint riding his donkey. The customs inspector, intent on nailing Nasirudin, would feverishly search the contents of the hung baskets, finding nothing but straw. Years go by, the search routine continues, and Nasirudin grows richer and richer.

Now old, Nasirudin retires from smuggling. One day he meets the customs inspector, now also retired, in a coffee shop.

"Tell me, Nasirudin," pleads his former adversary, "now that you have nothing to hide, and I have nothing to find, what is it that you were smuggling all these years?"

Nasirudin smiles. "Donkeys, of course!"

What lessons, if any, does Nasirudin's donkey story have for scholars and practitioners of global health? In the present chapter, we argue that the implications of the Nasirudin story are profound, and we detail why such might be the case. Simply put: this story illustrates that too often the reality, the answer, the solution, lies right in front of our eyes. However, we are unable to see it. Our expertise incapacitates us to see the donkeys. A customs inspector is trained to "look inside baskets," an affliction called "occupational psychosis" or "trained incapacity."

In the present chapter, we analyze the positive deviance (PD) approach to social change, arguing that often the solutions to intractable health problems stare us in the face, should we choose to notice them. We begin by defining the positive deviance approach and then we analyze the application of PD to address two highly complex problems in two different settings: (1) combating malnutrition in Vietnam, and (2) reducing maternal and newborn mortality in Pakistan. We conclude by arguing that the effectiveness of the positive deviance approach in these two real-life applications is

The Handbook of Global Health Communication, First Edition. Edited by Rafael Obregon and Silvio Waisbord.
© 2012 John Wiley & Sons, Inc. Published 2012 by John Wiley & Sons, Inc.

steeped in a variety of communicative practices, and that insights gleaned from our analysis hold important implications for scholars and practitioners of global health.

The Positive Deviance Approach

The positive deviance (PD) approach is premised on the argument that in every community there are certain individuals or groups whose uncommon behaviors and strategies enable them to find better solutions to problems than their peers, while having access to the same resources and facing worse challenges. However, these people are ordinarily invisible to others in the community, and especially to expert change agents (akin to Nasirudin's donkeys). "Positive deviants," against overwhelming odds, find ways to solve problems in a more effective manner than their peers. They are "deviants" because their uncommon behaviors are not the norm, and they are "positive" because they have found ways to effectively address the problem, while most others have not. The PD approach to social change enables communities to self-discover the positively deviant behaviors amidst them, and then find ways to act on them and amplify them (Pascale, Sternin, and Sternin, 2010; Shafique, Sternin, and Singhal, 2010; Singhal, 2010; Singhal, 2011; Singhal, Buscell, and McCandless, 2009; Singhal, Buscell, and Lindberg, 2010; Singhal, Sternin, and Durá, 2009).

Case 1: Combating Malnutrition in Vietnam

In December 1990, Jerry Sternin, accompanied by his wife Monique arrived in Hanoi to open an office for Save the Children, a US-based NGO. Their mission: to implement a large-scale program to combat childhood malnutrition in a country where two-thirds of all children under the age of five were malnourished (See Singhal, Sternin, and Dura, 2009).

The Vietnamese government had learned from experience that results achieved by traditional supplemental feeding programs were not sustainable. When the programs ended, the gains usually disappeared. The Sternins were challenged to come up with an approach that enabled the community, without much outside help, to take control of children's nutritional status. And quickly! They had six months to show results!

Necessity is the mother of invention. As traditional methods of combating malnutrition do not yield quick and sustainable results, the Sternins wondered if the concept of positive deviance, developed a few years previously by Tufts University nutrition professor Marian Zeitlin might hold promise (Zeitlin, Ghassemi, and Mansour, 1990).

The concept of positive deviance was first broached in the nutritional literature in the 1960s. Zeitlin explored the idea in some depth in the 1980s as she tried to understand why some children in poor households, without access to any special resources, were better nourished than others. What did they know and what were they doing that others were not? Might combating malnutrition take an asset-based approach? That is, identifying what's going right in a community, and finding ways to amplify it, as opposed to the more traditional deficit-based approach – focusing on what's going wrong in a community and fixing it.

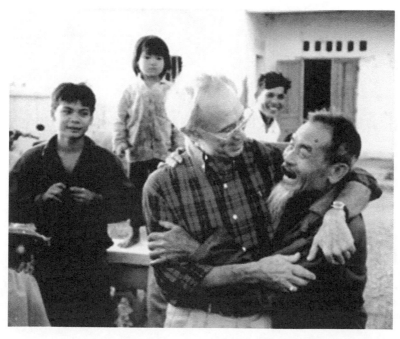

Figure 24.1 Building trust: Jerry Sternin with a village elder in Quong Xuong district, Vietnam.
Source: Monique Stemin, used with permission.

Self-discovering solutions

Positive deviance sounded good in theory but, to date, no one had used the concept to design a field-based nutrition intervention. Would it work in a community-setting? The Sternins had no roadmaps or blueprints to consult. Where to begin?

Starting close to Hanoi, where they were based, made sense. Childhood malnutrition rates were high in Quong Xuong District in Thanh Hoa Province, south of Hanoi. The Ho Chi Minh trail, a supply route for the guerilla fighters during the Vietnam War, snakes through Quong Xuong, so suspicion of Americans was palpably high. The Sternins needed to build trust with community members, especially the elders.

After several days of consultation with local officials, four village communities were selected for a nutrition baseline survey. Armed with six weighing scales and bicycles, health volunteers weighed some 2,000 children under the age of three in four villages in less than four days. Their locations were mapped and a growth card for each child, with a plot of their age and weight, was compiled. Some 64 percent of the weighed children were found to be malnourished. No sooner was the data tallied than, with bated breath, the Sternins asked: Are there any well-nourished children who come from very, very poor families? The response: Yes, indeed, there are some children from very poor families who are healthy! They are few in number but they do exist.

These poor families in Thanh Hoa that had managed to avoid malnutrition without access to any special resources would represent the positive deviants – "positive" because their children were well-nourished, and "deviants" because they were doing some things

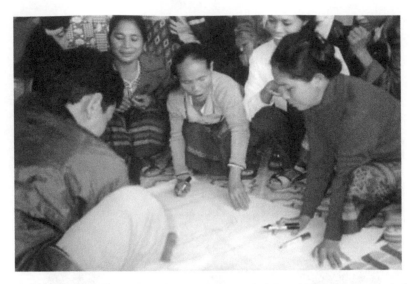

Figure 24.2   Community members mapping the nutritional status of children in their communities.
Source: Monique Sternin, used with permission.

differently. What were these PD families doing that others were not? To answer this question, community members visited six of the poorest families with well-nourished children in each of the four villages. If the community self-discovered the solution, they were more likely to implement it. Their discovery process yielded the following key practices among poor households with well-nourished children:

- Family members collected tiny shrimps and crabs from paddy fields and added them to their children's meals. These foods are rich in protein and minerals.
- Family members added greens of sweet potato plants to their children's meals. These greens are rich in essential micronutrients.

Interestingly, these foods were accessible to everyone, but most community members believed they were inappropriate for young children. Further,

- PD mothers were feeding their children smaller meals three to four times a day, rather than the customary big meal twice a day; and
- PD mothers were actively feeding their children, rather than placing food in front of them, making sure there was no food wasted.

Acting one's way

With best practices discovered, the natural urge was to go out and tell the people what to do: by means of household visits, attractive posters, informational and educational sessions, among other things. However, from past experience with development

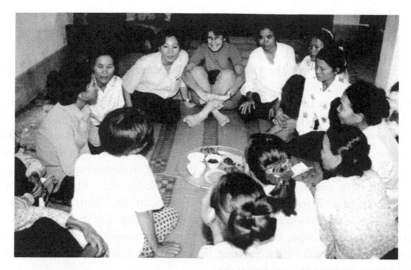

Figure 24.3 Cooking sessions that emphasized the importance of acting one's way into a new way of knowing. Monique Sternin (center).
Source: Monique Sternin, used with permission.

work in several countries over two decades, the Sternins knew "best practice" solutions almost always engendered resistance from the people. In spite of some modest adoption of these best practices, most of the poor households in Quong Xuong District had not adopted them.

The Sternins, local health volunteers, and community leaders felt they were hitting a brick wall of resistance. They wondered how to get around it. One evening, as the discussion was winding down, a skeptical village elder observed: "A thousand hearings isn't worth one seeing, and a thousand seeings isn't worth one doing."

On the car ride back to Hanoi, the Sternins talked about the sagacity of the elder's remark. Could they help design a nutrition program which emphasized *doing* more than *seeing* or *hearing*?

In the next few weeks, a two-week nutrition program was designed in each of the four intervention villages. Mothers whose children were malnourished were asked to forage for shrimps, crabs, and sweet potato greens. Armed with small nets and containers, mothers waded into the paddy fields. The focus was on action, picking up the shrimps and crabs, and shoots from sweet potato fields. In the company of positive deviants, mothers of malnourished children learned how to cook new recipes using the foraged ingredients. Again, the emphasis was on doing.

Before these mothers fed their children, they weighed them, and plotted the data points on their growth chart. The children's hands were washed, and the mothers actively fed the children. No food was wasted. Some mothers noted their children seemed to eat more in the company of other children. When returning home, mothers were encouraged to give their children three or four small meals a day instead of the traditional two meals.

Such feeding and monitoring continued for two weeks. Mothers could visibly see their children becoming healthier. The scales were tipping! After the pilot project, which lasted two years, malnutrition had decreased by an amazing 85 percent in the PD communities. Over the next several years, the PD intervention became a nationwide program in Vietnam, helping over 2.2 million people, including over 500,000 children, improve their nutritional status. A later study showed successive generations of impoverished Vietnamese children in the program villages were well-nourished (Mackintosh, Marsh, and Schroeder, 2002).

The sustained success of Save the Children's nutritional initiative in Vietnam was attributed, in part, to the combination of the positive deviance approach, in particular the PD inquiry, with the hearth model (see Wollinka *et al.*, 1997), which organizes volunteers for actionable intervening at the neighborhood level. Other components that contributed to its sustained effectiveness included an revolving loan program that allowed for ongoing community engagement, knowledge sharing, and self-help, and the establishment of a "living university" in several locations, through which neighboring village leaders, cadre workers, health volunteers, and aspiring mothers could witness and experience the actionable PD practices, engage in cooperative learning with their local counterparts, and take that learning back to their communities to implement a culturally appropriate nutritional program.

Born out of necessity, this pioneering experience in Vietnam, with all its struggles and lessons, paved the way for other PD applications to follow. Skeptics argued that PD may have worked in the field of nutrition as it was a noncontentious issue (who would not want their children to be healthy?), where programmatic ideas were easily trialable, and the results highly observable. Could the PD approach be applied to a highly intractable problem where the topic was highly sensitive, deeply ingrained in traditional structures of patriarchy and gender roles, and where prevailing beliefs and behaviors were closely connected to the harsh physical and social environment? The PD experience in Pakistan helped answer these questions.

Case #2: Reducing Maternal and Newborn Mortality in Pakistan

Nineteen-year old Rahima had just entered her ninth month of her pregnancy when she felt a sharp painful twitch in her abdomen (see Shafique, Sternin, and Singhal, 2010). Had her labor pains begun four weeks prematurely, she wondered?! As the cold wind blew outside her sparse two-room home in Bagra village, located in the mountainous Haripur District of Pakistan's Northwest Frontier Province (NWFP), Rahima's anxiety climbed. Of the last eight births in Bagra village, two newborns did not make it past the first 40 days. Would her firstborn beat the one-in-four odds of survival in this harsh physical environment that was notorious for harboring one of the highest rates of infant mortality in the world?

The odds for Rahima's firstborn to face pregnancy complications were stacked high. She had received no antenatal care leading up to her impending delivery, no iron or vitamin supplements, and no tetanus toxoid vaccination. Her workload was heavy, and she tired easily cooking, cleaning, and caring for her in-laws, her husband, and his younger unmarried brothers. While Rahima's body needed more food and nutrients for the growing fetus, her mother-in-law limited her food portions so that the newborn would not be too big and would be easily delivered. Rahima's husband, Mushtaq, a small-time farmer, was looking forward to becoming a father, wishing for the birth of a male child who could carry on the family name. Although a conscientious husband, Mushtaq, like most other husbands in Bagra Village, was not involved in his wife's pregnancy and antenatal care. Mushtaq had no cash savings and made no preparation for any emergencies or pregnancy-related complications for Rahima. Further, as per Bagra's social norms, pregnancy, delivery, and child care were exclusively in the women's domain. Mushtaq's mother, Shakila Bano, who with her experience of birthing 13 children (10 of whom survived), was Rahima's primary resource for maternal and newborn care.

With the blistering winds howling, calling the *dai*, the traditional birth attendant, from a neighboring village was not possible. Shakila would help Rahima deliver the baby with the help of a neighboring aunt. Some jute bags were spread on the cold floor of the animal shed where Rahima squat holding on to a *charpoy*, a four legged bed, for support. Writhing in pain, Rahima pushed and pushed until her firstborn – a daughter – was delivered. Shakila sawed the umbilical cord with a bamboo stick and tied a traditional thread around it. A dressing of *desi ghee* (clarified butter) was applied to keep the cord moist and lubricated. The aunt laid the premature newborn girl on the cold floor as Shakila delivered Rohima's placenta. Mushtaq brought in a bucket of tepid water heated in haste over a wood stove and the aunt bathed the shivering newborn in an attempt to remove the vermix. The baby was then wrapped in a rag-tag blanket and handed to Shakila so she could administer the child *ghutti*, a homemade pre-lacteal concoction made from green tea, buffalo milk, *ghee*, and sugar. The thick colostrum, *keer*, flowing out of Rohima's breasts, full of antibodies to boost a newborn's immunity, was discarded, deemed unfit for the newborn's consumption. For the first hours, the *ghutti* would suffice. With the newborn washed, wrapped, and fed, Mushtaq's father, the elder male, was summoned to whisper *azan*, a prayer from the Holy Quran, in the newborn's ear on the threshold of the room where Rahima delivered.

Rahima prayed silently that her tiny premature baby girl would survive, if not thrive, against overwhelming odds.

PD comes to Haripur

Between 2001 and 2004, the positive deviance approach was implemented in a phased manner in eight villages of Haripur District in Pakistan's North West Frontier Province to deliver better health outcomes for the likes of Rahima and their newborns. Among the thousands of Rahimas, Shakilas, and Mushtaqs of Haripur District, were there a handful of individuals, whose uncommon practices resulted in better health outcomes for the mothers and their newborns? Initiated by Save the Children as part of their Saving Newborn Lives (SNL) Initiative in Pakistan, the PD process was first introduced in two experimental villages – Bagra and Banda Muneer Khan, followed by a pilot phase in Kaag and Chanjiala villages, where various PD processes, tools, and strategies were further refined. A larger four-village PD intervention was implemented in Garamthone, Nilorepaeen, Bhaira, and Chambapind villages. Baseline and endline data were collected in these four interventional villages and in four comparison control villages to assess the effects of the PD intervention.

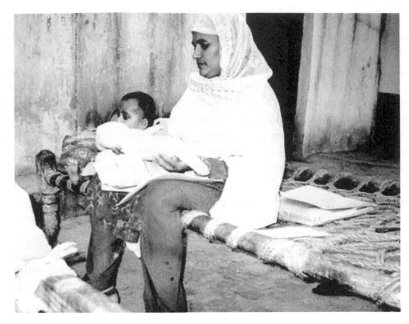

Figure 24.4 Women used dolls to demonstrate how the newborn was handled during the delivery and post-delivery.
Source: Muhammad Shafique, used with permission.

The use of the PD approach in these eight communities of Haripur District followed an iterative process in two phases. In phase one, activities were initiated to foster community dialogue about the problem of newborn mortality and morbidity among community members (separately between male and female groups) in order to identify PD newborns and their families, discover their demonstrably successful strategies (through a PD inquiry), and develop a plan of action. Phase two was dedicated to community action via community-designed neighborhood activities undertaken by both male and female groups.

As safe motherhood, pregnancy, and delivery, are highly taboo subjects in the NWFP, various participatory activities such as transect walks, focus group discussions (FGDs), social network maps, newborn mapping, and in-depth interviews were employed. During the community orientation and feedback sessions, facts and local figures about newborn and maternal care were shared, including powerful, emotive testimonies from family members who had lost a newborn or a wife, daughter-in-law, or niece during labor and delivery.

A baseline about newborns in the community was established working with both women's and men's groups. A newborn mapping activity was conducted by both groups to determine how many babies had been born the year before, how many had been stillborn or died immediately after birth, after seven days, after 28 days and within 40 days. Concurrently, explorations of common practices with women's groups around pregnancy, delivery, and immediate and subsequent postpartum care were explored using stuffed dolls as props. The dolls provided a visual representation of how the newborn was handled during the delivery, and post-delivery.

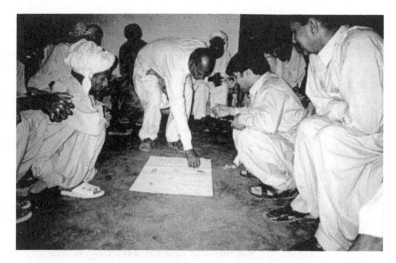

Figure 24.5 Men engaged in mapping newborn and maternal mortality in Haripur District.
Source: Muhammad Shafique, used with permission.

The PD inquiry was initiated to enable the community to discover the uncommon yet effective behaviors and strategies amidst them, and to develop a plan of action to promote their adoption among community members. The PD team – composed of village leaders, self-identified volunteers (activists), and the NGO staff – defined a positive deviant (*misali kirdar*) newborn as one who survived against heavy odds because of poverty, prematurity, and maternal health history (e.g. miscarriages, anemia, and/or age of mother). Besides the newborn, family members related to the newborn were identified as PD persons, such as a father who saved money in case of obstetric emergency at delivery, a mother-in-law who prepared a delivery kit for the arriving newborn, a *dai* who successfully resuscitated newborns that were not breathing and practiced clean cord cut and appropriate cord care.

The PD inquiry helped discern household behaviors that increased the chances of newborn survival e.g. the administration of tetanus toxoid vaccination and antenatal care for the mother, delivery preparedness on part of mother-in-laws and *dais*, emergency-preparedness on part of husbands, the use of clean surface for delivery, clean hands while delivering, clean cutting of umbilical cord, thermal care of newborn, exclusive breast-feeding, timely care-seeking for premature or sick babies, paternal involvement in spouse and childcare, increase in postpartum maternal diet, and others.

The PD inquiry also yielded rich insights on messaging strategies used by the *misali kirdars* (positive deviants). For example,

- A religious leader noted: "We don't need to bathe the baby for *azan* as when we listen to *azan* (a prayer from the Holy Quran) five times a day, we are not clean most of the time, so in the same way babies need not be bathed before saying azan in their ears." This religious leader, and his message about delaying the bathing rituals of a newborn, was then given play in *mohallah* (neighborhood) sessions and in community healthy baby fairs, thus multiplying its effects.

Table 24.1 Some positive deviance behaviors related to maternal and newborn care.

Maternal and Newborn Care Issues	*Observable PD Practices*
Pregnancy, Delivery, and Immediate Newborn Care	• A pregnant mother sought antenatal consultation and tetanus toxoid injection. • A husband asked the *dai*, the traditional birth attendant, to see his wife in her 9th month of pregnancy although she was well. • A husband increased the food intake of his wife during pregnancy, especially in the last 2 months. • A husband arranged to hire transport in case of a delivery emergency. • The family hand-stitched a small mattress (*gadeila*) for the baby to have a clean and warm surface immediately following delivery. • A husband gave the *dai* a clean blade. • A mother-in-law placed a clean sheet of plastic under the mother for delivery. • A husband ensured that nothing was applied on the umbilical cord after it was cut and tied.
Breastfeeding	• A sick and premature baby was exclusively breast-fed with no supplements and no *ghutti* (a homemade prelacteal concoction).
Nurturing	• A father realized that his newborn son was weak and small, and therefore a special child (*khas batcha*), requiring special care. The baby was kept warm by wrapping, and his nappies were changed frequently. The child was exclusively breastfed and the quality and quantity of food for the mother were increased. The mother was made unavailable to the rest of the household so that she could exclusively care for the baby.

• A father who strongly advocated paternal involvement in maternal health pre- and post-delivery noted: "Giving *panjiri*, a nutritionally rich protein bar, to the pregnant woman can lead to a healthy baby and also keep the mother's life out of danger. If we provide food for the mother, it will ensure the health of the baby."

• A mother-in-law explained the benefits of exclusive breastfeeding to her daughters-in-law: "The baby has no disease in the mother's womb. If breast milk were dangerous, the baby would become ill in the womb. So mother's milk is safe for the baby because it comes from the mother's body."

The PD messages were reinforced and repeated through different media, including religious and secular leaders, popular street theater, neighborhood meetings, and other means. However, the PD methodology focuses not just on the message delivery but also creates an enabling environment at the household level by involving husbands, mothers-in-law, the village health committee members, and members of Village Action Team (VAT), who collectively can facilitate and support the process of behavior change.

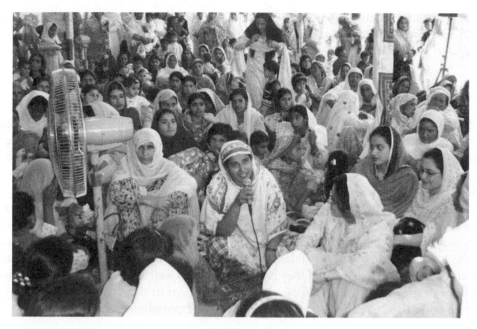

Figure 24.6 A PD mother sharing her practices in a *mohallah* session.
Source: Muhammad Shafique, used with permission.

PD inquiry to Implementation

The PD practices that were discovered were openly shared with community members. Because of cultural mores, male and female members were approached separately. Here the community members had an opportunity to discuss the PD behaviors, seeing their relevance, usefulness, and practicality. Village action teams developed a six-monthly plan, deciding that in cooperation with the community members a plethora of activities would be undertaken at the neighborhood level with regular bimonthly group interaction *mohallah* sessions. These meetings were facilitated by local social activists, who volunteered to carry out the community action plan. Each bimonthly session was focused on a newborn and maternal care topic and highlighted certain specific PD behaviors and strategies that had been discovered during the recent PD inquiries.

One of the fun activities in the male *mohallah* sessions was to set up a mock bazaar where men were asked to buy what they considered a clean delivery kit for pregnant women. Discussion on each participant's purchase followed and resulted in men declaring, some anonymously, that a new razor blade was the best tool for cutting the umbilical cord. The community's respect and open support for the men's contributions and decisions helped enhance their self and collective efficacy, leading to the emergence of a new and innovative leadership. Scores of new male volunteers signed up to run the *mohallah* sessions initiative.

In the female *mohallah* sessions, community volunteers also set up a bazaar, laying out several objects on a table and asking pregnant mothers, mothers-in-law, and *dais*, to select the five or six objects (e.g. soap bar, clean blade, clean plastic sheet, etc.) that were essential for a clean delivery kit. The selection of each object, essential or nonessential, sparked a healthy discussion about the object's relevance in delivery preparedness. New leadership emerged from these sessions to serve as volunteers and activists in improving the quality of lives of newborns and their mothers.

Involving men

Dialogue with community members from day one unequivocally revealed that male involvement in maternal and newborn care was minimal. In this dominant Pashtun culture of patriarchy, male bonding with infants or caring for one's wife is perceived as not being "manly."

Several interactive games and simulated role plays were employed in the PD process to help the local Pashtun men become more involved in the care of their wives and newborn children. One of the games used to pass on responsibility to the male village action team was the balloons-as-newborn game. Men were told that newborns are happy and alive as long as the balloons are afloat, but if they fall to the ground that means they are sick and may die. So, what could they do individually, as well as collectively, to minimize newborn deaths? By floating balloons, and keeping them in the air, they were "acting" on their collective communal, parental, and spousal responsibilities.

Overcoming odds

A pre-/post-interventional control research design involving both PD and non-PD villages pointed to significant gains in maternal and newborn care indicators. In comparison to control villages where the gains were insignificant, in the intervention villages

- the percentage of pregnant mothers visting antenatal clinics increased significantly from 45 percent to 63 percent;
- the percentage of fathers who saved money and arranged for transport to tackle pregancy emergencies increased significantly from 45 percent to 62 percent;
- the percentage of families that used a new blade to cut the baby's cord increased significantly from 19 percent to 33 percent;
- the percentage of newborns whose cords did not receive unhygenic homemade remedies increased significantly from 7 percent to 19 percent;
- the percentage of mothers giving homemade prelactal feeds in the first three days decreased significantly from 70 percent to 25 percent;
- the percentage of families that bathed the baby after waiting for 24 hours post-birth increased significantly from 18 percent to 32 percent.

Conclusions

In the present chapter, through an analysis of two case studies in global health, we argued that often the solutions to intractable health problems lie locally and with ordinary people. This alternative conceptualization of local, wisdom-centered health

Table 24.2 Key communicative practices embedded in the positive deviance approach.

Communicative Practices	*Illustrative Examples from Vietnam and Pakistan Cases*
Listening, trust-building, stakeholder dialogue, horizontal communication, and alliances with opinion leaders	• Horizontal communication between PD implementers and community members in both locales • Participation of local health officials, cadres, and community volunteers in Vietnam • Engagement and involvement of elders, men, and neighborhood activists in Pakistan
Reframing, self-discovery, and dialogic inquiry	• Reframing deficit-based assertions to asset-based *questions* • Facilitating self-discovery of endogenous, already-existing solutions in both locales • Encouraging community dialogue to define the problem, identify solutions, and amplify them through culturally appropriate actionable practices
Social proof and action-based learning	• Emphasis on learning by doing with community peers who represent social proof that PD behaviors are actionable, e.g. cooking sessions with caregivers in Vietnam; role-playing, fun, interactive games amongst community maternal and newborn care in Pakistan

solutions is known as the positive deviance (PD) approach – a process of change *that enables communities to discover the wisdom they already have, and find a way to amplify it*. The PD approach is now being used to address diverse issues such as childhood anemia, the eradication of female genital mutilation, curbing the trafficking of girls, increasing school retention rates, reducing hospital-acquired infections, and promoting higher levels of condom use among commercial sex workers (Pascale, Sternin, and Sternin, 2010; Singhal, Buscell, and Lindberg, 2010; Singhal and Durá, 2009).

As with most health communication campaigns, PD implementation is anchored in locally based communicative practices, community assets, and facilitative skills. The change agent in the PD approach bows to the wisdom that lurks within the community and is a humble learner and active listener. In this respect, the PD approach differs from most health communication campaigns derived from the diffusion of innovations or social marketing traditions that are premised on the notion that new health information or ideas come from the outside, are promoted by a change agency through expert change agents, and use top-down persuasive communication strategies to educate their client audience. The PD approach flips these long-standing tenets, positing that innovative ideas are often lurking within the system, so that the role of the change agents is to facilitate a process whereby the community can self-discover these ideas, and where dialogue and social proof result in an organic spread of the desirable health practices (see Table 24.2).

The PD approach questions the traditional role of outside expertise, believing that the wisdom to solve the problem lies inside the community. The expert's role is to employ participatory methods to help the community find the positive deviants, identify their uncommon but effective practices, and design a community intervention to make these practices visible and actionable.

The assumptions behind this initial shift in thinking depend heavily on the effective management of intercultural, interpersonal, and horizontal communication processes. These techniques are used to build relationships with local officials, opinion leaders, and community members whose support is needed at the beginning for trust-building and towards the end for program sustainability and scaling. Further, horizontal communication is the driving notion ensuring that the inquiry, dialogue, and program implementation are participatory and endogenous.

As the Vietnam and Pakistan cases demonstrate, the PD approach relies on culturally appropriate activities and learning techniques to communicate the social proof of immediately actionable, desirable behaviors. In the PD approach, change is led by internal agents who, with access to no special resources, present the social behavioral proof to their peers. Social proof is a psychological phenomenon in which people come to believe that they can adopt a different practice because they discover people like them, in their own community, using the practice. If they can do it, others can too. As the PD behaviors are already in practice, the solutions can be implemented without delay or access to outside resources.

Once social proof is presented and accepted, the PD approach challenges conventional implementation practices. Conventional learning theories assume that knowledge will change attitudes, which will in turn change practice. PD reverses that idea. PD practitioners have found action is the first step in changing attitudes. As opposed to subscribing to the notion that increased knowledge changes attitudes, and attitudinal changes change practice, PD is rooted in changing practice, as can be seen in the cooking sessions that took place in Vietnam and gender-based role-playing organized by the community in Pakistan. PD is premised on the notion that people change when that change is distilled from concrete action steps.

The PD approach holds important implications for scholars and practitioners of global health. It is an innovative method used to address seemingly intractable problems, especially when other approaches have failed. PD is paradigmatically situated in stark contrast to the traditional deficit-based, expert-driven message diffusion approaches. The approach is more sustainable because the community defines the problem, self-discovers the solutions, and is able to implement them right away without access to special resources. This way, solutions are likely to be sustained. Further, an approach based in local wisdom perspectives makes intuitive sense. As we systematically codify the PD approach, and gather a body of evidence to demonstrate the conditions under which it is most effective, PD is bound to make headway into uncharted territories.

Acknowledgments

The present chapter is informed by, and draws upon, the co-authors' work with the PD approach over the past six years (Singhal and Greiner, 2007; Singhal and Durá, 2009; Durá and Singhal, 2009; Singhal, 2010). We thank Jerry and Monique Sternin, Muhammad Shafique, Curt Lindberg, Prucia Buscell, and other collaborators for their wisdom and co-construction with us of many of the PD narratives. The present work also draws upon, and builds upon, the ideas presented by author Singhal in Singhal, Buscell, and Lindberg (2010).

References

Frost, R. (1942). The secret sits. A poem in *The Witness Tree*. Retrieved from http://wondering minstrels.blogspot.com/2001/01/secret-sits-robert-frost.html

Mackintosh, U., Marsh, D., and D. Schroeder (2002). Sustained positive deviant child care practices and their effects on child growth in Viet Nam. *Food and Nutrition Bulletin 23*(4), 16–25.)

Pascale, R. T., Sternin, J., and Sternin, M. (2010). *The Power of positive deviance: How Unlikely Innovators Solve the World's Toughest Problems*. Boston, MA: Harvard University Press.

Shafique, M., Sternin, M., and Singhal, A. (2010). Will Rahima's firstborn survive overwhelming odds? positive deviance for maternal and newborn care in Pakistan. *positive deviance wisdom series, number 5* (pp. 1–12). Boston, MA: Tufts University, positive deviance Initiative. Retrieved from http://www.positivedeviance.org/pdf/wisdom%20series/FINALPakistan WisdomSeries05.27.10.pdf

Singhal, A. (2010). Communicating what works! Applying the positive deviance approach in health communication. *Health Communication, 25*(6), 605–606.

Singhal, A. (2011). Turning diffusion of innovations paradigm on its head. In A. Vishwanath and G. Barnett (Eds.), *The Diffusion of Innovations: A Communication Science Perspective* (pp. 192–205). New York: Peter Lang Publishers.

Singhal, A., Buscell, P., and Lindberg, C. (2010). *Inviting Everyone: Healing Healthcare through positive deviance*. Bordentown, NJ: PlexusPress.

Singhal, A., Buscell, P., and McCandless, K. (2009). Saving lives by changing relationships: positive deviance for MRSA prevention and control in a U.S. hospital. *positive deviance wisdom series, number 3*, pp. 1–8. Boston, MA: Tufts University, positive deviance Initiative.

Singhal, A., and Durá, L. (2009). *Protecting children from exploitation and trafficking: Using the positive deviance approach in Uganda and Indonesia*. Washington D.C.: Save the Children.

Singhal, A., Sternin, J., and Durá, L. (2009). Combating malnutrition in the land of a thousand rice fields: positive deviance grows roots in Vietnam. *Positive deviance wisdom series, number 1*, pp. 1–8. Boston, MA: Tufts University, positive deviance Initiative.

Wollinka, O., Keeley, E., Burkhalter, B.R., and Bashir, N. (Eds.) (1997). *Hearth Nutrition Model: Applications in Haiti, Vietnam, and Bangladesh*. Arlington, VA: USAID. Retrieved from http://pdf.usaid.gov/pdf_docs/PNACA868.pdf

Zeitlin, M., Ghassemi, H., and Mansour, M. (1990). *Positive deviance in Child Nutrition*. New York: UN University Press.

25

Health Promotion from the Grassroots
Piloting a Radio Soap Opera for Latinos in the United States

María Beatriz Torres

Introduction

Worldwide several public health interventions using entertainment-education (EE) strategies through different media (radio, television, printed materials, posters, theater, and music) in combination with interpersonal means (dialogue with experts, visits, training, community meetings, community groups, listening groups, etc.) have successfully produced increased knowledge and attitude and behavior change with respect to topics such as HIV/AIDS (Bosch, 2006; Do and Kincaid, 2006; Goldstein *et al.*, 2005; Porto, 2007; Smith, Downs, and Witte, 2007; Sood, Shefner-Rogers, and Sengupta, 2006; Vaughan *et al.*, 2000), safe sex (Horner *et al.*, 2008), family planning (Boulay, Torey, and Sood, 2002), breastfeeding practices (Maxwell, Borwanker, and Gonzalez Yucra, 2003), and men's involvement in safe motherhood (Shefner-Rogers and Sood, 2004), to name but a few. EE is a strategy used to promote social change through creating media messages that entertain and educate. This strategy has been around for at least three decades (Singhal and Rogers, 2003). One of the major reasons for EE's success is that it appeals to its audience's emotions through narratives and stimulates interpersonal communication about a variety of topics (Boulay, Torey, and Sood, 2002; Goldstein *et al.*, 2005; Shefner-Rogers and Sood, 2004; Singhal and Rogers, 2003; Sood, Shefner-Rogers, and Sengupta, 2006).

In the United States, EE has been used to introduce health information in various TV sitcoms, dramas, and PSAs. Results of these interventions showed moderate to low success in producing behavior change (Hether *et al.*, 2008; Valente *et al.*, 2007; Wray *et al.*, 2004, among others) compared with the effectiveness such initiatives have demonstrated in developing countries. Some of the reasons for that difference may be due to cost, the feasibility of coproductions, and the saturation of the media environment in the United States (Valente *et al.*, 2007).

A few health initiatives have used EE to reach Latinos[1] in the United States. Perez and colleagues (2008) examined the impact of 63 radio spots and found them to be moderately successful at raising awareness about child obesity with Hispanic target groups. Similarly, Willkin *et al.* (2007) reported that viewers of the soap opera *Ladrón de Corazones* increased their knowledge and understanding of breast cancer therapies based on information introduced in its storyline by health promoters. Viewers' identification with characters in the soap opera triggered interpersonal communication about this topic.

Based on the above evidence, our pilot project identified the potential for reaching, from the grassroots, the dispersed Hispanic diaspora in south-central Minnesota through a radio soap opera aimed at increasing knowledge of, and interpersonal communication about, their health, prevention measures, and resources available in the community. Before detailing the specifics of the project, it is necessary to consider why this minority group is particularly deserving of attention. More specifically, in the section that follows, I explain the significance of this project and/or its potential to address the health knowledge gap of this minority group in the United States, and the steps that were taken to create and evaluate a radio soap opera.

Why Latinos?

The US Bureau of Census (2010, p. 2) estimated that Hispanics had reached "50.5 million" "or 16 percent of the estimated total US population of 308.7 million." Those figures make Hispanics the largest minority ethnic group in the US surpassing African Americans. They are also the fastest-growing group. Frates, Bohrer, and Thomas (2006) maintain that the new Hispanic immigrants are transient and possess a low level of knowledge about the complexity of the health care system in the United States. Hispanics also tend to have higher mortality rates than any other ethnic group (Willkin *et al.*, 2007).

In the state of Minnesota, 3.8% of the foreign-born residents are Hispanic (American Community Survey 2005–2006, US Census Bureau). This population is expected to grow exponentially by the year 2025. Of this group, 71 percent of Hispanics are from Mexico and located mostly in greater Minnesota – the central, southwest, and southeast regions of the state (http://www.clac.state.mn.us). Many of these immigrants are illiterate or possess low literacy levels and do not speak English fluently (http://www.clac.state.mn.us).

There is little research about Latinos in Minnesota. Smaida and colleagues (2002) found that Latinos experienced a lack of preventive health care due to numerous health disparities. Among those disparities are: economic constraints (housing, transportation, and money), differences in cultural beliefs (in expectations about doctors' visits and health beliefs), and language barriers impacting the quality of the health care they receive. As a result, they also lack an understanding of the health care system in the United States. Therefore, increasing outreach campaigns, training professionals to understand the Latino population, and expanding the use of materials in Spanish would be of help (Smaida *et al.*, 2002). Participants in another study, using eight focus groups in the metropolitan area (Twin Cities) and greater Minnesota (Willmar and Rochester), manifested a need for more education on diabetes, heart disease, cancer, sexual transmitted diseases, teenage pregnancy, alcoholism, and mental health (http://www.clac.state.mn.us).

Very little is known about what knowledge (and perceptions) Latinos hold regarding specific conditions and what resources are available to them. Research is this area is needed. However, the growing number of undocumented Latino immigrants in Minnesota (estimated at between 55,000 and 80,000 according to http://centrocampesino.net) makes data collection challenging. Surveys or self-reports are not feasible due to low literacy levels, and lack of trust in completing written documentation (due to their legal status) or even speaking to someone they do not know well. This limitation affects how much formative baseline research can be done unless different, nontraditional approaches are used (Dutta-Bergman, 2005; McLean, 1997; McKinley and Jensen, 2003, among others).

Services to Latinos in the Minneapolis-Saint Paul area are well covered by various organizations (e.g., CLUES, *Comunidades Latinas Unidas en Servicio* – Latino Communities United in Service, a nonprofit organization, and the Chicano Latino Affairs Council – a state government agency). They offer health services and health education (CLUES) and/or act as advocates for affordable health care, medical assistance, culturally competent services and prevention (see Chicano Latino Affairs Council, 2009).

Two main nonprofit organizations in south-central Minnesota work with Latinos. One of them, La-Mano, offers interpreting services, crime victim support programs, leadership, and cultural consultations (http://lamanomn.com). The other, Centro Campesino, serves migrant workers (those who come during harvest season to Minnesota) and focuses on community organizing, education, and advocacy. Centro Campesino (http://centrocampesino.net) trains community leaders to become health promoters within their migrant communities. However, these efforts only reach migrant workers from four communities.

In sum, south-central Minnesota lacks a comprehensive approach to health prevention programs targeting Latinos. The goal of this pilot project was to think of ways to work more effectively and creatively and reach the Latino community's health needs. So, now I briefly describe the start of this process, the target audience, and the preferred communication channel to engage Latinos in the area.

Starting from the Grassroots

The project began in fall 2008, when I became a board member of La-Mano. During meetings I had with the director, she emphasized the lack of health prevention programs for Latinos in the area and the need to diffuse health-related information. Among its projects, La-Mano uses *La Hora Comunitaria* (*The community hour*), a three-hour Spanish radio program for Latinos aired every Saturday through KMSU FM. The program features general information about the crime victims' program, immigration issues, sports, events in the community, and Hispanic music.

Although Spanish television, radio, and newspapers are widely available through the Web and on cable, most of them offer general information and are not locally produced. Dutta-Bergman (2004), Frates *et al.* (2006), and Willkin *et al.* (2007) concurred that health campaign planners should use television and radio, as they tend to be consumed by less health-oriented and less educated individuals. Others claim that Latinos prefer television over other media and prefer media in their native language (Frates, Bohrer, and Thomas, 2006; Perez *et al.*, 2008; Willkin *et al.*, 2007). Local television programming does not target Latinos in Minnesota.

The Twin Cities area is well covered by Spanish-language newspapers (*Gente de Minnesota, La Prensa de Minnesota, La Voz Latina, VidaySabor,* and *El Cambio* – http://www.echo-media.com) and private commercial radios (*La Mera Buena, La Invasora,* and *Radio Rey*). Outside the metropolitan area, media in Spanish are scarce. Only two radio stations (one religious station in Saint James and a station in Mankato-KMSU) offer programs in Spanish. KMSU (from Minnesota State University) has Spanish programming on Saturdays. This radio is accessed by "approximately 500–600 Latinos" (Victoria Salas, Director of La-Mano Inc. Personal communication, March 5, 2010) throughout south-central Minnesota.

Curiously, radio has been widely and effectively used by national governments in Latin America for informational and persuasive purposes (McKinley and Jensen, 2003). The benefit of using the radio is that it can reach dispersed audiences in rural places (Maxwell, Borwanker, and Gonzalez Yucra, 2003), produces higher identification and emotional involvement than television (Smith, Downs, and Witte, 2007), and provides people with social cohesion and cultural identity (Ramos Rodríguez, 2005).

Due to the fact that Latinos are spread over south-central Minnesota, possess low literacy levels, and rely on the community radio for local information, we decided to focus on new ways to use La-Mano's Saturday program to get to this audience. Reed and Hanson (2006) maintain that community radios present "localism and access" (p. 215) to smaller communities. In their view, community radios offer a voice to the locals, who have a say in the programming decisions and operation of the radio. La-Mano embodies such voice for the Latino community.

Numerous meetings were arranged with community members and organizations from several counties, the radio host (and staff of La-Mano), board members and members of *Las Comadres* (a social support group from La-Mano) to explore health information needs within the Latino community and to examine possible ways to use the radio program. In the next section, I share how the process of defining needs and goals was collectively discussed and shaped with input from community members.

The Planning Stage: Involving the Community

Before creating messages to diffuse health information, health communication scholars underline the importance of conducting formative research to determine the audience characteristics and "guide strategy choices" (Dutta-Bergman, 2006, p. 11). Through several meetings with La-Mano's staff, board members, Latino Mother-Daughter conference members, opinion leaders, and Centro Campesino, I investigated the health needs of Latinos and issues more frequently present in the community. Extensive notes were taken during these meetings. Diabetes, high blood pressure, alcoholism, and teenage pregnancy were the most common and serious conditions affecting this population.

I then attended three meetings with *Las Comadres* in order to gain a better understanding of the community and its members. *Las Comadres* organizes various preventative and educational activities for the community. Among the activities are children's drawing competitions with the theme of ending domestic violence, gatherings such as women and families for a healthier youth, and soccer tournaments, just to name a few. Many of these activities involve creating a space for interpersonal connections, which, according to Dutta-Bergman (2004), is a way to obtain and share health-related information. Although *Las Comadres* use La-Mano's radio program to announce their events, they confirmed the need to engage the Latino audience more systematically.

Las Comadres and I explored ways in which the radio could be used to support the group's educational activities. Members voiced the need to raise awareness and provide knowledge of health conditions experienced locally and resources available in the community. Participants then prioritized topics and made a list of the conditions they felt affected the Latino community more deeply. Much like the previously mentioned list, the topics included diabetes, alcoholism, domestic abuse, heart problems, teenage pregnancy, and depression. Interestingly, storytelling dominated most of this task of creating this list: stories of alcoholic parents or in-laws; daughters of friends becoming pregnant at a young age; the physical wounds of abuse intertwined with their own migrant experiences. I realized these stories were filled with role models and collective healing.

Fisher (1984) states that "humans are essentially story tellers" (p. 2) and explains that stories possess a persuasive and a literary force that serve to give meaning and order to human experience. During this process, for example, one of the *Comadres* asked if diabetes was contagious. This comment triggered other members to openly asked questions such as "what is diabetes?", "how do I know if my child has it or may be predisposed to it?" Knowledge about diabetes and community resources was shared by a member dealing with the illness.

Las Comadres confirmed that the Latino community needed more information presented in a way that could be entertaining. These conversations extended to La-Mano staff, board members, and other community leaders. During these conversations, I shared ideas of different ways the radio could be used: invitations to experts, audience calls, drama, etc. I also explained the success of using drama to increase people's knowledge of health issues. In the end, the group agreed that creating a radio soap opera would be the best way to educate the community, as they felt people would be able to identify themselves through the stories.

The goal of this project was to pilot the use of a radio drama to present the audience with real stories, create identification with the characters, and generate interpersonal communication on and about the health issues present in the episodes. It was decided that on each Saturday, one hour of *La Hora Comunitaria* would be used to air an episode of the radio soap opera. After it was aired, the radio host would invite respected Latino professionals to address issues presented in the story. Experts would offer advice and additional information on community resources and encourage audience members to call in with their questions and comments.

The project began to take shape. La-Mano staff, board members, *Las Comadres*, and I agreed on a plan for this pilot project and for evaluating later its effectiveness in reaching the community. The plan included searching for health stories, experts and resources available, and leaders in different communities; planning and executing logistical aspects of radio production (selection of actors/actresses, rehearsals, recording in studio, post-production, and advertisement); and evaluating the impact of the drama based on calls to the radio, short surveys, and focus groups. Steps were then taken for acquiring IRB approval for the project. In the following section, I briefly explain how and why entertainment education works, and the uniqueness of our project.

The Making: A Community Process

Freimuth and Quinn (2004) pointed out that entertainment media are a good strategy to use with minority audiences "who are heavy consumers of this type of media" (p. 2054). Singhal and Rogers (2003) explain that entertainment education (EE) "can influence audience awareness, attitudes and behaviors toward a socially desirable end" (p. 289) and can influence the external environment at the interpersonal, social, and public levels. The success of EE lies in its narrative format, which allows the audience to follow a story/plot and transport themselves "from their real-life situations into a hypothetical situation" (Singhal and Rogers, 2003, p. 292). This format appeals to the audience's emotions, involving them with the story, and triggering interpersonal communication on and about the lifestyles of the characters. Furthermore, EE permits audiences to talk in public about topics that may be taboo. The strength of EE is that it allows audiences to enjoy a program while learning about a topic.

Our EE project is unique in five ways: (1) We started the project from the grassroots, directly involving and mobilizing community members in this process (Dutta-Bergman, 2005). (2) As with Horner and colleagues (2008), our data collection helped as a basis for developing a radio soap opera to creatively introduce knowledge, clarify misunderstandings, and trigger interpersonal communication. (3) Like *Bienvenida Salud* (McKinley and Jensen, 2003), a health initiative targeting 65 indigenous communities in the Peruvian Amazon, we used radio dramas to reach our audience. However, in the Peruvian initiative, ideas were taken from the audience, but a team of creative professionals shaped the content and format of the messages in accordance with the sponsor agency's objective to provide information about reproductive health. The content of our episodes followed audiences' real stories and were more participatory in nature. (4) The soap opera episodes were in Spanish acted by Latinos and for Latinos. (5) We used the local community radio to reach this dispersed ethnic minority.

Members of *Las Comadres* helped locate potential interviewees. Then, using a snowball technique, interviewees connected me with others willing to share their personal stories about health/healing. The process of informed consent was sought before each interview. Participants signed a consent form in Spanish and kept a copy of it.

Interviews were conducted in Spanish (the author's mother tongue), audio-taped and transcribed verbatim. In two instances, two women asked for a conjoint interview. The rest of the stories came from in-depth individual interviews. Interviews started with one open-ended question, "what is your story?" Interviewees spoke freely. I added a few probing questions (when needed) to expand on the role relationships played in their stories and why they thought their story would be important for the Latino community. They were encouraged to re-create dialogues and circumstances surrounding their stories. Data was collected between February-May 2009. Eight interviews were initially collected (102 pages of transcripts) for this pilot. I interviewed five women (9) and a man (1). All interviewees, except one, were born in Mexico and came to the United States as adults; one woman was Mexican American.

After transcriptions were completed, the author[2] drafted radio soap-opera episodes based on the interviews (moving from a synopsis, to a skeleton of the script, and finally to a fully developed script). Scripts followed real stories containing verbatim the dialogues re-enacted by participants during the interview process. I added, when needed, a few fictional aspects, grounded in the contexts and characters provided through the interview, to help with the narration of the story.

All eight copyright episodes, lasting 23–26 minutes, included: (1) an opening and closing of the radio soap opera (program title; episode's name; credits); (2) a disclaimer indicating how the author had changed personal information to protect the identity of those who shared their stories. It was, however, stated that the story was real. (2) A narrator's voice used to start and end each episode and to provide transitions throughout the story. The first season focused on: leukemia, domestic abuse, diabetes (affecting the kidneys), alcoholism, sexual marital problems, diabetes (producing blindness), congested heart failure, and teenage pregnancy (see Box 25.1).

Feedback from community members was sought to help the author make changes to improve the quality, cohesiveness, and culturally appropriate expression of the scripts. The author read the script to either the members of *Las Comadres* and/or the interviewees, whenever available.[3] Participants stopped the reading of the script to clarify meanings, change words, and/or suggest things what could be cut or expanded. As a final precaution, the author sought feedback from a Spanish soap-opera writer from Latin America.

Then the radio host from La-Mano, one member of *Las Comadres*, and a couple of volunteers helped with the logistics involved in the production. KMSU radio offered support with recording and post-production studio time. The initial contact and search for actor/actresses were channeled through *Las Comadres*. To be an actor/actress, the person had to be either Latino or Chicano, read fluently in Spanish, and be willing to volunteer their time.[4] Starting in October 2009, the actors who had been recruited met three times to rehearse the scripts. Attendance varied during those three days (from 20 to 14 people) as did their reading level. During rehearsals, I explained the characters involved in each episode, their personalities, the emotional tone, the emphasis of each scene, etc. At the third rehearsal, the acting crew was reduced to 14 people (6 men and 8 women[5]). I divided up the episodes, characters, dates, and times of our recordings. We recorded on eight days for approximately 2 ½ to 3 hours each day in the evening after work. More acting directions were given during the recordings. Then I post-produced each episode adding openings, closings, music, and sound effects. Each episode took approximately 3 hours of postproduction.

A couple of brainstorming sessions with *Las Comadres* and the actor/actresses were completed to find a proper title for the radio soap-opera. Ideas were pieced together

---

Box 25.1 Episodes in the first season

Title of episode	Main topic	Synopsis
1. "I don't want to die alone"	Leukemia	Juan Antonio's journey to bring his family to the United States as his quest for medical treatment.
2. "Please, don't hit me!"	Domestic abuse	María Lidia's story as she seeks support and abandons her abusive husband.
3. "Oh holy God!"	Type II diabetes	Roberto Carlos discovers his diabetes has led to kidney failure. His story of denials, family pressures and his road to awareness.
4. "One more drink will calm my worries"	Alcoholism	What led Pedro to alcoholism, how it impacted his and his family's life.
5. "I love you but I won't do that!"	Sexual problems	María Viviana experienced sexual problems with her newlywed husband.
6. "None of that could be true!"	Type II diabetes	Miguel Angel leaves his diabetes type II uncontrolled. His journey into blindness and recovery.
7. "I can't leave you, my love!"	Congestive heart failure	This story shows how Juan Gabriel seeks treatments, negotiates advance directives, and accepts death.
8. "How much is a little?"	Teenage pregnancy	Claudia Patricia's struggle as a 15 year-old mother with dreams of going to college.

---

until the title was formed: "Pruebas del destino: Historias de amor, dolor y sanación" [Test of destiny: Stories of love, suffering, and healing]. Radio announcements, flyers, and word of mouth were used to publicize the program. The first season ran November–December 2009. The same season was rerun starting March 6, 2010. In February 2010, succinct information about the soap-opera's episodes was posted on La-Mano's web site, with a calendar of new emissions and a link to the radio.

In the next section, I explain how each radio episode was intended to produce vicarious learning and the identification of the audience with the plot and characters.

Theories Behind the Project

The goal of each episode was to persuade the audience to identify with the characters and plot of each story and to introduce information (i.e. what a battered woman should do; what diabetes means and how it can affect your health, etc.). First, each story fit the major principles behind social learning theory (Bandura, 1977), later called social cognitive theory (Bandura, 1986). Bandura (1977) states that human behavior can be explained as "a continuous and reciprocal interaction between cognitive, behavioral, and environmental determinants" (Preface). In his view, individuals learn from observation and direct experience from other "people's behavior and its consequences for them" (Bandura, 1986, p. 19). This learning is internally processed serving as a model that guides future behaviors. Bandura (1977) explains that individuals learn from "association patterns" (p. 24). These models influence what "people will observe and which they will disregard" (p. 24). The functions of modeling, Bandura (1986) continues, are for individuals to learn "new patterns of behaviors, judgmental standards, cognitive competencies, and generative rules for creating new behavior" (p. 49); to strengthen or discard certain observed behaviors; to provide examples of behaviors the learner has not yet performed; and to act as "prompts for similar action" (p. 50). Nevertheless, mere exposition is not an absolute condition for producing observational learning, as the reinforcement of those observational models is needed. Sometimes this reinforcement is obtained when the behavior is perceived as producing positive and beneficial rewards (punishment/reward).

Each episode contained positive, negative, and neutral characters (Sabido's methodology cited in Greiner, Singhal, and Hurlburt, 2007). Positive characters served to model the behavior or educational objective (e.g., the benefits of following a diet and exercising to control the diabetes; inquiry about birth control methods; etc.); negative characters were those who rejected a healthy behavior or educational objective (e.g., Pedro continues drinking; María Lidia's husband and his friends talk about how to control their women; having unprotected sex, etc.). Neutral characters were those who were middle ground but transitioned at the end towards the positive behavior (e.g., the children of Roberto, in Episode 3, slowly realized the importance of diet, exercise, and doctor's consultations to control their dad's diabetes; Claudia realizes the importance of safe sex and family planning in Episode 8). The invitation of a community expert after each story served to reinforce the positive behaviors reflected in the story, in addition to providing more information and indicating community resources available. For example, during the episode on domestic violence a toll-free number for abuse and crime prevention was given repeatedly for people to call if they were victims of abuse or violence.

In the health context, Bandura (2004) argues that *knowledge of health benefits and risks* of a specific health practice is one of the core determinants, and first step for change. Unless individuals understand how a specific behavior or lifestyle is unhealthy, they will not be motivated to change it. For example, in Episodes 3 and 6, the main characters did not realize how their lifestyle (eating habits, lack of exercise, stress, and lack of prevention) left their type II diabetes uncontrolled, producing serious consequences (renal failure, blindness). This realization was the first step for change. Similarly, knowledge about resources for battered women and how to report violent incidents to the police were important steps in Episode 2 to prepare the character for a change. However, knowledge is not enough to produce change. Bandura states that "Beliefs of personal efficacy play a central role in personal change" (2004, p. 144). The perception that one has *self-efficacy*, meaning the capacity to control one's health habits and therefore to produce positive effects, appeared in each of the stories of the soap opera. For example, in Episode 7 the characters try to control their situation by seeking treatments to improve Juan Gabriel's congested heart failure condition.

"*Outcome expectations*," which are a person's expectations regarding the benefits and costs of changing the behavior are another important aspect of moving individuals to action, according to Bandura (2004, p. 144). The outcomes may be social approval or disapproval, material and affective losses, as well as positive and negative reactions towards one's health status. Unable to stop her husband from beating her and her children, María Lidia (Episode 2) realizes she has lost everything and decides to take action.

Health goals also play an important role in motivating people to take action and produce changes in their health status (Bandura, 2004). The desire to stay alive to see their children grow motivated the characters with type II diabetes to change their lifestyles; similarly to the characters in Episodes 1 and 7.

The last determinant, Bandura (2004) states, is "*the perceived facilitators and social and structural impediments* to the change they seek" (p. 144, italics in original). Characters in many of the episodes experienced lack of health insurance, lack of money, illegal status, discrimination, lack of English fluency, and lack of transportation as the major impediments to their treatment/healing. However, these characters sought help and found resources available in their communities. Experts invited after the airing of each episode, were also used to share information about community resources available.

Second, each episode was intended to produce identification between the audience, plot and characters (Cohen, 2001). *Identification* is a powerful persuasive tool. Cohen (2001) explains that identification focuses on "feeling with the character rather than about the character" (p. 251), which implies an emotional and cognitive connection with the character. According Cohen, the outcomes of identification "may include liking or imitation [… or] negative feelings" (p. 252). He also states that narrative genres are more likely to produce identification. The more similar the audience thinks they are to the character, the more likely that identification will occur. Similarly, Cohen explains that some scholars have hypothesized that "perceived realism of a character will promote identification" (p. 259). Some evidence that identification between audience members and the characters occurred came from our initial assessment. This identification might be triggered by the fact that the soap opera episodes came from real, culturally bound stories based on topics Latinos perceived to be important for their community.

Evaluating the Project

Several methods were used to obtain feedback from the audience. We created an online survey with 10 questions, available through La-Mano's web site. The survey contained demographic information (gender and age), three closed-ended questions to determine the number of episodes listened to, and how the person knew about the soap-opera, and who they listened the soap-opera with, and six open-ended questions regarding favorite episode. More specifically, what they recalled about the episode, if the episode made them think about their personal life, what they learned from the episode, and who (if applicable) they talked to about this episode and what they talked about.

In addition, we created an anonymous 22-question printed survey available at the La-Mano's office for the general public. The survey expanded the questions from the online survey to determine message exposure, message comprehension, and identification with the stories/characters (Is there any aspect of the episode/s that reminds you of your own life? Why?). In addition, we were interested in determining topics they would like to learn more about and why.

Not surprisingly, the responses to surveys were scarce. Only one online survey and two printed surveys were completed. Two of these surveys were completed by women. These participants were between 37 and 50 years of age and self-identified as Hispanics. They listened to soap opera via the radio and the Web. Each of the participants identified a different episode of their preference (*leukemia; domestic abuse and diabetes*). When asked what impacted them from the stories, responses varied depending on what episode they preferred: "how important it is to live," "diabetes is a condition that is not easy to control," "the spouse that abuses his wife, and that there is help in the community."

When asked if there was anything in the episodes that reminded them of their own life, participants responded: "yes. Coming to this country alone without my family," "men think that they can abuse their woman." When asked what they learned from the story, respondents explained "how to search for help or clinics," "not to be afraid to ask for help," "resources available for battered women." The two women listened to the radio program with their families. One of them talked to her children about the episode and about the importance of valuing life. The man listened to the program with his workmates and commented with them "that we'd better think what we are doing." Only one of the participants mentioned she would like to hear more about heart problems.

Another method used was a five-question phone survey[6] to be used with those radio callers who self-identified as listeners to the soap opera. Questions included demographic information (gender, age, and county) followed by "Did you listen to the radio soap opera?" (yes or no); "Who did you listen it with?" (alone, with family, with friends, with coworkers); "What did you learn?" (open-ended); "evaluation of the episode" (excellent, very good, not interested); and finally a space for additional comments. Around 25 percent of the general calls each Saturday were about the soap opera.

Results showed a total of 30 callers (16 men and 14 women)[7]: all self-identified as Latinos; most of them listened to the program with family (12), friends (7), coworkers (5), or alone (6). It is noteworthy that two of those callers were from Texas, as they accessed the radio online. Nineteen callers thought the soap opera was "excellent" while 11 rated it as "very good." Callers claimed to have learned different things. Some comments focused on the value of information and the educative quality of the soap opera. "I am an old person and I hope younger people listen to these stories"; "The information presents things similar to a case in real life"; "It offers us information that we should take into consideration. We should seek information"; "In Mexico I used to watched soap operas about love and violence but these ones are more educative." "The topic is very sad. Therefore I need to enjoy life" (referring to Episode 7).

Others were more specific about what they learned from the episodes: "I listened to the episode about alcoholism when we were driving. With my friends we talked about it and wondered how the actors had the courage to participate. I wish that all of us listeners had more respect"; "I really like the radionovela because it is very educative. I have to pay more attention to my diet due to the topic of diabetes"; "this is the first time I listened to the novela. I learned that diabetes can ruin your health"; "I have to find recipes to cook better food"; "I learned to respect women more." "I have to teach my girls to talk about topics related to sexual education"; "Nobody ever talked to me about sex education"; "Youngsters should learn about these types of topics and one – as a parent – should talk to our children about them too"(referring to Episode 8).

Others expressed general opinions about it or what they would do with the information: "All my friends and I were talking about the episode and made comments about it"; "The novelas make sense about our own lives ..."; "I always listen to the soap operas"; "Thanks to God I have not experienced the things that happened to the people in the novela." One of the callers established a clear connection with the characters stating that she learned "the experience of life. I love listening to them. I cry when I see children involved or when an adult dies." A female caller asked that more information about sex education for boys be given.

Do and Kincaid (2006) argue that entertainment education, in particular, is expected to trigger interpersonal communication. This idea was reflected by additional comments some people made about their intention to talk to others about the soap opera, for example, "I will tell my neighbors to listen to it"; "I will recommend this program to other people"; "I will share this information with my friends." All of these instances involved talking about the topic of the radionovela with someone else, reflecting the collective self-construals of Hispanics (Oetzel *et al.*, 2007); in some instances some level of identification has occurred (Cohen, 2001).

It was clear that individuals found some information useful and intended to talk to someone about it. A couple of focus groups were scheduled after the second-running of the season. However, none of them were accomplished due to a lack of organizational capacity from this NGO. In the following section, I address what was learned from this project in terms of its opportunities and obstacles, and offer recommendations.

Discussion and Implications: Opportunities, Obstacles, and Recommendations

EE is a communication strategy aimed at promoting knowledge and attitude and/or behavior change through the use of media that simultaneously entertains and educates (Singhal and Rogers, 2003). As aforementioned, EE was utilized successfully in many health interventions around the world; nevertheless, few health initiatives in the United States have employed EE. A few of those interventions targeted Latinos accomplishing moderate success (Perez *et al.*, 2008; Willkin *et al.*, 2007).

Our goal was to find more creative ways to reach the widely dispersed and largely illiterate Latino population of southern Minnesota through a local Spanish radio show *La Hora Comunitaria* (*The Community Hour*). This population experiences many barriers to accessing healthcare and education about preventative health. Thus, we created an EE project that included a soap opera (based on a real story) and a space for dialogue about the health issues presented in the episodes, conversations led by credible professionals from the community and the radio hosts. Our purpose was to communicate health knowledge through real stories and experts, to create audience identification with the stories, and to trigger interpersonal communication on and about the episodes. Ultimately, we created a virtual space for Latinos, outside of mainstream media, to voice their concerns and discuss health-related issues and behaviors, and learn about resources available in the community.

Our audience responded positively to the soap opera pointing out its educative value and emotional connections to stories. To generate this virtual space, following the advice of Dutta-Bergman (2005), we used the culture-centered approach. In his view, "instead of speaking for the subaltern, the culture-centered approach focuses on creating conduits for the expression of the subaltern voice" (pp. 116–117). This project accomplished that; functioning as a conduit and/or giving voice to participants' health stories and allowing them to share those stories with members of the Latino community. Each drama reflected many of the various factors that affect the health of Latinos along with their cultural attitudes towards health, illness, and healing (Freimund and Quinn, 2004). The health stories were embedded in participants' experiences as immigrants, and their struggles to adapt to a new cultural milieu while maintaining important Hispanics collective values (such as family, religion, trust, sympathy, etc.).

Soap opera stories fit the major principles behind social learning theory, later called social cognitive theory (Bandura, 1977, 1986). The stories were filled with role models, recognition of benefits and risks of certain health behaviors, and discussions about structural elements that helped/hindered characters' change (Bandura, 2004). Do and Kincaid (2006) pointed out four ways in which EE can be successfully applied to drama. Those four suggestions were present in this project which included – (1) appropriate health information, (2) persuasive messages about new ideas, (3) the modeling of desired health behavior, and (4) the integration of desired behaviors within the plots of our soap opera episodes via character interactions and/or relationships. More to the point, the soap opera stories contained fear messages, messages from family and friends directly from participants' own life experiences, which made the episodes more credible to audience members and suitable for varied levels of acculturation (Oetzel *et al.*, 2007).

As a way of enhancing the learning process, we used both *homophily* (through a Latino's story) and *heterophily* (through an expert opinion) (Rogers, 1995) to successfully reach our audience. More specifically, we invited respected professionals (Hispanic family doctors, a psychologist, a case worker, and several advocates) after each soap opera episode was aired, to offer more explanations about specific conditions, recommendations, and the availability of local resources. It was our hope to generate dialogue about these issues with family and friends. Evidence shows this happened.

This project included the active participation of more than 40 community members who volunteered their time, resources, and connections to support this initiative (e.g., members of *Las Comadres*, board members, radio staff, interviewees, experts, and community actors/actresses). Mobilizing the Latino community in this area illustrates what Dutta-Bergman (2005) stated about bridging the theory and practice of health prevention from a grassroots and culture-centered perspective – creating a design that reflected the needs of the Hispanic community. We tried to make this process as participatory as possible and shaped by various community members. Working from the grassroots and using small media offer a unique opportunity to mobilize an interesting variety of organizations serving Latinos and the potential for creating synergy among their objectives and collective activities. Again, most importantly, it also enabled members of this minority group to have a voice and create community.

The assessment demonstrated that the program reached Latinos from Blue Earth, Le Seur, Faribault, Freeborn, Nicollet, Olmstead, Rice, Sibley, Steele, Waseca, and Watonwan counties in Minnesota. In general, listeners gave very positive evaluations, which seems to support what Dutta-Bergman (2006) stated, that audience members choose media programs and content that is congruent "with existing beliefs, attitudes, and behaviors" (p. 12). We found evidence that audience members learned information about a health condition or available resources from the program. For the future, it will be important to know what learning occurred through this project and what prior knowledge was reinforced. This said, the phone survey questionnaire requires revision so that callers can more clearly state what they recall from the episodes and what new information was learned. We also need to add to our evaluation a few questions to assess what people learned from expert sources.

Next, as stated earlier, the organization (*La-Mano*) was unable to coordinate focus group interviews that would have allowed us to access richer data. Similar to Boulay *et al.* (2002), Shefner-Rogers and Sood (2004), Sood *et al.* (2006) and others, we know that, based on callers' feedback[8], interpersonal communication occurred during and after the broadcast. We also hope to learn more about how communication regarding the episodes occurred and what people talked about. We also found evidence that the stories triggered the audience's emotional connection with the plot. Callers stated that the stories made them cry, made them respect others/life, and/or simply reminded them of their own life stories.

Third, the design included only the use of the radio, which has the potential to reach this dispersed audience. However, we did not account for other ways to process and reinforce messages. For instance, several successful health interventions (Bosch, 2006; Maxwell *et al.*, 2003; McKinley and Jensen, 2003, and others) designed ways to engage the audience through interpersonal means. Shefner-Rogers and Sood (2004) state that interventions need to "go beyond direct exposure to evaluate the effects of mass media interventions" (p. 256). Along with using the radio, we need to establish ways to process the information in this EE with audience members and/or work with churches, nonprofit and/or governmental organizations to foster dialogue among the Latino communities they serve.

Lastly, one of the major challenges experienced, however, was to work on the design, implementation, and evaluation of this pilot within the context of a small nonprofit organization and with limited resources. Our project was solely sustained by volunteers. Wray *et al.* (2004), after evaluating the results of a violence prevention intervention by means of a radio drama became "skeptical of voluntarism as a means of assuring substantial exposure to social messages" (p. 49). They found that campaign drama spots were not aired as planned. During our rerun, we encountered several obstacles (e.g., inability to air one episode due to technical problems; lack of community experts to speak after episodes were aired; lack of training on how to survey the audience, etc.). Voluntarism is neither sustainable nor desirable. We believe there is local capacity if we work cooperatively with other organizations, but not if we continue the project in isolation. Resources should be sought in order to continue and expand this pilot.

In sum, there is an untapped potential for reaching the scattered Latino audience of rural southeastern Minnesota and giving them voice through radio and EE. According to O'Guinn and Meyer (1984), Spanish-language radio "offers an opportunity for Hispanics to maintain, reestablish, or simply be reminded of a cultural or subcultural identity" (p. 14). Ramos Rodriguez (2005) concurred that music and stories in the native language help create "a self-worth of one's own culture" (p. 165). Our project was unique in that it started within this ethnic minority community, it was based on people's real stories, it was performed by Latinos and for Latinos, and through a small media it created a virtual space that was nonexistent before. We believe that working cooperatively among varied Latino community organizations and resources could move our project forward.

Notes

1   The terms Latinos and Hispanics are used interchangeably referring to those with ethnic origins from Central and South America, the Caribbean, and/or Spain.
2   The author has experience in script writing and soap opera production.
3   On three occasions the interviewees were unavailable to provide feedback on the script.
4   One European American actor, a volunteer from La-Mano, was used to help with scenes representing American professionals.
5   Two Mexican Americans, 6 Mexicans, 1 Colombian, 1 Guatemalan, 1 Honduran, and 1 European American.
6   The phone survey was implemented during the rerun.
7   General calls to the radio program varied from 15 up to 22 per Saturday. Callers solicited music, sent varied greetings to relatives or friends, inquired about information, or made comments about the radionovela.
8   Twenty-four out of 30 callers listened to the episodes with family, friends, or coworkers.

References

Bandura, A. (1977). *Social Learning Theory.* Englewood Cliffs, NJ: Prentice-Hall.

Bandura, A. (1986). *Social Foundations of Thought and Action: A Social Cognitive Theory.* Englewood Cliffs, NJ: Prentice Hall.

Bandura, A. (2004). Health promotion by social cognitive means. *Health, Education and Behavior, 31*(2), 143–164.

Bosch, T. E. (2006). "AIDS is gold. HIV is platinum": Bush radio use of the entertainment education strategy. *Postamble, 2*(2), 28–44.

Boulay, M., Torey, J. D. S., and Sood, S. (2002). Indirect exposure to a family planning mass media campaign in Nepal. *Journal of Health Communication, 7,* 379–399.

Chicano Latino Affairs Council, State of Minnesota (2009). A Latino health report. Identifying barriers and solutions to reduce health care disparities. Retrieved from http://www.clac.state.mn.us/pdf/CLAC%20Health%20Report.pdf

Cohen, J. (2001). Defining identification: A theoretical look at the identification of audiences with media characters. *Mass Communication and Society,* 4(3), 2450–2464.

Do, M. P., and Kincaid, L. (2006). Impact of an entertainment-education television drama on health knowledge and behavior in Bangladesh: An application of propensity score matching. *Journal of Health Communication, 11,* 301–325.

Dutta-Bergman, M. J. (2004). Primary source of health information: Comparisons in the domain of health attitudes, health cognitions, and health behaviors. *Health Communication, 16*(3), 273–288.

Dutta-Bergman, M. J. (2005). Theory and practice in health communication campaigns: A critical interrogation. *Health Communication, 18*(2), 102–122.

Dutta-Bergman, M. J. (2006). A formative approach to strategic message targeting through soap operas: Using selective processing theories. *Health Communication, 19*(1), 11–18.

Echo Media Print Media Solutions. (2010). Hispanics. Retrieved from http://www.echo-media.com/targetcat.asp?TargetType=ETHNI

Fisher, W. R. (1984). Narration as a human communication paradigm. The case of public moral argument. *Communication Monographs, 51,* 1–22.

Frates, J., Bohrer, G. G., and Thomas, D. (2006). Promoting organ donation to Hispanics: The role of the media and medicine. *Journal of Health Communication, 11,* 683–698.

Freimuth, V. S. and Quinn, S. C. (2004). The contributions of health communication to eliminating health disparities. *American Journal of Public Health, 94,* 2053–2055.

Golstein, S., Usdin, S., Scheepers, E., and Japhet, G. (2005). Communicating HIV and AIDS, What works? A report on the impact evaluation of Soul City's fourth series. *Journal of Health Communication, 10,* 465–483.

Greiner, K., Singhal, A. and Hurlburt, S. (2007, May). "With an antenna we can stop the practice of female genital cutting": A participatory assessment of *Ashreat al Amal,* an entertainment-education radio soap opera in Sudan. Paper presented at the 57th Annual Meeting of the International Communication Association, San Francisco, CA. Retrieved from http://manglar.uninorte.edu.co/handle/10584/1039

Hether, H., Huang, G. C., Beck, V., Murphy, S.T. and Valente, T. W. (2008). Entertainment-education in a media-saturated environment: Examining the impact of single and multiple exposures to breast cancer storylines on two popular medical dramas. *Journal of Health Communication, 13,* 808–823.

Horner, J. R., Romer, D., Vanable, P. A. *et al.* (2008). Using culture-centered qualitative formative research to design broadcast messages for HIV prevention for African American adolescents. *Journal of Health Communication, 13,* 309–325.

La-Mano Inc. (2010). History. Retrieved from http://www.lamanomn.com

Maxwell, K., Borwanker, R., and Gonzalez Yucra, O. (2003). Evaluation of a Bolivian radio broadcasting campaign: "For stronger and healthier children." Paper presented at the 53rd Annual Meeting of the International Communication Association, San Diego, CA, May 27.

McKinley, M. A. and Jensen, L. O. (2003). In our own voices: Reproductive health radio programming in the Peruvian Amazon. *Critical Studies in Media Communication, 20*(2), 180–203.

McLean, S. (1997). A communication analysis of community mobilization on the Warm Springs Indian reservation. *Journal of Health Communication, 2,* 113–125.

Oetzel, J., DeVargas, F., Ginossar, T., and Sanchez, C. (2007). Hispanic women's preferences for breast health information: Subjective cultural influences on source, message, and channel. *Health Communication, 21*(3), 223–233.

O'Guinn, T. C. and Meyer, T. P. (1984). Segmenting the Hispanic market: The use of Spanish-language radio. *Journal of Advertising Research, 23*(6), 9–16.

Perez, F., Dena, S., Witherspoon, P. *et al.* (2008). Entertainment education in a radio spot campaign: Hispanics and childhood obesity in El Regalo de Salud. Paper presented at the 58th Annual Meeting of the International Communication Association, Montreal, Canada. May 22–26.

Porto, M. P. (2007). Fighting AIDS among adolescent women: Effects of a public communication campaign in Brazil *Journal of Health Communication, 12,* 121–132.

Ramos Rodriguez, J. M. (2005). Indigenous radio stations in Mexico: A catalyst for social cohesion and cultural strength. *The Radio Journal – International Studies in Broadcast and Audio Media, 3*(3), 155–169.

Reed, M. and Hanson, R. E. (2006). Back to the future: Allegheny mountain radio and localism in West Virginia community radio. *Journal of Radio Studies 13*(2), 214–231.

Rogers, E. M. (1995). *Diffusion of Innovations.* New York: Free Press.

Shefner-Rogers, C. and Sood, S. (2004). Involving husbands in safe motherhood: Effects of the SUAMI SIAGA campaign in Indonesia. *Journal of Health Communication, 9,* 233–258.

Singhal, A. and Rogers, E. (2003). *Combating Aids. Communication Strategies in Action.* New Delhi, India: Sage Publications.

Smaida, S. A., Blewett, L. A., Carrizales, P. J., and Robert, R. A. (2002). Disparities in health access: Voices from Minnesota's Latino community. Retrieved from HACER http://www.hacer-mn.org/downloads/English_Reports/DisparitiesHealthAccess.pdf

Smith, R. A., Downs, E. and Witte, K. (2007). Drama theory and entertainment education: Exploring the effects of a radio drama on behavioral intentions to limit HIV transmission in Ethiopia. *Communication Monographs, 74*(2), 133–153.

Sood, S., Shefner-Rogers, C. L. and Sengupta, M. (2006). The impact of a mass media campaign on HIV/AIDS knowledge and behavior change in North India: Results from a longitudinal study. *Asian Journal of Communication, 16*(3), 231–250.

US Bureau of Census (2010). The Hispanic Population: 2010. Census brief. Retrieved from http://www.census.gov/prod/cen2010/briefs/c2010br-04.pdf

US Bureau of Census (2009). *American community survey 2005–2006.* Retrieved from http://www.census.gov/

Valente, T. W., Murphy, S., Hunag, G. *et al.* (2007). Evaluating a minor storyline on ER about teen obesity, hypertension, and 5 a day. *Journal of Health Communication, 12,* 551–566.

Vaughan, P. W., Rogers, E. M., Singhal, A., and Swalehe, R. M. (2000). Entertainment-education and HIV/AIDS prevention: A field experiment in Tanzania. *Journal of Health Communication, 5,* 81–100.

Willkin, H. A., Valente, T. W., Murphy, M. *et al.* (2007). Does entertainment-education work with Latinos in the United States? Identification and the effects of a telenovela breast cancer storyline. *Journal of Health Communication, 12,* 455–469.

Wray, R. J., Hornik, R. M., Gandy, O. H. *et al.* (2004). Preventing domestic violence in the African American community: Assessing the impact of a dramatic radio serial. *Journal of Health Communication, 9,* 32–52.

26

"Children can't wait"
Social Mobilization to Secure Children's Rights to Social Security

Shereen Usdin and Nicola Christofides

Introduction

The Alliance for Children's Entitlement to Social Security (ACESS) was formed against the backdrop of new government programs in South Africa that were offering some social security to the most vulnerable of children. The provisions were far from sufficient and – for a range of reasons – not easily accessible to the majority of targeted children. ACESS is a coalition of over 1,500 organizations in South Africa mobilizing for a comprehensive package of social security for children that will secure their constitutional rights.

Alliance building was the hallmark of the anti-apartheid struggle, often described as one of the most powerful social mobilization efforts of the late twentieth century. The defeat of apartheid was the result of the combined efforts of the liberation movements, the mass mobilization of ordinary South Africans, together with trade unions, professional and academic groupings, nongovernmental organizations, faith- and community-based organizations, arts, cultural, sporting, and other sectors as well as international solidarity actions, such as sanctions, with the global anti-apartheid movement. ACESS has continued this tradition of combining "people power" with more centralized organizational forms to mobilize successfully for the constitutional rights of children in the post-apartheid era.

This chapter describes the social mobilization experience of ACESS together with that of one of its founder organizations, the Soul City Institute for Health and Development Communication (Soul City Institute). It explores some of the complexities involved in the social mobilization process, including challenges specifically related to mobilizing in the context of an alliance.

The Handbook of Global Health Communication, First Edition. Edited by Rafael Obregon and Silvio Waisbord.

Children's rights to social security

Millions of children in South Africa face harsh circumstances despite living in a middle-income country. Apartheid left a legacy of grinding poverty and inequity. Although many gains have been made since the advent of democracy, a range of factors have combined to deepen inequality with South Africa having the highest Gini Coefficient in the world. In 1999, there were 10.2 million children (0–18 years) in South Africa, 60–70 percent of whom were living in poverty. One in four households experienced food hunger, and one in five children was stunted due to malnutrition.

The critical role of social security in alleviating some of these challenges has been widely recognized. There is strong evidence that the Child Support Grant (CSG) in particular, results in increases in height-for-age (an important indicator of child well-being) and in the level of school enrolment both for the immediate child beneficiary and other children in the household.[1] Children who receive the CSG are more likely to stay in school, concentrate in class, and pass exams. Without it, many children cannot pay for transport, food, books, or stationery. Additionally, grants have proven to have a developmental effect, promoting economic engagement and financing job seeking as opposed to the often widely held view that they promote dependency (Posel, Fairbairn, and Lund, 2004). Social grants play a major role in realizing a range of children's rights enshrined in our constitution, including the right to social assistance, equality, education, food, health, housing, water, dignity, and protection from abuse and neglect.

The CSG was introduced by the new democratic government for destitute caregivers of children under seven years old. However, millions of children (defined by the Convention on the Rights of the Child as young people up to 18 years) over seven years old were also destitute. Tragically, even eligible children faced substantial barriers to accessing the CSG. Of the three million eligible children under seven, only 40 percent accessed the grant. The most significant of these barriers was, and remains, the lack of identity documents and birth certificates, both necessary to obtain the CSG. At the time, only 51 percent of all children had birth certificates (Smart, 1999). To get these documents, caregivers often have to wait years, incurring unaffordable costs including multiple trips to faraway government offices and suffering bureaucratic delays and corruption at the same time. Yet, as meager as the grant is, it has the potential to provide a lifeline for millions in the context of massive unemployment.

Government's adoption of a neoliberal macroeconomic policy has been blamed in large part for the growing inequality in South Africa. The AIDS epidemic has been a major cofactor. With a prevalence rate of over 11 percent and more than five million people living with HIV, the country's epidemic has impacted substantially on children. Pushing millions of families deeper into poverty, it places children at risk of HIV transmission through lowered physical immunity related to malnutrition. Income inequality also increases the likelihood of the early onset of sexual activity. This sexual activity is often linked to high rates of transactional sex and multiple concurrent sexual partnerships – all recognized as drivers of the epidemic in South Africa. Additionally, when caregivers living in poverty become sick with AIDS, it is often their children, in the absence of sufficient social and health services, who must care for them. Relatives and other community members are often the only safety net for children who have lost both parents to AIDS. Taking children into their own homes often deepens their poverty and impacts on the existing children in their households.

The birth of ACESS

In 2001, the Soul City Institute for Health and Development Communication, a South African NGO, initiated a program to support children infected and affected by HIV and AIDS. Formative research identified social security grants as critical to address both immediate and longer term development needs of children living in poverty and those made vulnerable by the epidemic.

The Soul City Institute's strategy is based on a socio-ecological model. Its programs operate at multiple levels that focus on the individual, the broader community, as well as the sociopolitical environment. It combines the use of edutainment programming (weaving social issues into prime time television and radio drama and reality shows) with advocacy for healthy public policy. Social mobilization is also a key component of its strategy. Social mobilization functions both as a policy advocacy tool as well as an intervention in its own right to support communities to take control over matters affecting their health as active agents of change. Going beyond simple "information transfer," mass media programs role-model positive behavior and inspire local communities to take action to solve health and social problems.

The Soul City Institute's programs reach over 80 percent of South Africans through a range of different platforms, including prime time television and radio dramas, a TV reality "community makeover" show, radio talk shows, booklets and life-skills material for schools (Shisana *et al.*, 2009). Its social mobilization initiatives include Kwanda Communities and Soul Buddyz Clubs at schools as well as training communities in media advocacy. (These initiatives are described in boxes below.) The Soul City Institute's operating principle is to form partnerships with other organizations involved in social mobilization to deepen and sustain its social change programs. The formation of ACESS arose in part through this approach.

In developing its HIV and AIDS initiative, the Soul City Institute sought the support of the Children's Institute (CI) and the Children's Rights Centre (CRC), to explore ways to address children's access to social security. The CI is a policy research and advocacy unit at the University of Cape Town, and the CRC is an NGO with specific experience in mobilizing child participation, an important ACESS principle.

The CRC and CI were already engaged in debates to influence the Taylor Committee of Inquiry into a Comprehensive Social Security System to address the plight of South Africans living in poverty. There was a concern that the Taylor Committee's work had not focused sufficiently on children. At the request of the above three organizations, the Committee funded a national consultative summit of organizations working to support children's rights to help formulate its policy recommendations. The summit brought together key stakeholders – from nongovernmental organizations (NGOs), Community Based Organizations (CBOs), faith-based organizations (FBOs), service providers, and members of Parliament. This was the genesis of ACESS. The summit recommended the formation of an alliance of the broad array of civil society role-players to promote a comprehensive social security system for children. The three convening organizations were mandated to build ACESS to ensure the summit's recommendations were incorporated into the Committee's report. Ultimately, the organizations were to ensure the implementation of these recommendations through the passage of appropriate policy and legislation, resource allocation and service delivery. Most of the Summit's recommendations found their way into the Taylor Report, which was published in 2001. ACESS produced a simple summary of the Report for its members so that they could begin to advocate for its translation into law.

This marked the beginning of ACESS members' lengthy struggle to secure a comprehensive social security system for children. Almost a decade since its formation, ACESS has grown into a national alliance of more than 1,500 children's sector organizations and activists and is now a registered NGO, legally able to fundraise for its activities. Member organizations are drawn from across South Africa; small and large, urban and rural, CBOs, FBOs, NGOs, social security service providers, academic institutions, and research bodies. They are all working towards a comprehensive social security package that fulfills children's constitutional rights. Members also include grass roots social movements such as the New Women's Movement (NWM) and the Treatment Action Campaign (TAC) which advocates, inter alia, for universal access to treatment for AIDS.

ACESS campaigns

ACESS has a number of campaigns that run concurrently. The two described in this chapter illustrate the alliance's approach to social mobilization. These campaigns are:

- To increase the age of eligibility of the CSG in the existing Social Assistance Act to cover all children in need, up to age 18.
- To remove barriers in the regulations to the Social Assistance Act to increase access for those already eligible.

Government argued that it could not afford to extend the existing CSG provisions and should rather focus its expenditure on stimulating economic engagement. Economic growth would benefit the poor in the longer term and be more sustainable. Challenging this, ACESS's campaign to increase the age of the CSG to 18 came together under the slogan "Children Can't Wait." ACESS argued that, historically, "trickle-down economics" have not delivered and that children can't wait. Childhood deprivation causes irreversible harm and children's rights to social security are enshrined in South Africa's Constitution.

The campaign approach combined a "partnership" with government to improve existing grant delivery as well as more confrontational tactics such as public protest and litigation. It also brought together the combined impact of inputs from various members, all bringing unique contributions to the campaign.

Social Mobilization Activities

Social mobilization activities relating to the ACESS campaigns operated at multiple levels. There was community based action orchestrated by ACESS members at the grass-roots as well as national and provincial level efforts. There were also mass media components that served as a catalyst for wide-scale mobilization. All these levels were mutually reinforcing and combined in a manner such that the impact of its "whole was greater than the sum of its parts".

Mobilizing through prime time dramas and children's clubs

Information on grants was woven into all Soul City Institute mass media initiatives to create both awareness and demand. The dramas were also designed to inspire audiences to mobilize for these rights. ACESS campaign demands were also integrated into the activities of the Soul Buddyz Club project. The club project mobilizes children to be active agents for social change and is modeled on the story of the Soul Buddyz television and radio drama series.

The series is about a group of children who form a club at their school to try to right the many wrongs they see in their communities. They do this through adventures, detective work, and other collective activities. The notion of child activism resonated powerfully among children, and they started writing in large numbers to the Soul City Institute to find out how to form real clubs in their schools. There are now over 6,000 such Clubs throughout the country, with over 110,000 participating children. The clubs meet weekly and the Soul City Institute provides learning and motivational materials to the clubs that mesh with the dramas and brings together club members through district, provincial and national meetings. The children initiate and run their club themselves. (See Box 26.1 for an example of how children mobilized around grants in their community).

Mobilizing children and members to tell their stories in support of the campaigns

The Children's Rights Centre led a process to help children relate their own experiences of grant access. Hundreds of children across South Africa were mobilized by ACESS member organizations to contribute their stories to a book to give to politicians. Representatives were nominated by the children to travel to parliament to present the book and to persuade parliamentarians to influence social security legislation.

Later, the Children's Institute collated ACESS members' experiences of the barriers to grant delivery into case studies which were sent out to major stakeholders and opinion leaders in government and civil society. These case studies were used in ACESS litigation activities (see below).

Reality shows and social mobilization

Kwanda is a community "makeover" reality television show developed by Soul City Institute, in partnership with the Department of Social Development (DSD) and a development agency called Eventually Africa. On Kwanda, communities mobilize to transform their environments for the better. They participate in a process known as the Organization Workshop, which was developed by the Latin American development

Box 26.1   Children's mobilizations around grants

Soul Buddyz Club action for the right to the CSG

The Ntuthuko Primary School Soul Buddyz Club is situated in a remote rural area in South Africa. One of the Club members stopped attending school and her fellow club members discovered that she was sick with AIDS. They also found out that her grandmother could not afford to care for her properly and had sent her to live with nuns in a nearby mission. She had tried unsuccessfully for over five years to get the CSG for her grandchild. As part of its contribution to the ACESS campaigns, the Soul City Institute asked Clubs to submit ideas around social grant action and the best ideas would be broadcast on national television. One of the Ntuthuko Primary School Club's ideas was to help their friend's grandmother access the CSG. Their plan was to use the presence of the cameras to "shame" the government officials into speeding up the grant process. At the Home Affairs office, backed up by the camera crew, the Buddyz Club explained to the government officials why they were there. The officials had no choice but to expedite the process. The Club members' collective efforts had set a precedent for speeding up other grant applications in their community. Their story was broadcast on national television inspiring viewers to mobilize and get government departments to deliver on their rights.

Buddyz Club Letter Campaign to the President

The Soul City Institute also encouraged Buddyz Clubs to conduct research in their communities around grant access and to write letters to the South African President about their findings and their concerns. The Soul City Institute organized for the Club with the winning letter to meet the President and to present their issues directly to him. The winning letter is included below:

Sesalong Primary School, Box 32, Bochum, 0790

Hi Mr President

We are the "Small Buddyz". We live in Buffelshoek in Limpopo Province. We once so (sic) you when you visited our place in 2001. But we were very young. As you have seen, our area ... needs a lot of improvement. We hope you will be the one to come to our rescue. We seriously need your help.... People are suffering from poverty because most of our people have no jobs, housing, food, health care and some of the children are unable to go to school......................Our school starts at 07H45 and we come home at 15h00 without something to eat nor drink. Can we concentrate in class. No! We will be hungry and thirsty. It is said that applying for the Child Grant is free. We have to pay R40 to the Tribal Office for application forms to be filled. As such, the following children had to suffer...... Their mother can not apply for the grant because she does not have R40. Their father is ill. They only rely on her grandmother for food and she has a lot of responsibility as all her grandchildren live with her.

Can you also please consider the increasing of the age to at least 14? Our friend [....] is 8 years...her grant just stopped when she turned seven. Now it is a problem. Her mother is not working and she has seven children to support....Must we suffer because we are eight years old? Please look at it and do something.

We know you love us and you will act to our benefit. Hoping to see you soon,

Yours faithfully
The Small Buddyz

* The names of the children have been removed to protect their rights.

activist, Carlos de Morais. The workshop generates organizational skills amongst elected community representatives. They then mobilize their broader community for an "extreme makeover." While the communities organize around already defined areas such as grant access, the ultimate aim of the program is to promote long-term community activism. The show attracts and inspires audiences of millions to adopt similar social mobilization initiatives in their own communities.

Media advocacy and social mobilization

Media advocacy is defined as the "strategic use of mass media to support community organizing to advance a social or public policy initiative" (Berkley Media Studies Group, 2011). In this approach, a distinction is made between "media for education," which focuses on narrowing a gap in information, and "media advocacy," which focuses on narrowing the power gap, as communities use the news media as a tool to bring about social change (Wallack and Dorfman, 1996).[2] The Soul City Institute trained ACESS members in media advocacy skills. These include constructive ways to engage the news media and frame their stories in ways more likely to get coverage. Also important is framing the content so that activists can shape the debate in a way that will help reflect their viewpoint. So, for example "framing for content" involved redefining grants away from the conventional view that grants "create dependency amongst the undeserving poor" and "divert resources which could be better used to stimulate economic growth" towards showing how "grants are powerful poverty alleviation mechanisms that save lives" and that "grants themselves are capable of stimulating economic engagement."

Using these skills ACESS activists succeeded in achieving a sustained media presence for the campaign through national and community radio, television and newspapers. When talk shows were secured (often with ACESS representatives and politicians as studio guests), ACESS mobilized its members to phone in and speak about the ACESS campaigns. Media exposure was timed to coincide with key decision-making periods. For example, when parliament was debating social security legislation and the African National Congress

---

Box 26.2   Media advocacy: putting social security on the public agenda and framing the debate

As an ACESS member, the Soul City Institute, pitched a disturbing story to the "Special Assignment" prime time investigative journalism program on national television. ACESS members brought to the fore research conducted by the University of the Western Cape on the situation of children in Mount Frere, a rural community in the Eastern Cape. Malnourished children were being discharged from hospital upon recovery, with instructions on how to access the CSG as one mechanism to prevent a recurrence. A few months later, most of the children were readmitted with malnutrition. Their caregivers were unable to obtain the CSG due to lack of identity documents and birth certificates. The journalists covered the story in a moving episode that held the Departments of Social Development and Home Affairs to account. ACESS members were interviewed, with the opportunity to draw attention to the campaigns. Immediately after broadcast, the Minister of Social Development flew down with a "crack team" to investigate the matter and to fast-track solutions to grant access in the area. A special session in parliament debated the high profile program and contributed to the overall pressure placed on government to remove the documentation barriers to access.

(ANC – South Africa's governing political party) was convening decision-making meetings. ACESS members orchestrated a number of visually powerful public protests to attract the media such as supporting children to make their own presentations to parliament.

Mobilizing through Community Events

The Soul City Institute and ACESS, together with key government departments, cohosted community events called "Grant Jamborees" to increase grant uptake in remote areas. The Jamborees brought together all government agencies in a "one-stop shop" to process grant applications particularly in marginalized rural communities. The police service was present to take affidavits from people who did not have the necessary documents so that officials at the next table from the Department of Home Affairs could process applications for identity documents. Grant applications were submitted at the same venue to the Department of Social Development for processing. Photocopiers, cameras, and fingerprinting equipment were on hand. Radio stations broadcasting Soul City dramas agreed to promote the events, giving listeners detailed information about what they should bring to the Jamborees in order to apply for grants. ACESS members went door to door to spread news of the event. Soul City celebrity actors and musicians provided entertainment at the Jamborees. Safe spaces were provided for children to play while their caregivers were in the application tents.

While the Jamborees were used to support the government's grant uptake drive, they were also used strategically to mobilize local ACESS members within the community to advocate with local government for the campaign demands. Government ministers were

---

Box 26.3   ACESS's grant workshops

Following an ACESS workshop a member mobilized community volunteers to work daily in the local clinic to facilitate birth certificates applications shortly after the birth of all babies. The ACESS member then delivered these forms herself every week to Home Affairs and simultaneously collected for caregivers the birth certificates from the previous week's applications.

ACESS members used the workshops to formulate their own localized strategies in support of the campaign. The following letter was written to ACESS central office:

How can we [ACESS members in the Umkhanyakude district in rural KwaZulu Natal]….thank you for your support through your trainings, workshops, dialogues, and advocacy and lobbying campaigns. They have paved a smooth way for us and created a space for almost all stakeholders … to plan, implement, monitor and evaluate our work together towards social security for children. Through our Ward Aids Councils which we have established in the 19 municipal wards made up of four traditional authorities, we will be able to have monthly meetings with all stakeholders doing what you have trained and capacitated us on in identifying children's needs and planning for sustainable interventions at a ward level ….having all stakeholders reporting on their progress in making children's lives better. And what is good is the commitment they have shown and allocation of their [government] responsible staff members for each ward. As community organizations we have aligned this to the provincial flagship program which calls for responsibility and accountability by all stakeholders especially the [local government departments].

---

invited to speak, which helped ACESS secure meetings with key government officials to find solutions to improve service delivery in the area and to put forward ACESS campaign demands. The success of the Jamboree initiative is evident not only in the documented increase in grant uptake around the period of the events, but also in the subsequent adoption by government of the "one-stop-shop" jamboree model itself.

Grant workshops – supporting social mobilization

ACESS held workshops for its members across the country to raise awareness, support members with grant access challenges, and to assist members to formulate their own social mobilization strategies to advocate for the ACESS campaigns. The workshop process was driven by the ACESS central office, but the outcomes were decided upon and driven by local membership. During the workshops government officials were invited to engage with ACESS members to help resolve local concerns.

Protest action

Grassroots ACESS members such as the New Women's Movement (NWM) mobilized their membership to protest outside key parliamentary and political events in support of

---

Box 26.4   The New Women's Movement

Interview with Chairperson of the NWM and Board Member of ACESS - Mama Dalina Tyawana

The New Women's Movement (NWM) was formed in 1995 after South Africa's first democratic elections. Based largely in the Western Cape province, grassroots activists in the women's movement, who had fought alongside other structures in the struggle for democracy, decided that a new structure was necessary post apartheid to ensure attention to women's rights. Launched in 1997, the NWM members total over 3000 women. Most of its members are the poorest of the poor, mainly unemployed women, living in shacks and largely uneducated. Many of the members are farm workers – often the most exploited workers in South Africa. Many are grandmothers who are often the only caregivers of children in their communities, having lost their own children and the parents of their grandchildren to AIDS. Many run informal crèches providing food and care to vulnerable children. The issue of social grants is central to their daily concerns and, as an ACESS member, the NWM has thrown its weight behind ACESS's campaigns. There are 14 branches primarily around Cape Town. However, many members are "semi-migrants" with strong links to the rural areas of the Eastern Cape where their extended families also live in poverty. Members tackle burning community issues and find ways to support one another. It is not uncommon, for example, to find women arriving en masse at courts to support survivors of rape. The NWM has mobilized its membership in support of ACESS campaigns and has encouraged leaders of other organizations in their communities to do the same.

---

the campaign. For example, women from the NWM came in hundreds from around Cape Town to protest outside the annual policy conference of the ANC to support a conference resolution to extend the CSG. People brought ACESS banners and campaign T-shirts, and danced outside the conference from early morning, when delegates began to arrive, singing freedom songs and talking to the media and the public about the campaign. ACESS members had also collected a petition with thousands of signatures to extend the CSG to age 18 and a delegation presented the petition and a memorandum of demands to the ANC leadership and to the Minister of Social Development. The delegation secured a meeting with the minister immediately after the conference to discuss the campaign demands. This pressure contributed to the ANC passing the relevant resolution to increase the age of the CSG to children up to 14 years and this later became law in 2003 (Budlender, Proudlock, and Jamieson, 2008). Soon after the conference, government also committed itself to intensify its work to reach all those eligible for the grants. It was during this period that government adopted the ACESS/ Soul City Institute Jamboree model, rolling the process out in many parts of the country, often with ACESS and Soul City Institute support.

Other mass organizations such as the Treatment Action Campaign integrated the ACESS campaign into its own program of action to secure universal access to anti-retroviral treatment for people living with AIDS. Its mass protests also included calls for the extension of the CSG to 18 years.

Successes

Winning the CSG Extension to 18 years

After the 2003 victory, when government announced an increase in the CSG to 14 years, the CI, in collaboration with ACESS members, began monitoring the extension. A hotline was set up for caregivers and ACESS members to report administrative problems with the extension. Members also collected evidence of experiences in their communities. The information was compiled into monthly case alerts that were sent to government decision makers, parliamentarians, service providers, civil society and the media to ensure ongoing vigilance around implementation (Budlender, Proudlock, and Jamieson, 2008). All the while ACESS continued to campaign to increase the CSG to 18 years.

By 2006, there was extensive support within the DSD itself for a full extension of the CSG to 18years and the DSD commissioned the Children's Institute to assist in the formulation of a memorandum on the proposed extension which the DSD would submit to Cabinet.

In February 2007 the President of South Africa acknowledged publicly the need to look at policies to support older children, and a high-level government meeting in July 2007 reportedly discussed how better to provide for 14 to18-year-olds. The ANC Policy Conference in July 2007 and its National Conference in December 2007 also came out in support of an extension to 18 years. In February 2008, the Minister of Finance announced that the CSG would be extended to age 15 from January 2009 (Budlender, Proudlock, and Jamieson, 2008). Later that year, government announced the extension of the CSG to 18 years.

Over the years many individual members of the ANC as well as officials within the DSD expressed support for the increase, but political dynamics within the governing party resulted in a dominance of the opposing forces which included a reluctant Treasury. The final victory was facilitated in large part by seismic changes in the ANC which radically altered its internal power dynamics, allowing those in support of the extension to gain ascendency. However, the role of ACESS in influencing the ANC and other key stakeholders to support the increase is widely acknowledged.

Removing barriers to CSG access

Throughout this period ACESS's second campaign, to remove the barriers to access for those already eligible for the CSG, was ongoing. The requirement for ID documents and birth certificates was onerous given the poor functioning of the Department of Home Affairs in processing the applications for these documents. Initially, the Social Assistance Act's 1998 Regulations allowed officials to use their discretion in accepting alternative forms of proof. However, this clause was ignored and most caregivers without these documents were turned away. The ACESS campaign applied pressure on government to ensure adherence and also undertook large-scale information drives to create public awareness of this provision. However, the Regulations were later amended to remove this clause with government citing widespread fraud. ACESS and government itself conducted research, which consistently found that most of the fraud came from within government itself. In 2005 the regulations were again amended to re-include the discretionary clause, but government did not publicize this and applications continued to be rejected. Lack of birth certificates and identity documents were still excluding potentially up to 20 percent of eligible children from accessing their rights (Budlender, Proudlock, and Jamieson, 2008). ACESS mobilized members to intensify their efforts. However, having exhausted all other forms of advocacy, it later reluctantly decided to litigate government. ACESS collated evidence from a range of sources, including CI's primary research of ACESS members' experiences. On the day of the hearing, government announced that the 2005 regulations to the Social Assistance Act were, in effect, repealing the amended 1998 regulations. To create legal certainty, the Court ordered the 2005 regulations to officially come into effect and that, if the Department were to change them by removing the discretion again, the court case would continue. The Court also ordered the government to implement the use of alternative forms of identity and to give a detailed statistical report later that year on its progress in giving CSGs to children and caregivers without identity documents. The court order was a victory for children: even if they were unable to produce the official identify document, as long as they could provide alternate proof they would be assisted in accessing the grant. In the meanwhile, government would assist them to secure the official ID documentation (Hall and Proudlock, 2008).

While ACESS had finally achieved its major campaign goals, as with most advocacy ongoing vigilance is necessary. Although the necessary legislation is in place, implementation of the age extension is still in question, and many children still do not access their grants due to lack of documents. In 2011, at the time of writing this chapter, ACESS continues to mobilize its members to ensure government delivers on its promises.

Lessons and Challenges

Mobilizing across diverse membership

ACESS member organizations are autonomous, and there are often debates around conflicting positions on issues related to social security. It is within the nature of alliances that they must strive for strategic compromise and consensus without weakening the alliance or the individual member organizations' objectives. For example, TAC had thrown its weight behind the ACESS campaign for the CSG but was also a member of the Basic Income Grant (BIG) Coalition, which wanted to see every individual regardless of age or income getting a monthly grant. Higher earners would subsidize the grant through a "claw back tax." The BIG Coalition was concerned that ACESS's more limited demands would undermine its campaign. Children would be seen as more "deserving" and hence extending the CSG to 18 would be more palatable to government and particularly to a hostile Treasury Department than the BIG. While ACESS members recognized the value of a BIG as a socially just measure of huge benefit for children too, they were reluctant to drop the call for an increased CSG age limit. Many saw BIG as unwinnable in the short to medium term. Shelving the CSG call would leave children wholly unprotected while the debates around BIG could be used to delay action on all fronts. ACESS and the BIG Coalition agreed to formulate their demands in mutually reinforcing ways. Both coalitions reframed their demands to a unified call for "the increase of the CSG to 18years as the first phase of the implementation of a BIG for all." This consensus resulted in all BIG coalition members, including the largest trade union and umbrella church bodies in the country, joining in the social mobilization efforts to increase the CSG to 18 years.

In another example, the New Women's Movement was preparing to take the government to the Constitutional Court in order to increase the CSG amount. As a member of ACESS, the New Women's Movement dropped the case, deciding to support the alliance consensus to favor more children getting less, rather than less children getting more.

Strength in diversity

Alliances bring together the diverse strengths and abilities of their members. Different ACESS members made important and often unique contributions in support of a common goal. The Soul City Institute brought its large mass communication vehicle and network of children's clubs to raise awareness to catalyze social mobilization through inspiring stories of community action. Its media advocacy expertise made an important contribution to the social mobilization process.

Members specializing in research such as the Children's Institute and university academics, as well as service providers and advocacy organizations such as the Black Sash, were able to provide the alliance with sound evidence for its demands and were highly articulate in advocating for the campaign demands. Organizations with legal expertise such as the Department of Public Law at the University of Stellenbosch and the Legal Resources Centre, played a critical role in litigation.

Members' firsthand experiences strengthened the campaigns by providing accounts of poor grant delivery. ACESS organizations with mass grassroots membership played a critical role in positioning ACESS as an alliance with a substantial constituency, a factor of particular concern to politicians. The diversity of ACESS membership enhanced its legitimacy and increased its ability to apply pressure.

At the same time, the ability of ACESS through its membership to support government in increasing grant uptake resulted in the alliance being seen as a resource and a partner. As described previously, government even adopted the Jamboree model for grant delivery. Behind the scenes, some government officials encouraged ACESS to increase the pressure for the age extension in order to strengthen their own advocacy with less supportive government departments such as the National Treasury.

Using community-based activities to mobilize

Education and awareness-raising activities, such as the Jamborees and Grant Workshops, served an important mobilizing function. They were used to educate communities on grants and facilitate access to them, but they also provided an opportunity for local community activists to formulate and implement their own campaign strategies with local government.

This was vital not only to affect change at local level but also at a national level, as certain bills, if dealing with policy areas in which national and provincial government share authority, must go through provincial government for ratification, before being passed into law at the national level.

The need for sustained action

Legislative and policy victories are hollow without ongoing vigilance to ensure hard won gains are sustained and enforced. In ACESS's case, its legislative campaign objectives were achieved after many years of mobilization but it continues to mobilize to ensure effective implementation of policy and legislation including the allocation of the necessary resources.

ACESS governance and social mobilization

In carrying out its mandate from the Children's Sector Summit, three nongovernmental organizations drove ACESS's initial activities including building the alliance, with the understanding that, ultimately, it would be driven democratically through its membership. Initially members' ongoing mandate was solicited through meetings, fax, phone and email. With time, and as the Alliance grew, the ability to consult members in a timely manner became more difficult. The need to revisit the original mandate from its constituency and to find ways to decentralize decision making became more urgent. A mass meeting of ACESS membership was convened to debate the structure of the alliance and to renew its mandate. In an attempt to ensure greater member representation and accountability, the meeting elected office bearers to an ACESS board and members unable to attend the meeting voted via telephone, fax and email. This was envisaged as the first of many such member gatherings.

However, ACESS has grappled with sustaining this decentralized approach. Attempts to establish provincial "branches" worked initially in some provinces with active members but not in others. Over time, the elected board moved even further away from its vision of a democratic structure with branches and elected officials toward a more formal Alliance NGO, able to raise donor funds and employ staff. This transition resulted in part from inadequate funding to support regular mass meetings and multiple branches across the country. It was also due to the difficulties of functioning nimbly within a dynamic advocacy environment where far reaching decisions often needed to be made urgently. It also been a challenge to sustain a bottom-up, community-driven approach in the context of a diverse community and a protracted struggle for children's rights that has spanned close on a decade and has required national and provincial level organizational planning, implementation capacity, and funding.

Ongoing direction was sought through strategy meetings, working groups, and workshops involving more proactive members, rather than through an organized grassroots mobilization effort with for example, formalized voting mechanisms to ensure "bottom up" member control. Debate is ongoing within ACESS as to the best governance options to deepen membership engagement.

Defining Social Mobilization in the Context of Alliances

Community mobilization has been clearly defined as strategies that facilitate a "collective response to community-defined social and health needs and give communities an effective voice in program delivery, service, and policy" (Fawcett *et al.*, 2000, cited in Kim-Ju *et al.* 2008, p. S3). The community in these initiatives is often defined by a geographical location and is therefore able to be community driven or controlled. The definition of social mobilization, on the other hand, is less clear cut. Many use the terms "community mobilization" and "social mobilization" interchangeably. However, at a societal level, there is diversity and heterogeneity which makes collective control more challenging to achieve. As a result of this diversity, partnerships, alliances and coalitions have a critical role to play in mobilizing different groups and constituencies to have a voice around a common ideal or goal.

The role of partnerships and alliances has been acknowledged in definitions of social mobilization. UNICEF, for example, defines social mobilization as "a process of inter-sectoral coalition building and action by which social actors come together to raise awareness about specific issues, raise demand, support service delivery, and strengthen local participation" (UNICEF, 2003). This was echoed by Obregon and Waisbord (2010, p. 25) who state that "Social mobilization has been a strategic component of the polio eradication initiative and a form of intersectoral collaboration." The ACESS case study provides a useful example of how alliances were able to mobilize diverse groups around a common goal and at the same time, to strengthen local participation.

Participation was particularly evident in the marches led by the New Women's Movement and in the Soul Buddyz club, where children mobilized local stakeholders to facilitate community members acquiring the necessary documentation to enable them to access child grants.

While bottom-up control is a key characteristic of community mobilization it is worth exploring the extent to which this is possible in the context of wider social mobilization. Given the diversity and heterogeneity of society overall (where the definition of community becomes contested), the goal of social change cannot be attained without leadership. This leadership can be both "external" and come from within communities.

Obregon and Waisbord (2010, p. 42) see these two situations as "mutually exclusive" concluding that "centralized strategies [externally defined] hardly amount to social mobilization." "Bottom-up micro-planning" is seen as essential to social mobilization. However, the governance structure of ACESS is best described as a hybrid of "bottom-up" and "centralized" and requires a more nuanced definition of what constitutes genuine social mobilization.

In the case of ACESS, the alliance is a "collective" of stakeholders in the children's sector all coming together to mobilize in unison. It is a community of communities. It must act on the mandate of its membership. The broad mandate initially given to ACESS – to advocate for social security for children – remains its driving force. It is for changes in its strategies and tactics that ACESS seeks an ongoing mandate.

This raises the question of how one gets an ongoing "bottom-up" mandate from over 1500 diverse members spread over sectors and geography. Is it through geographical branches with voting rights? Branches would themselves be required to develop consensus from their own memberships of diverse communities. This would require a robust set of democratic structures that potentially creates its own bureaucracy and would be difficult to fund. Membership fees would be unlikely to sustain ACESS given that most of its members would not be in a position to contribute substantively.

The South African historical context created a conducive environment for the formation of alliances as an integral part of mobilization for social change, with an active civil society present when ACESS was formed. However, dimensions highlighted by this case study could be transferred to other settings.

As a powerful alliance, ACESS has helped coordinate, direct, and facilitate the social mobilization efforts of its membership and alliance partners in support of a commonly defined goal – to secure children's rights to social security. In relation to social grants, it has had major successes albeit over close on a decade of struggle.

Conclusion

As a powerful alliance, ACESS has helped coordinate, direct, and facilitate the social mobilization efforts of its membership and alliance partners in support of a commonly defined goal – to secure children's rights to social security. In relation to social grants, it has had major successes, albeit over close on a decade of struggle.

ACESS can be described as a "community of communities" that engages in social mobilization but does not fit easily into many of the current definitions. Despite the original intention to be democratically driven through its membership, it has evolved into a hybrid of a nongovernmental organization that functions as a central driver constantly struggling to find ways to retain meaningful "member direction." ACESS's experience illustrates the complexity of definitions specifically in the context of alliances. Is there a "one size fits all" definition that can be used to describe "genuine" social mobilization, or is it better thought of as a continuum where different definitions of social mobilization apply depending on the context? ACESS's experience points to the need for nuanced definitions of social mobilization that take into account the complexities of development and realities on the ground.

Notes

1   See Budlender, Proudlock, and Jamieson (2008), who cite numerous studies to this effect.
2   Both Charlotte Ryan and Lawrence Wallack have written extensively of the practice of "media advocacy." Ryan describes the practice developed with organized labour in her seminal work *Prime Time Activism* while Wallack and colleagues (1993) describe it in relation to public health, media advocacy and public health.

References

Berkley Media Studies Group (2011). *Media Advocacy 101.* Retrieved from http://www.bmsg. org/resources/media-advocacy-101

Budlender, D., Proudlock, P., and Jamieson, L., (2008). *Developing Social Policy for Children in the Context of HIV/AIDS: A South African Case Study. No 3.* Cape Town: Children's Institute, University of Cape Town and Community Agency for Social Enquiry.

Fawcett, S. B., Francisco, V. T., I-Lyra, D. *et al.* (2000). Building healthy communities. In A. R. Tarlov and R. F. St. Peter (Eds.), *The Society and Population Health Reader: Vol II : A State and Community Perspective* (pp. 75–93). New York: New Press.

Hall, K. and Proudlock, P. (2008). "Litigating for a better deal", *Children's Institute Annual Report, 2007/2008.* Retrieved from http://www.ci.org.za/depts/ci/pubs/pdf/general/ annual/report08/litigating.pdf

Kim-Ju, L., Mark, G. Y., Cohen, R. *et al.* (2008). Community mobilization and its application to youth violence prevention. *American Journal of Preventive Medicine, 34*(3, Supplement), S5–S12.

Obregon, R. and Waisbord, S. (2010). The complexity of social mobilization in health communication: Top-down and bottom-up experiences in polio eradication. *Journal of health Communication, 15*(Supplement 1), 25–47.

Posel, D., Fairburn, J., and Lund, F. (2004). *Labour Migration and Households: A Reconsideration of the Effects of the Social Pension on Labour Supply in South Africa.* Forum paper 2004. Retrieved from http://www.tips.org.za/files/Labour_Migration_and_Householdsposel_ fairburn_lund.pdf

Shisana, O., Rehle, D., Simbayi, L. *et al.* (2009). *South African National HIV Prevalence, Incidence, Behaviour and Communication Survey 2008: A Turning Tide among Teenagers?* Cape Town: HSRC Press

Smart, R. (1999). *Children Living with HIV and AIDS: A Rapid Appraisal.* Pretoria: Department of Health and Save the Children (UK).

UNICEF (2003). *A Critical Leap to Polio Eradication in India* (Working Paper). New Delhi, India: UNICEF Regional Office for South Asia

Wallack, L. and Dorfman, L. (1996). Media advocacy: A strategy for advancing policy and promoting health. *Health Education Quarterly 23*(3), 293–317.

Wallack, L., Dorfman, L., Jernigan, D. H., and Themba-Nixon, M. (1993). *Media Advocacy and Public Health: Power for Prevention.* Thousand Oaks, CA: Sage Publications.

Part IV

Crosscutting Issues

27

Capacity Building (and Strengthening) in Health Communication
The Missing Link

Rafael Obregon and Silvio Waisbord

Capacity development has moved to the center stage of the agendas of development organizations. Substantial sums are being invested in capacity-building programs. Yet, their design and management leave much to be desired. Marred by untested, unrealistic assumptions, the results of many programs fall short of their goals and expectations.

(LaFond and Brown, 2003, p. 5)

Introduction

The Paris Declaration on Aid Effectiveness (2005, see OECD, n.d.), one the most influential statements that multilateral, bilateral, and private international development organizations and donors have issued in the recent past, provided a strategic platform for international development aid programs. Its focus on issues that are perceived as critical for the effectiveness of international development – that is, harmonization of efforts, increased focus on results, and capacity building – has coincided with, and contributed to, a number of important shifts in the international development agenda. One of the Declaration's key areas of emphasis concerned capacity development as a vital component in achieving better development results, and particularly in the attainment of the Millennium Development Goals.

The signatories of the Declaration stated that capacity development should "be responsive to the broader social, political and economic environment, including the need to strengthen human resources" (OECD, n,d,, p. 12). The Paris Declaration and the subsequent Accra Agenda for Action (2008, see OECD, n.d.), underscore the renewed importance of capacity development as a critical component of international development programs. Furthermore, in the health sector several documents and initiatives have also emphasized the centrality of capacity strengthening to international development and health. In particular, the 2006 World Health Report epitomizes that aspect, as it called for a concerted effort aimed at addressing the global crisis in health human resources. Yet, when it comes to capacity building and strengthening (CBS) in health communication at international level, we do not see the same impetus found in other related areas.

The overarching objective of this chapter is to call for greater attention to CBS efforts in global health communication from researchers and academics. The lack of peer-reviewed publications and academic works that document, assess, and critically discuss CBS in health communication is alarming, contrary to what is found in other fields that have similar academic and practical interests such as health promotion. The specific objectives of this chapter are twofold. First, to discuss the role of capacity building (and strengthening)[1] as an integral component of global health communication programs. Second, to emphasize collaboration with higher education institutions as a critical dimension of sustained and long-term efforts aimed at building a critical mass of individuals and organizations with the required competencies in health communication.

The chapter is organized as follows. First, we briefly discuss the conceptual history and evolution of CBS in international development, followed by a brief overview of CBS in health promotion and communication. We present examples of previous and ongoing collaborative efforts with higher education institutions as a means to support long-term capacity development in health communication. We then describe and discuss an example of a university and competency-based capacity building and strengthening program in health communication, which provides important lessons for further action. In our conclusions we (1) stress the importance of CBS in global health communication, (2) put forth strategic recommendations that may contribute to efforts aimed at developing greater capacity in global health communication through competency and university-based programs, and (3) call for increased dialogue and collaboration between health promotion and health communication scholars and practitioners involved in CBS efforts.

Understanding Capacity Building: Definitions, Approaches, Issues

The term "capacity building" (CB) is widely found in the international development literature (Lebel *et al.*, 2006; Blagescu and Young, 2006; LaFond and Brown, 2003; Degnbol-Martinussen, 2002: Bolger, 2000; Lusthaus, Adrien, and Perstinger, 1999; Morgan, 1998; Cohen, 1993), with seemingly general consensus that capacity building is a key component in the success of international development programs (Battel-Kirk *et al.*, 2009; Lebel *et al.*, 2006). Most multilateral and bilateral development agencies have developed principles and models that guide their capacity building and strengthening programs (UNDP, 1997; DFID, 2002; LaFond and Brown, 2003). References are also commonly found to the importance of accelerating capacity building efforts toward the attainment of the Millennium Development Goals (Whyte, 2004).

Capacity is defined as the set of "activities, approaches, strategies, and methodologies which help organizations, groups and individuals to improve their performance, generate development benefits, and achieve their objectives over time" (Bolger, 2000, p. 1). Capacity development refers to the approaches, strategies, and methodologies used by developing countries, and/or external stakeholders, to improve performance at the individual, interpersonal, organizational, network/sector or broader system level (Flaman *et al.* 2011; Bolger, 2000, p. 3). Other perspectives emphasize the political nature of CB, its impact on the organizational culture, the time required in investing in such initiatives, and the complexity of the process (Teskey, 2005), as elements that capacity development programs must take into account for effective implementation and optimal results.

Capacity building has been used interchangeably with such terms as capacity development, institutional development, institutional building, and capacity strengthening. For some authors, this elasticity in the definition of CBS has contributed to a lack of consensus and coherence on what CBS ultimately means (Lusthaus, Adrien, and Perstinger, 1999). For instance, although some development organizations have developed their own definitions and learning principles of CBS, there is little agreement on what approaches to capacity building work best – a finding consistent with other literature reviews of capacity building (e.g., Blagescu and Young, 2006; Light and Hubbard, 2004; McKinsey & Co., 2001). Lack of agreement is due, in part, to historic inattention to capacity building in the nonprofit sectors (Light and Hubbard, 2004), that capacity building is a long-term process, often unpredictable and difficult to track (Morgan, 1998), and because organizations often pay less attention to monitoring and evaluation of capacity building efforts (Blagescu and Young, 2006). Lack of agreement is also due to the use of multiple frameworks and models from many disciplines which makes it difficult to answer the questions as to what works best and why, and to the lack of frameworks and models to structure programs, which make it challenging to understand what guided choices and how outcomes relate to those choices.

However, beyond the obvious questions and challenges that this lack of coherence might raise, there is ample evidence that capacity building and strengthening has regained a prominent place in international development. In response to the Paris Declaration's guiding framework and recommendations for its implementation put forward by the Accra Agenda for Action, capacity building and strengthening is highly visible in policy documents and the agenda of multilateral and bilateral technical cooperation agencies for development. Yet, critical assessments of CB have shown that many initiatives have not delivered the promised results. Merely providing skills training and equipment "in the name of 'capacity building' was failing to address the real needs, was a waste of scarce resources, and at worst helped bolster systems which were corrupt and harmful to those they were supposed to assist" (Potter and Brough, 2004, p. 337). Lavergne and Saxby (2001, p. 4), for instance, characterized CBS as the "increased ability to use and increase existing resources, in an efficient, effective, relevant and sustainable way", and recognized "the primacy of learning by doing, a holistic approach that recognizes the interdependence of actors and systems, and (the pursuit to) balance the need for short term results in satisfying social needs with the need for long-term improvements in capacity."

CBS is generally defined as a continuous and dynamic learning process that takes a long time and should be applied at multiple levels for it to be effective and sustainable.

The conceptual evolution of CB over the last three decades shows a shift from a focus on building individual capacity in the 1970s, primarily through training and skills development, to an emphasis in the redesign and restructuring of organizations in the 1980s (DFID, 2002; Lavergne and Saxby, 2001). When these perspectives also failed, international development agencies started to acknowledge that increasing organizational capacity was not enough either. There was a realization that greater focus had to be placed on reforming formal institutions (e.g., the legal system, property rights, the relationship of the executive to the legislature, etc.) and informal institutions (norms and values that influence individual and collective behavior). Several scholars subscribe to the perspective that, with some minor variations depending upon the author, building and strengthening capacity requires work at individual, organizational, sectoral/networks, and institutional levels (Lebel *et al.*, 2006; Lavergne and Saxby, 2001; Borger, 2000; Morgan, 1998). This holistic view echoes the need to focus on facilitating an enabling environment that encourages individuals and organizations to apply what they have learned, and provides opportunities to do so (Fukuda-Parr, Lopes, and Malik, 2002).

Scholars argue that two broad lines of thinking have dominated CBS programs: CBS as an approach (process), and CBS as a goal (objective) (Lavergne and Saxby, 2001; Lusthaus, Adrien, and Perstinger, 1999). As an approach, CB seeks to promote a systematic process that stresses the intangible dimensions of development – the "core" capabilities – that enable individuals and groups to use resources effectively, efficiently, and sustainably. These capabilities can help groups and individuals internalize clear principles and engage in actions that range from developing a sense of purpose to assessing performance and adjusting to new challenges. By contrast, CB as a goal seeks to identify gaps and challenges in human resource capacity that need to be addressed in order to ensure effective program implementation and the achievement of results. Health and development programs conceptualized from this perspective may focus on infrastructure, education, training, and organizational development. These activities by themselves, however, may not constitute CBS efforts necessarily, unless they are implemented as part of a broader initiative whose primary aim, emphasis, or center of gravity is capacity development. However, CBS efforts often draw from both approaches (Lusthaus, Adrien, and Perstinger, 1999).

One common expectation of CBS work is that it should foster independence instead of perpetual dependency on institutions; nevertheless, many conventional CBS practices, particularly those of large of NGOs, have been criticized as being "ultimately about retaining power, rather than empowering their partners" (Eade, 2007, p. 630). Because of these weaknesses, there have been efforts aimed at developing new paradigms for technical cooperation that give more value to learning, empowerment, social capital, and an enabling environment. For global health communication such new focus is critical given the long-term health challenges that need to be addressed, a response that requires density (presence of a critical mass of qualified professionals) in health communication capacity.

Lastly, a critical issue in CBS, as in any other development-related area, is monitoring and evaluation (M&E). Few capacity development programs have been systematically and thoroughly evaluated and reported in the extant literature (Horton *et al.*, 2003;

Lessik and Michener, 2000). This calls for more thorough and systematic evaluations of capacity building. Most capacity measurement tends to emphasize capacity assessment rather than M&E. Assessment normally takes place at the beginning of an intervention as part of an organizational diagnosis or formative design process. Evaluators can learn a great deal from capacity assessment tools. However, capacity- building M&E differs from assessment by virtue of its explicit focus on measuring change (Brown, LaFond, and Macintyre, 2001), which makes M&E an important challenge in CBS programs (World Bank, 2005; LaFond and Brown, 2003).

Arguably, CBS has progressively moved toward more holistic and systemic perspectives that take into account multiple levels of intervention. In particular, the literature shows that CBS efforts need to pay attention to different levels (individual/organizational; sectoral/network; institutional), that these levels have a high degree of interaction and interdependency, and that CBS is complex and demands flexibility and adaptation (Folke *et al.*, 2002; Crisp, Swerissen, and Duckett, 2000). These aspects are essential to our understanding of CBS, and to further assessment of CBS efforts in health communication and promotion. To what extent have CBS needs in health communication been addressed? We discuss this issue in the next section of the chapter.

Capacity Building in Health Promotion and Communication

The Paris Declaration's framework is reflected in a number of international development initiatives, including capacity development in health. In 2005, the United Nations General Assembly adopted a resolution reiterating the urgency of enhancing capacity building in global public health given the potential global impact of new epidemics (e.g., avian flu and severe acute respiratory syndrome (SARS)), and the existing concern with infectious diseases such as HIV/AIDS, tuberculosis, and malaria (United Nations General Assembly, 2005). In this resolution, the UN asserted the need to strengthen public health systems through further integrating public health into member countries' national economic and social development strategies, awareness raising, active international cooperation among countries, and the improvement of global public health preparedness and response systems among others. This sense of urgency was further underscored by the 2006 World Health Report's focus on the health human resources crisis. The Report called for a global response to the crisis in health human resources. This was a paramount example of the increasing need to accelerate efforts aimed at strengthening local capacity in the health sector. The Report noted that:

> Skill mix and distributional imbalances compound today's problems. In many countries, the skills of limited yet expensive professionals are not well matched to the local profile of health needs. Critical skills in public health and health policy and management are often in deficit. Many workers face daunting working environments – poverty-level wages, unsupportive management, insufficient social recognition, and weak career development. Almost all countries suffer from maldistribution (of health personnel) characterized by urban concentration and rural deficits, but these imbalances are perhaps most disturbing from a regional perspective (WHO, 2006, p. 6).

The WHO 2006 report also made several references to the role of information and communication technologies, risk communication, and the role of health workers in reaching out to communities in order to promote healthy lifestyles and behaviors. However, it was disconcerting that, while several professions and occupations were specifically highlighted throughout the report as key to the world's response to the crisis, the report did not make specific references to health promotion and health communication. Our interest in examining CBS efforts in health communication is amplified by the fact that the academic and peer-reviewed literature provides limited examples of CBS efforts in health communication, while documented examples are found primarily in technical reports and documents from international development and nongovernmental agencies, some of which we summarize later. Yet, we frequently hear expressions such as "communication is critical to the success of public health programs," or "communication capacity needs to be strengthened in order to increase demand for services, or change behaviors or social conditions that impact health outcomes."

This reality contrasts with the fact that over the past few decades health communication has become a key component of public health programs, whether to promote and increase demand for services, mobilize communities and societies in order to respond to public health challenges, create awareness about emerging or reemerging diseases, fight stigma and discrimination, promote positive changes in attitudes, behaviors, and norms, or reinforce positive ones, stimulate people's participation and public debate on health policy making and implementation, and many other aspects that require communication strategies and interventions in support of both small and large-scale public health programs. Such a range of objectives and outcomes does demand and require strong technical capacity in health communication.

It is also true that training opportunities in health communication are widely present in health and development programs (Waisbord, 2006). Arguably, capacity building and strengthening is inherently embedded in any health and development communication program. Most international development organizations would agree that the process of designing, implementing, and evaluating health communication strategies at country level necessarily contributes to strengthening local capacity. Also, most international health programs include some capacity-strengthening component, which is often operationalized through short-term and on-the-job training activities. A number of regional training organizations offer short-term health communication courses (e.g., the African AIDS Regional Training Network and the Center for African Family Studies (CAFS) have been set up in the past few years (Chikombero, 2009; Weiner, 2009).

Unlike health communication, health promotion is a field with a much richer literature on capacity building and strengthening, and particularly on the development of core competencies (Battel-Kirk *et al.* 2009). This might be due to two factors. First, health promotion, a key area of public health, has been a central feature of international health for several decades, partly as a result of statements included in influential documents such as the Ottawa Charter for Health Promotion and WHO official declarations. Second, to a large extent, health promotion and health communication often overlap. For instance, some scholars discuss health and behavior change communication as a subset of health promotion (Onya, 2009; Nyamwaya, 2003). Third, many CBS efforts in health promotion often include health communication, or, at the very least, behavior change communication, components. Capacity building in the health promotion literature has been defined as "an approach to the development of sustainable skills, organizational structures, resources and commitment to health improvement in health and other sectors, to prolong and multiply health gains many times over" (Barry, 2008, p. 1). Capacity building in health promotion is commonly regarded as a set of strategies that can be applied both within and across systems to lead to a greater capacity of people, organizations and communities to promote health (Heward, Hutchinson, and Keleher, 2007; Labonte and Laverack, 2001). These perspectives reflect the complexity and multi-level approach to CBS discussed earlier in this chapter.

There is a considerable amount of peer-reviewed literature that discusses and examines different projects, programs and interventions that seek to build and strengthen capacity in health promotion, including collaboration with higher education institutions. Such initiatives range from efforts aimed at strengthening research capacity of African universities (Airhihenbuwa *et al.*, 2011; Lansang and Dennis, 2004), at improving practices in health promotion through international collaboration (Van den Broucke *et al.*, 2010), and at helping health promoters provide client-centered information and advice on key health issues (Wills and Rudolph, 2010). Private-sector-led initiatives that seek to strengthen the capacity of NGOs that work in health issues, particularly HIV/AIDS, also have been documented (Hartwig, Humphries, and Matebeni, 2009). Lessons learned from these initiatives highlight common issues in CBS such as the need to take a collaborative approach, the challenge of evaluating CBS programs, the importance of creating an enabling environment, and a broader focus that goes beyond training activities only. For instance, Wills and Rudolph reported that "it is also clear that training alone is insufficient when the context for health promotion in primary health care settings is unsupportive. A focus on simply building skills among individual practitioners alone will not lead to effective health promotion practice without strong support from the organization within which they work" (2009, p. 34).

Because the focus of CBS programs has gravitated toward short-term and in-service training and skills development, large NGOs or training units of government organizations have typically led those programs. However, over the past two decades there has been an increasing shift toward greater collaboration with universities and higher education institutions (i.e., the Earth Institute's Masters in Development Practice) that particularly emphasize identification of core competencies and minimum training standards as a mechanism to better define the type of professional needed in development, and the possibility of establishing long-term programs that do not depend upon the availability of funds of short-lived projects. In the case of health promotion, the 2008 Galway Consensus Report, which convened a number of experts and leading academics in health promotion, is a collaborative attempt to strengthen capacity in health promotion through the development of "health promotion core competencies and common approaches to academic programme accreditation, continuing professional development and the development of professional standards" (Barry *et al.*, 2009, p.7). The Galway Report puts forward a number of competency areas that are recommended for the design of training programs in health promotion. Those competencies include catalyzing change, leadership, assessment, planning, implementation, evaluation, advocacy, and partnerships (Barry *et al.*, 2009; Onya, 2009; Shilton, 2009).

While the Galway Consensus Report acknowledges that greater efforts need to be made to identify and incorporate efforts aimed at strengthening health promotion capacity in Africa, Asia, and Latin America, there is evidence of similar interest in some of those regions. For instance, Arroyo (2009) writes that for more than a decade the Inter American Consortium of Universities and Training Centers for Health Education and Promotion (CIUEPS) has worked toward facilitating the creation of networks, university programs, and other CBS activities. Similarly, Onya (2009) posits that, despite little progress, various countries in Africa have made important efforts aimed at developing capacity in health promotion, including South Africa, Nigeria, Botswana, as well as organizations such as the African Medical and Research Foundation (AMREF) in Kenya. Nyewmania (2003) had called for a serious effort of CBS in health promotion in Africa in order to end the "undeclared war" that organizations – national and international – involved in health promotion and health communication-related areas are engaged in, primarily as a result of their own interests in accessing resources.

CBS in Health Communication: A Competency Focus

While the academic literature consistently shows that there is a clear focus on the importance of CBS in health promotion and that important advocacy efforts have been, and continue to be, made to maintain CBS issues on the agenda of international health organizations, such a strong emphasis and level of advocacy is not found in the literature on CBS in health communication, nor are there many documented examples of systematic efforts with that focus. It is not our intention to discuss in this chapter the reasons for such a lack of interest or limited dissemination, although that is an important question that must be addressed at some point. In the next few lines we describe some examples of health communication CBS initiatives. These examples include regional initiatives that focus on CBS through higher education institutions, regional and global nongovernmental organizations that seek to strengthen the capacity of their partners, and regional training institutions whose mandate is to develop capacity in health development, including health communication-related areas, through short-term training programs.

Between 1997 and 2002, the Pan American Health Organization (PAHO) led an initiative that sought to strengthen the health communication capacity of university-based programs in Latin America. The purpose of this initiative was to mainstream health communication within a group of universities in the region, strengthen their research capacity, and build a network of higher education institutions with a common interest in making health communication an important component of their training programs. This initiative included two phases. The first phase involved a group of twelve universities from nine countries in the region that conducted research on media coverage of health issues (Alcalay and Mendoza, 2000). The second phase, with the participation of thirteen universities from eleven countries, focused on how adolescents consumed, used, and negotiated meanings of media content on health issues (Collignon *et al.*, 2003). This CBS initiative triggered the creation of an informal network of universities with interest in health communication, and eventually contributed to the insertion of health communication content in the curricula and course offerings of participating universities, the creation of specialized courses and seminars, and the creation of at least two post-graduate programs in health communication.

In the early 2000s, a collaborative effort led by the US Agency for International Development (USAID), PAHO, the Rockefeller Foundation, and the Change Project (Irigoin *et al.*, 2002) resulted in a competency map in communication for development and social change (CFSC), a global effort to develop and propose a common set of competencies deemed necessary for communication for development and social change practitioners to design, implement, and evaluate theory-driven and evidence-based communication strategies, through participatory approaches (Irigoin *et al.*, 2002). The primary concern in this process was the belief that, given the proliferation of schools of communication around the world (in Latin America there are more than 1,400 media and communication programs) there was an urgent need to identify a set of competencies and standards to define who a communicator for social change was and what that communicator needed to know and do. A year later, several international agencies met in Ica, Peru, including universities, national and international NGOs, international cooperation agencies, and ministries of health from several countries in Latin America, with the purpose of adapting the CFSC competencies and identify and develop key competencies in health communication.

The outcome of the meeting was the development of a competency map for health communication training and the design of various training options for different audiences (professionals; health providers; community workers) at university and in-service levels (Castro, Waisbord, and Coe, 2003). Competency is defined as the set of knowledge, skills and values/attitudes that individuals and organizations must have in order to effectively solve and respond to real life situations (Irigoin *et al.*, 2002). The competency map in health communication identified the key functions of a health communicator: promotion of individual and community empowerment for health management and activities, facilitation of dialogue and consensus building among social actors and government institutions in order to facilitate social management and to promote healthy behaviors, advocacy for favorable public health policies, development of communication interventions that contribute to creating favorable conditions for individual and collective healthy behaviors, and understanding and analysis of determinants of health and disease, and the diversity of responses in specific realities and settings in order to provide strategic guidance in health communication interventions (Waisbord, 2003).

Between 2002 and 2005 the USAID-funded Change Project implemented an innovative program in collaboration with a consortium of Peruvian universities, which included Universidad de Lima, Universidad Cayetano Heredia, Universidad Católica, and Universidad del Pacifico, which had expertise in communication, public health, social sciences, and business administration respectively. The Change Project implemented a series of capacity-building activities derived from a national assessment of health communication capacity and needs. Activities included training of NGO practitioners in mid-size cities and rural areas of the country, internships for on-site, experiential, and peer learning, and strengthening of communication networks. The project also had a clear interest in strengthening capacity at rural and local levels, given the increasing administrative decentralization of the country. As a long-term component of this process, an MA program that drew on the health communication competency framework developed in Ica, Peru, was designed with the participation of the four universities involved in the program. Waisbord (2006) identified five key lessons that included the importance of focusing on strengthening institutional capacity, building local ownership for sustainability, ensuring institutional commitment of involved partners, involving university institutions for long-term work, and approaching capacity development in a way that does not reduce it "to a series of isolated, haphazardly programed workshops and other activities. Just because workshops are offered and materials are produced year after year, a stronger capacity would not be the final result" (p. 235).

In Africa, with support from the Johns Hopkins University's Center for Communication Programs, The African Network for Strategic Communication in Health and Development (AfriComNet), an association of HIV and AIDS, health and development communication practitioners who reside, work, or have a primary interest in Africa, has worked over the past decade to engage universities on the continent to offer health communication training programs. Formerly known as the Regional HIV and AIDS Behaviour Change Communication Network (BCC Network), AfriComNet was established in October 2001 in recognition of the severity of the region's HIV and AIDS pandemic and the need for high-quality strategic health communication to respond to the crisis.

AfriComNet's strategic objectives are to promote effective strategic communication practices; increase recognition of strategic communication as critical to effectiveness of health and development programming; strengthen organizational capacity, credibility, and visibility of AfriComNet (www.africomnet.org). At a meeting held in 2011 in Kigali, Rwanda, faculty from 15 universities from nine countries reported progress on their health communication programs and activities, which included short courses and seminars on strategic health communication, research, monitoring and evaluation, and interpersonal communication, amongst other topics, with an increasing interest in the creation of master's level programs that would ensure greater institutionalization of these programs. While AfriComNet has not directly drawn on the health communication competency map, its training materials do reflect a similar set of competencies.

Some organizations have undertaken their own internal initiatives to build and develop the capacity of their staff and/or partners in health communication areas. Population Services International (PSI), a social marketing organization that works in Africa, Asia, Europe, and Latin America has implemented since 2007 the Results Initiative (RI), a 12-country regional capacity building project. It aims at increasing the regional and country capacity of PSI's social marketing affiliates and partners in Southern Africa (Angola, Botswana, Lesotho, Madagascar, Malawi, Mozambique, Namibia, South Africa, Swaziland, Uganda, Zambia, and Zimbabwe). RI was designed to build capacity in health impacts, behavior change, sustainability, and stakeholder satisfaction to address the HIV/AIDS epidemic. RI strategically built capacity in four main areas: operations, research, marketing, and management and leadership, which were identified based on an assessment of capacity needs by each of the participating country offices (Larson and Obregon, 2007).

A comprehensive capacity-strengthening package developed for this program included: distance education, university courses led by a full-time instructor; annual regional workshops, which reinforced distance education courses, and regional networks for communication/support and to share experiences; annual customized technical assistance visits to help improve job-related performance and outputs; cross-border exchange visits coupled with technical assistance visits; mini-grants and on-the-job training; expert-driven and peer-facilitated strategies; peer-led lunch box discussions with peer modeling; toolkits, case studies, and assigned readings; weekly, consistent, and timely feedback, follow-up, guidance, mentoring, and coaching; development of partnerships to build platform capacity; and dissemination of existing capacity building tools (Larson and Obregon, 2008). A mid-term assessment of this initiative showed significant improvements in many areas, for example, better use of research data in strategic communication plans, and highlighted the importance of institutional support to facilitate learning and application. In terms of recommendations, participants overwhelmingly concurred on the need to provide accreditation for this type of training, which was later addressed through collaboration with the University of South Florida.

The Soul City Institute for Health and Development Communication, a well-known and reputable nongovernmental organization that uses edutainment, advocacy and social mobilization to address health and development issues, has moved into the CBS arena by establishing a number of partnerships with local NGOs in nine countries in Southern Africa (Weiner, 2009; see also www.soulcity.org.za). Through a collaborative process that seeks to build and ensure local ownership through implementation of activities at local level, on-site technical support and training activities, and masters level training for some of the organization's staff (through collaboration with the University of Witwatersrand and other partners as discussed later), Soul City has progressively strengthened the capacity of its partners in the region.

Rimon and Sood (see Chapter 28 in this volume) discuss in detail efforts undertaken to institutionalize health communication in international health. The authors report how, through a series of systematic and integrated efforts, that includes a well-established three-week workshop in strategic health communication, the Center for Communication Programs at Johns Hopkins University has contributed to institutionalization of health communication at regional and country levels. The authors report on a number of indicators that range from resource allocation to health communication activities, to focused short-term training programs, to the creation of regional networks of trained health communication practitioners.

Yet, despite the increasing emphasis that many donors and agencies have placed on capacity building and strengthening in international development and global health, reflected in some of the examples listed above, systematic and long-term initiatives that specifically focus on capacity strengthening in health communication are rare. As stated earlier, it is assumed that all or most health communication interventions have an intrinsic CBS component. Most interventions typically involve some form of training and technical support; often, it is believed that the collaboration between practitioners with significant field experience in health communication and those who are new to the field naturally leads to some form of learning and knowledge and skills acquisition. However, for sustained capacity in health communication to be achieved, we argue that more systematic and longer-term efforts are needed.

Who Should Build and Strengthen Capacity in Health Communication?

In his analysis of the Peruvian experience of capacity strengthening in health promotion and communication, Waisbord (2003) introduces an important question in regard to whether universities, NGOs, or private voluntary organizations are in a better position to lead capacity building and strengthening efforts in health communication, a question that also might be relevant to other technical areas in international development. Waisbord summarizes advantages and disadvantages that apply to either universities or NGOs/PVOs (pp. 232–233).

- NGOs and PVOs typically have more field experience than universities, but are not always designed to be long-term, capacity-development institutions. Universities are expected to offer training opportunities, but generally are not sufficiently involved in applied work.
- NGOs are more likely to have expertise working with donors and international organizations (partially because their finances are closely dependent on development projects), but they may lack sufficient time and resources to conduct specific tasks. Universities might have a cadre of experts, but institutional mandates tend to restrict their participation in development work and social outreach.
- NGOs tend to have a wealth of hands-on experience, but they lack time to reflect upon and impart lessons learned. The presence of universities does make a difference in terms of the quality and expertise of local professionals. Universities are generally not designed to plan and conduct training programs in a short amount of time for key audiences (e.g. MOH staff).
- Despite their size and number of staff, NGOs generally have a structure that is better suited to implement capacity projects on the ground in a relative short amount of time than universities, which have a more complex and slow-moving decision-making process.

Waisbord's summary aptly captures the technical, operational, and managerial advantages and disadvantages of each type of organization. We argue that university-based training offers additional important advantages. First, universities can offer formal accreditation of health communication training, including postgraduate degrees. For many practitioners this option is particularly important for them to embrace formal education. Accreditation also contributes to addressing questions about the legitimacy and professionalization of the field, especially in light of the historical focus on short-term courses (see Fox, Chapter 3, and Rimon and Sood, Chapter 28, in this volume). Second, and connected to the previous point, given the elasticity and often blurred lines amongst various areas of communication training (e.g., public relations; media relations) and health communication (and the particular competencies needed for applied work), university programs can contribute to greater demarcation of what specialized training in health communication is about and higher standards. Third, short-term courses tend to be short-lived and dependent upon project funding or the initiative of individuals and organizations. University-based programs, particularly those at masters or diploma level are more likely to contribute to institutionalization and long-term commitment to health communication training. Lastly, institutionalized programs at university level can contribute to greater advocacy before other disciplines in the health and social sciences, particularly through the interaction amongst students and faculty, and the ability to produce new knowledge through thesis and research projects that can enrich the literature in this field.

Against this backdrop, in the next section we focus on an example of university and competency-based CBS in health communication. We describe and discuss the ongoing experience of C-Change (Communication for Change), a USAID-funded initiative that has the mandate to strengthen capacity at various levels. We draw on our own involvement with C-Change, provide a brief description of the program, highlight its key components and activities with a particular focus on its university-based component, and summarize lessons learned to date.

Building and Strengthening Capacity through Institutionalization of Health Communication at University Level

Communication for Change (C-Change) is a five-year initiative (2007–2012) supported by the US Agency for International Development that works across sectors (and across USAID bureaus) to improve the effectiveness and sustainability of communication as an integral part of development efforts. C-Change brings together a partnership of US-based and Southern organizations with extensive experience in communication for global health and development. The lead partner is FHI 360[2] (Family Health International), which has worked with other Southern partners to institutionalize competency-based programs in SBCC (social and behavior change communication). SBCC is a particular approach within development and health communication that seeks to address change at individual, community, and social level through integrated communication strategies. Strengthening local capacity in communication for health and development is a central goal of the C-Change Project. C-Change aims to transfer health and development communication skills and knowledge to developing country institutions. Its goals include the promotion and support of system-wide and long-term changes by strengthening communication capacities in health and development systems, facilitation of organizational synergies, and mobilization of existing resources to improve local capacity to deliver top-quality and relevant technical support in communication for health and development.

C- Change's conceptual approach rests upon three central elements: strengthening core competencies in communication applied to specific technical sectors, supporting and enhancing institutional networks committed to CBS through a system-wide approach (working at individual, organizational, sectoral, institutional levels and toward capacity distributed across different actors); and ensuring an exit strategy that facilitates local ownership of CBS efforts. As stated earlier, the competency-based model refers to the combination of skills, knowledge, and attitudes required to perform effectively in

SBCC-CAT

Step 1: Assessing SBCC capacity

Component 1: Understanding the context through situation analysis					
Sub-component 1: Evidence-based and theory or model-driven planning and design					
A situationan alysisis a systematic review of social, cultural, political, and behavioral data to identify internal and external determinants of a situation, such as immediate and underlying causes and effects.					
How does your program gather and analyze information to guide the planning and design process for SBCC programs?					
Question	1	2	3	4	Score
1.1 Do you conduct a situation analysis before designing SBCC programs?	Programs do not analyze the social and behavioral issues	Programs rely on their own networks and experience to analyze social and behavioral issues	Programs involve key informants in the analysis of social and behavioral issues	Programs involve multiple perspectivesto analyze social and behavioral issues	☐ = 1 ☐ = 2 ☐ = 3 ☐ = 4
1.2 Do you use theories or models for situation analysis or communication strategy design?	Programs do not use theories or models	Programs use elements of theories or models but they cannot be traced back to specific theories or models	Programs use relevant theories or models for situation analysis or communication strategy design	Programs always use relevant theories and models for both situation analysis and communication strategy design	☐ = 1 ☐ = 2 ☐ = 3 ☐ = 4
1.3 Do you use research data to assist with SBCC program design?	Programs do not collect data because design is pre-determined	Programs rely on their own sources of information to design programs	Programs use data from existing research to design programs	Programs use data from both existing and original research to design programs	☐ = 1 ☐ = 2 ☐ = 3 ☐ = 4
1.4 Do you review the activities of stakeholders during a situation analysis?	Programs do not review stakeholders' activities	Programs review stakeholders' activities or share program plans and ideas	Programs review stakeholders' activities and share program plans and ideas	Programs review stakeholders' activities, share program plans, and collaborate to reduce replication of services and overlap of activities	☐ = 1 ☐ = 2 ☐ = 3 ☐ = 4

Figure 27.1 The first section of a CAT.
Source: Produced by C-Change and funded by USAID.

different work settings. A competency-based approach incorporates organizational expectations in the definition of competencies and training. Just as C-Change addresses the enabling environment to promote healthy behaviors and social change in its programs, the competency model similarly integrates contextual demands and institutional variables that affect the utilization of skills and knowledge. It is crucial to ensure that individuals learn what they can effectively use and that CBS programs match the needs and expectations in different work settings.

The basic premise of C-Change's approach is that strengthened communication capacity of local actors is necessary to ensure long-term sustainability and impact of programs. CBS aims to expand technical competencies and resources at local, national, and regional levels, so that more individuals and institutions based in Southern countries will be able to own and lead the planning, implementation, and evaluation of future activities. With work in several countries in Africa, Asia, Eastern Europe, and Latin America, C-Change developed a capacity-strengthening toolkit that includes a competency-based capacity assessment tool (CAT), which allows for the identification of SBCC needs at organizational level (Figure 27.1 and Figure 27.2 provide examples of two sections of CAT); a series of SBCC training modules for on-site and online learning; a series of tools and resources for focused training in areas such as interpersonal communication, and community-based dialogue; and several online resources that provide access to training tools and evidence of SBCC impact. Some of these resources and tools

SBCC-CAT

Component 4: Implementing & monitoring change processes					
Sub-component 4: Frameworks and mechanisms					
How do you monitor your SBCC programs?					
Question	1	2	3	4	Score
4.9 Do you develop M&E plans for your SBCC programs?	Programs do not have M&E plans	Some of the programs have M&E plans	Nearly half of the programs have M&E plans	A majority or all of the programs have M&E plans	☐ = 1 ☐ = 2 ☐ = 3 ☐ = 4
4.10 Do you develop indicators for SBCC programs that are linked to your communication objectives?	Programs do not have indicators for their SBCC programs	Programs have some indicators but they are not clearly linked to the communication objectives	Programs have process and output indicators that are linked to the communication objectives	Programs have process, output, and outcome indicators that are linked to the communication objectives	☐ = 1 ☐ = 2 ☐ = 3 ☐ = 4
4.11 Do you have tools to monitor implementation of SBCC programs?	Programs do not monitor SBCC programs	Programs create tools to monitor SBCC programs as needed	Programs have standardized tools to monitor indicators	Programs always use standardized tools to monitor indicators	☐ = 1 ☐ = 2 ☐ = 3 ☐ = 4
4.12 Do you have a system in place to make sure high quality M&E data is collected and analyzed?	Programs do not have a data collection and analysis plan	Programs have a data collection and analysis plan	Programs have trained or hired people to implement thedata collection and analysis plan	Programs have trained or hired people to implement the data collection and analysis plan and conduct data quality checks	☐ = 1 ☐ = 2 ☐ = 3 ☐ = 4

Figure 27.2 A further section of a CAT.
Source: Produced by C-Change and funded by USAID.

have been used to guide various capacity strengthening efforts at country level. For instance, in Namibia a CAT-based capacity assessment was conducted with 13 organizations working in HIV/AIDS. That assessment led to the identification of SBCC areas and competencies that needed to be strengthened, and to a series of training and onsite mentoring activities. Similarly, in Guatemala the CAT has been used to guide capacity strengthening activities. In South Africa, the HIV Community Dialogue toolkit was used to strengthen the capacity of NGOs working with low literacy populations.

Within the broad range of capacity building and strengthening activities that C-Change has implemented, its work with universities is of particular interest to us. C-Change has collaborated with six universities in three continents. The University of Witwatersrand (Wits University) in South Africa, in cooperation with C-Change's Southern partner the Soul City Institute of Health and Development Communication, the University of Tirana in Albania, the Universidad del Valle in Guatemala, the University of the West Indies in Jamaica, and Cross River State University of Technology (CRUTECH), and University of Calabar (UNICAL) in Nigeria. We focus primarily on the experience of Wits University and Soul City.

Through collaboration with its Southern-based partner, the Soul City Institute of Health and Development Communication, C-Change has supported the creation of a division of social and behavior change communication within the masters of public health (MPH) at Wits University's School of Public Health. The creation of a division essentially means that the MPH now offers an SBCC field (area of concentration), in addition to the other five fields it has traditionally offered. This initiative evolved from Soul City's realization that the SBCC capacity needs in South Africa and Southern

Africa demanded a longer-term focus and higher-level capacity development beyond short-term and continued education courses only. With support from the UK Department of International Development (DFID) and later from the Centers for Disease Control (CDC), and based on a thorough assessment of the need for such a program and where to establish it, a decision was made to work with Wits University on the basis of its strong record in quality education and research on public health and health promotion, and its focus on health, human rights, and social justice.

One of the advantages of health communication as a field is its interdisciplinary character. While areas of emphasis might vary, health communication programs can be equally run out of schools of communication, public health, or even other schools or departments (for instance, in Albania an MA program has been set up in the School of Social Work and Public Policy). There are multiple examples in the United States of such programs based in schools of communication or media, or public health and medicine. However, an additional advantage at Wits University is the opportunity the SBCC field offers for dialogue and engagement with other fields within the MPH program (i.e., Health Systems and Policy; Rural Health; Maternal and Child Health; Occupational Hygiene), which is critically important to continue positioning SBCC and mainstreaming it within the larger health and development field.

The design of the Wits SBCC program followed a series of steps that provided a strong foundation. A consultative meeting that convened existing health and development-related communication programs (e.g., University of KwaZulu Natal, South Africa; Ohio University, USA; Roskilde University, Denmark), NGOs and international organizations that work in social and behavior change communication-related issues (e.g., Soul City; Population Services International; C-Change; Johns Hopkins University's Center for Communication Programs), and members of various academic units at Wits university allowed for inputs from various key players. The meeting also led to the definition of key competency areas for the Wits University program (drawing on the competencies developed at the Ica, Peru, regional meeting) that served as foundation for the development of SBCC curriculum and content. The competency-based curriculum (focused on skills, knowledge, and attitudes/values) includes courses in Applying Social and Behavior Theory to Practice; Communication, Media and Society; Social and Behavior Change Communication Approaches; Planning and Implementing Social and Behavior Change; and Research, Monitoring and Evaluation of SBCC.

The Division of Social and Behavior Change at Wits University was officially launched in May 2010. In the first year of the program, 42 practitioners applied for admission into the MPH program with SBCC as their field (out of more than 120 who applied for other fields). A total of 14 students from seven countries in Southern Africa, seven of them females and seven males, were admitted into the program, although only 13 eventually enrolled in it. Such a strong response is, in no small measure, an indication of the tremendous interest that this program has generated in the region. In addition, because the Wits University program is offered in the form of block release courses (one week) students not admitted into the MPH program can enroll in the SBCC courses listed above as certificate courses only. As of 2011, more than 150 participants had enrolled in certificate courses, with many participants having enrolled in two or more courses. More importantly, the majority of participants in the program, both MPH students and certificate course students, are typically affiliated with nongovernmental and governmental institutions (e.g., ministries of health; national HIV/AIDS councils), who see in the SBCC program an opportunity to hone and strengthen a number of skills they have either learned or been introduced to on the field, and to become accredited SBCC professionals. This also ensures that CBS is focused on a group of practitioners who can more easily contribute to greater legitimacy and professionalization of the field.

Participants in the Wits SBCC program also have been introduced to a virtual community of practice that seeks to create a space for knowledge and information sharing, networking, debate, and collaboration on issues of common interest in SBCC. Ongoing support through virtual communities of practice provides participants in the SBCC program with the opportunity to engage in an open dialogue outside their regular work environments, and ongoing reflection and learning. Thus, the Wits SBCC program exemplifies an example of a solid university-based program that can serve as a reference for similar efforts.

Lessons Learned

While it is still too early to evaluate the contribution and long-term effects of the Wits University SBCC program, as well as the other university programs we have cited, they represent promising examples of longer-term efforts that might effectively address challenges in health communication. We now summarize a number of issues that we believe add value to this type of effort, mainly as a result of the Wits University experience and also applicable to the ongoing experience of the other universities involved in similar SBCC programs.

First, the institutionalization of the Wits SBCC program offers hope that it will contribute to the creation of a critical mass of highly qualified SBCC practitioners. While the existing short-term courses that many organizations and universities offer are necessary to address immediate needs, diploma and masters level courses are only possible if institutional commitment and support is available (Waisbord, 2006). Second, the Wits SBCC program is also a prime example of successful collaboration between international development agencies, local nongovernmental organizations, and higher education institutions. While this collaborative approach carries some logistical and administrative complexity, the Wits SBCC program is an example that such collaboration, which has made the program more feasible and stronger, is possible. Openness to collaboration and respect amongst participating partners is essential to the success of these programs (Airhihenbuwa *et al.*, 2011). In addition, through this collaboration participating partners have also benefited by strengthening their own staff and faculty. Third, the SBCC program will address a felt need for the accreditation of SBCC training, particularly in Africa. While short-term courses often lead to a certificate of completion or participation, the Wits SBCC program certifies participants in a way comparable to other programs and fields. In particular, the fact that students receive an MPH degree also adds to the legitimacy of the SBCC field.

Fourth, the competency focus of these programs can provide a much needed impetus for a renewed emphasis on CBS in health communication. Other than the efforts we have summarized above, we did not find any other recent or ongoing regional or global initiatives focused on CBS in health communication. If the crisis in human resources and the sense of urgency declared by the WHO 2006 World Health Report translates into action across all areas of global health, then health communication also should have an important place in those efforts. Fifth, because the Wits SBCC program is located within the School of Public Health it has created opportunities for dialogue with other public health fields. For instance, one of the authors of this chapter presented on SBCC research at a weekly forum that convenes students and faculty across the Wits School of Public Health. Similarly, some students from other fields of the MPH program have elected to enroll in some of the SBCC field courses. Sixth, these types of programs should contribute to greater empowerment of local institutions as they can count on the availability of human resources with higher qualifications.

Lastly, even though it is still too early to measure the impact of the programs we have discussed in this chapter, it is critically important to emphasize the need to develop systematic evaluations that might provide strong evidence of the contributions of such programs to the field of health communication at individual, organizational, sectoral, and institutional levels. There is an intrinsic evaluation measure in the Wits SBCC program – and of the other programs – on the basis of the delivery of a trained workforce in this field. However, more importantly, the impact that the qualification of the students will have on health and development programs, how SBCC graduates will more largely influence the field and the organizational environment in which they operate, their ability to advocate for greater mainstreaming of SBCC, and the perception of SBCC amongst professionals and decision makers in the health and development field, are potential indicators that might provide a true measure of the contribution of these programs.

Traditionally, training has been synonymous with instruction and much of the emphasis has been placed on design and delivery, and on the evaluation of individual capacity. These remain important components of CBS programs. But the concept of what constitutes effective training and capacity development, particularly competency-based training in the context of CBS programs, has broadened to consider the interpersonal, social, and structural characteristics that influence the relationship of the trainee and the training program to the broader organizational and institutional contexts. In other words, measuring the success of university and competency-based programs that are part of larger CBS initiatives will require evaluation approaches that take into consideration the larger social, cultural, organizational and institutional context in which participants are immersed.

Conclusions and Recommendations

In this chapter we have sought to discuss the role of capacity building (and strengthening) as an integral component of global health communication programs, and to emphasize collaboration with higher education institutions as a critical dimension of sustained and long-term efforts aimed at creating a critical mass of individual and organizations with the required competencies in health communication. Our analysis reveals that capacity building and strengthening has regained a prominent role in international health and development. However, that prominence comes with additional demands, particularly the need to more effectively evaluate the contribution of CBS to health and development work.

It is also clear that the discourse on CBS has found a niche within the international health agenda with a particular emphasis on strengthening human resource capacity. Efforts developed in the health promotion field are a prime example of that. We identified in the literature strong evidence of the degree of attention that is paid to CBS in health promotion, and the strong advocacy that different institutions have made toward increased efforts CBS in health promotion. Conversely, that is not the case in health communication today. Some of the initiatives that took place in the 1990s and early 2000s have faded away and current efforts are rather limited. Nevertheless, there are some interesting examples of advocacy and CBS in health communication. The SBCC program at the University of Witwatersrand is a recent and interesting example of how such programs can make a contribution to CBS efforts in health communication. However, we believe that more focused efforts and investment are needed in order to revitalize capacity building and strengthening initiatives in health communication.

The overarching purpose of this chapter is to raise greater awareness about the importance of examining CBS issues in health communication. By documenting the current state of CBS efforts in health communication and contrasting it with similar efforts in health promotion, we have exposed a tremendous need for more work in that area. We advocate greater dialogue with higher education institutions, health organizations, and academics and researchers involved in CBS efforts in health promotion and health communication. While each field must retain its own identity, the similarities between the two provide interesting opportunities for further dialogue and potential collaboration.

We now put forward some recommendations derived from our previous analysis. First, it is clear that a holistic perspective on CBS is needed. CBS initiatives should articulate efforts at different levels (individual, organizational, sectoral, and institutional). The recent emphasis of international organizations on CBS provides a tremendous opportunity for further enhancement of work in this area. Health communication initiatives should reflect these trends as well, with particular attention to rigorous evaluation of these programs. Second, articulation of various efforts in CBS in health communication might maximize the existing limited efforts. This should be reflected through collaboration at international and regional level. For instance, the C-Change project has initiated collaboration with AfriComNet, which should contribute to greater positioning of CBS in health communication in Africa. Third, greater collaboration between academic institutions and established NGOs and organizations that do effective work in health communication is desirable and should be more frequent. As explained earlier, NGOs and universities have different strengths and abilities. In an area where so much work needs to be done, such synergies are critical for enhancement of CBS efforts. The collaboration between the Wits University SBCC program and the Soul City Institute of Health and Development Communication in South Africa is a good example of that approach.

Fourth, greater presence of health communication programs and courses at university level is essential. While some universities in Africa and Latin America have taken steps in that direction, the reality is that there is significant gap in this area. In Latin America, as stated earlier, there are more than 1,400 schools of communication and media, but only a handful of them offer health communication programs, which contrasts with the extensive list of schools that run health promotion programs (Arroyo, 2009). In Colombia, where there are more than 70 schools and/or programs of media and communication, hardly five institutions offer health communication programs, and another handful occasionally offer health communication courses as electives. Fifth, curricula of current and potentially new health communication programs would benefit from a competency-focused approach. The demands that health and development work places on health communication can be best met by professionals trained through programs that subscribe to a competency-based curriculum, which also might contribute to better evaluation of capacity development in this area. Sixth, new technologies offer new opportunities for innovation in the delivery of CBS programs in health communication. Online platforms should provide new alternatives for greater reach.

Despite the important progress made in international health communication over the past two decades, particularly its visibility in public health and development programs, capacity building and strengthening work in health communication has been highly fragmented and has lacked continuity. For global health communication to grow as a field in the long run, CBS efforts must be strengthened over the next few years.

Notes

1 The authors favor the term capacity strengthening based on the assumption that in any given context some capacity exists on the ground, particularly in the health field.
2 C-Change was previously run by the Academy for Educational Development.

References

Airhihenbuwa, C., Shisana, O., Zungu, N. *et al.* (2011). Research capacity building: A U.S.–South Africa Partnership. *Global Health Promotion, 18*(2), 27–35.

Alcalay, R. and Mendoza, C. (2000). *Proyecto Comsalud: Un Estudio Comparativo de Mensajes Relacionados con Salud en los Medios Masivos Latinoamericanos* [A comparative study of health-related message sin Latin American media]. Washington, DC: Organización Panamericana de la Salud.

Arroyo, H. (2009). La formación de recursos humanos y el desarrollo de competencias para la capacitación en promoción de la salud en América Latina [The training of human resources and the development of competencies for health promotion in Latin America]. *Global Health Promotion, 16*(2), 66–72.

Barry, M. (2008). Capacity building for the future of health promotion. *Promotion and Education,15*(4), 56–58.

Barry, M., Allegrante, J., LaMarre, M. *et al.*, (2009). The Galway Consensus Conference: International collaboration on the development of core competencies for health promotion and health education. *Global Health Promotion, 16*(2), 5–11.

Battel-Kirk, B., Barry, M., Taub, A., and Lysoby, L. (2009). A review of the international literature on health promotion competencies. *Global Health Promotion, 16*(2), 12–20.

Blagescu, M. and Young, J. (2006). *Capacity development for policy advocacy: Current thinking and approaches among agencies supporting Civil Society Organisations.* London: Overseas Development Institute. Retrieved 4/21/06 from http://www.odi.org.uk/cspp/Publications/Index.html.

Bolger, J. (2000). Capacity development: why, what, and how. *CIDA Capacity Development Occasional Series, 1*(1), 1–8. Retrieved from http://portals.wi.wur.nl/files/docs/SPICAD/16.%20Why%20what%20and%20how%20of%20capacity%20development%20-%20CIDA.pdf

Brown, L., LaFond, A., and Macintyre, K. (2001). Measuring capacity building. *MEASURE Evaluation.* University of North Carolina at Chapel Hill: Carolina Population Center. Retrieved from http://www.heart-intl.net/HEART/Financial/comp/MeasuringCapacityBuilg.pdf

Castro, A., Waisbord, S. and Coe, (2003). *Comunicacion en Salud: Lecciones Aprendidas y Desafios en el Desarrollo Curricular* [Communication and health: Lessons learned and challenges in curricular development]. Washington, DC: Organización Panamericana de la Salud/Proyecto Change.

Chikombero, M. 2009. Existing development and health curricula and training materials in selected countries in Africa. Unpublished report submitted to Ohio University/C-Change.

Cohen, J. M. (1993). *Building Sustainable Public Sector Managerial, Professional, and Technical Capacity: A Framework for Analysis and Intervention.* Harvard Institute for International Development, Harvard University. Development Discussion Papers, no. 473.

Collignon, M., Valdez, M., Obregon, R. *et al.* (2003). *Medios y Salud: La Voz de los Adolescentes* [Media and health: The voice of the adolescents]. Washington, DC: Organización Panamericana de la Salud.

Crisp, B., Swerissen, H., and Duckett, S. (2000). Four approaches to capacity building in health. *Health Pomotion International, 15*(2), 99–107.

Degnbol-Martinussen, J. (2002). Development goals, governance and capacity building: aid as a catalyst. *Development and Change, 33*(2), 269–280.

DFID (Department for International Development) (2002). *Capacity Development: Where Do We Stand Now?*London. Retrieved from http://info.worldbank.org/etools/docs/library/114227/CD%2DDFID%2DWhere%20Do%20We%20Stand%20Final.doc

Eade, D. (2007). Capacity building: who builds and whose capacity? *Development in Practice, 17*(4&5), 630–639.

Flaman, L., Nykiforuk, C. Plotnikoff, R., and Raine, K. (2010). Exploring facilitators and barriers to individual and organizational level capacity building: outcomes of participation in a community priority setting workshop. *Global Health Promotion,17*(2), 34–43.

Folke, C., Carpenter, S., Elmqvist, T. *et al.* (2002). Resilience and sustainable development: Building adaptive capacity in a world of transformations. *AMBIO: A Journal of the Human Environment, 31*(5), 437–440.

Fukuda-Parr, S., Lopes, C. and Malik, K. (2002). *Capacity for Development. New solutions to old Problems.* New York: United Nations Development Program and Earthscan Publications.

Hartwig, K., Humphries, D., and Matebeni, Z. (2008). Building capacity for AIDS NGOs in Southern Africa: Evaluation of a pilot initiative. *Health Promotion International, 23*(3), 251–259.

Heward, S., Hutchins, C., and Keleher, H. (2007). Organizational change – Key to capacity building and health promotion. *Health Promotion International, 22*(2), 170–178.

Horton, D., Alexaki, A., Bennet-Lartey, S. *et al.* (2003). *Evaluating Capacity Development: Experiences from Research and Development Organizations around the World.* Retrieved from http://www.crdi.org/en/ev-31556-201-1-DO_TOPIC.html

Irigoin, M., Whitacre, P., Faulkner, D. and Coe, G. (2002). *Mapping Competencies for Communication for Development and Social Change: Turning Knowledge, Skills, and Attitudes Into Action.* USAID: Washington, DC.

Labonte, R. and Laverack, G. (2001). Capacity building in health promotion, Part 1: For whom? And for what purpose? *Critical Public Health, 11*(2), 111–127.

LaFond, A. and Brown, L., (2003). Defining capacity-building monitoring and evaluation: A guide to monitoring and evaluation of capacity-building interventions in the health sector in developing countries. *Measure Evaluation Manual Series, No. 7.* University of North Carolina at Chapel Hill: Carolina Population Center. Retrieved from http://gametlibrary.worldbank.org/FILES/610_M&E%20of%20Capacity%20Building%20Interventions.pdf

Lansang, M. and Dennis, R. (2004). Building capacity in health research in developing countries. *Bulletin of the World Health Organisation, 82*(10), 764–770.

Larson, S. and Obregon, R. (2008). Mid-term evaluation of the Results Initiative: A report submitted to Population Services International. Athens, OH: Ohio University.

Lavergne, R. and Saxby, J. (2001). Capacity development: Visions and implications. *CIDA Capacity Development Occasional Series, 3,* 1–12.

Lebel, L., Anderies, J. M., Campbell, B. *et al.* (2006). Governance and the capacity to manage resilience in regional social-ecological systems. *Ecology and Society, 11*(1), 19. Retrieved from http://www.ecologyandsociety.org/vol11/iss1/art19/

Lessik, A., and Michener, V., (2000). Recent practices in monitoring and evaluation: Measuring institutional capacity (TIPS). *USAID Center for Development Information and Evaluation.* Washington, D.C. Retrieved on 4/10/06 from http://pdf.dec.org/pdf_docs/PNACG612.pdf

Light, P. and Hubbard, E. (2004). *The Capacity Building Challenge Part I: A Research Perspective.* New York: Foundation Center.

Lusthaus, C., Adrien, M. H., and Perstinger, M. (1999). *Capacity development: Definitions, Issues, and Implications for Planning, Monitoring and Evaluation.* Universalia Occasional Paper No. 35. Montreal: Universalia.

McKinsey & Co. (2001). *Effective Capacity Building in Nonprofit Organizations.* Retrieved from http://vppartners.org/learning/reports/ capacity/toc.pdf

Morgan, P. (1998). *Capacity and Capacity Development – Some Strategies.* Hull: Policy Branch, CIDA.

OECD (Office of Economic Development) (n.d.). *The Paris Declaration on Aid Effectiveness and the Accra Agenda for Action.* Retrieved from http://www.oecd.org/dataoecd/11/41/34428351.pdf

Onya, H. (2009). "Health promotion competency building in Africa: A call for action. *Global Health Promotion, 16*(2), 47–51.

Nyamwaya D. (2003). Health promotion in Africa: Strategies, players, challenges and prospects. *Health Promotion International, 18*(2), 85–87.

Potter, C. and Brough, R. (2004). Systemic capacity building: A hierarchy of needs. *Health Policy Planning, 19*(5), 336–345.

Shilton, T. (2009). Health promotion competencies: providing a road map for health promotion to assume a prominent role in global health. *Global Health Promotion, 16*(2), 42–46.

Teskey, G. (2005). *Capacity Development and State Building: Issues: Evidence and Implications for DFID.* London: DFID.

UNDP. (1997). *A Synopsis of General Guidelines for Capacity Assessment and Development.* New York: UNDP.

United Nations General Assembly (2005, January 14). Resolution enhancing capacity building in global public health. 59th session A/RES/59/27. Retrieved from http://www.worldlii.org/int/other/UNGARsn/2003/50.pdf

Van den Broucke, S., Jooste, H., Tlali, M. *et al.* (2010). Strengthening the capacity for health promotion in South Africa through international collaboration. *Global Health Promotion, 17*(2), Supplement 6–16.

Waisbord, S. (2006). When training is insufficient: Reflections on capacity development in health promotion in Peru. *Health Promotion International, 21*(3), 230–237.

Weiner, R. (2009). *Report on the Consultative Meeting on Social and Behavior Change Communication.* Johannesburg: School of Public Health, University of Witwatersrand.

Whyte, A. (2004). *Human and Institutional Capacity Building: Landscape Analysis of Donor Trends in International Development,* report to the Rockefeller Foundation. New York: Rockefeller Foundation.

WHO (World Health Organisation) (2006). *Working Together for Health,* The world health report 2006 (Overview). Retrieved from http://www.who.int/whr/2006/06_overview_en.pdf

Wills, J., and Rudolph, M. (2010). Health promotion capacity building in South Africa. *Global Health Promotion, 17*(3), 29–34.

World Bank (2005). *Capacity Building in Africa: An OED Evaluation of World Bank Support.* The World Bank: Washington, DC.

28

Institutionalizing Communication in International Health
The USAID–Johns Hopkins University Partnership

Jose Rimon II and Suruchi Sood

Introduction

The primary question of interest for funded health communication programs is "Did the intervention have an effect?" This interest has fueled considerable research on the efficacy and effectiveness of health communication interventions. In 2003, Snyder, Diop-Sidibe, and Badine, completed a meta-analysis of 39 different Family Planning communication campaigns in developing countries, all of which were supported by the Center for Communication Programs (CCP), to examine the effectiveness of these campaigns. The results from the meta-analysis indicated that, although several campaigns had high baseline levels of knowledge, these levels continued to increase due to the campaigns. Overall, positive effects of campaign exposure were noted on several ideational factors, such as partner communication about family planning ($r = 0.10$), approval of family planning ($r = 0.09$) and behavioral intentions ($r = 0.07$). The rates of change for knowledge and interpersonal communication were somewhat larger than for behavior change, at the same time consistent with the hierarchy of effect model, the meta-analysis concluded that the campaigns had a positive effect on the use of modern methods of family planning ($r = 0.07$).

While much is known about the effectiveness of health communication relatively little attention is focused on the broader dissemination, uptake, and diffusion of public health promotion interventions (Oldenburg *et al.*, 1999). This requires asking follow-on questions of specific interest to funders such as "Did the effect last, will the behaviors sustain themselves?" and "Will the intervention program endure?" (Thompson and Winner, 1999).

Several synonyms – institutionalization, incorporation, sustainability, capacity building, and durability – are used to focus on these follow-up questions. While these terms

The Handbook of Global Health Communication, First Edition. Edited by Rafael Obregon and Silvio Waisbord.
© 2012 John Wiley & Sons, Inc. Published 2012 by John Wiley & Sons, Inc.

are used interchangeably, sometimes, especially in the case of institutionalization and sustainability, there are nuances in their meaning (Thompson and Winner, 1999). Institutionalization, which is more commonly used in the United States, has been defined as developing community and organizational support for interventions such that they become an integral part of a larger system and remain viable in the long term (Goodman *et al.*, 1993). Sustainability on the other hand, which is more commonly used outside of the United States, refers to the ability of an intervention to deliver activities and benefits after external assistance ends (Lefebvre, 1992; Scheirer, 2005; St. Leger, 2005; Swerrisen and Crisp, 2004; Thompson and Winner; 1999).

Over the last 20 years, the term "institutionalization" has elicited great interest among public health researchers and practitioners alike. The goal of health communication programs is often to reinforce or promote behavior change at various levels. Long-lasting behavior maintenance, especially involving changes in social norms and social systems associated with health, is a complex process. Organizations require concerted time and effort to integrate and implement innovative approaches (Goodman *et al.*, 1993). For behavior change to be sustained and the lessons learned shared with the larger community, the importance of institutionalization therefore, cannot be overstated.

This chapter traces the trajectory of funding, programs, and research at the Johns Hopkins University Center for Communication Programs (JHU/CCP: see www.jhuccp.org) supported by USAID (United States Agency for International Development) from 1982, when Population Communication Services 1 (PCS 1) was first implemented, through 2008, when the Health Communication Partnership (HCP), ended. While this chapter refers mostly to PCS and HCP, both projects were part of a larger institution CCP, which is housed within the Johns Hopkins Bloomberg School of Public Health. In addition, both PCS and HCP were partnerships with several domestic and international agencies. Specifically PCS 1–4 partners included: Academy for Educational Development (AED), Save the Children, Prospect Associates, Program for Adaptation of Technology in Health (PATH), Center for Development and Population Activities (CEDPA), and Porter and Novelli. The core partners under HCP were Academy for Educational Development (AED), Save the Children, The International HIV/AIDS Alliance, and Tulane University School of Public Health. For purposes of this chapter, whenever the collective experience of the PCS and HCP projects are referred to, it will be called the Program, for easier reading.

First, we will examine the literature on institutionalization, specifically in terms of measurement of the construct of institutionalization. This will form the basis of the key areas this chapter will explore. USAID's efforts to institutionalize communication will rely on three strands of information pertaining to funding, programs, and research. This chapter will conclude with a summary of key learnings from the Program.

Institutionalization: Description and Measurement

As noted above, institutionalization is the most commonly used term to connote maintenance of intervention activities (Thompson and Winner, 1999). An understanding of the process of diffusion, which culminates in institutionalization involves, among other things, formalized organizational and structural support, appropriate and targeted funding, formal monitoring of research activities and its dissemination, and ongoing training for both researchers and practitioners (Nutbeam, 1996).

While several measures of institutionalization exist, the most notable is the levels of institutionalization (LoIn) measure, first proposed by Goodman and Steckler in 1989 and later codified by Goodman, McLeroy, Steckler, and Hoyle in 1993. The LoIn measure has been tested for validity and reliability and formed the basis for several studies on institutionalization (Shediac-Rizkallah and Bone, 1998; Johnson *et al.*, 2004; Barab, Redman, and Froman, 2004; Pluye, Potvin, and Denis, 2004). According to the LoIn, organizations consist of four subsystems: production, maintenance, supportive, and managerial. Institutionalization occurs when a project becomes embedded into these subsystems (Goodman and Steckler, 1989) and when a project's innovations diffuse into a larger social system (Rogers, 1995).

The production subsystem refers to the product-directed activities and includes implementation. The maintenance subsystem is concerned with personnel and examines items such as recruitment and retention of staff. Both the production and maintenance subsystems are internally directed. The supportive subsystem, on the other hand, refers to the creation of an enabling environment and includes funding and housing for project activities. The last managerial subsystem is "the lubricant which controls, coordinates, and directs all of the other subsystems' operations" by formal assignment of roles and responsibilities, routinization of progress reports, and integration of evaluation into the project (Goodman *et al.*, 1993, p. 165).

Since its creation, the LoIn measure has been utilized primarily as a data collection tool to examine the institutionalization of several programs within an institution or one program within several institutions (Shediac-Rizkallah and Bone, 1998; Johnson *et al.*, 2004; Barab, Redman, and Froman, 2004; Pluye, Potvin, and Denis, 2004). Studies of institutionalization have not focused on the processes leading to institutionalization, a gap that this chapter tries to fill by applying a LoIn framework to study *post hoc* the level of institutionalization achieved through USAID's long term commitment and funding of the Program.

From PCS to HCP: An Overview

The academic study of communication devolved out of the social sciences in the post-World War II era (Rogers, 1994). However, the organized integration of communication strategies within the field of public health is relatively new. PCS was established in 1982 with funding from USAID through a competitive procurement. Prior to this time, "family planning communication was underfunded, undervalued by policy makers, and largely devoid of strategic thinking" (Rogers as quoted in Piotrow *et al.*, 1997). The history of the Program in many ways mirrors the history of the field of health communication, which has been characterized as passing through four big-picture but distinct eras (Figure 28.1).

As Figure 28.1 shows, the field of global health communication has evolved over time from a medical and supply-oriented model to one that is integrative and focuses on

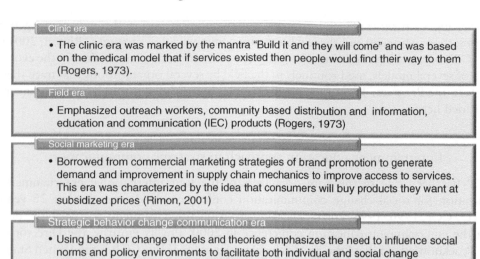

Figure 28.1 Eras in global health communication.
Source: Rimon (2001), adapted from Everett Rogers.

Table 28.1 JHU/CCP projects and years of operation.

Project	Term	Award Date	Completion	Extended To
PCS 1	5-year term. Renewed in 4 years	Sept. 30, 1982	Sept. 30, 1987	
PCS 2	5-year term. Renewed in 4 years	Sept. 1, 1986	Aug. 31, 1991	
PCS 3	5-year term. Ceiling increased, term extended	July 18, 1990	July 15, 1995	July, 15 1997
PCS 4	5-year term, 2-year extension option exercised	Nov. 7, 1995	Nov. 6, 2000	Nov. 6, 2002
HCP	5-year term, with Associate Awards option	July 24, 2002	Jan. 31, 2008	8 Associate Awards in Egypt, Jordan, Zambia, Ethiopia, Uganda, India, Mozambique and South Africa

Note: The PCS 3 cooperative agreement included the PIP Project during FYs 1993–1997.
Source: Piotrow *et al.* (2003).

individuals and communities as producers of their own health. The period for the five projects included in this chapter (Table 28.1), reflect to a large extent the development in thinking about program design, implementation, and evaluation as characterized by the era during which they functioned. Based on lessons learned from over a 25-year period, our current thinking about "strategic health communication" is one of integration: of demand and supply as well as multiple channels each serving its own niche but reinforcing each other. Finally, strategic communication occurs through convergence among those who send and those who receive communication messages (Rimon, 2001).

CCP's overarching commitment to strategic communication has resulted in the evolution of several models, used routinely in the field by several organizations that trace their roots to the Program. Two of the many examples spearheaded through the Program are provided here.

Entertainment-education approach to strategic communication

CCP has been one of the core organizers of the four international entertainment-education for social change communication conferences held over the last 25 years (JHU/CCP, 1990, 1998, 2001). Speaking at a panel titled "strategic partnerships" during the entertainment-education conference in 2000, Phyllis Piotrow, the Director of CCP, acknowledged that "the most valuable partner for JHU/CCP is the United States Agency for International Development, which is a long term partner that has funded many projects (JHU/CCP, 2001, p. 24)." Under PCS 3, some 43 entertainment-education programs were implemented, under PCS 4 this number increased to 64. An exact count of the total number of entertainment-education projects during HCP is not available, since the approach was considered mainstreamed and not specifically tracked. However, some 89 projects during HCP resulted in testing of innovative intervention approaches. This makes it likely that using entertainment as a medium for promoting behavioral and social change continued in the positive direction. In addition, of note is the fact that the entertainment-education approach outlined by CCP set an example for other organizations, for example, the Soul City Institute based in South Africa.

While primarily a demand-generation tool, the Program has been successful in using entertainment-education to improve the supply side dynamic related to interpersonal communication and counseling, public expectations about attributes of quality services, and health care systemic change. One robust example of the use of entertainment-education to improve supply is the Nepal Radio Communication Project, which involved the development of an entertainment-education distance education radio drama for community-level providers in Nepal and ran from 1994 through 2004. Implemented simultaneously with a radio drama program aimed at a low literate audience, the expectations on both the health providers side as well as the client side being made public through radio, created an atmosphere of improved client–provider interactions at the clinic level (Storey *et al.*, 1999).

GATHER approach to interpersonal communication and counseling

The Program successfully argued that improvements in client–provider interactions (CPI) are essential to sustained behavior change and systemic quality. The conceptual models that have been at the center of this debate include the GATHER approach and the role of CPI in the Maximizing Access and Quality (MAQ) initiative of USAID's Office of Population and Reproductive Health. The GATHER approach focuses on the six elements of counseling. Each letter in the word GATHER stands for one element

(G = Greet, A = Ask, T = Tell, H = Hear, E = Explain, R = Return). The success of this simple mnemonic device is evident in that the first Population Reports counseling guide was used around the globe for 10 years and subsequently updated in 1998 (Rinehart, Rudy, and Drennan, 1998). Over time, working in close collaboration with the MAQ initiative, the Program focused its attention on CPI, which encompassed improved provider skills, client roles and responsibilities, and also changes at the health-system level. Notably, the quick investigation of quality (QIQ) system, a rapid assessment tool to measure progress in quality of care, included specific indicators to examine CPI (Rudy *et al.*, 2003).

Institutionalization of the Program

Table 28.2 below highlights the four subsystem domains for institutionalization and the key information gleaned from published and gray literature from JHU/CCP written archives and from the CCP website (www.jhuccp.org). This information is designed to

Table 28.2 Institutionalization: Measures by subsystem.

Institutionalization subsystem	*Description*	*Measures*
Production	Concerned with product-directed activities and includes implementation.	1. SOs and IRs 2. No. of countries 3. No. of projects 4. Topics covered 5. Implementing partners Baltimore 6. Implementing partners field 7. South –South Collaboration 8. Awards
Maintenance	Concerned with personnel and examines items such as recruitment and retention of staff.	1. Recruitment of staff 2. Retention of staff 3. Organizational setup
Supportive	Concerned with funding and housing for the project activities and the creation of an enabling environment	1. Funding 2. Evolution of project housing from headquarters to the field
Managerial	Concerned with formal assignment of managers and research dissemination.	1. Training and capacity building 2. Research and valuation (including dissemination) 3. Leadership/champions

Source: Population Communication Services November 7, 1995 to March 31, 2003. Final Report. Johns Hopkins Bloomberg School of Public Health, Center for Communication Programs, Baltimore, MD; HCP Final Report 2007 (2008). The Health Communication Partnership. Annual Report. Johns Hopkins Center for Communication Programs, Baltimore, MD.

highlight the extent to which PCS 1 through PCS 4 were successful in meeting their overall goal of changing knowledge, attitudes, and behaviors in reproductive health while working in over 42 countries across the globe (Piotrow, Rimon, Payne-Merritt and Saffitz, 2003), as well as how HCP contributed to strengthening public health communication organizations and practice in the 25 countries in the developing world through strategic communication programs (HCP Final Report, 2008).

Production institutionalization

The first question regarding institutionalization at the production level requires a review of the overall achievements under the intermediate results of the Program. The critical achievements under the PCS 4 project between 1995 and 2000 are provided in Figure 28.2. The HCP strategic objective was "Communication employed effectively to improve health, stabilize population, and advance a health competent society." The specific

Increased access, quality and demand for FP/RH services

- 44 Multimedia campaigns
- 48 Community mobilization campaigns
- 78 Sets of IEC materials for specific audiences
- 43 IPC/C training manuals
- 64 Entertainment-education programs
- 714 Technical assistance trips

Enhanced capacity for sustainable FP/RH programs

- 24 National IEC task forces established
- 8 International and 265 national/regional (including 2–3 day local) educational programs and SCOPE workshops
- 66 LDC institutions with improved IEC training capacity

Improved policy, increased resources

- 50 National or sub-national IEC strategies developed/being implemented
- 12 IPC/C sections in national medical standards

New improved technologies, approaches, strategies, knowledge

- 43 Innovations in: communication technology, research training, programs
- 17 International/regional specialized conferences/meetings
- 193 Major publications, articles, reports, working papers etc...
- 135 Professional presentations (research and evaluation division only)

Figure 28.2A PCS 4 (1995–2000) Intermediate results with key achievements.
Source: Population Communication Services November 7, 1995 to March 31 2003. Final Report. Johns Hopkins Bloomberg School of Public Health, Center for Communication Programs, Baltimore, MD.

IR1: Strengthened in country capacity for strategic health communication.

- 150+ local implementing partners that, adopt, and/or implement a national or sub-national health communication strategy
- 350+ local implementing partners that use evidence-based nodels or tools
- 20+ countries in which HCP has increased capacity of institutions, coalitions, or groups to design, implement, and evaluate strategic health communication programs

IR2: Effective health communication implemented at scale.

- 33 national or sub-national communication programs having interventions reaching over 50% of the intended audiences.
- 400+ national or sub-national organizations involved in HCP program implementation
- $16,000,000+ (126% of required cost share) leveraged

IR3: Communication integrated into a broad range of programs that improve health

- 27 programs that address multiple strategic objectives (SOs)
- 29 programs which address multiple domains
- 14 programs in which communication is integrated into a new health or nonhealth SO program (for that country)

IR4: Research used to guide and advance health communication

- 86 programs in which research is used to test innovative intervention approaches or key questions that advance health communication
- 132 programs in which research is used as basis for program design or adjustments
- 200,000+ sample materials distributed by the Media Materials Clearinghouse
- 143 peer-reviewed journal articles
- 12 "communication impact" publications
- 4 "communication insights" publications
- 47 evidence-based tools and products completed and/or disseminated to advance health communication knowledge

Figure 28.2B HCP (2002–2007) Intermediate results with key achievements.
Source: HCP Final Report 2007 (2008). The Health Communication Partnership. Annual Report. Johns Hopkins Center for Communication Programs, Baltimore, MD.

achievements under each of these intermediate results are also summarized in Figure 28.2a and Figure 28.2b.

There are some critical linkages between the two projects. For example, both projects included in their stated goals the critical need to build local capacity. In addition, both projects focused on diffusing state-of-the-art communication programs. Table 28.3

Table 28.3 Institutionalization of the production subsystem.

	PCS 1 – PCS 4	HCP
Countries of operation	42	25
Topics covered	Family planning, reproductive health, HIV/AIDS and STD prevention, safe motherhood, child survival, breastfeeding, nutrition, environment, democracy and governance related to heath	FP/RH, HIV/AIDS, child survival, safe motherhood, malaria, TB, hygiene and sanitation, safe water, avian influenza, SARS, safe injections, smoking, obesity, exercise, nutrition, and democracy and governance
Implementing partners	Academy for Educational Development (AED), Save the Children, Center for Development and Population Activities (CEDPA), Prospect Associates, Program for Adaptation of Technology in Health (PATH), Porter and Novelli	Academy for Educational Development (AED), Save the Children, The International HIV/AIDS Alliance, Tulane University
Awards and citations	20 awards between 1996 and 2002 at various local and international venues including the global media awards for multiple projects in several countries including Tanzania, Jordan, Indonesia and Bolivia	19 awards in various film and media festivals across the globe. Including among others the New York Film and Video Festival, the US International Film and Video Festival, the Telly Awards and the International Association of Web Masters and Designers, these projects came from several countries such as South Africa, India, Zambia, Pakistan, Jordan and Bangladesh and covered topics such as HIV/AIDS, adolescent reproductive health, family planning and reproductive health.

Source: Population Communication Services November 7, 1995 to March 31, 2003. Final Report. Johns Hopkins Bloomberg School of Public Health, Center for Communication Programs, Baltimore, MD; HCP Final Report 2007 (2008). The Health Communication Partnership. Annual Report. Johns Hopkins Center for Communication Programs, Baltimore, MD.

provides a short summary of selected awards and citations indicating the accolades and appreciation for the quality of communication products created through the Program.

There are also, however, some important distinctions. For example, HCP reflects a growing diversification of content areas beyond FP/RH to include other public health and development issues, as USAID realized (and the Program argued) that the principles of good communication are largely similar whether applied to family planning or other health concerns such as HIV/AIDS, maternal and child health, malaria, water and sanitation, or democracy and governance. In addition, rather than information, education, and communication (IEC), the HCP project was couched within a broader health communication framework. Third, the HCP project was committed to bringing projects to scale. Last, there was a strategic shift in the framing of communication from an activity- or program-based approach to a holistic establishment of communication as part of the national or subnational strategy. This is evident in the fact that in PCS 4 there were some 50 national communication strategies developed and/or implemented. HCP worked with some 150 local partners to produce, adopt, and/or implement national or subnational communication strategies.

Maintenance institutionalization

The maintenance subsystem comprises elements such as recruitment and retention of staff and is critical for the internal functioning of an organization. Figure 28.3 below provides information on project staffing during PCS 4.

Of note in Figure 28.3 is the growing global institutionalization over the course of PCS 4. In 1996, some 45 percent of the staffing was field–based, but by 2002, that number had grown to 78 percent. This rapid growth in field staff, composed mostly of local nationals, is telling in the context of the fact that the goal of these projects was to improve capacity at the country level. Moreover, the early realization that the program was global and therefore would need to recruit "the best and the brightest" from the developing world resulted in more than 20 nationalities working on the Program. Retention of staff is another key indicator of maintenance. The official reporting of PCS 4 staffing indicated that over 30 percent of the senior staff in headquarters had been with CCP for over 10 years and an additional 25 percent had been with CCP for at least 5 years. A review of human resources data, conducted by CCP from a core group of 51 management, program, research, training, and administrative staff, indicates that the average length of time with CCP among this core group was 15 years, considered by independent evaluators for USAID as quite remarkable compared to other similar organizations. Figures 28.4 and 28.5 include the organizational charts for PCS and HCP, both of which are fairly detailed with clear role and responsibility demarcations. One feature that comes to the fore is that the HCP organizational chart is considerably more complex in terms of the structure as a

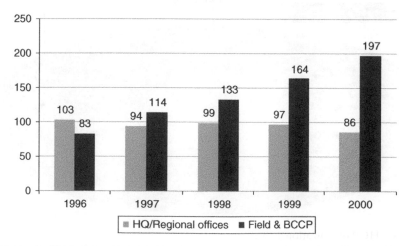

Figure 28.3   Staffing of the PCS 4 Project.
Source: Johns Hopkins Bloomberg School of Public Health, Center for Communication Programs, Baltimore, MD.

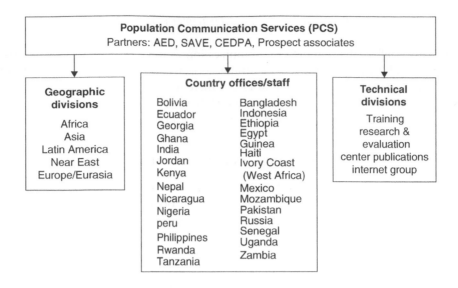

Africa: Ghana, Kenya, Nigeria, Rwanda, Tanzania, Ethiopia, Guinea, Ivory Coast, Mozambique, Senegal, Uganda, Zambia.

Asia: India, Nepal, Philippines, Bangladesh, Indonesia, Pakistan.

Latin America: Bolivia, Ecuador, Nicaragua, Peru, Mexico, Haiti.

Near East: Jordan, Egypt.

Europe/Eurasia: Georgia, Russia.

Figure 28.4 PCS 4 organizational chart.
Source: Johns Hopkins Bloomberg School of Public Health, Center for Communication Programs, Baltimore, MD.

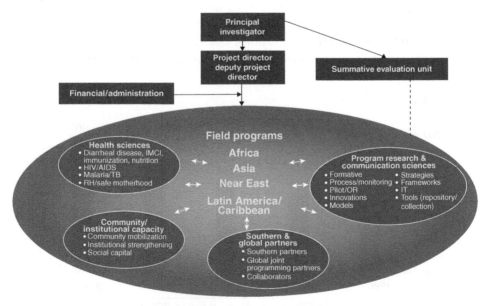

Figure 28.5 HCP organizational chart.
Source: Johns Hopkins Bloomberg School of Public Health, Center for Communication Programs, Baltimore, MD.

whole and the organizational units contained within it. As with PCS 4, during HCP, the geographical program divisions continued to be at the core of the Program. However, the HCP organizational chart reflects the growing understanding that field programs and the headquarters staff worked as a seamless whole. Therefore, in the HCP organizational chart the field programs in Africa, Asia, the Near East, and Latin America/Caribbean were placed front and center. Another testament to the growing global institutionalization of HCP projects is the attention on Southern and Global partners.

One human resource element that is not self-evident from the organizational charts is the strategic choice of the Program early on to primarily recruit staff with communication expertise supported by technical content experts, and not the other way around. Over time, this strategic choice proved itself a wise decision with the growing realization both within the program and with USAID that the core principles and expertise required in communication are largely similar whether these are applied to family planning, HIV/AIDS or democracy and governance. Topical expertise was translated into the HCP organizational chart through the inclusion of a health sciences group that brought together experts from various health fields. Finally, the continued emphasis on research and evaluation of health communication is reflected in the inclusion of an external summative evaluation unit in the HCP project.

Supportive institutionalization

The supportive subsystem consists of two key elements: housing project activities and funding. Information on the housing of project activities is reported above in terms of the strategic shift in staffing from headquarters to the field. In addition to this shift, increasing local sustainability of projects was evident in the creation of independent local NGOs that evolved from country offices. One of many such examples is the Bangladesh Center for Communication Programs (BCCP), which was established in 1996 as a non-profit, nongovernment communication organization. BCCP's 2007–2008 annual audit report indicates yearly expenditures of approximately $1.5 million, a testimony to its robust existence as a lead organization in health communication in the country long after it became an independent organization (see http://www.bangladesh-ccp.org/).

Another aspect housing of project activities is apparent in the ability to work closely with established and new partners in the field. The PCS 4 final report (2003) documents relationships with 64 local public and private-sector agencies. The HCP project worked with over 300 local partners worldwide. The HCP project further consolidated working with new partners and institutions that traditionally did not focus on health issues. For example: Ministries of Education, new faith-based institutions, sports groups including national Olympic committees.

Table 28.4 shows the increase in the budget over time from an original ceiling of $9,895,000 under PCS1 to $117,026,748.60 under HCP. The HCP ceiling does not include the Associate Awards provided by the USAID Missions, therefore a more realistic estimate of the total HCP funding including core and USAID mission buy-ins total over $190 million. The nature of the increase also reflects the increasing demands placed on the programs resulting in increased budgets and ceilings to accommodate demand from USAID field missions. For example, under PCS 3 the original budget ceiling of

Table 28.4 Supportive institutionalization: Funding.

	Original Ceiling	Final Funding
PCS 1	$9,895,000	$9,863,845
PCS 2	$30,000,000	$29,749,867
PCS 3	$60,000,000	$96,995,580
PCS 4	$108,351,269	$143,868,380
HCP^	$117,026,748.60	$190,000,000*

Notes: ^ Funding leveraged $16,000,000. This represents a cost share of $3,3000,000 and was 126% of the HCP-required cost-share amount. * This is the most conservative documented estimate available. Additional funding added to the Associate Awards, indicates that the actual final total is even higher.
Source: Population Communication Services November 7, 1995 to March 31, 2003. Final Report. Johns Hopkins Bloomberg School of Public Health, Center for Communication Programs, Baltimore, MD; HCP Final Report 2007 (2008). The Health Communication Partnership. Annual Report. Johns Hopkins Center for Communication Programs, Baltimore, MD.

$60,000,000 was raised by over 60 percent, ending in the final ceiling of $ 96,995,580. At the same time, under PCS 1 country and regional field support provided by USAID field Missions constituted some 27 percent of the total budget. In PCS 3, this increased to 43 percent of the total budget. Under PCS 4, field support funds made up 68 percent of the total funds obligated. Subsequently, under HCP, this proportion increased to 87 percent. The growing overall budget and, more importantly, the ever-increasing proportions provided by USAID Missions through their country programs (as differentiated from core funds provided by USAID Washington) represent the ability of USAID/ Washington to create a mechanism for addressing the growing needs in the field and the US Missions' growing understanding and appreciation of investing in strategic communication to help them achieve their objectives.

Managerial institutionalization

The managerial subsystem is concerned with formal assignment of managers and research dissemination. In addition, the presence of a "program champion" also plays a critical role. Goodman and Steckler (1989) describe a champion as a person who serves as a catalyst to bring coalitions of actors together. The existence of a strong managerial subsystem is implicit in the formal management structure illustrated in the organizational charts above. The institutionalization of this subsystem is evident in the relative stability in the top leadership of the CCP, from PCS-1 to PCS-4 and HCP, from the Directors, to Deputy and Divisional Directors and Senior Program Officers. Additionally, it is important to discuss the presence of two crosscutting divisions that worked closely with all geographic programs: training and capacity building and research and evaluation.

Training and capacity building

Training and capacity building is inherent in all of the Program's work. It would be hard to identify a single project that has not involved some level of local project-specific training and capacity building. A formal commitment to training and capacity building is

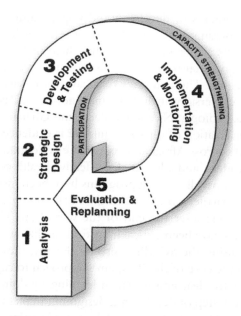

Figure 28.6 The P-Process.
Source: HCP (2003).

evidenced through the Training and Capacity Building division, which was formally established under PCS 3 with the goal of providing high-quality communication training and developing both communication skills and a cadre of public health professionals well versed in strategic communication.

A model workshop titled the Advances in Family Health Communication has been held in Baltimore and in many developing countries annually since 1989. Since 1996, the Advances trainings have included over 3,000 participants from over 35 countries. While originally designed for family planning, over time the Advances workshop curriculum has been adapted to other health arenas, such as Safe Motherhood and HIV/AIDS and to many cultural and country situations. The workshop is based on the P-Process (see Figure 28.6) communication framework. The P-Process is a systematic road map that leads health professionals from a loosely defined concept about changing behavior to a strategic and participatory program with a measurable impact on the intended audience.

One driving force behind the popularity and demand for the workshops, despite the fact that they were not free, has been the SCOPE software, which was first developed in 1992. SCOPE stands for Strategic Communication Planning and Evaluation and serves as an online and interactive representation of the P-Process. A standard implementation of SCOPE has been used for training purposes in over 30 countries in 5 languages for over 10 years.

In response to the growing need for global leadership in health communication, an additional training program co-funded by the Gates Institute for Population and Reproductive Health at Johns Hopkins University was designed specifically for leaders to address the leadership elements of designing and implementing effective crosscutting health communication programs. Since its inception, the leadership program has included more than 270 participants at the annual workshop held in Baltimore. In addition, an average of three international customized workshops has created additional alumni of 500 leaders across the globe. The countries that have hosted workshops and acquired expertise in designing local versions include China, Indonesia, Pakistan, Nepal, Nigeria, the Philippines, Uganda, Ethiopia, Nicaragua, Peru, and Ghana.

The overall institutionalization of capacity building is evidenced in many ways. First, through alumni networks across Africa and Asia that enable graduates of workshops to remain in contact, share ideas, and advocate for effective health communication policies and strategies. Second, almost all training programs have been institutionalized through collaborations with local partners, thus ensuring that the training remains effective and can be delivered locally long after the end of the workshop. Third, the training and capacity-building activities have been critical in institutionalizing specific approaches, for example, the P-Process using the SCOPE software. Finally, these training events were designed to supplement the core of the Program's approach to capacity building, which focused around collaborative learning in which learning by doing and technical assistance are infused into every step of developing, designing, implementing, and evaluating communication programs. One example of collaborative learning is the annual Advances in Family Health and Social Communication that BCCP has conducted for over 8 years and trained over 400 Bangladeshis in the P-Process approach. As a result, a professional association has been created called the Bangladesh Association of Social Communicators, which meets annually to exchange information and advance strategic communication.

Research and Evaluation

A unique strength of the Program was its housing within one of the premier public health schools in the world, which resulted in a close merger between research and practice. The role of research in health communication is clearly an area that set the Program apart from other players in the field. The staffing of the research and evaluation division with Ph.D.-level researchers trained in different disciplines, spanning public health, demography, communication, economics, and sociology resulted in a uniquely multidisciplinary perspective.

The existence of an evaluation group, which was internal and worked closely with, but at the same time remained relatively independent of, program units, allowed for formative research to design effective, audience- or "receiver-oriented" strategic messages, enabled monitoring to make sure the programs were implemented as planned, and finally helped in conducting independent impact evaluation to measure effects. Research and evaluation was integrated within practice as a matter of course, resulting in rapid uptake of research findings and lessons learned because the researchers did not need to advocate to program staff on the importance of theory and research-based programming.

The research and evaluation division can also be credited with the evolution of more and more rigorous research and evaluation methodologies to show scientifically the impact of communication. The voluminous number of publications in peer-reviewed forms (journal articles and book chapters) accompanied with detailed project reports and

Table 28.5 Institutionalization of the managerial subsystem: Research dissemination.

Research Dissemination	PCS 3	PCS 4	HCP
Peer-reviewed journal articles	Not available	40	143
Book chapters	Not available	9	19
Project reports /country reports/ field reports	9	26	55
Special papers	–	22	
Working papers	–	5	
In-house publications			
Communication impact	7	15	12
Communication insight	Not applicable	Not applicable	4
Evidence-based tools (How to Manuals)	3	8	47

Source: Population Communication Services November 7, 1995 to March 31, 2003. Final Report. Johns Hopkins Bloomberg School of Public Health, Center for Communication Programs, Baltimore, MD; HCP Final Report 2007 (2008). The Health Communication Partnership. Annual Report. Johns Hopkins Center for Communication Programs, Baltimore, MD.

easily digested summaries such as the "Communication Impact Series" is testament to the importance given to evaluation within the Program. Information on the research dissemination within the Program is presented in (Table 28.5).

According to Nutbeam (1996), one important intermediate measure of the institutionalization of an innovation is for research findings to be appropriately disseminated, in particular, by their publication in peer-reviewed journals. The large number of articles published is even more relevant in the context of the wide variety of disciplines represented by these publications. As Table 28.5 shows, there was a dramatic increase in the number of peer-reviewed journal articles published during the HCP, with 143 peer-reviewed journal articles in comparison with PCS 4 when 40 articles were published.

In addition to the peer review journal articles are of specific note are book contributions: Piotrow, Kincaid, Rimon, and Rinehart (1997) and McKee, Bertrand, and Becker-Benton (2004), several reports and a special issue of the Journal of Health Communication (Bertrand and Hutchinson, 2006) devoted to the topic of cost-effectiveness of health communication interventions.

It is also important to note the use of innovative research methodologies ranging from qualitative techniques drawing from anthropology, linguistics, and the humanities and involving multiple forms of narratives, pictorial, and videotaped data to large-scale quantitative studies utilizing experimental and quasi-experimental designs.

From humble beginnings that included the establishment of sentinel sites to examine the effectiveness of exposure to communication messages using post-only exit interviews and surveys, CCP staff have over time, studied the impact of communication using sophisticated research designs and cutting-edge analysis techniques such as: (1) sociometric analysis to study social networks and understand indirect effects of communication. (2) multivariate causal attribution to estimate precisely the contribution of communication interventions to behavior change and consequently cost-effectiveness of communication interventions. (3) propensity scoring as applied to communication to approximate the internal validity of a randomized control trial while examining a full-coverage program and (4) sensitivity analysis to generate prediction models. Two specific methodologies that are currently at the forefront of health communication research, propensity scoring and multiple level analyses are described below.

Propensity scoring is a statistical method that allows for matching respondents in a survey not exposed to a communication intervention on various demographic and economic variables with respondents who are actually exposed to the intervention. For full-coverage communication programs where control groups are impossible to replicate the use of propensity scoring is the most appropriate research design as it strengthens the argument for causal attribution by reducing self-selection (Do and Kincaid, 2006; Babalola and Vondrasek, 2005). Another advantage of the propensity score matching is that by eliminating the need for a baseline survey, this method provides considerable cost-savings. The Program has used the propensity score matching for impact assessments in Egypt, Nigeria, Jordan, Bangladesh, and the Philippines (HCP Final Report, 2008).

Multiple level analysis (MLA) provides the means to examine the impact of communication interventions across a variety of domains, ranging through the individual, family, community, and institutional to the policy level. Based on the understanding that individuals exist within a social-ecological framework, MLA provides a means to analyze the effects of one level on changes at another level. The MLA report has most recently been used in examining the effectiveness of the Egypt Communication for Healthy Living program described later in this chapter (HCP Final Report, 2008).

There are many leadership champions within the Program as well as at USAID who contributed to the institutionalization efforts described above. It is outside the scope of this chapter to mention all of these individuals. For the purposes of this chapter, we chose instead to ask a series of questions of Dr. Duff Gillespie. Dr. Gillespie, was in senior management positions within USAID from 1982 through 2002, when he was the Senior Deputy Assistant Administrator at the Global Health Bureau, the most senior career position in the health sector. Dr. Gillespie was involved with the PCS and HCP projects in various capacities. As Associate and Deputy Director he approved all project descriptions (PDs) and funding decisions for PCS. Additionally, he reviewed and/or was briefed at least annually on PCS. For HCP, as Senior Deputy Assistant Administrator (SDAA) he approved various preliminary documents as well as the final budget for the HCP project.

Dr. Gillespie attributed his championship for the cause of strategic communication within USAID to his reading of Everett M. Rogers "Diffusion of Innovations," which he indicated "opened up a new world" and "has remained my guiding principle to this day." When asked how he championed the need for strategic communication within USAID, Dr. Gillespie noted that the original PCS approach demonstrated a "new way of doing business" and mirrored his own views on how to diffuse family planning innovations. He further mentioned that PCS was initiated in an environment that was favorable to the idea that a critical mass of knowledgeable and trained individuals in communication was needed to expand family planning programs and increase contraceptive use. In a modest summary of his role, Dr. Gillespie wrote: "How I championed strategic communications was pretty straightforward: I simply set aside money for it and encouraged the relevant staff to work up a project."

In line with the Program's contributions to communication research discussed above, Dr. Gillespie's role as a champion included his commitment to ensuring that rigorous research and evaluation form the backbone of the Program. In Dr. Gillespie's words, "Over the course of several years, Hopkins became a leader in assessing the impact of communication campaigns in terms of both attitudinal and behavioral change."

In discussing barriers he faced in supporting the Program, Dr. Gillespie responded by stating that much time was spent on having to defend its long-term relationship with JHU/CCP (even though PCS1, 3, 4 and HCP were competitively bid out), due to fears that long-term institutional relationships between the government and con-tract/grantees results in the perpetuation of programs irrespective of their merits. Dr. Gillespie also indicated that the conventional belief is that competition inherently leads to superior products. The field of international health, Dr. Gillespie mentioned "is not large enough to support a truly competitive marketplace" but, given that "competitive solicitations are the norm, we now have relatively few organizations competing for a limited number of solicitations, each with accompanying opportunity costs (writing proposals rather than providing services). The end result is an unhealthy project-driven network of organizations without a sustained critical mass of experi-ence and expertise." He elaborated on this point by indicating that "if a contract is awarded to a new organization, the organization almost invariably has to retool and recruit new staff, often from the losing bidders. Moreover, since there is practically no core or programmatic funding (as most of the funds have to be generated from the USAID field missions), it is difficult to create an environment among contractors that encourages contemplation and innovation." In summarizing the key contributions of the Program in advancing the field of health communication at the global level, Dr. Gillespie stated: "these two projects (PCS and HCP) basically defined the field of health communication, initially for family planning and now for other health sectors, especially HIV/AIDS. The main contribution is the break from previous IEC approach that was little more than primitive messages, similar to World War I recruitment post-ers. These projects developed more appealing and sophisticated messages and messag-ing that were well received, effective, and even entertaining. These approaches were also well documented and evaluated. In summary, these projects professionalized the field."

Lessons Learned

Piotrow, Rimon, Payne-Merritt, and Saffitz (2003) in a report titled "Advancing Health Communication: The PCS Experience in the Field" provided a list of 52 key lessons learned. These lessons were categorized into eight groups and further accom-panied with five overarching conclusions. The eight categories covered formative ele-ments, including the need to learn about local needs and have a clear strategy to start with. They also addressed production institutionalization by focusing on implementa-tion issues such as the importance of addressing key program issues, specifically decen-tralization, integration of services, quality of care, and gender, as well as the role of

Health communication programs can be effective.

- A meta-analysis of 39 international programs, found an influence of 7 percent could occur in the desired behavior because of large-scale communication campaigns (Hornik, 2002; Snyder, Diop-Sidibe, and Badine, 2003).

Impact is directly proportional to program reach

- Comprehensive programs employing mass media, interpersonal communication and counseling, advocacy and community mobilization are more effective than small-scale efforts. While one on one personal contact may be more effective on a case by case basis, economies of scale achieved by full-coverage programs determine success from a public health perspective (Piotrow *et al.*,1997; Hornik, 2002).

Entertainment-education is a creative way to reach many people including those who are otherwise hard to reach

- CCP has been at the forefront of the entertainment-education programming since this format was first popularized in the early 1980s. Based on Bandura's Social Cognitive theory (1986), the entertainment-education approach posits that role models allow for vicarious learning (Singhal and Rogers, 1999; Singhal *et al.*, 2004).

Sustained individual and social change is more likely to occur through participatory programs that allow communities to be engaged in designing, implementing and monitoring efforts.

- While participatory programs require more effort to implement, the results from such programs are more sustainable in the long run (Figueroa *et al.*, 2002; Howard-Grabman & Snetro, 2003).

Programs must satisfy all their constituencies, including program beneficiaries, local partners and implementers, and sponsors and donors.

- Effective programs are possible only through continuity of support from all three elements.

Figure 28.7 PCS Four overarching conclusions.
Source: Piotrow *et al.* (2003).

community participation and having the foresight to be able deal with controversy. Two of the eight categories dealt with research and evaluation issues that fall within the managerial subsystem of institutionalization, including the need to measure how the program worked and the importance of sharing results and credit. The last category focused on the issue of capacity building and sustainability, thereby linking the internally driven maintenance with the externally driven supportive sub-systems of institutionalization. In addition to the eight categories noted above Piotrow *et al.* (2003) also provided five overarching conclusions summarized with examples of each in Figure 28.7.

HCP lessons learned: 10 big ideas

Similar to the PCS experience documentation, the HCP project final report concludes with "10 big ideas" for the future of behavior change communication. These ideas are summarized along with examples in Table 28.6.

Table 28.6 Ten big ideas for the future of behavior change communication (HCP Final Report 2008).

The more communication, the better the impact: The Egypt Communication for Healthy Living (CHL) program utilized public, private, and NGO partners by integrating messages under a single unifying communication platform "Your Health is Your Wealth," while using all available channels – mass media, outreach, community, and service delivery systems as well as large-scale publicity events, roaming transit events, and televised local entertainment. Impact assessment indicated that there were more health behaviors on average with increase in campaign recall, from an average of 3.2 behaviors at the lowest levels of recall to 5 behaviors at the highest levels of recall

Impact should be measured with precision.

The impact of health communication on behavior can be predicted.

Measure both direct and indirect effects of communication.

Secondary analysis extends the life and lessons learned from programs: All of these big ideas relate to research and evaluation, an area that clearly sets the Program apart. HCP programs have served as a global laboratory for advancing health communication science. HCP researchers have developed and refined numerous theoretical frameworks (ideation, indirect effects, bounded social norms) and research methods including propensity scoring, multi-level analysis and sensitivity analysis.

Measure both direct and indirect effects of communication: PCS and HCP have spearheaded the use of the ideation model, which refers to new ways of thinking and the diffusion of these new ways of thinking by means of social interaction in local, culturally homogeneous communities (Cleland and Wilson, 1987). Factors such as knowledge, attitudes, efficacy, social influence, and social norms therefore serve as ideational "mediators" of actual use. The impact of communication interventions on ideational factors and contraceptive use has been previously examined with data from five countries including Nepal, the Philippines, Honduras, Tanzania, and Egypt, which confirmed that ideation increased the odds of family planning use by 1.2 to 1.3 times, even after controlling for a wide variety of other socioeconomic factors (Kincaid *et al.*, 2006). Ideation suggests that communication influences behavior directly and indirectly through these mediating factors, therefore, providing credence to the need to measure both direct and indirect impact.

For sustainable impact, change social norms: Social norms are part of the indirect pathway to behavior change in the ideation model. The Program has been in the forefront in the conceptualization and operationalization of social norms (Rimal and Real, 2003, 2005; Lapinski and Rimal, 2005; Rimal *et al.*, 2005). In addition, Kincaid (2004) described the "bounded normative influence" (BNI) effect, which explains how new ideas take root and grow in a given community. The groundbreaking BNI effect was utilized to study sustainability of family planning behaviors in Indonesia by Schoemaker (2005). The BNI effect has also been studied from the context of how communication campaigns can be instrumental in the creation of new norms (Storey and Kaggwa, 2009).

(Continued)

Table 28.6   (*cont'd*).

Go to scale now to achieve cost-effectiveness: The HCP project sought to overcome the paucity of information on "cost-effectiveness" by commissioning a special issue of the *Journal of Health Communication* to build a more robust evidence base. The special issue consisted of eight articles, four of which were empirical studies. All the empirical studies prove the cost-effectiveness of communication interventions that covered mass media, entertainment-education dramas, and interpersonal communication and counseling across a spectrum of health behaviors.

Use communication to transcend physical, economic and cultural gaps: This axiom has been applied to various projects, utilizing television, work-sites, community networks and the private sector. For example, it is estimated that using a TV satellite channel in South Africa, Mindset Health Channel provided both service providers and clients with HIV information, reached over 2.2 million clients, and won the 2006 Development Gateway award of $100,000. The Jordan Health Communication Partnership leveraged private sector resources and established Jordan's Arabic language portal (www.Sehetna.com) to serve the health needs of Jordanians and other Arabic-speaking populations throughout the Middle East. This health portal was awarded the Golden Award in the Pan-Arab Awards, contest in the health services domain. In addition to country projects, the Health Communication Materials Network links over 1,000 communication professionals worldwide via email to discuss special topics identified by network members. Finally, the Media Materials Clearinghouse which consists of over 46,000 materials, is the first choice in a Google search for "health communication materials."

Institutions are best built through collaborative learning, not training by experts: Serves as a guiding principle for projects across the board. These include among others: the "Ankoay" program in Madagascar that transformed youth groups into instruments for community leadership in the fight against AIDS; using communities to design radio programs in Nepal and using Village Health Committees (VHC) in Egypt as a conduit for male leader meetings called *Dawars* in charge of monitoring and evaluating project activities. The commitment to community empowerment is further evident in the creation of a "Participation Guide," wherein a group of 70 HCP trained professionals from across three continents participated in the development of a Participation Guide to accompany the P-Process. The participation guide provided practical tips for involving beneficiaries directly in all stages of designing, implementing and evaluating health communication interventions (Tapia, Brasington, and Van Lith, 2008).

Communication can impact gender equity as a gateway to multiple health behaviors: This is evidenced by Africa Transformation (AT), which was produced by HCP in collaboration with the Center for Development Foundation in Uganda. The AT included a series of nine profiles of women and men who overcame gender barriers and challenges in their own lives, thus becoming role models for others. Results from a post-test only control group design indicated that participation in AT was positively and significantly (after controlling for socioeconomic variables) associated with equitable gender normative beliefs, shared decision making and propensity to take part in community activities to eliminate harmful gender traditions. Another good example of how gender norms serve as a gateway to other behaviors was seen in research conducted in Ethiopia. This research, while testing the validity and reliability of the Gender-Equitable Men (GEM) scale developed by USAID's Horizon's Project, noted how beliefs about masculinity were associated with or predicted a range of behaviors, supporting the notion that gender norms act as a gateway and impact multiple behavioral outcomes.

The 10 big ideas for the HCP project are culled from the five years of HCP experience across the globe and also relate to the four measures of institutionalization. The production subsystem refers to the product-directed activities and includes implementation. The following big ideas: *The more communication, the better the impact* and *Go to scale now to achieve cost-effectiveness,* and *Communication can transcend physical, economic, and cultural gaps* fall within the production subsystem of institutionalization, by including innovative, full–coverage, and multilevel activities implemented by the Program at scale.

A second cluster of big ideas: *Impact should be measured with precision,* and *The impact of health communication on behavior can be predicted,* and *Measure both direct and indirect effects of communication,* and *Secondary analysis extends the life and lessons learned from programs,* all have to do with research and evaluation and as such they relate to the managerial subsystem of institutionalization a fundamental part of that is the extent to which monitoring and evaluation are integrated into the project design.

The supportive subsystem is concerned with the creation of an enabling environment. In general, this subsystem is internally directed and focuses on issues of staffing and retention. However, this subsystem also deals with the ability of the Program to create an enabling environment for its key beneficiaries. Therefore the big ideas that: *For sustainable impact, change social norms,* and *Communication can impact gender equity as a gateway to multiple health behaviors,* and *Institutions are best built through collaborative learning, not training by experts* are testament to the ability of the Program to create and foster an enabling environment for its key constituents, the people for whom the interventions were designed. Much of the Program's work required the creation of enabling environments at several levels including within individuals, families, communities and all the way to advocacy at the policy level. The level of supportive institutionalization is also evidenced in the programmatic, capacity-building and research focus on the normative dimensions of the ideation framework and in the implicit inclusion of gender equity and community involvement in intervention design and implementation as a matter of course.

Conclusions

This chapter summarizes the manifold contributions of the Program to the landscape of global health communication from the perspective of funding, program innovations, and research. The Program witnessed increase in funding allocations over time. Of special note are the increases in allocations from USAID field-based budgets as opposed to core funding. This highlights the success of the programs in the global context, in that the major source of funding was from a multitude of USAID Missions voting to invest in communication with their budgets. A further institutionalization of these programs, from the content perspective, is evident in the diversification of program topics from a narrow focus on population and family planning in the beginning to an all-encompassing emphasis on "health" as a whole. This diversification was clearly based on a growing understanding that the principles of good communication apply to health topics as a whole. Last but not the least is the institutionalization that the Program engineered by establishing a rigorous research agenda, evidenced in the body of peer reviewed literature in the field of global health communication.

None of these achievements would be possible without the sustained support and commitment of USAID managers and leaders from many organizations that realized the wisdom of investing in health communication and in turn served as champions in this field. USAID commitment is evident in Dr. Gillespie's assertion that the Program was instrumental in defining and professionalizing the field of health communication. Interestingly, the Program was part of a larger organization CCP, which was established by D. A. Henderson, partly because he recognized from his groundbreaking work in smallpox eradication that good communication was a crucial element in public health.

In recent years scholars have questioned whether sustainability, when measured in terms of an intervention delivering activities and benefits after external assistance ends, is possible or perhaps an unattainable ideal in health promotion (Scherier, 2005; St. Leger, 2005). This chapter does not attempt to make claims of sustainability but chose instead to examine the extent to which USAID funding of PCS and HCP allowed for institutionalization of health communication at the international level. The Paris Declaration 2005 and the Accra Agenda for Action (AAA) 2008 both endorse the commitment of the international aid community to focus on bottom-up institutionalization, while at the same time setting up systems to monitor and measure the success of their efforts. Of note is the fact that both the Paris Declaration and subsequently the AAA, while emphasizing the role of donors and aid recipient nation states, do not elaborate on the role of technical assistance in promoting international development. The USAID–Johns Hopkins University Partnership, on the other hand, shows how global and local expertise can be harnessed to promote best practices in the field of health communication. Perhaps those attempting to translate the ideas reflected in the Paris Declaration and the AAA into reality can use the case study chronicled in this chapter as a blueprint for future international aid efforts. Since HCP ended in 2008, CCP has continued to expand its programmatic, research and funding portfolios in the field, thus providing further proof of institutionalization that continues to occur long after PCS and HCP ended. Strategic health communication endures.

Acknowledgments

None of this work would have been written if it were not for Phyllis Piotrow, the Founding Director of CCP, who was the pioneering and visionary leader through most of the life of PCS and HCP. This chapter is a testimony to her inspired leadership. The authors would like to thank Susan Krenn, current CCP Director, for her valuable suggestions in the preparation of this chapter and for being so generous with our requests for data and reports. The feedback we received from D. Lawrence Kincaid and Ben Lozare on earlier drafts was valuable in writing specific sections of this chapter. There are literally hundreds, if not thousands, of actors who made possible the collective work of advancing health communication. We cannot acknowledge them all. Therefore, we apologize in advance for any omissions to the list below: We owe a debt of gratitude to senior management at CCP, specifically Jane Bertrand, Patrick Coleman, Alice Payne Merritt, and Gary Saffitz. We would like though to thank all the Program's core partner organizations mentioned in the text as well as cited in the attachments. We acknowledge the support and intellectual contributions to the Program by leaders at USAID including Duff Gillespie, Joe Speidel, Liz Maguire, Margaret Neuse, and Steve Sinding, and the Cognizant Technical Officers: Al Bernal, Sandra Buffington, Gloria Coe, Joanne Grossi, Roy Jacobstein, Earle Lawrence, Chloe O'Gara, Marshal Roth, and Clay Vollan, and many colleagues both at USAID missions in the field and in Washington DC too numerous to mention here. From the Johns Hopkins Bloomberg School of Public Health we thank W. Henry Mosely, Bernard Guyer, Robert Blum, and David Holtgrave. Finally, we salute the work of all CCP staff whose dedication, imagination and entrepreneurship made possible this incredible work and helped save lives and alleviate suffering worldwide.

References

Babalola, S. and Vondrasek, C. (2005). Communication, ideation, and contraceptive use in Burkina Faso: An application of the propensity score matching method. *Journal of Family Planning and Reproductive Health Care, 31*(3), 207–212.

Bandura, A. (1986). *Social Foundations of Thought and Action: A Social Cognitive Theory.* Englewood Cliffs, NJ: Prentice-Hall.

Barab, S. A., Redman, B. K., and Froman, R. D. (1998). Measurement characteristics of the levels of institutionalization scales: Examining reliability and validity. *Journal of Nursing Measurement, 6*(1), 19–33. Retrieved from www.scopus.com

Bertrand, J. and Hutchinson, P. (Eds.) (2006). Special issue: Cost-effectiveness analysis. *Journal of Health Communication, 11*(2), 1–173.

Cleland, J. and Wilson, C. (1987). Demand theories of fertility transition: An iconoclastic view. *Population Studies, 41*(1), 5–30.

Do, M. and Kincaid, D. L. (2006). Impact of an entertainment-education television drama on health knowledge and behavior in Bangladesh: An application of propensity score matching. *Journal of Health Communication, 11*(3), 301–325.

Figueroa, M., Kincaid, D. L., Rani, M., and Lewis, G. (2002). *Communication for Social Change: An Integrated Model for Measuring the Process and Its Outcomes.* Working Paper Series No. 1. Rockefeller Foundation and Johns Hopkins University, Center for Communication Programs. Retrieved from http://www.communicationforsocialchange.org/pdf/socialchange.pdf

Goodman, R. M., McLeroy, K. R., Steckler, A., and Hoyle, R. H. (1993). Development of Level of Institutionalization (LoIn) Scales for health promotion programs. *Health Education Quarterly, 20*(2), 161–178.

Goodman, R. M. and Steckler, A. (1989). How to institutionalize health promotion programs. *American Journal of Health Promotion 3*, 34–44.

HCP (Health Communication Partnership) (2003). The New P-Process: Sepes in Strategic Communication. Retrieved from http://www.jhuccp.org/sites/all/files/The%20New%20P-Process.pdf

HCP (Health Communication Partnership) Final Report 2007 (2008). *The Health Communication Partnership. Annual Report.* Baltimore, MD: Johns Hopkins Center for Communication Programs.

Hornik, R. (2002). *Public Health Communication. Evidence for Behavior Change.* Mahwah, NJ: Lawrence Erlbaum Associates.

Howard-Grabman, L., and Snetro, G. (2003). *How to Mobilize Communities for Health and Social Change.* Field Guide. Johns Hopkins Bloomberg School of Public Health, Center for Communication Programs. Retrieved from http://www.jhuccp.org/node/1256

JHU/CCP (Johns Hopkins University Center for Communication Programs) (1990). *Proceedings from the Enter-Educate Conference. Entertainment for Social Change.* March 29–April 1, 1989. Baltimore, MD: JHU/CCP.

JHU/CCP (Johns Hopkins University Center for Communication Programs) (1998). *A Report on the Second International Conference on Entertainment-Education and Social Change.* Baltimore, MD: JHU/CCP. Available at: http://www.jhuccp.org/node/1087

JHU/CCP (Johns Hopkins University Center for Communication Programs) (2001). *A report on the Third International Conference on Entertainment-Education and Social Change.* Baltimore: JHU/CCP. Available at: http://www.jhuccp.org/node/1085

Johnson, K., Hays, C., Center, C., and Daley, C. (2004). Building capacity and sustainable prevention innovations: A sustainability planning model. *Evaluation Planning, 27,* 135–149.

Kincaid, D. L. (2004). From innovation to social norms. Bounded normative influence. *Journal of Health Communication, 9*(Supplement 1), 37–57.

Kincaid, D. L., Storey, D., Figueroa, M. E., and Underwood, C. (2006). Communication, ideation and contraceptive use. The relationships observed in five countries. Paper presented at the World Congress on Communication for Development, Rome, Italy, October 2006.

Lapinski, M., and Rimal, R. (2005). An explication of social norms. *Communication Theory, 15*(2), 127–147.

Lefebvre, R. (1992). Sustainability of health promotion programmes. *Health Promotion International, 7,* 239–240.

McKee, N., Bertrand, J., and Becker-Benton, A. (2004). *Strategic Communication in the HIV/ AIDS Epidemic.* New Delhi, India: Sage Publications.

Nutbeam, D. (1996). Achieving "best practice" in health promotion: Improving the fit between research and practice. *Health Education Research, 11*(3), 317–326.

Oldenburg, B. F., Sallis, J. S., French, M., and Owen, N. (1999). Health promotion research and the diffusion and institutionalization of interventions. *Health Education Research, 14*(1), 121–130.

Piotrow, P. T., Kincaid, D. L., Rimon, J. G., II, and Rinehart, W. (1997). *Health Communication Lessons from Family Planning and Reproductive Health.* Westport, CT: Praeger.

Piotrow, P. T., Rimon, J. G., II, Payne-Merritt, A. and Saffitz, G. (2003). *Advancing Health Communication The PCS Experience in the Field.* Retrieved from http://www.jhuccp.org/ node/1058

Pluye, P., Potvin, L., and Denis, J. (2004). Making public health programs last: Conceptualizing sustainability. *Evaluation and Program Planning, 27*(2), 121–133. Retrieved from www.scopus.com

Rimal, R. N., Lapinski, M., Cook, R., and Real, K. (2005). Moving toward a theory of normative influences: How perceived benefits and similarity moderate the impact of descriptive norms on behaviors. *Journal of Health Communication. 10*(5), 433–450.

Rimal, R. and Real. K. (2003). Understanding the influence of perceived norms on behaviors. *Communication Theory, 13,* 184–203.

Rimal, R. and Real. K. (2005). How behaviors are affected by perceived norms. A test of the theory of normative social behavior. *Communication Research, 32,* 389–414.

Rimon, J. G., II (2001). Behavior change communication in public health. In *Beyond Dialogue: Moving Toward Convergence.* Presentation at the United Nations Roundtable on Development Communication, Managua, Nicaragua.

Rinehart, W., Rudy, S., and Drennan, M. (1998). *GATHER Guide to Counseling. Population Reports, Series J, No. 48.* Baltimore, MD: Johns Hopkins University School of Public Health, Population Information Program.

Rogers, E. M. (1973). *Communication Strategies for Family Planning.* New York: The Free Press.

Rogers, E. M. (1994). *A History of Communication Study. A Biographical Approach.* New York: The Free Press.

Rogers, E. M. (1995). *Diffusion of Innovations.* New York: The Free Press.

Rudy, S., Tabbutt-Henry, J., Schaefer, L. and McQuide, P. (2003). *Improving Client–Provider Interaction. Population Reports, Series Q, No. 1.* Baltimore,MD: Johns Hopkins Bloomberg School of Public Health, the INFO Project. Retrieved from http://www.populationreports.org/Q01/

Scheirer, M. (2005). Is sustainability possible? A review and commentary on empirical studies of program sustainability. *American Journal of Evaluation,* 26 (3), 320–347.

Schoemaker, J. (2005). Contraceptive use among the poor in Indonesia. *International Family Planning Perspectives, 31*(3), 106–114.

Shediac-Rizkallah, M. and Bone, L. (1998). Planning for the sustainability of community-based health programs: Conceptual frameworks and future directions for research, practice, and policy. *Health Education Research, 13,* 87–108.

Singhal, A., Cody, M. J., Rogers, E. M., and Sabido, M. (2004). *Entertainment-Education and Social Change. History, Research and Practice.* Mahwah, NJ: Lawrence Erlbaum Associates.

Singhal, A. and Rogers, E. M. (1999). *Entertainment-Education a Communication Strategy for Social Change.* Mahway, NJ: Lawrence Erlbaum Associates.

Snyder, L., Diop-Sidibe, N., and Badine, L. A. (May, 2003). Meta-analysis of the impact of family planning campaigns conducted by the Johns Hopkins Bloomberg School of Public Health/Center for Communication Programs. Paper presented at the International Communication Association Annual Meeting, San Diego, CA.

St. Leger, L. (2005). Questioning sustainability in health promotion projects and programs. *Health Promotion International, 20*(4), 317–319.

Storey, D., Boulay, M., Karki, *et al.* (1999). Impact of the Integrated Radio Communication Project in Nepal, 1994–1997. *Journal of Health Communication, 4,* 271–294.

Storey, D. and Kaggwa, E. (2009). The influence of changes in fertility-related norms on contraceptive use in Egypt, 1995–2005. *Population Review, 48*(1), 1–21.

Swerissen, H. and Crisp, B. (2004). The sustainability of health promotion interventions for different levels of social organization. *Health Promotion International, 19*(1), 123–130.

Tapia, M., Brasington, A. and Van Lith, L. (2007). *Participation Guide Involving Those Directly Affected in Health and Development Communication Programs.* Baltimore, MD: Health Communication Partnership based at the Johns Hopkins Bloomberg School of Public Health/Center for Communication Programs. Retrieved from http://www.jhuccp.org/hcp/pubs/tools/participationguide.pdf

Thompson, B. and Winner, C. (1999). Durability of community intervention programs: definitions, empirical studies and strategic planning. In N. Bracht (Ed.), *Health Promotion at the Community Level* (pp. 137–154). Thousand Oaks, CA: Sage.

29

Communication and Public Health in a Glocalized Context
Achievements and Challenges

Thomas Tufte

As health communication as a formal and internationally recognized discipline approaches its 40th birthday, and its success seems evident, it is worthwhile stopping and asking two fundamental questions: What are the achievements of health communication? and What are current challenges in health communication?

As a scientific discipline health communication has grown enormously since it was formally recognized as a subdiscipline to communication in 1975, when the Health Communication Division was first recognized at the International Communication Association (Freimuth, 2004, p. 2053). Today it is a well-established discipline, mostly in schools of public health, and to a lesser degree in schools of media and communication. It is also a discipline with very particular characteristics. The *Journal of Health Communication* conducted a review of the first 10 years of its own publishing of health communication research (1996–2006). It was a review that revealed a very clear profile of what health communication is, and is not. The study comprised 321 articles, and the profile of the published material was as follows:

> Its primary author is a US academic. It probably focuses on smoking, HIV=AIDS, or cancer. It is an empirical research study, more likely to use quantitative, specifically survey, methods, rather than qualitative methods. It probably is not driven by theory. It is much more likely to examine mass media communication than interpersonal communication. Its purpose is just as likely to be audience analysis as message design, as evaluation of a planned communication intervention. If its purpose is to evaluate a planned communication intervention however, that intervention is almost certainly a successful one (Freimuth, Massett, and Meltzer, 2006. p. 11).

This characteristic is further deconstructed in the opening section of this chapter where I reflect upon the characteristics of the discipline, presenting core achievements

The Handbook of Global Health Communication, First Edition. Edited by Rafael Obregon and Silvio Waisbord.
© 2012 John Wiley & Sons, Inc. Published 2012 by John Wiley & Sons, Inc.

in health communication, also identifying and discussing what hasn't been achieved. This is done based on a more recent article reviewing the field published in *The Lancet* in 2010.

One significant characteristic of health communication, as represented both in the *Journal of Health Communication* review and the review in *The Lancet*, is the significant absence of social sciences, in particular sociology, anthropology, media studies, and political science. As I argue in the second section of the chapter, it has as a consequence that some of the overall processes of globalization, the development of a risk society and the changing social relationships that are having significant implications for the health, well-being, and everyday life of ordinary citizens are overlooked. This is to a degree, I argue, that calls for a fundamental rethinking of global health communication today and for an inclusion of these subject areas and scientific disciplines. My basic point here is that a much stronger interdisciplinary approach is needed in health communication in order to grasp the complexity of contemporary health challenges and the health communication responses to these.

Thirdly, and in recognition of the interdisciplinarity of the field, I explore health citizenships and in particular how two stronger societal development trends are influencing the articulation of health citizenships. These development trends are mediatization and globalization. On the one hand, our world is increasingly mediatized, which is setting a whole new agenda regarding the formation of norms, values, and lifestyles. On the other hand, the multidimensional challenge of globalization is challenging national frameworks for responses to public health problems and emphasizing the need for transnational collaboration. In order to understand the social determinants and the rights of ordinary citizens, we therefore need to complexify our conceptual approach to health communication, exploring the processes and challenges of mediatization and globalization.

Finally, I wrap up this chapter by formulating three statements that, hopefully, can help us advance the research agenda of global health communication in the future.

Achievements

The discipline of health communication has in recent years reached a significant peak as a subdiscipline of both communication and communication for development (when it comes to global health). As the critical mass of health communication campaigns and research grows, it is relevant to ask ourselves: what are the main achievements of health communication?

A recent review article in *The Lancet*, "Use of mass media campaigns to change health behaviour" (Wakefield, Loken, and Hornik, 2010) contributes to shedding light on this question. This article reviews key English-language scientific production relating to the use of mass media campaigns to change health behavior. It makes a thorough analysis of full-text review articles as well as notable nonreviewed studies published from 1998 onwards. The criterion for selection was articles representing what the authors "judged to represent advances in assessment methods or substantial increments in knowledge" regarding the use of mass media campaigns to change health behavior (p. 1261).

The article starts out from the premise that health communication initiatives should be viewed from a behavioral perspective, with success based on the ability to persuade audiences to change their behavior, and, furthermore, takes the standpoint that exposure to the messages from these campaigns is generally passive. Wakefield, Loken, and Hornik state: "The great promise of mass media campaigns lies in their ability to disseminate well defined behaviorally focused messages to large audiences repeatedly, over time, in an incidental manner, and at a low cost per head" (p. 1262). The problem, the authors argue, is that this promise is far from always realized due to unmet audience expectations, inadequate funding, fragmented media environments, poorly researched and inappropriate formats, or a combination of reasons: "homogeneous messages might not be persuasive to heterogeneous audiences: and campaigns might address behaviors that audiences lack the resources to change" (Wakefield, Loken, and Hornik, 2010, p. 1262). The authors distinguish between direct and indirect methods of effecting behavior change, where the direct methods are about effecting decision-making processes at the individual level, while the indirect "routes" speak about an increase in interpersonal discussion as a reinforcement mechanism to individual behavior change, as a tool to influence peers, and finally as a manner of prompting public discussion as a pathway to achieving change in public policy (Wakefield, Loken, and Hornik, 2010, p. 1262).

This review article stands as a good example of the dominant line of thought and communicative practice seen within health communication:

Firstly, the scientific approach which informs not only the review article but also the core framework within which the scientific debate primarily navigates, is rooted in the behavioral sciences and based on a conceptualization of mass communication as a tool for persuasion. The methodologies used are overwhelmingly quantitative, that is, surveys with randomized controls, experimental designs, assessing reach, exposure, changes in knowledge, norms, and the beliefs and practices of individuals. These characteristics connect well with the post-positivist perspective in health communication which Zoller and Dutta (2008) refer to as the dominant discourse in health communication.

A series of challenges and limitations outlined in Wakefield, Loken, and Hornik's *Lancet* article speak to the limitations of this dominant scientific framework, reinforcing the need for other approaches. For example, its authors find that "smoking prevention in young people seems to have been more likely when mass media efforts were combined with programmes in schools, the community or both" (p. 1262). This illustrates the need to approach the health challenge from a holistic perspective, embedding the pursuit for solutions in broader contexts of social networks and lived community life.

Secondly, the need for more socially and culturally embedded research is reinforced by the recurrent challenge of not being able to isolate the "effect" of the particular intervention: "almost all assessed mass media campaigns have included multiple programme components (e,g., other community, school, worksite interventions) and therefore the effects of mass media campaigns are difficult to isolate" (Wakefield, Loken, and Hornik, 2010, p. 1266). The challenge here points towards a discrepancy between the complexity of the interventions and the methods used to evaluate how multimedia campaigns are made sense of. This speaks to the need for both interpretive and culture-centered approaches. In methodological terms, it calls for a palette of qualitative approaches. Particularly, it calls for media ethnographic approaches, a discipline well established with qualitative audience studies (Tufte, 2000, 2001; Ginsburg, Abu Lhugod, and Larkin, 2002; Spitulnik, 1993, 2002) but still very disconnected from the discipline of health communication. Ethnography can help deconstruct the practices of everyday life, and media ethnography is the art of understanding how media flows into everyday life, contributing, as one of many mediators, to processes of sense making, identity formation, and social action. Wakefield and colleagues also touch upon the challenge of understanding one particular health communication intervention in the context of the general media outlet to which people are exposed: "separation of the effects of exposure to modern values through ordinary media content from effects of exposure to specific procontraceptive campaign content is not always clear-cut" (Wakefield, Loken, and Hornik, 2010, p. 1266). Again, media ethnography could suggest a relevant methodological response to this challenge (Tufte, 2004). Another approach to conceptualizing the interventions is to understand them from the perspective of narration, deconstructing the relation between behavior change narratives and their audiences, something which Petraglia (2007, 2009) and Galavotti and colleagues (2008) have extensively analyzed.

Thirdly, there is the policy challenge. Dutta and Zoller (2008, p. 20) state that health policy is "the most newly emergent trend in health communication." Wakefield, Loken, and Hornik (2010, p. 1268) do bring the policy challenge up in their article: "the creation of policies that support opportunities to change provides additional motivation for change, whereas policy reinforcement can discourage unhealthy or unsafe behaviours." However, they don't address how health policy can connect to the underlying conditions influencing issues such as youth violence, intimate partner violence, or child maltreatment. They do not address the relation between mass media campaigns and the issues of power, injustice, inequality, and poverty. The contributors to Zoller and Dutta's book do bring these issues up, but without any deeper analysis of the complex relation between media flow, consumption and sense-making, articulation of civic engagement, and possible health policy outcomes. Most often, what is seen are either studies of the "receiver" side of health communication interventions, *or* the specific advocacy communication addressing more exclusive policy agendas.

In rounding up this first section, some of the challenges for health communication identified as emerging from the Wakefield review, speak to the following:

1 Difficulty in providing clear-cut results when multimedia campaigns are in question. There is a lot of work pending to explore further the synergetic effects between different interventions as well as to develop an understanding of, and a methodology to capture, the creation of enabling discursive and/or policy environments as forms of outcome from health communication;

2 Narrowly defined evaluations not enabling deep analysis of the reasons for change or lack of change nor exploring all avenues of changes. Tools such as "outcome mapping" and "EAR" (ethnographic action research) place single interventions in broader contexts of activities, stakeholders, and sociocultural practices. There are promising pathways ahead, but, in research terms, evaluations have a lot yet to gain from connecting more deeply with the softer sides of social sciences (anthropology and sociology), as well as with qualitative audience studies and some of the growing trends within political science;

3   The limited evaluation of nonmedia components speaks to the above-mentioned evaluation challenge, as do the difficulty and limits in assessing social class differences as identified by Wakefield and colleagues.

Most of the above issues address the relationship between agency, structural conditions, and the media intervention in a health communication intervention. To capture the complexities of some of these issues a much more elaborate interdisciplinary approach to health communication is required. This is a call which has been underway for some years now, and I find that Zoller and Dutta's 2008 book, *Emerging Perspectives in Health Communication*, is one of the most articulate proposals for a new research agenda for health communication. It sheds light on the growing body of research which takes on questions of sense-making processes, the roles of culture, and the challenge of the often very important but not so explicitly targeted power relations that make health communication difficult.

However, despite some significant advancement, I would like in the following section to highlight three dimensions of "an interdisciplinary approach to health communication" which remain still to be further conceptualized:

- *The notion of development and social change.* Most often in health communication writings there is no explicit mention of how the case studied or the authors writing conceive development. What is the implicit understanding of change that informs the study? What is it assumed should change on the basis of a health communication intervention? How is the expected change process assumed to happen? Theory of social change and theory of development can help answer these questions, while the field of media and communication for social change can provide a solid basis for understanding the role of media and communication in development and social change (Gumucio-Dagron and Tufte, 2006; Obregon 2010)
- Understanding *the relation between globalization and questions of identity, subjectivity, sense making, and action* (both as individuals and collectivities). Although the subject is mentioned in, for example, Zollner and Dutta's book (2008. pp. 5 and 20), there is a growing need to analyze and establish more clarity as to how processes of social, cultural, and economic globalization influences the "agency" of people as well as influencing global health policy and practice (see the next section).
- *Reconceptualizing the media as more than merely carriers of messages* to rather being a constitutive social institution providing opportunities for ordinary citizens to speak out, voice their concerns, engaging in public deliberation and social critique (see the next section).

In the following I discuss these three perspectives.

Challenges

Drawing especially on four social scientists – Ulrich Beck, Anthony Giddens, Zygmunt Baumann, and Arjun Appadurai – the fundamental aim and underlying ontology of health communication are offered a stronger sociological and anthropological basis.

Beck's notion of a "risk society," Giddens' concept of ontological security, Baumann's notion of liquid modernity and the flexibilization of social relationships, and Appadurai's theory of rupture and the production of unstable modern subjectivities in the world today – all these concepts can assist us in identifying a whole new set of communicative challenges that exist between governments or health-focused organizations on one side, and their publics, citizens, or audiences, on the other.

These scholars' social theories inform how we can identify the conditions in society that influence processes of identity formation, feelings of citizenship, and people's general sense of *agency* today – also basic preconditions for any action to be taken or behavior change to occur. My studies of South African youth's sense making around HIV/AIDS communication has shown that a number of inconsistencies and what I elsewhere have called "communicative disconnects" exist between, on the one side, the existential feelings of anxiety, the material conditions of poverty, the social instability, and the ontological insecurity that characterize the lived experience of many people today, and on the other hand the way governments and organizations communicate to their publics (Tufte, 2006, 2012). My claim is that health communication practices sometimes end as disempowering processes rather than empowering processes in society. These shortcomings to health communication interventions remain largely unknown, given that natural interest in organizations' (self-)evaluation or donor-driven evaluations is to document all the positive outcomes of the communicative intervention.

Drawing on a proposal for a "communication for peace" sketched by the Colombian media scholar Clemencia Rodríguez (2004) my argument is that communication today is a poorly explored societal force. Used appropriately – based on principles such as open access, multiplicity of voice, improved room for dialogue and difference of opinion – the large area of organizational health communication, in the form of public and private noncommercial communication strategies, can become an important societal force in developing citizen-driven strategies to strengthen or rebuild the social fabric of society and thus stimulate the general health and well-being of people.

What I am arguing points towards the need for a more explicit social vision and societal ambition in health communication. It is an argument in favor of a broader-based interdisciplinary communication paradigm, where modernity, globalization and social change is well theorized, where the mediatization of society is analysed and understood, and where the principles of open access to the media, voice and visibility in the media, recognition of difference, and room and time for dialogue and debate guide our global health communication practice.

Let me now elaborate on the four social theorists' core concepts.

Globalization and unstable subjectivities

What is happening in the field of health communication these days is tied to the fundamental rethinking of the field of communication for development. This I see as the discipline's response to what Polish sociologist Zygmunt Baumann has termed "an epochal shift" in the constitution and dynamics of society. We are living in a time of strong economic and cultural globalization, a process which the Indian anthropologist, Arjun

Appadurai, has sought to capture and understand from 1996 in his "theory of rupture." In formulating this theory, Appadurai explores the relation between globalization and modernity. In so doing he emphasizes two issues that are characteristic of the current transformation of society: one is *mass migration* and the other is the *electronic mediation of everyday life.*

Appadurai sees these two phenomena as interconnected, with both affecting the "work of the imagination" as a constitutive feature of modern subjectivity (Appadurai, 1996, p. 3). He argues that the electronic media "offer new resources and new disciplines for the construction of imagined selves and imagined worlds." Juxtaposed with the both voluntary and forced mass migrations, the result, Appadurai argues, is "a new order of instability in the production of modern subjectivities" (1996, p. 4). In this new order, social roles and relations are disembedded, people's projections to the future change, values and ontologies are challenged. In these processes of transformation, the consequence for many individuals is what I have previously termed as "the articulation of ontological *in*security" (Tufte, 2006, 2011). While a natural process of human activity is to strive for ontological security, emphasizing our need for belonging and for fundamental and existential security (Giddens, 1991), Appadurai's theory of rupture seems to indicate a process contrary to this.

This ontological insecurity came through in a noteworthy fashion in my study of young South Africans and how they produced meaning from their exposure to HIV/ AIDS prevention campaigns (Tufte, 2006). In a media ethnographic analysis I conducted, including essays written by youth from five schools in different socioeconomic strata in the town of Grahamstown in the Eastern Cape, South Africa, a few points can be highlighted: it was very striking how all the key messages from numerous campaigns came through both in the essays as well as in my everyday talk with youth and in the in-depth interviews I conducted. However, this "knowledge" deeply contrasted with the deep-felt problems of stigma, fear, and lack of social support systems that also came through in the same data. Two handfuls of excerpts from essays on the subject "How do you experience HIV/AIDS in your community?" can provide an illustration: "the great thing is to talk about it" (M17); "And to the youth, they must stick to one partner and be protected, the condoms are there for safe sex" (M17); "Use a condom because HIV/ AIDS is a killer disease" (M18); "I think the solution is to condomize" (M19); "The solution to this disease is to use condoms" (M20); "There is only one cure. Condom." (M21); "In order to get help about this you have to talk about it" (M22 – Mtwisita Ayanda); "Young people must use condom – is the easy way to protect our life" (M24); "Message: Please, 'don't compromise, condomize, people' and 'AIDS kills our people so we must fight it'" (N23 – M? Loyi); "Don't be shy, talk about it, eat good food, especially fruit and vegetables, and drink juice, not alcohol" (N25 – Buwi); "Wrap it or Zip it" (K13 – M). On the one hand the slogans illustrate the fact that the campaigns are reaching the target groups, are being listened to and watched and even discussed in the community. The big problem arises when you start contrasting this apparent success with the other findings identified: deep-felt experience of being stigmatized, fear of acquiring the virus let alone disclosing your status, and the lack of support systems (Tufte, 2006). What appeared in my analysis was parallel discourses – one of handling information in everyday discourse, the other revealing deep levels of ontological insecurity, fear and uncertainty (Tufte, 2006). Although it may seem difficult to connect these findings with processes of globalization, the connect appears when the analysis is set in the light of global discourses on HIV/AIDS prevention campaigns, communicating the messages of ABC in HIV/AIDS (Abstain, Be faithful, and use a Condom) and with the lives of these youth, many suffering the socioeconomic constraints of a postapartheid South Africa adapting to a new economy and global competition.

Risk society

Appadurai's analysis of cultural globalization and social transformation resonates well with Ulrich Beck's point about the emerging "risk society" having fundamental consequences on peoples way of thinking and acting (Beck, 1992, 2009). Beck's notion of our contemporary society as a risk society refers to the emergence of a new notion of risk; it is human-made, transnational, and often invisible and imperceptible to the senses – it refers to risks such as nuclear energy, pollution, environmental insecurities, and health hazards. Compared to the perceived risk in early industrial societies, the risks of today are of a fundamentally different nature. The existence of these hazards and insecurities in what Beck calls the "second modernity," are impacting upon our way of thinking and acting, he argues. Many people are feeling anxious and unsure about current processes of development, and these feelings often transcend clashes between tradition and modernity and have more to do with the ability or not to control the conditions of one's own everyday life.

The emergence of the risk society provides both a risk and an opportunity with regard to the sense of "agency" and ability to act amongst people. Beck explains that while the "first modernity" (the industrial era) was characterized by a clear sense of social structure that guided and put order into people's lives, where people's experiences were "contained, ordered and regulated," the structures of the emerging risk society are largely dissolved (Beck and Willms, 2004, p. 8). In the risk society lives are disembedded, but are not re-embedded into new orders and regulations. This process articulates different experiences of instability, flow and feelings of "liquidity" in both social roles and relationships (Beck and Willms, 2004, p. 63–65). He speaks of an increased individualization. John Urry explains this concept:

> There is a radicalization of individuals who are forced by social and cultural change to live more varied, flexible, and fluid lives. Beck shows how globalization coerces people to live less role-centered lives, lives that involve extensive negotiation and dialogue and where people have themselves to accept responsibility for their actions as they try to work them out with others in their network (Urry, 2004, p. 9)

This produces a double-sided process – on one hand the risk of being "lost – socially and ontologically – in the process of change" – this resulting in a variety of personal, social, and political instabilities, varying from depression to acts of violence or conflict. On the other hand, this process of individualization is leading to increased possibilities of agency, action, and mobilization. The dramatic rise of NGOs, transnational advocacy networks, and citizen-driven activities is an example of this, and most contemporary examples may well be found in the current uprisings of young angry citizens in Northern Africa and the Middle East – young unemployed people with nothing to lose and a lot to gain. Or, stated bluntly, the ruptures and transitions experienced in the contemporary processes of modernization are leading to significantly new situations in which to live our lives and project ourselves towards the future.

In the context of health communication, an illustrative example can be found in Tanzanian reality. A successful NGO, Femina HIP, has for more than 10 years now used popular culture in the form of glossy magazines, TV talk shows, and radio drama to create an enabling environment in which young Tanzanians are provided with the relevant information to make informed choices on their sexual and reproductive health and rights. Femina HIP also stimulates their overall civic engagement. The challenge for the organization has been to work in a societal context where their target audience, the youth, are facing the challenges of a young democratic society that has recently moved out of many years of one-party rule (1967–1995), adapting to market economy, but being challenged by enormous youth unemployment rates, massive migration to the urban areas, shortages of electricity, exclusion from the formal economy (only 12% of the adult population has a bank account), and prospects for the future that are somewhat bleak for the large majority. In this challenging context, Femina HIP's health communication response is not just to position its communication initiative as a response to sexual and reproductive health challenges, but to place this challenge in the context of *a livelihood perspective*. Consequently, Femina HIP connects public health challenges with the financial constraints that youth face, as well as being attentive to engaging youth, promoting their civic engagement, and encouraging them to speak out in public and participate in the general development of their society. This broader embedded approach to public health marries very well with the Alma Ata and Ottawa Charters, and speaks to the more holistic approach not very present in the achievements of, and approaches within, health communication identified at the outset of this chapter. This is Femina HIP's response to the risk society experienced by many young Tanzanians.

The ambivalence of human relations

While Ulrich Beck's work focuses on deconstructing the risk society, Zygmunt Baumann delivers an interesting analysis of social relations and networks. Baumann has written extensively on globalization, community, and social change, and some years ago launched the term "liquid modern world" (Baumann, 2003). In his 2003 book he describes how human relationships are undergoing profound changes. Basically, what we are seeing, Baumann suggests, is increased flexibilization of relationships: relationships are becoming shorter-lived, less committed, and possible to change for other relationships. Relationships continue to be the center of the security of togetherness and belonging, which we always have seen, but they are also the burden that causes strain because many feel limited by the freedom they need – ironically – to relate. The *ambivalence of human relationships* is at the core of Baumann's book *Liquid Love* and at the core of what he describes our time as: a liquid modern world (Baumann 2003, p. viii). The relevance here of bringing Baumann's analysis of the fluidity of social relationships into the discussion, is that it speaks to a core problem in our contemporary experiences of rupture and transition, and not least in situations of violence and conflict: it is that the social fabric upon which our society is built is strained, roles are changing and in transition, and, in the most violent cases, the social fabric is being destroyed. Wakefield, Laken, and Hornik (2010, p. 1268) touch briefly upon a similar category of social health problems, but they leave the question open as how to respond to it in communication terms.

The fundamental question in this context is exactly that: how we can use communication strategically, as a tool in the process of repairing or weaving new social networks and thus renewing societal foundations where such foundations have been lost or eroded. The challenge for social scientists engaged with health communication is to rethink the role of media and communication in support of a development process and a public health vision where the media – including mainstream media – can better serve the contemporary health concerns of citizens.

Health Citizenship in Contexts of Mediatization and Globalization

A central challenge for health communication from an interdisciplinary, social-science-oriented perspective is how to configure and articulate health citizenships. This challenge is not new in the public health debate, but has often been neglected in the practice of public health. It resonates well with the longstanding international discourse on public health, which emphasizes the social determinants and the rights of the citizen. This has been seen already in the Alma Alta Declaration of 1978, it was very elaborate in the Ottawa Charter of 1986, and the focus on rights and citizenship was reemphasized and argued strongly in the final declaration from the UN conference in Cairo in 1994, emphasizing sexual and reproductive health and rights. Later, this rights-based and citizen-oriented approach to public health was also emphasized in more communication-focused international encounters, such as the UN Roundtable on Communication for Development held in Managua in 2001, where HIV/AIDS was the issue discussed.

One problem in many health communication interventions has been that they do not connect interventions on one level with interventions on another level in society. Thus, it is often seen that there is either a focus on mainly national policy development or on more limited local project activity. The interconnection and need for coordination between levels can create synergies and also lead to stronger coherence in communication processes, and thus to stronger impact. Most public health- and health communication-oriented practice points to narrow health issues that require focused interventions emphasizing individual behavioral change often dissociated from tackling the broader socioeconomic and political determinants – the so-called post-positivist approach (Zoller and Dutta 2008). The fact that most health communication interventions do not target issues of power inequality, gender relations, sexual and reproductive rights, the voices of marginalized groups and their access to media and information services, points towards the argument made eloquently by Zoller and Dutta, that of bringing interpretive, critical, and culture-centered approaches on board in health communication theory and practice.

While I can only endorse the Zoller and Dutta arguments and positions, let me highlight two dimensions of the emerging interdisciplinarity of health communication. The first is that of understanding media better and in particular the way in which mediatization influences and even determines human behavior and interaction; the second is the more concrete challenges of globalization for public health.

Understanding media and mediatization

While media studies have expanded, diversified, and grown enormously in the past two or three decades, many of the insights are not fully incorporated into the practice of health communication and its use in promoting healthy lifestyles, changing human behaviour, and promoting public health. Big advances have been achieved in understanding how audiences make use of communication, analyzing the political economy of the media, developing media content analysis, and increasingly taking on studies of social media as a phenomenon challenging traditional models of communication and media. Also, a stronger emphasis has developed on connecting studies of media and communication practices with studies of cultural practices and popular culture. Lately, we have seen a growing interest in studying the increasing *mediatization* of our everyday lives and how this relates to our formation of norms, values, and lifestyles. The mediatization of everyday life will, beyond doubt, come to constitute a dominating factor of life to the degree that health communication interventions and evaluations will need strong conceptual frameworks to understand the changing role of the media in society and the generalized mediatization of everyday life.

Informed by the growing insights into the interplay between popular culture, mediated social practices, audience sense making, and mediated ways of life and identity formation, a growing epistemological recognition can be observed amongst some health communication scholars to connect to these fields of media studies. It is a type of thinking that increasingly points to the need to address media sociology contexts and media institution analysis and to carry out media ethnographies amongst audiences of health communication.

Challenges of globalization

Having identified the already existing broad understanding of health and health citizenship within the international declarations on public health, another big challenge remains to be reflected upon: the multidimensional challenge of globalization in promoting public health. Why should we, and how should we, deal with the many dimensions of social, cultural, political, and economic globalization in our public health policies, and in our health communication practice in particular? Zollner and Dutta mentioned globalization in passing (Zollner and Dutta, 2008, pp. 5 and 20) and a couple of the cases in their book speak to the issue. However, it largely remains an unarticulated analysis and debate, both at the conceptual level, as discussed earlier in this chapter, and empirically, as I will briefly mention in the following. As stated earlier, Appadurai's analysis of globalization shows us how cultural globalization is producing instability in our processes of identity formation and thus in our behaviors. His analysis of cultural globalization carries in it the core argument that justifies the need for public health systems and health communication strategists to broaden their perspective and take on the challenge of dealing with globalization in policies and strategies. The empirical evidence of globalization, both as a social, cultural, economic and political process can be illustrated with a few examples:

1 *Epidemics travel.* They always have, throughout history. But we have a growing number of recent cases, such as HIV/AIDS, SARS and Avian Flu, where outbreaks have challenged national frameworks and invited stronger international cooperation. International agencies are increasingly defining local agendas from a global perspective and starting out from the need for collaboration, something that is certainly creating tensions but also opportunities.

2 *Media development.* With new technologies, satellite communication, and Internet-based networks, the symbolic worlds people have access to and navigate within are expanding tremendously. Ideas, norms, and values are formed in an increasingly mediatized and globalized symbolic universe where local and global discourses mix and hybridize. How is this influencing our perceptions of health and our human behavior?

3 *Social movements and transnational advocacy networks.* In the last decade, social movements have established strong transnational advocacy networks and platforms, seen in a multitude of examples across the globe (Downing, 2010). They are appearing both as a new civil society platform of agency (seen around the Social Fora) and also as very loose movements mobilizing around single cases as well as broader development challenges. The point to make here is that there is a clear global dimension to most of these efforts indicating that agency potentially has a global outreach.

4 *New economy.* The "New Economy" based on liberalized, market-driven, globalized principles is setting the agenda as the logic of production, organization, and service provision. How is this impacting upon the public health sector? Are alternative economic models feasible? The New Economy is also influencing the logic and function of the media, seen most clearly in the global trend of deregulation of the media.

5 *Diasporic public spheres.* With migration, increased mobility, and the proliferation of social media, people are reorganizing the ways in which they, in their diasporic communities, are organizing themselves and communicating with each other. How do we communicate with people organized, in terms of norms and values, *both* along national boundaries and in diasporic communities, cutting across the more classical sociological categories of age, gender, and profession?

6 *Global conflicts, catastrophes, and environmental challenges.* The world we are living in is increasingly influenced by a range of new forms of risk: global terrorism, international conflict, and transnational environmental risks. How is this impacting upon our mobility, identity formation, and sense of security? And is it impacting upon our behavior and well-being?

7 *Migration, urbanization, and social exclusion.* Connected to a variety of reasons inherent in the above-mentioned characteristics of contemporary processes of globalization, we are experiencing not only massive urbanization, but a growing number

of economic refugees, a growing number of poor people, and an increased social polarization in the world. What are the public health consequences, and how are we to face these challenges in our health communication interventions?

The list of change processes associated with globalization that have public health implications is very long, and the above simply pinpoints some of them. The examples basically serve to illustrate my point: as researchers in global health communication, we need to develop a much stronger awareness and analysis of global development trends and how they relate to locally lived lives. Communication and public health increasingly occurs in a globalized context (see Hemer and Tufte, 2005, or Robertson, 1992 for further elaboration of the concept of glocalization).

An Emerging Health Communication Agenda

To conclude, I will synthesize the above analyses and discussions by formulating three statements which, I hope, can serve the further development of an increasingly interdisciplinary health communication research agenda.

Statement 1: The center of public health lies outside the public health system.
This hypothesis paraphrases an old quotation from the German critical sociologist and media researcher Oscar Negt, who in the early 1970s reflected upon the role of the media and the public sphere. Negt said that "the center of the media lies outside of the media." His point was that media content, access to the media, control of the media, as well as debates within the mediated public sphere were all determined by structural and political conditions that lie outside the media and media system itself. His vision was consistent with the strong emphasis upon the development of media policies that was a substantial part of media and communication research in the 1970s and early 1980s (the debate around the New World Information and Communication Order, NWICO).

My point here is that the situation is similar for the public health system. Many problems of public health for citizens and communities nowadays do not originate in the public health system, but relate to broader issues of citizenship, empowerment, socioeconomic status, culture, power relations, and policy priorities. The Alma Ata Charter, the Ottowa Charter, and the Cairo Declaration point towards these contextual factors and their role in attaining global public health. This hypothesis continues that discourse, inviting health communication researchers to broaden the basis of the field in pursuit of more comprehensive health communication strategies and public health solutions.

Statement 2: The forces of globalization are at the heart of the challenges that we must understand and relate to in order to achieve a "healthy" society.
This hypothesis follows the line of arguments about globalization put forward in Arjun Appadurai's writings on the cultural dimension of globalization. Appadurai's theory of rupture works from the premise that mass migration and the electronic mediation of everyday life offer a new order of instability in the production of modern subjectivities, subjectivities that, by default, are at the center of social processes of communication.

Therefore, although globalization *is* an extremely broad concept, it does encompass a range of the societal constraints under which locally embedded everyday lives unfold. We thus need to connect our health communication challenges – when relevant – to these developments. While national public health is not passé, it is at least insufficient to address global health risks and challenges.

Statement 3: (Global) Health Communication is a discipline in urgent need for a more interdisciplinary epistemological, theoretical and methodological basis.
The international debate on health communication in recent years has challenged the attitude of "business as usual" in this field. The continuously severe situation regarding public health challenges such as HIV/AIDS, tuberculosis, malaria, and the growing problems of obesity and diabetes are just some of the indicators of health communicators not doing a good enough job. This calls for a critical review of our discipline. As argued throughout this chapter, to advance the theory and practice of health communication will require a philosophical and epistemological base that takes into consideration some of the development processes, changing mediascapes, and altered subjectivities that constitute contexts of health communication today. As health communication researchers, we need to further develop our subdiscipline of health communication, producing the called for solid interdisciplinary understandings of – but also the relevant communicative strategies to approach – the broader health challenges we face in our globalized world.

References

Appadurai, A. (1996). *Modernity at Large. Cultural Dimensions of Globalisation.* London and Minnesota: University of Minnesota Press.

Baumann, Z. (2003). *Liquid Love.* Cambridge: Polity Press.

Beck, U. (1992). *Risk Society: Towards a New Modernity: Theory, Culture and Society.* London: Sage.

Beck, U. (2009). *World and Risk.* Cambridge: Polity Press.

Beck, U. and Willms, J. (2004).*Conversations with Ulrich Beck.* Cambridge: Polity Press.

Downing, J. (Ed.) (2010). *Encyclopedia of Social Movement Media.* London: Sage.

Dutta, M. J. and Zoller, H. M. (2008). Theoretical foundation: Interpretive, critical, and cultural approaches to health communication. In H. M. Zoller and M. J. Dutta (Eds.), *Emerging Perspectives in Health Communication. Meaning, Culture, and Power* (pp. 1–38). London: Routledge.

Freimuth, V. (2004). The contributions of health communication to eliminating health disparities. *American Journal of Public Health, 94*(12), 2053–2055.

Freimuth, V. S., Massett, H. A., and Meltzer, W. (2006). A descriptive analysis of 10 years of research published in the *Journal of Health Communication. Journal of Health Communication, 11*(1), 11–20.

Galavotti, C., Kuhlmann, A. K., Kraft, J. M. *et al.* (2008). From innovation to implementation: The long and winding road. *American Journal of Community Psychology, 41*, 314–326.

Giddens, A. (1991). *Modernity and Self-Identity: Self and Society in the Late Modern Age.* Cambridge: Polity Press.

Ginsburg, F. D, Abu-Lughod, L., and Larkin, B. (Eds.) (2002). *Media Worlds. Anthropology on New Terrain.* Berkeley: University of California Press.

Gumucio-Dagron, A. and Tufte, T. (2006). *Communication for Social Change Anthology: Historical and Contemporary Readings.* South Orange, NJ: Communication for Social Change Consortium.

Hemer, O. and Tufte, T. (Eds.) (2005). *Media and Glocal Change. Rethinking Communication for Development.* Göteborg: Nordicom.

Obregon, R. (2010). Un panorama de la investigación, teoría y práctica de la comuniación en salud [A panorama of investigation, theory and practice in health communication]. *Folios, 23,* 13–32.

Petraglia, J. (2007). Narrative intervention in behavior and public health. *Journal of Health Communication, 12*(5), 493–505.

Petraglia, J. (2009). The importance of being authentic: persuasion, narration, and dialogue in health communication and education. *Health Communication, 24*(2), 176–185.

Robertson, R. (1992). *Globalization – Social Theory and Global Culture.* London: Sage.

Rodríguez, C. (2004). Communication for peace: Contrasting approaches. *The Drum Beat, 278*(December 5, 2004). Retrieved from http://www.comminit.com/drum_beat_278.html

Spitulnik, D. (1993). Anthropology and mass media. *Annual Review of Anthropology, 22,* 293–315.

Spitulnik, D. (2002). Mobile machines and fluid audiences. rethinking reception through Zambian radio culture. In F. D. Ginsburg, L. Abu-Lughod, and B. Larkin (Eds.), *Media Worlds. Anthropology on New Terrain* (pp. 337–354). Berkeley: University of California Press.

Tufte, T. (2000). *Living with the Rubbish Queen. Telenovelas, Culture and Modernity in Brazil.* Luton: University of Luton Press.

Tufte, T. (2001). Entertainment-education and participation – assessing the communication strategy of Soul City. *Journal of International Communication, 7*(2), 25–51.

Tufte, T. (2004). Soap operas and sense-making: Mediations and audience ethnography. In M. Cody, A. Singhal, M. Sabido and E. Rogers (Eds.), *Entertainment-Education Worldwide: History, Research and Practice* (pp. 417–434). New York: Lawrence Erlbaum Associates.

Tufte, T. (2006). Your future gets stuck! Challenges for HIV/AIDS communication. *Media Development, 3,* 25–29.

Tufte, T. (2011). Mediapolis, human (in)security and citizenship communication and *glocal* development challenges in the digital era. In M. Christensen, A. Jansson and C. Christensen (Eds.), *Online Territories: Globalization, Mediated Practice and Social Space* (pp. 113–131). New York: Peter Lang Publishers.

Tufte, T. (2012). Facing violence and conflict with communication – Possibilities and limitations of storytelling and entertainment-education. In S. R. Melkote (Ed.), *Development Communication in Directed Social Change: A Reappraisal of Theories and Approaches.* AMIC, Singapore.

Urry, J. (2004). Introduction: Thinking society anew. In U. Beck and J. Willms, *Conversations with Ulrich Beck* (pp. 1–10). Cambridge: Polity Press.

Wakefield, M. A., Laken, B. and Hornik, R. C. (2010). Use of mass media campaigns to change health behavior. *The Lancet, 376,* 1261–1271.

Zoller, H. M., and Dutta, M. J. (Eds.) (2008). *Emerging Perspectives in Health Communication. Meaning, Culture, and Power.* London: Routledge.

Part V

Conclusions: Rethinking the Field

Toward Social Justice in Directed Social Change
Rethinking the Role of Development Support Communication

Srinivas R. Melkote

"The biggest enemy of health in the developing world is poverty." Kofi Annan (Former Secretary General, United Nations)[1]

The chapters in this volume have explored in detail theories, models, programs, and practices in health communication, especially at the global level. As Waisbord and Obregon attest in the introductory chapter, the field of health communication has its roots in theories and models related to socioeconomic development as well as in concepts grounded in social-psychological theories and media effects research. It is not my objective to rehash the arguments made in the earlier chapters on the applicability or superiority of the transmission models of communication over participatory ideas or vice versa. According to Storey and Figueroa in Chapter 4, at different times and in varied contexts the information diffusion models and the participatory/empowerment models have made, and continue to make, valuable contributions to theories and models in health communication. Another strain of thought present in this book is the argument that health communication theories and practices have focused too much on national or regional issues and contexts and not enough attention has been paid to the global context. In this chapter, I wish to focus on the larger issue of directed social change (in which health is an important concern) and dwell on my concern about systemic injustice in our global communities and discuss what communicative actions should do to address this.

As we entered the twenty-first century, the challenge of unequal development in our communities and in our world continued to be intractable. The Millennium Development Goals (MDGs), approved by the United Nations, which were then adopted by most countries in the year 2000, present us with a blueprint of the pressing priorities in development in the next decade. The MDGs constitute the centerpiece of the Millennium

The Handbook of Global Health Communication, First Edition. Edited by Rafael Obregon and Silvio Waisbord.

Declaration of the United Nations and serve not only as an important milestone in the history of the development agenda for most countries, but also remind us of the formidable development-related challenges that lie ahead. MDGs, which provide basic guidelines on eight development goals to be achieved by the year 2015, address and highlight the needs of the poorest and the most marginalized individuals and groups in the world today. The eight goals are: (1) eradication of extreme poverty; (2) achieving universal primary education; (3) promoting gender equality and empowering women and girls; (4) reducing child mortality; (5) improving maternal health; (6) combating HIV/AIDS, malaria, and other major diseases; (7) ensuring environmental sustainability; and, (8) developing a global partnership (see UNDP, 2010). The MDGs constitute the benchmarks that serve as signposts for leaders and other decision makers in national governments, civil society, NGOs, and other significant groups concerned with unequal development in communities worldwide. For example, MDGs 4, 5, and 6 focus on specific health-related challenges facing the world today. MDG 6 puts the spotlight on the pandemics of malaria, HIV/AIDS, and tuberculosis. According to the World Health Organisation (WHO), at the end of 2009, 33.3 million people around the world were living with HIV. That same year about three million people were newly infected, and about two million died of AIDS, which included 260,000 children. The problem is endemic in sub-Saharan Africa, where 68 percent of people living with AIDS are concentrated. Here, there are an estimated 10.6 million people needing antiretroviral therapy. WHO reports that malaria has made a comeback in many parts of the Third World but especially in Africa, South Asia, and Southeast Asia. It kills nearly one million people a year, a majority of whom are children below 5 years of age in Africa. On average, a child succumbs to malaria every 30 seconds. Meanwhile, tuberculosis (TB) has been rampant in many parts of the world, especially the Third World countries. There were approximately 9.4 million new cases of TB in 2009 and an estimated 1.7 million deaths, making TB a deadly infectious disease (WHO, 2011a, 2011b). It is not a coincidence that these deadly diseases are rampant in the poorer parts of the world and affect the most poor and vulnerable populations.

Development communication, as an area of scholarship and practice, has been engaged in finding a niche in the efforts to tackle the formidable problems of underdevelopment and marginalization of millions of people and thousands of communities worldwide through a process of directed social change. What should be the mission of the field of development support communication in the face of contemporary realities and challenges? What are the ways in which we can visualize and reconstruct the mission and role of media and communication in directed change, including health-related changes? This chapter attempts to explore these issues.

Reappraisal of Development Communication Scholarship vis-à-vis Contemporary Realities

What is the extent of deprivation and marginalization of millions of the poorest individuals and communities in the world today? Below, a few highlights of the health-related challenges are sobering (World Bank, 2011):

- There are more extremely poor people today. Millions of individuals worldwide, but especially in the developing countries, still earn less than US$1.25 per day.
- In the developing countries, one out of four children under five years of age is underweight.
- In sub-Saharan Africa and parts of south Asia, rates of children completing primary schools are lower than 69 percent, in many cases under 50 percent.
- Thousands of children do not live to see their fifth birthday. The child mortality rate in much of Africa is over 100 per 1,000, and nearly 30,000 children (under five years of age) die each day in developing countries from preventable causes.
- Communicable diseases strike 30 million children often resulting in blindness or deafness and killing more than 600,000 a year.
- Ninety-nine percent of maternal deaths occur in developing countries. In many poor African countries, one mother dies for every 100 children born.
- Even today, tuberculosis kills about 1.8 million people per year.
- Nearly one billion people still lack access to reliable source of clean water and nearly 2.5 billion are still in need of improved sanitation services.

In addition to these grim statistics, there are other formidable challenges that include lack of food security affecting millions of people including children, and environmental and habitat destruction or unsustainability. The list goes on.

Today, the challenge is not just to achieve a certain level of development, but, importantly, to identify the reasons for its unequal spread and suggest theories, models, and strategies to eradicate or at least minimize the ravages of unequal development in societies worldwide. Many today would prefer to reconstruct the challenge of directed social change; it is unconscionable to justify the present inequality between people on issues so basic as food security, clean drinking water, basic education, and health care. The foci of development communication should be not just to facilitate development, but also to look at the present state of unequal development among global communities, document its negative consequences on people and communities, and identify reasons for such an unequal spread of development benefits. Following this exercise in deconstruction, the scholarship in development communication should be better able to reconceptualize and reoperationalize the real meaning and goal of development. This, in turn, would provide a better understanding of the real constraints to achieving development thus providing scholars with opportunities to incorporate models and theories that are most relevant and germane to the task of achieving equitable development.

Reconceptualization of Development

The articulation of the Millennium Development Goals by the United Nations (UN) is itself a testament to the stark differences among individuals and global communities in areas basic to human survival (World Bank, 2011). Over the last 70 years, since development was adopted as a goal by the UN and many countries around the world, it has become increasingly evident that, while the process of development did produce development in many countries and communities, its spread has been uneven leaving many individuals and communities behind. Some suggest that it is the nature and process of development (as it has been conceptualized and operationalized), which is associated with increasing inequality among global communities on indicators very basic to human survival and growth such as adequate food and nutrition, clean drinking water, basic education, and basic health care. True, many individuals and communities have benefitted from the development process; their standards of living and consumption have risen. However, for millions of individuals around the world today, the outcomes have been continued incapacity and incapability to lead effective lives. The relative state of countries today and stratification of people within them on basic human development indicators are an indication of a process of development that has failed a very large section of people and communities (World Bank, 2011; Berger, 1974) around the world. It is the poor, the marginalized, and the vulnerable who are worst affected by inadequacies in health care and the ravages of killer diseases. WHO reports that malaria disproportionately affects poor people who are not in a position to pay for the treatment or have limited access to health care, thus "trapping families and communities in a downward spiral of poverty" (WHO, 2011c). The World Health Organisation states:

> Poverty is associated with the undermining of a range of key human attributes, including health. The poor are exposed to greater personal and environmental health risks, are less well nourished, have less information and are less able to access health care; they thus have a higher risk of illness and disability. Conversely, illness can reduce household savings, lower learning ability, reduce productivity, and lead to a diminished quality of life, thereby perpetuating or even increasing poverty. (WHO, 2011c)

In a scathing report, WHO states that it is the poorest of the poor around the world who suffer from the worst health conditions. Within many countries, the data indicate that in general the lower an individual's socioeconomic position, the worse off is his/her health. "There is a social gradient in health that runs from top to bottom of the socioeconomic spectrum. This is a global phenomenon, seen in low, middle and high income countries" (WHO, 2011c).

Ultimate Goal

Increasingly, the idea of establishing *social justice* is finding common ground among development scholars. I agree with this view and conceptualize development as a process of directed social change with the establishment of social justice as its ultimate goal. The achievement of social justice should serve as an anchor for development communication theory and propel social transformations in global communities. At the conceptual level, the term *social justice* helps to create a common platform for scholars and practitioners from myriad different disciplines and professions that constitute development communication. While the term *social justice* connotes a common understanding in the conceptual domain, its operationalization has been a challenge. The main reason why unequal development prevails around the world is because the operationalization of development has not captured all facets of social justice.

What is *social justice* in directed social change and what are the ways in which it may be operationalized? In Table 30.1, I present a tabular model in which the achievement of social justice or the elimination of injustice is the ultimate goal of directed social change (in level 1). The model operationalizes the indicators of social justice through the outcomes desired at national and community levels (in level 2); it then presents the outcome desired by development support communication (in level 3), which would constitute the means by which outcomes articulated at national and community levels may be achieved; and, in turn, the model lists the principal communicative means by which the outcome desired by development support communication may be achieved (in level 4). All through the model, the interactivity between the different levels and between national and community contexts is stressed. The role and place of development support communication are highlighted as it addresses the challenges at both the national and community contexts. The overlapping and reinforcing nature of the principal actions of development support communication (as indicated by the double-edged arrow) between the macro and micro contexts is a contribution that this model makes to highlight its utility across national and local contexts.

In Table 30.1, the elimination of injustice is the ultimate goal of directed social change. Achieving social justice would constitute the elimination of persistent and endemic deprivation of individuals and communities in areas basic to human survival and enhance the capacity and capability of people to live effective lives. These would include sustained access to resources such as adequate food and basic health care to live healthy lives, basic education to be able to function effectively in society, access to land or income generating employment, access to clean drinking water and sanitary living conditions, political participation, and basic civil rights. This list is not exhaustive, but it is a good beginning. Since elimination of social injustice is central to the process of directed social change, media and communication processes and actors attempting to bring about social change must be committed to this goal. Therefore, the assessment of the contribution of development support communication must be in terms of its success in eradicating the egregious forms of injustice in societies. The model in Table 30.1 also suggests that elimination of injustice (in level 1) could be instrumental in helping toward the achievement of outcomes desired at level 2 and vice versa. This interrelationship is evident and empirically verifiable between the different levels in Table 30.1; they feed each other through symbiotic relationships.

It is evident from the preceding discussion that the context of directed social change efforts should not be confined to the Third World or the countryside. Today, the applicability and application of development support communication is in all environments and contexts punctuated by social injustice. Thus the location could be the depressed urban communities in Detroit, USA, marginalized communities in Haiti, the hinterland of Bangladesh, or any other location where people and communities are victims of injustice.

Outcomes at national and community levels

At the national level, the state and civil society are the main agencies or avenues and, therefore, should share the primary responsibility of protecting and strengthening the welfare of their citizens. Specifically, these agencies would include the governments from

Table 30.1   Model for reappraisal of the role of media and communication in directed social change in multiple contexts.

Social Justice

Expected Outcomes (National Level)	**Expected Outcomes (Community Level)**
Social, political, economic, media structures/policies that foster/ sustain equity (including health equity)	Social, political, economic, cultural arrangements/structures/ conventions/practices that foster/ sustain equity (including health equity)
>Structures and policies, which establish equity in claims & access to resources & rights of communities and other stakeholders	>Structures, arrangements, practices, and rules, which value equity in claims and access to resources and rights of all local stakeholders
>Structures and policies, which value choices, opportunities, enhance capacity and capability of communities and other stakeholders	>Structures, arrangements, practices & rules, which value choices, opportunities, enhance capacity & capability of all local stakeholders

Outcomes from Communicative Actions	**Outcomes from Communicative Actions**
Vibrant public sphere	Social norms that are compatible with equity
Active public discussion and debate	Democratic participation of members
Public/mass media support	Empowered community/Building of social capital
Empowered communities, groups and coalitions	

Principal Communicative Actions	**Principal Communicative Actions**
Social mobilization: expand/ sustain public spheres and public communication, participation, and debate;	Create/change social norms to be compatible with notions of equity in social, political, economic, cultural, and informational arenas/ resources;
Media mobilization: influence public opinion; raise awareness, win public support;	Create, expand, sustain agency/ power of the community;

(*Continued*)

Table 30.1 (*cont'd*).

Advocacy communication: raise awareness of issues, win support of important constituencies; influence policies;	Create, strengthen democratic participation of all local stakeholders;
Social Movements/Resistance communication: organize resistance to structures and policies that foster inequity;	Community mobilization: expand, sustain public participation, debate, and discussion; grassroots organizing; use of local media and mobile technologies;
Networking: build coalitions; strengthen partnerships between stakeholders.	Create, expand, sustain networking of all local stakeholders;
	Participatory action/ communication approaches; Co-Equal knowledge sharing approaches.

Source: Melkote and Krishnatray (2010).

the federal to the local levels; public institutions such as schools and courts; political parties; market structures; media systems; legal systems; professional associations; as well as NGOs, social service organizations, cooperatives, and others. Together, these entities in a society influence the social, political, economic, and cultural laws, policies, arrangements, and conventions that have a bearing on individual opportunities, capabilities, capacities, and welfare.

What should be the primary normative concerns in a society that is sensitive to the ravages of inequality in directed social change? What are the facets of social justice that all people in a society must be guaranteed? At the most elementary level, all females and males should have access to basic education, basic health care, and to land or sustainable and gainful employment opportunities. Individuals must have claims to social safety nets such as social security, unemployment benefits, etc. during times of distress – and guarantees of individual safety at all times. In addition, there should be opportunities for people to participate in a market system that is monitored by the state to provide avenues for production, exchange, and consumption (Sen, 2000). Importantly, all citizens should have claims and access to civil rights, which include free expression of speech, autonomous mass media, and a guarantee of transparency in all public transactions that are open to public and media scrutiny. In other words, what is needed is a pervasive will to establish and sustain social, political, economic, and media structures/policies that foster/ sustain equity, including health and gender equity. Inequities in health care or inadequate health behaviors and skills are not just due to poor knowledge/attitudes of individuals but are largely due to oppressive structural obstacles. As Campbell and Scott emphasize in Chapter 8 in this volume, what is needed are enabling social environments. Writing about the evaluation of social change communication for HIV/AIDS in Chapter 14, Byrne and Vincent posit that the challenge of effective multilevel programming may be traced to structural issues, thus leading to an examination of the social determinants of

HIV. They present challenges at the macro level (social characteristics that affect people's lives such as racism, sexism, and discrimination); the intermediate level (infrastructure and service availability, neighborhood characteristics, and local resources); and individual micro-level factors. Hess, Meekers, and Storey emphasize in Chapter 18 that individuals and households become health-competent when they can successfully access or mobilize the resources they require such as information, social factors, and empowerment-related factors to make health decisions and achieve positive health outcomes.

Table 30.1 highlights the interconnections between the different levels. For example, the elimination of injustice (in level 1) could be instrumental in helping toward the achievement of outcomes desired at the institutional and local levels and, in turn, the elimination of inequities in society (in level 2) could help in facilitating social justice. In addition, there are interlinkages between the different factors within the expected outcomes. The learning of literacy and numeracy skills through education helps improve a person's economic participation and productivity, while access to adequate health care will have a positive impact on individual productivity, which in turn helps economic growth. While a free and robust market is the engine of development, its beneficial effects on the entire society is contingent upon equitable social and political policies, laws, and arrangements. It has also been demonstrated that access to education for females has had a positive impact on fertility rates and female empowerment (Sen, 2000). These interconnections and others have been empirically verified and further reinforce the practical advantages that would accrue from a concern to eradicate the major sources of injustice in a society.

Outcomes Expected by Development Support Communication

At level 2 in Table 30.1, we see the different roles and responsibilities of the state and civil society in protecting and strengthening individuals and communities from the ravages of social injustice. This perspective, however, does not imply that I visualize communities or individuals as passive recipients waiting for societal institutions to play the roles of benefactors and protectors. People and the groups they belong to or the communities of which they are members should have the active task of making the social/ political/ economic structures and policies in a society more appropriate and effective in establishing social justice through directed social change. The outcome desired by development support communication, then, should be to create, expand, and sustain the agency of communities, organizations, and individuals in directed change. This indicates a move from a passive "patient" to an active "agent" of change. The new avatar of development support communication should be one that encourages and pursues an agent-oriented view (Sen, 2000) for individuals and communities engaged in directed social change. Individuals and communities must have the capacity and opportunity to play an active role in articulating and shaping the kind of change they desire. This could be aided by communicative actions at the larger societal level by creating or strengthening: a vibrant public sphere, active public discussion and debate, empowered communities, groups, and coalitions, and supportive public/mass media. At the community level, communicative actions should strengthen social norms that are compatible with the notion of equity in the distribution of resources and rights, democratic participation of all local stakeholders, and the countervailing power of the community and its constituents. Again, there is an active link between levels 2 and 3. While the outcomes in level 2 help in strengthening the capacities and capabilities of individuals and communities to craft the kinds of change they desire, the active agency of individuals and groups outlined in level 3 aids in the quest for creating a more just society and, concomitantly, a more equitable spread of the benefits of directed change.

However, the task of creating active agency at the larger societal, community or individual levels will not be successful unless the lack of economic, political, and social power among individuals or communities in contemporary societies is addressed. Any meaningful discussion of unequal development must address issues of the inequitable spread of power in a society. The reality of the social and political situation in most societies is such that the urban and rural poor and other oppressed communities, women and others at the grassroots, are entrapped in a dependency relationship in highly stratified and unequal socioeconomic structures that are also punctuated with sharp inequities in countervailing power. Therefore, power inequities in societies are posited as major impediments to creating active agency on the part of the marginalized people and communities.

The World Health Organisation warns that the social determinants of health are crucial for the poor, oppressed, and marginalized populations. "The social determinants of health are the conditions in which people are born, grow, live, work and age, including the health system. These circumstances are shaped by the distribution of money, power and resources at global, national and local levels, which are themselves influenced by policy choices. The social determinants of health are mostly responsible for health inequities - the unfair and avoidable differences in health status seen within and between countries" (WHO, 2011d). In 2005, in response to the persistent and wide inequities, the World Health Organisation set up a body called the Commission on Social Determinants of Health (CSDH) to provide guidelines on meeting the growing inequity in health between the haves and the have-nots. In 2008, the Commission issued its report, which contained important recommendations such as: improve daily living conditions, and tackle the inequitable distribution of power, money, and resources (WHO, 2011c).

Principal means of development support communication

Social mobilization

If directed social change is to have any relevance to the communities and people who need it most, it must start where the real needs and problems exist, that is, in the rural areas, urban slums, and other depressed sectors in society. People and communities living in such peripheries must perceive their *real* needs and identify their *real* problems. Identification of needs and constraints are, to a great extent, impacted by the nature of public participation and dialogue. To a large extent, these people and communities have lacked agency due to an absence of genuine participation in change strategies ostensibly set up to ameliorate their problems. Alternatively, bottom-up communication strategies have often turned out to be mere clichés lacking in substance. The bottom line is the issue of the lack of power of people in having a voice in effecting the type of social change they need to live the kinds of life they desire. Therefore, the new task of development support communicators should be directly linked to the building and exercise of social power (Speer and Hughey, 1995) of individuals and communities who are regarded merely as "targets" by change agencies in directed social change programs. Individuals and communities that have been affected by societal injustice should be able to participate in crafting what they want and have reason to accept. This civil right should not be the prerogative of just political, economic/business, or religious leaders. Public participation and discussion are necessary for creating transparency and for making responsible social choices, which are fundamental to policy making in the social arena. Besides, it can create shared norms especially on many social and cultural issues, which can then have a beneficial effect on public policies, arrangements, and conventions relating to these matters and concerns (Sen, 2000). Other communicative actions would include the mobilization of public media in influencing public opinion, raising awareness, and winning public support for issues and projects that involve systemic social injustice.

Social Movements

Social movements have always played an important role during times of great change in societies around the world throughout history. Many observers are now visualizing a new post-development phase in which social movements can serve as radical alternatives working on behalf of the marginalized and against the dominant knowledge structures, ideology, etc. in a society (Wilkins, 2008; Escobar, 1995). In the postindustrial societies of today, social movements are seen as vehicles to craft political identities, challenge dominant social norms, and serve as channels of resistance (Atkinson, 2010; Steeves, 2003). Examples of social movements include those against environmental destruction, against global capitalism or big government, and for greater human rights including women's rights (Wilkins, 2003). While social movements may desire outcomes in many different areas, what should be of interest to scholars in development support communication are social movements that sensitize the people and the media to issues of unequal and unjust development structures and policies, and lead the fight against the power structures that desire to maintain the status quo. This may be done in many ways, by collecting and sharing pertinent information, framing issues, building coalitions with allies, targeting media attention, and generally acting as vehicles of social mobilization at the community, national, or transnational levels. Recent events in Egypt, Tunisia, Syria, China, and other places have also shown that using mobile communication technologies can be very effective in "crowd sourcing" and bringing pressure to bear on authorities and create global media awareness of structures and polices that sustain systemic injustice.

Advocacy communication

Advocacy communication has been regarded by some as separate from the work of development support communication (Mefalopulos, 2008). However, the new avatar of development communication must include advocacy communication to raise awareness of issues, win support of constituencies, and influence policy debates especially on matters relating to unequal distribution of development's benefits in a society.

The World Health Organisation recommends the following: health equity must become a marker of a government's performance; public sector leadership in the provision of essential health-related goods/services and control of health damaging commodities should be strengthened; civil society should be enabled to organize and act in a manner that promotes and realizes the political and social rights affecting health equity; health care systems should be based on principles of equity, disease prevention, and health promotion with universal coverage, focusing on primary health care.

Grassroots participation

Many scholars over the past four decades, including several authors in this volume[2], have favored active participation of the people at the grassroots. On the surface, these signaled a positive departure from the earlier overly top-down and prescriptive change approaches. However, the structure of elite domination was not disturbed in these approaches. Diaz-Bordenave (1980) noted that in these approaches the participation that was expected was often directed by the sources and change agents. Thus the people were induced to participate in change efforts, but the agenda and the solutions to alleged problems were controlled and selected by the external change agencies. People at the grassroots were co-opted in so-called participatory activities that were directed and controlled by agencies external to the local communities. Participation, therefore, was a means to an end; the end being greater dependence of the local people and communities on external agencies, both national and international. This remains the case even today in many traditional social marketing projects.

True participation should go beyond such tactics to involve the people and communities in social and political action. The participatory model that I envision would incorporate the framework of critical social change and involve social mobilization at the community level. The goal should be to facilitate *conscientization* of marginalized people and communities to the unequal social, political, economic, and spatial structures in their societies. It is through conscientization and collective action that people can perceive their needs, identify constraints to addressing the needs, and plan on overcoming problems and constraints. Paulo Freire (1970) first introduced the concept of conscientization. He was disappointed with the educational systems in Brazil and Chile and advocated their replacement with a type of pedagogy that would be more receiver-centered and involve the experience of the people, especially of their existential situations, reflection, and dialogue. He called this process "conscientization." Armed with the new knowledge of their existential situation, the people could then come up with action plans to liberate themselves from their dependent and exploited status. This was truly empowerment pedagogy and contrasted sharply with the "banking" education practiced by the authorities wherein exogenous prescriptive information was "deposited" into the heads of passive recipients. Especially among the marginalized individuals and groups who were victims of societal injustice, the process of action/experience and reflection on their unequal power situation led to a critical consciousness with respect to pertinent situations and set them on a path to social change where they could serve as risk-taking agents and not merely as targets (Cadiz, 2005; Tufte, 2005).

The participatory communication model provides a heuristic role for development support communication. It is a clean break from the role it played in the modernization paradigm as transmitter and disseminator of exogenous messages; instead the development support communicators in the participatory model serve as facilitators of empowered local communities, strengthening local knowledge, experiences and narratives and encouraging active agency at the grassroots in the process of social change. As Campbell and Scott put it in Chapter 8 of this volume, individuals need to engage in critical reflection and dialogue and understand the debilitating consequences of unequal social relations, which limit their health and other opportunities. Development support communicators will need to further work with these individuals and communities so that they can enter the social, economic, and political arenas in their societies as active agents of change.

Participatory Action Research

This model has been influenced by the methodology of Freire. It has emerged as a forceful methodology cum action approach, principally as a reaction to the degradation of the economic and social conditions of poor and marginalized groups. It is dedicated to resuscitating both the power of marginalized people and their knowledge. The knowledge that Participatory Action Research (PAR) attempts to generate is specific, local, non-Western, and nonpositivist. Importantly, it is used to initiate collaborative social action to empower local knowledge and wrest social power inherent in knowledge away from the privileged (Friesen, 1999).

The basic ideology of PAR is that endogenous efforts and local leaders will play the leading role in social transformations using their own praxis. It encompasses an experiential methodology. In this process, the people on their own develop methods of consciousness-raising or critical awareness of their existential situation; their knowledge is generated or resuscitated by collective and democratic means; and this is followed by reflection and critical self-evaluation leading to endogenous participatory action. This, in essence, forms the praxis (Rahman, 1991). PAR takes place in a local context, uses local material/nonmaterial inputs, and is dominated by local people and their organizations. PAR displaces the external agents of change with internal agency and successful PAR efforts will lead to the acquisition of countervailing power by the people's organizations and groups. In Latin American and Asia where land and other resources have been keenly contested and where class and ethnic divisions have been sharp, marginalized groups and their organizations have used PAR for macro-level empowerment-related movements and outcomes.

Co-Equal knowledge sharing model

The symmetric (subject to subject) relationship articulated in the participation models as opposed to the asymmetric (subject to object) communication relationship in the modernization paradigm allows for exchange of information between equals. The emphasis is on symmetric knowledge sharing rather than top-down information transmission or teaching (Ascroft *et al.*, 1987; Ascroft and Masilela, 1989). The communication model set up for this kind of interaction is interactive. It incorporates multiplicity of ideas, decentralization, deprofessionalization, deinstitutionalization, and symmetrical exchange with interchange of roles between senders and receivers. This orientation of the new communication model, contrary to the oligarchic communication models of the past, is fundamentally two-way, interactive, and participatory. The pluralistic nature of this model fits well with the *multiplicity in one world* (Servaes, 1985) idea; it also implies a more dialectic social mobilization, thus complementing the Freirian approach.

Communication on a co-equal basis is ethically preferable and practically more relevant and useful. By promising a more democratic forum for communication, it supports the *Right to Communicate*, a basic human right recognized by the UN charter affording access to communication channels to all people at all levels. It builds active agency at the grassroots besides being practically relevant. It provides access to the storehouse of information and ideas of people and communities at the grassroots. However, in communication models and practices of the modernization paradigm, the experts and policy makers have often neglected to listen, understand, and incorporate the innate wisdom and knowledge of the rural and urban poor concerning their environment. The diffusion of innovations models and research reinforced the stereotype constructed earlier by modernization theories that the people at the margins had little useful knowledge or skills to contribute to directed social change. Newer approaches such as the Positive Deviance model, which Singhal and Durá elaborate in Chapter 24 of this volume, question the assumption of the superiority of exogenous ideas and knowledge over the local. Often, local knowledge and practices have proved very useful in solving development problems. Sengupta and Elias (Chapter 23 in this volume) provide an instructive example of local knowledge and wisdom related to an understanding of a healthful life. Working among Amazonians, they interrogated the local stakeholders on their ideas of a healthy lifestyle only to discover that it was not as constrictive as the biomedical idea of being free of illness, but a holistic and grounded version of reality, which also looked at other environmental factors such as good interpersonal relationships and a life free from damaging forces such as domestic violence, disharmony with nature, discrimination, etc. People's ideas of good health are related to their perceived identities, experiences, and membership in their communities and a tapping of local knowledge enriches our understanding of a healthy life. Knowledge sharing on a co-equal basis will mobilize the large knowledge resource in local communities, be they rural or urban, which has remained underutilized. The elevation of the knowledge of local communities, then, could not only provide active agency but also serve as a countervailing power to the presumed superiority of outsiders' knowledge in directed social change processes.

Communication for empowerment

While the radical variants in participatory communication models have advocated empowerment and social action on the part of the downtrodden and marginalized individuals and communities, other development communication models especially in the modernization paradigm have ignored the systemic barriers erected by societies that permit or perpetuate inequalities among individuals and communities. Elimination of social injustice in directed social change is not possible unless the crucial problems in society are confronted, namely the lack of economic, political, and social power among individuals at the grassroots and other marginalized groups (Steeves, 2000). Individuals are impoverished or sick or often slow to adopt useful practices that better their lives not because they lack knowledge or reason, but because they do not have reasonable access to appropriate or sustainable opportunities to improve their lives. This is an issue of unequal power. The focus on unequal power dynamics has a direct consequence for development support communication. The objective of development support communication professionals should be to work with individuals and communities at the periphery of society so that they eventually enter and participate meaningfully in the political and economic activities/processes in their societies. This calls for grassroots organizing and communicative social action on the part of people at the grassroots, meaning women and others who have been marginalized in the process of social change. Greater importance will need to be directed to the use of communication in empowering citizens. The new focus in development support communication then should be to assist in the process of empowerment.

Therefore, I advocate a *social system change* model as opposed to the *social equilibrium model* of the modernization paradigm. This is not an easy task. It not only requires dealing with enclaves of power and influence that are deeply anchored in global and national structures, but also the active participation of individuals and communities in intervention efforts affecting their welfare. However, it is the right thing to do if we are truly interested and working toward the elimination of injustice in directed social change.

The concept of empowerment is heuristic in understanding the complex constraints in directed social change. The empowerment-oriented outcomes in this paradigm (i.e., increased access of all citizens to social, economic, political, cultural resources through social mobilization, social movements, and other types of communicative social action; honing of individual and group competence; leadership skills; useful life and communication skills; honing of critical awareness skills; and empowered local organizations and communities) provide a useful niche for development support communication.

While the construct of empowerment has been mentioned quite often in the social change literature, the terms, best practices, levels of analysis, and outcomes have not been thoroughly explicated. Table 30.2 attempts to articulate elements for a conceptual framework of development support communication. A reading of Table 30.2 reveals that the phenomena of interest in the empowerment communication model are vastly different from the modernization paradigm and so are the underlying beliefs about underdevelopment. The bias in the modernization paradigm was to favor exogenous ideas and innovations over the local. In the absence of participation by local people, such exogenously introduced ideas most often resulted in social engineering by the government or the elite. The differences between the two frameworks are stark when it comes to the communication models used. An examination of the communication model in the empowerment framework brings into sharp relief the differences with the model used in the modernization paradigm. Communication models in the modernization paradigm looked at communication as a process of moving a message through some channel with the hope that it would reach the receiver and have an impact. The process was usually linear, top-down, prescriptive, preachy, and quite often technical in nature. The transmission approach or the delivery of technical information (as in the modernization paradigm) will be insufficient for the task because empowerment requires more than just information delivery and diffusion of technical innovations.

Table 30.2 Development support communication in an empowerment paradigm.

Goal: Empowerment of people and communities; social justice; building capacity and Equity.

Belief: Unequal development due to lack of access to economic, political, social, and cultural resources; unequal development due to lack of power and control on the part of people and communities especially those at the margins.

Bias: Cultural proximity, ecological, diversity in standards; change directed and controlled by endogenous actors and ideas; open-ended and ongoing process of change; system blame hypothesis; group or community is paramount.

Context: Urban and rural settings; cognizant of power inequities and systemic constraints.

Level of Analysis: Individual, group or organization, community.

Role of Change Agent: Collaborator, facilitator, participant, advocate, risk taker, activist.

Communication Model: Nonlinear, participatory, convey information as well as build organizations, symmetrical relationship (subject–subject), horizontal and bottom-up flows of communication.

Type of Research: Participatory action research, quantitative and qualitative research, longitudinal studies.

Exemplars: Activate social support systems, social networks, mutual-help and self-help activities; participation of all actors; empowerment of community voices and narratives; facilitating critical awareness; facilitate community and organizational power; communication used to strengthen interpersonal relationships.

Outcomes Desired: Increased access of all citizens to social, economic, political, cultural resources; honing of individual and group competence, leadership skills, useful life and communication skills; honing of critical awareness skills; empowered local organizations and communities.

Conclusion

If the ultimate outcome in directed social change is achievement of social justice for all, the objective of media and communication processes is not just to serve as vehicles for information delivery and diffusion of technical innovations, but rather to work with individuals and communities, especially those at the peripheries of a society, so that they eventually have a voice and agency in political, economic, and ideological processes in their societies. This creates a useful niche for development support communication professionals. Campbell and Scott (Chapter 8 in this book) have alluded to this as "bridging social capital" by communication professionals acting as liaisons for local stakeholders with the powerholders. In Table 30.2, we can see that the new role of a development support communication practitioner is to serve as a collaborator, facilitator, participant, advocate, risk-taker, and even an activist.

Social change is inherently nonlinear and quite often chaotic. This understanding cautions us against putting all our faith in models of communication and evaluation that are essentially linear and deterministic. Lessons learnt from participatory approaches, and tenets of complexity science (see Lacayo, Chapter 10 this volume) applied to the strategies of directed social change will provide us with more open-ended and non-deterministic models to work with. In terms of an overarching theory, the communitarian theory emphasizes preservation of community and emancipation from oppression at all levels

(Tehranian, 1994). Liberation, feminist, environmental and some Third World social movements have made arguments consistent with communitarian theory. It appears that communitarian theory offers potential as a general framework that could ground participatory and empowerment-oriented perspectives in directed social change.

Notes

1   See WHO web site at http://www.who.int/hdp/en/index.html
2   See the chapters by Greiner (17); Campbell and Scott (8); Sengupta and Elias (23); Singhal and Dura (24); and Byrne and Vincent (14).

References

Ascroft, J. with Agunga, R., Gratama, J., and Masilela, S. (1987). Communication in support of development: Lessons from theory and practice. Paper presented at the seminar on Communication and Change, The University of Hawaii and the East-West Center, Honolulu, Hawaii.

Ascroft, J. and Masilela, S. (1989). From top-down to co-equal communication: popular participation in development decision-making. Paper presented at the seminar on *Participation: A Key Concept in Communication and Change*. University of Poona, Pune, India.

Atkinson, J. (2010). *Alternate Media and Politics of Resistance*. New York: Peter Lang.

Berger, P. L. (1974). *Pyramids of Sacrifice*. New York: Basic Books.

Cadiz, M. (2005). Communication for empowerment. In O. Hemer and T. Tufte (Eds.), *Media and Glocal Change*. Göteborg: Nordicom.

Diaz-Bordenave, J. (1980). Participation in communication systems for development. Unpublished paper. Rio de Janeiro.

Escobar, A. (1995). *Encountering Development: The Making and Unmaking of the Third World*. Princeton, NJ: Princeton University Press.

Freire, P. (1970). *Pedagogy of the Oppressed*. New York, NY: The Seabury Press.

Friesen, E. (1999). Exploring the links between structuration theory and participatory action research. In T. Jacobson and J. Servaes (Eds.), *Theoretical Approaches to Participatory Communication* (pp. 281–308). Creskill, NJ: Hampton Press.

Mefalopulos, P. (2008). *Development Communication Sourcebook*. Washington, DC: World Bank.

Melkote, S. and Krishnatray, P. (2010). Development support communication in directed social change: A reappraisal of theories and approaches. Paper presented to the 19th annual conference of the Asian Media and Information Center (AMIC), Singapore, June 20–23.

Rahman, M. A. (1991). The theoretical standpoint of PAR. In O. Fals-Borda and M. A. Rahman (Eds.), *Action and Knowledge: Breaking the Monopoly with Participatory Action-Research* (pp. 13–23). New York: Apex Press.

Sen, A. (2000). *Development as Freedom*. New York: Oxford University Press.

Servaes, J. (1985). Toward an alternative concept of communication and development. *Media Development*. Volume 32, 4/1985.

Speer, P. W. and Hughey, J. (1995). Community organizing: An ecological route to empowerment and power. *American Journal of Community Psychology, 23*(5), pp. 729–748.

Steeves, H. L. (2000). Gendered agendas: Dialogue and impasse in creating social change. In K. Wilkins (Ed.), Redeveloping communication for social change: Theory, practice, and power (pp. 7–25). Boulder, CO: Rowman and Littlefield.

Steeves, H. L. (2003). Development communication as marketing, collective resistance, and spiritual awakening: A feminist critique. In B. Mody (Ed.), *International and Development Communication* (pp. 227–244). Thousand Oaks, CA: Sage Publications.

Tehranian, M. (1994). Communication and development. In D. Crowley and D. Mitchell(Eds.), *Communication Theory Today* (pp. 274–306). Stanford, CA: Stanford University Press.

Tufte, T. (2005). Entertainment-education in development communication. In O. Hemer and T. Tufte (Eds.), *Media and Glocal Change* (pp. 159–176). Göteborg: Nordicom.

UNDP (United Nations Development Programme) (2010). Basic Facts about the Millennium Development Goals. Retrieved from http://www.undp.org/mdg/basics.shtml

WHO (World Health Organisation) (2011a). *MDG 6: Combat HIV/AIDS, Malaria and Other Diseases*. Retrieved from http://www.who.int/topics/millennium_development_goals/diseases/en/index.html

WHO (World Health Organisation) (2011b). *World Malaria report 2010*. Retrieved from http://www.who.int/malaria/world_malaria_report_2010/en/index.html

WHO (World Health Organisation) (2011c). Poverty. Retrieved from http://www.who.int/topics/poverty/en

WHO (World Health Organisation) (2011d). Social Determinants of Health. Retrieved from http://www.who.int/social_determinants/en/

WHO (World Health Organisation) (2011e). Closing the gap in a generation—how? Retrieved from http://www.who.int/social_determinants/thecommission/finalreport/closethegap_how/en/ index2.html

Wilkins, K. (2003). International development communication: Proposing a research agenda for a new era. In B. Mody (Ed.), *International and Development Communication* (pp. 245–257). Thousand Oaks, CA: Sage Publications.

Wilkins, K. (2008). Development communication. In W. Donsbach (Ed.), *The International Encyclopedia of Communication* (pp. 1229–1238). Oxford: Blackwell Publishing.

World Bank (2011). *Online Atlas of the Millennium Development Goals*. Retrieved from http://devdata.worldbank.org/atlas-mdg/

31

Conclusions
Why Communication Matters in Global Health

Silvio Waisbord and Rafael Obregon

The chapters featured in this book make individual and collective contributions to the field of global health communication. Individually, they provide updated and nuanced surveys of key issues in research, theory, and practice. Collectively, they put forward several important arguments to assess current and future directions in global health communication, which also have implications for international health and development research and practice.

The chapters demonstrate important theoretical innovations in the field in recent years. These innovations, as Tufte rightly argues in Chapter 29, have notably enriched the analytical toolkit. Several contributors to the book illustrate this process. Growing attention to issues that determine the nature of public health programs such as human rights and equity (Airhihenbuwa and Dutta; Sengupta and Elias), and community participation (Campbell and Scott; Manyozo); to emerging health areas that include risk communication (Chitnis), to new theoretical perspectives such as complexity science (Lacayo), social norms (Pulerwitz, Barker, and Verna), and social capital (Usdin and Christofides) reflects the expansion of theoretical horizons. These are welcome additions. They foreground critical dimensions of communication such as social resources, participation, interactivity, and identity. They direct our attention to the social and cultural embeddedness, as well as the political dimensions, of health communication. Communication is unthinkable outside specific sociocultural and political contexts. This should not be simplistically seen along the lines of superficial interpretations about local cultures and social mores affecting communication. Instead, they suggest that communication is constitutive of participation and identity-making processes (Martin-Barbero, 1993) as they relate to health. Various experiences in health communication reveal how groups and communities define and seek rights, empowerment, and recognition. Because these issues refer to social groups and communities, rather than to individuals, they push

The Handbook of Global Health Communication, First Edition. Edited by Rafael Obregon and Silvio Waisbord.
© 2012 John Wiley & Sons, Inc. Published 2012 by John Wiley & Sons, Inc.

the field in new directions (as discussed by Melkote). They renew traditional health communication concerns by focusing on analytical dimensions beyond psychological and informational processes, which have dominated the field for many years.

Also, several contributors subscribe to notions that emphasize social dimensions of communication such as trust, participation, and institutions. This invites us to rethink conventional communication concepts. The media are not simply platforms for information transmission; instead, as Manyozo discusses, they are community resources that are mobilized to problematize and transform health conditions. Likewise, people's attitudes and beliefs, such as trust and collective efficacy, are core components of the local social capital that can be tapped for positive transformations, as Ferrara, Roberto, and Witte suggest. Community knowledge should be broadly understood in terms of abilities and capacities that local populations have to assess problems and identify solutions through various participatory techniques, an argument convincingly made by Greiner. This emphasis also reflects greater or renewed interest in public health communication processes that take an asset-based communication perspective, in contrast to a needs-based approach.

The broadening of theoretical and methodological approaches doesn't mean that the field of global health communication is as comprehensive as it could be. Some issues remain notoriously underexplored. Among other gaps, the paucity of studies about the linkages between communication, mobilization, and health policy in international settings is remarkable. This gap is particularly noticeable considering that, despite the growing acceptance of socio-ecological approaches, we have limited knowledge about how communication strategies affect policies and structural/systemic factors, and, in turn, promote health changes. One can scarcely doubt that policies affect health conditions and opportunities through multiple and complex mechanisms. The quality of public health programs, government investments, taxation, systems management, treatment policies, legislation, and technical recommendations are just some critical policy issues with direct impact on health conditions and opportunities. Changes in policies may encourage or deter populations from health practices, reinforce health norms, encourage citizen participation in healthcare, and so on. Yet we need to know more, for example, about how mobilized publics advocate and interact with political elites, how policies are communicated, or how communication and social participation shape policy options. Investigating these issues is particularly relevant given growing mobilization around the world around a range of health issues. Citizens have mobilized in various ways to reduce social disparities and demand changes to insurance programs, service quality, access to treatments and drugs, research funding, and other critical aspects of health policies. Communication is at the center of public actions to redress power imbalances in decisions typically controlled by governments, health providers, and pharmaceutical companies. Although these issues have been studied by sociologists (Brown *et al.*, 2011; Hankin and Wright, 2010) and political scientists (Kaufman, 2004), attention from communication scholars remains limited. Communication analysis is crucial to understand how issues become public issues and policy priorities in the media, everyday conversation, and other spaces. Furthermore, comparative research is needed to assess similarities and differences in the linkages between communication and health policy issues across national and global contexts.

The analytical renovation in health communication should not be interpreted as the displacement of old approaches and interests in favor of new ones. Intellectual foci and disciplinary approaches have been broadened rather than completely shifted or narrowed. Global health communication is analytically rich and inclusive, a reflection of the diversity of disciplinary backgrounds and theoretical questions. As a "transdisciplinary science" (Kreps and Maibach, 2008), the field is a meeting point for academics and practitioners interested in various questions about health and communication. It resembles the architecture of old, well-preserved cities in which different styles are layered on top of each other.

Certainly, there are some common themes that attract attention from various theoretical and disciplinary traditions. Entertainment-education, as discussed by Brown, by Torres, and by Sengupta and Elias, is one of the best examples of analytical convergence around a specific set of questions and practical models. For several decades it has been a fertile ground for interdisciplinary dialogue and programmatic experiments. Increased sophistication about the theoretical premises and questions about edutainment, as well as implementation of nuanced interventions, are the result of the cross-pollination of theories and approaches. The coexistence of arguments about the value of edutainment to promote psychological changes that affect health behaviors as well as encourage community dialogue attests to its enduring appeal and conceptual flexibility. Edutainment is a relatively simple yet tremendously powerful and attractive idea to think about central issues in communication. It brings up questions about identification, para-social communication and interaction, message effectiveness, attitude change, public conversation, norming and shaming, and many other issues. Edutainment is also the subject of renewed thinking and approaches. Lacayo introduces the use of complexity science to understand how communication facilitates change on various health issues, through an edutainment-driven experience. Even though it is not the focus of their chapter, Sengupta and Elias discuss how edutainment serves as the central vehicle for a process that also addresses social determinants (e.g., education, income) that impact the health and well-being of women and their families in the Peruvian Amazon.

Another area of growing consensus is the need to adopt a broad, ecological perspective on health communication, as discussed in several chapters (Ahmed; Pulerwitz, Barker, and Verma; and Storey and Figueroa). This move, which points to greater convergence between public health and communication practice, represents the recognition not only that health is affected by multiple factors, but also that communication is present at several levels. This perspective is a valuable, integrated analytical model that seeks to bridge traditional divides, even though it doesn't meet conventional definitions of theory. It doesn't predict or explain; rather, it offers a roadmap to assess conditions that determine health outcomes and practices. It doesn't carry ostensible normative implications about desirable changes or communication approaches. Its usefulness lies in stimulating problem-based analysis and determining how communication contributes to maintaining health problems or, conversely, how it may successfully address various obstacles. These approaches represent a significant shift from the individual behavior focus that has dominated the field for the past decades. However, the new challenge is how to enrich socio-ecological approaches with theoretical inputs that provide greater guidance for program design and evaluation, and better understanding of individual and collective processes that determine health behavior.

Although edutainment and the socio-ecological model serve as meeting points for scholars and practitioners informed by different theoretical frameworks, the field remains fragmented in research and programmatic foci. There are still few questions to define a unified research agenda or serve as common guiding posts for scholars concerned with different questions. Whereas some scholars are interested in examining effective messages to promote new behaviors (Ferrara, Roberto, and Witte), others are primarily concerned with discussing integrated communication strategies (Hess, Meekers, and Storey). While some discuss the nature and broad impact of health news (Arroyave; Pirio), others are particularly interested in the strengths of social marketing and branding to promote specific behaviors (Evans and coauthors). In the spirit of inclusiveness and intellectual curiosity, this persistent diversity should not be seen negatively. Doubtless, it has contributed to a cacophony of concepts and theories that characterizes health communication and that, occasionally, engenders Babel-like situations. As frustrating at this may be, the superposition or, at times, parallel existence of theories and models are congenital to a field that draws on a broad range of disciplines. If health is a contested term, as demonstrated by extensive discussion about the impossibilities of defining health outside specific contexts and situations, communication is unquestionably a multivocal concept, perpetually subjected to multiple and contrasting definitions. Communication is associated with information and dialogue, participation and messaging, platforms and human contact, strategy and activism. How communication is understood is inevitably shaped by disciplinary loyalties and normative preferences. Resolving this ambiguity, rooted in the origins of rhetoric and democratic theory in Western thought, seems an endless task. Finding ways to bridge differences or identifying common questions seems more productive that insisting on settling definitional matters once and forever.

Another important issue implicitly raised by the chapters is the global dimensions of health communication. Put it simply, what does "global health communication" mean? Several plausible definitions can be suggested. Global health communication refers to multiple issues, processes, and perspectives. It includes globalized health and disease, transnational normative values, communication across boundaries and differences, and analyzing and producing arguments that are relevant beyond local settings. The handbook doesn't advance one single definition of "global health communication." Rather, our intention was to problematize this issue, and call attention to the many ways in which scholars typically approach the relation between health and communication in a global context.

One interpretation is that global health communication refers to how the world acts upon global challenges – that is, planetary health problems that affect everybody in the world. The health consequences of environmental degradation or infectious epidemics, like the case of avian influenza discussed by Chitnis, are examples of global health risks that disregard political, economic, and cultural borders. They are real and potential challenges that threaten millions of people around the world. Certainly, these are not new developments as the history of scourges such as smallpox, plague, and human influenza painfully demonstrates. Conquest, war, and commerce historically globalized disease and were responsible for decimating entire populations. The global intensification of human contacts in the past decades, however, has raised the specter of health threats that can quickly affect large populations around the world.

Another interpretation suggests that "global health communication" refers to how certain health issues are defined. Although they do not directly affect human civilization as a whole, and are rather concentrated in certain populations and territories, they are "global" because they affect fellow human beings. The social and geographical distribution of health and disease is well documented. Not everybody is likely to be affected by the same challenges. Socioeconomic and geographical factors are strong predictors of morbidity and mortality. Some problems, such as tuberculosis and maternal mortality, disproportionately affect poor and socially excluded people, particularly in the global South. The majority of annual cases of malaria and HIV are concentrated in sub-Saharan Africa. Yet, despite geographical and social concentration, these challenges are construed as global problems because they affect the quality of life of other human beings. Underlying this conception is the notion that global health implies the adoption of certain values, such as universal human consciousness, solidarity, and compassion that transcend national divisions. Global is about the definition of health problems as matters of collective interest rather than the particular distribution of disease or the conditions of health services.

One could also think about "global health communication" in terms of an analytical perspective – a way of asking questions and studying the intersection between health and communication. It is about addressing theoretical and empirical questions from multiple locations and experiences. Several chapters demonstrate such a "thinking globally" approach. Evaluation approaches analyzed by Bertrand, Babalola, and Skinner, and participatory interventions discussed by Greiner, are solidly informed by global experiences. Likewise, the study of health and interpersonal communication (Ahmed), the application of information technologies to health (Ratzan and Suggs; de Tolly and Benjamin), and the usefulness of concepts such "Positive Deviance" (Singhal and Dura) are grounded in broad, global perspectives.

Lastly, "global health communication" can also be defined by the types of issues that determine people's health and how communication contributes to addressing those factors. Just as avian influenza, tuberculosis, and other health issues have taken on a global dimension, a number of social, political, and cultural issues that determine individual and collective health also have become increasingly global. Issues such as human rights, equity, and community empowerment and engagement, to mention a few, are central to improving people's health whether in developing countries as illustrated in several chapters (Airhihenbuwa and Dutta; Sengupta and Elias; Campbell and Scott; Usdin and Christofides), or in more developed contexts as discussed by Torres. However, it is worth asking to what extent global health communication programs truly attempt to tackle these issues in an unquestionable fashion, or to what extent global health communication programs do not challenge or address existing inequities and disparities.

A global, comparative approach helps to overcome conventional divides in health communication in terms of the location of reflection and practice. Historically, the majority of theories, concepts, and intervention models in the field were developed in the West, particularly in the United States. Their application in non-Western contexts, expectedly, generated much controversy, as Storey and Figueroa point out. Critics believed not only that they were unfitting to explain health communication in largely different contexts, but also that they constituted acts of intellectual imperialism and academic patronizing. They argued that communication models embedded in psychological theories and notions about rationality and decision making grounded in Western social science did not apply to widely different cultural contexts. Non-Western models that reflected local conditions were better suited to study the reality of health communication.

Several authors (Airhihenbuwa and Dutta; Singhal and Dura; Tufte) are particularly sensitive to this debate and offer variegated ideas as to how to have a broad, culturally specific approach, a point convincingly argued since, whether interpersonal communication, as Ahmed argues, or mediated communication, as Manyozo, and Torres demonstrate in their chapters, health communication is firmly embedded in specific contexts. Recognition of the intertwined relations between culture and communication is fundamental to understanding the way people develop and maintain conceptions about health.

Context is not just a matter of acknowledging and addressing cultural differences. It also refers to social inequalities in health disparities. The challenges that have been historically prominent in the agenda of international health communication overwhelmingly affect poor people – populations marginalized by dominant power structures on the basis of class, gender, ethnicity, religion, and age. Health disparities and disempowerment are intertwined. Power articulates not only health conditions but also communication. Communication about health, as Campbell and Scott demonstrated in the case of community mobilization, and as Arroyave and Pirio argue in their chapters about health news, is inseparable from power structures and dynamics. Power is manifested in how health is constructed, represented, and publicly discussed. This is why addressing socioeconomic differences is critical to improve health opportunities. This demands communication approaches that tackle deep-seated inequalities in society at large or, as Sengupta and Elias show, in the micro-spaces of everyday life in the family and neighborhoods. Communication needs to be understood as collective efforts to redress power relations that affect health opportunities and conditions. Tufte's discussion of health citizenship nicely captures this political dimension of communication.

Other chapters tacitly address the issue of whether models grounded in Western and non-Western premises are relevant across settings by warning us to avoid the limitations of orthodoxies and, instead, encouraging researchers to be theoretically and analytically open-minded. Critical scholarship must interrogate the premises underpinning theories and explanations. The merits of models and arguments should not be simply assessed on the basis of their cultural provenance. Nor should we essentialize communication by simply assuming, rather than examining, cultural differences. Arguments need to be sensitive to particular settings, but they should aim to provide explanations that are relevant across contexts. What deters people from healthy behaviors may be different, yet what encourages them to overcome obstacles may be similar – care for family members, spiritual beliefs, social trust. Communities may participate in different ways around health, given local traditions, resources, and motivations, yet social mobilization may similarly contribute to strengthening access to health services. Analytical and methodological frameworks as well as specific interventions and strategies need to be probed in different contexts to determine their validity.

This is particularly important given the paucity of cross-national, cross-issue reflection in international health communication. The field has not escaped, unfortunately, the broad compartmentalization of global health in distinct and separated programs, a trend exacerbated by the issue-driven agendas of powerful donors. The earmarking of funds for particular programs has reinforced the much-discussed trends towards "silo-ization" of international health. Not surprisingly, this tendency has driven communication research and practice to focus on specific health issues rather than health communication more broadly. Certainly, the specialization of communication around specific health issues produced a wealth of valuable findings that laid the foundations of the field in the past decades, a legacy that Rimon and Sood carefully reconstruct in their chapter based on their experience with the US Agency for International Development, one of the major donors in the field. Recent studies about the communicative dimensions of child immunization and tuberculosis confirm that research focused on the unique epidemiological and social aspects of particular health challenges and diseases provides valuable insights into broad analytical themes. Yet it is important to think beyond specific diseases and problems by foregrounding broad communication questions. When does risk perception motivate people to action? When are social networks effective in promoting healthy practices or encouraging citizen participation? How does communication contribute to redressing power imbalances in couples, households, and communities that affect health? Similarly, issue-driven programs, usually well-funded, result in communication practice that subscribes to key health communication planning, implementation, and evaluation principles, and produces useful tools and lessons learned. Yet translating those principles, tools, and lessons to other health areas is not always an easy task. This challenge is clearly illustrated by the limitations of translating the successes of communication in vaccinations programs to other, arguably more complex issues such as HIV/AIDS and tuberculosis.

The globalization of health demands globalized reflection about communication – connecting ideas and probing conclusions across communities and health issues. Advocacy or social mobilization around specific issues in one community may offer valuable lessons for other communities. Popular soap operas that address family planning issues or youth sexual and reproductive health, as analyzed by Vega and Mendivil, offer ideas for planning communication and engaging communities with other health issues. Likewise, edutainment ideas implemented in programs with Latinos in the United States, discussed by Torres, share many points in common with the global experiences analyzed by Brown. Also, de Tolly and Benjamin show that innovative uses of mobile phones to support HIV/AIDS care and treatment could be applicable to other health programs. Pirio shows how insights from effective health news coverage, which utilize a diversity of sources and frames, can be incorporated across issues, while Arroyave warns how a number of social and political factors related to journalistic practice influence news framing of health issues.

Adopting a global approach to health communication that acknowledges the different definitions we have put forward earlier is needed given the globalization of health advocacy and participation. From child health to reproductive health, myriad health challenges have become matters of global attention due to combined actions and interests of international donors, technical agencies, national governments, and grassroots associations. Obviously, this is not entirely new. There is a long history of international action and communication around health issues. The recent multiplication of international organizations, increased levels of international aid, the ease of global connectivity, and transnational health social movements, have helped to consolidate global actions. International agencies and funders exert significant influence on health advocacy, policy agreements, and technical recommendations. Globally, nongovernment organizations, interest groups, faith-based associations, and activist groups provide health services, influence policy, and mobilize communities. Having a globally mobilized constituency is fundamental for any health issue to gain world visibility in international forums and the media, receive funding, and gain priority status. Regrettably, health problems are likely to remain largely unnoticed if they lack institutional entrepreneurs constantly pushing for global attention and investments. Aside from these dynamics, it is necessary to recognize the significance of communicative processes in the definition of health priorities in international politics and development aid as well as the formation of "strategic alliances," like the examples discussed by Campbell and Scott. The complexity of mobilized alliances, particularly at the local and national levels, is discussed in depth by Usdin and Christofides in the case of the Alliance for Children's Entitlement to Social Security in South Africa.

Thinking globally and broadly about health communication, then, is congruent with the affirmation of global actions and the multiple social dimensions of health and disease across the world. The chapters provide conceptual, theoretical and practical arguments.

Taking this approach to health communication research and practice is desirable not only to continue to produce quality studies and refine theories and methods. It is also needed given the institutional conditions of the field in international aid. The position and legitimacy of communication in global health programs and agencies are critical issues that, unfortunately, have not received sufficient attention. Communication scholars should consider perceptions and expectations about communication inside donors and technical organizations, as Fox argues. This is not simply a matter of intellectual curiosity, but rather a matter that profoundly affects the workings of communication programs and research agendas (Waisbord, 2008). Communication is hardly a priority, and is often confused with information and materials production and dissemination, or often it is assumed that it does not require specific competencies and professional training. Thanks to intensive internal advocacy, perceptions have changed – yet much still needs to be done to correct narrow views about communication and, as Rimon and Sood argue, institutionalize the contribution of communication to health and development. The fact that health communication is an interdisciplinary field naturally creates such challenges. However, that also means that a proactive approach should be taken to further strengthen and institutionalize this field.

Such efforts need to be cognizant that aid agencies have particular understandings about what constitutes "legitimate knowledge," including quality of evidence and effectiveness assessments. These perceptions are not inconsequential, obviously, for they affect the mission of communication (what it is expected to do) as well as staffing and funding decisions. These issues should be seriously considered for "rethinking," as Fox puts it, health communication in the particular contexts of practice. It's not just about what the academic community determines is sound, innovative knowledge, but also about institutional expectations grounded in the professional cultures of public health and medical professions. Rimon and Sood rightly insist that, for communication scholars and specialists, it is critical to understand such expectations and consider the priorities of aid programs and public health experts.

On this point, three chapters (Bertrand, Babalola and Skinner; Hess, Meekers and Storey; Byrne and Vincent) offer valuable insights. They present persuasive evidence about the impact of communication as well as state-of-the-art surveys of quantitative and qualitative methodologies used to produce rigorous evaluations. The chapters document impact across health issues, countries, and communication goals. Furthermore, they provide evidence about smart uses of communication whether to affect knowledge and attitudes or sustain local participation. The evidence presented provides examples of the kind of data, including triangulation approaches, needed to discuss the contributions of communication to the specific technical goals of various programs and aid agencies.

A related matter is the question of appropriate capacity for studying and implementing health communication, as we discuss in Chapter 27. In order to further develop the theory and practice of global health communication, vigorous and sustained efforts to build capacity are needed worldwide. The creation of a critical mass of health communication professionals and qualified practitioners is essential to strengthen the field. Obregon and Waisbord, with a focus on university-based efforts that draw on a competency-based (knowledge, skills, and values) approach, and Rimon and Sood, with a focus on in-service training, provide insights into the critical importance of advancing capacity development in health communication.

Public health programs tend to privilege technical solutions and evidence-based interventions. However, social reality is "messy," as Lacayo points out in her chapter. There are no easy solutions to issues that are determined by socially and culturally driven factors. Rather, understanding the complexity of those issues is critical to facilitating change processes driven by communities themselves. Lacayo's chapter on complexity science and the experience of Puntos de Encuentro in Nicaragua introduces a provocative approach that highlights the need to acknowledge the complexity and "messiness" of social reality as an entry point. This is not necessarily what donors and governments want to hear, but it is certainly a reality that scholars and practitioners need to grapple with. This handbook offers a diverse set of concepts, approaches, and strategies that can help in designing and evaluating global health communication efforts in a way that acknowledges such complexity.

Undoubtedly, global health communication is an evolving concept. Drawing on the many contributions to this handbook, we have attempted to provide some conceptual clarity, and identify key issues that characterize global health communication. However, given the rapidly changing world we live in, we acknowledge the need to continually engage in analysis and research that will allow us to assess short-term transformations and long-term trends in the field. Public health issues are amongst the most challenging for the international development and health community, as rightly discussed by Melkote through his emphasis on issues of social justice and empowerment. Communication will continue to play a central role in how we effectively think about and address those challenges.

References

Brown, P., Morello-Frosch, R., Zavestoski, S. _et al._ (2011). Health social movements: advancing traditional medical sociology concepts. In B. A. Pescosolido, J. K. Martin, J. D. McLeod and A. Rogers (Eds.), _Handbook of the Sociology of Health, Illness, and Healing: A Blueprint for the 21st Century_, Part 2 (pp. 117–137). New York: Springer.

Hankin, J. R. and Wright, E. R. (2010). Reflections on fifty year of medical sociology. *Journal of Health and Social Behavior, 51*, S10–S14.

Kaufman, R. (Ed.) (2004). *Crucial Needs, Weak Incentives: The Politics of Health and Education Reform in Latin America*. Baltimore, MD: Johns Hopkins University Press.

Kreps, G. L. and Maibach, E. W. (2008). Transdisciplinary science: The nexus between communication and public health. *Journal of Communication 588*, 723–748.

Martin-Barbero, J. (1993). *From Media to Mediations*. London: Sage.

Waisbord, S. (2008). The institutional challenges of participatory communication in international aid. *Social Identities 14*, 505–522.

Index

Accra Agenda for Action 559, 561
advocacy 89, 98, 413, 634
advocacy journalism 431
African Network for Strategic Communication
    in Health and Development
    (AfriComNet) 568
agenda-setting 195, 428
agency 632–637
AIDS *see* HIV/AIDS
alcohol abuse 121, 129, 130
    and entertainment-education 130–132
    and news 201
Alliance for Children's Entitlement to Social
    Security (ACESS) 539
    background 540–542
    campaigns 543–544
    and governance and social mobilization 552
Alma Alta Declaration 617
Arab Women Speak Out (AWSO) 84, 392–393
Australia 104, 258
avian influenza 53, 198, 402, 408–423

Bangladesh 130, 164–165, 410, 590, 596
behavior change 14, 20, 22, 107, 418, 423, 426
    community-based 474
Bienvenida Salud (Welcome to Health) 488
body 455
    perceptions 455–457

brand 330
    brand execution 331
    brand personality 331
    brand positioning 331
    research methods 332
brand equity 331–346
    research 331, 334, 338, 346
branding 330, 331
Brazil 63, 123, 469–486
breast cancer 198, 205
    and entertainment-education 132–133,
        276–278
Burkina Faso 419

C-Change project 73, 571–575
Cambodia 422
campaigns 99–100, 102
    cost-effectiveness 105
    effects 115
Canada 206
capacity 46, 63–64
capacity building and strengthening 63,
    560–578, 594–595
    competencies 559, 578
    definitions, approaches, issues 561
    in health promotion and communication 563
    media 427–428
causality 112–114

The Handbook of Global Health Communication, First Edition. Edited by Rafael Obregon
and Silvio Waisbord.
© 2012 John Wiley & Sons, Inc. Published 2012 by John Wiley & Sons, Inc.

Change Project 567
child activism 543
child health 17
children's rights 540
China 260
chronic disease 255
co-equal knowledge sharing model 636
collective action 421
collective efficacy 282–283
Colombia 201, 444–463
commercial sex workers 337
Commission on Social Determinants of Health (CSDH) 633
communication
  for avian influenza control 417–419
  definition 11
  democratization 234
  for empowerment 637
  for healthy living 375–403
  as iterative process 70
  for participatory development model 74
  for social change 247–248, 446
  as "transdisciplinary science" 644
community AIDS competence 301
community-based total sanitation 82
community competence 89
community development associations 84
community dialogue 74, 75, 180, 186
community health 74, 236
  and development 236–238
community health package 391–392
community involvement 525
community knowledge 643
community media 234–235
  and health communication 235–236
community mobilization 177, 391, 553
community participation 20, 22, 43
  see also health, activism 48, 187
complex adaptive systems 220, 298
complexity 216, 219, 297
condoms 336
  Madagascar Protector Plus (brand) 336–337
  use 477
Convention on the Rights of the Child 540
cost analysis 483–485
cost-effectiveness 105–106
cost-study 484
Costa Rica 123

courting 457–458
critical studies 20–21, 24, 44
cultural competency 36
cultural proximity 122
culture 11, 40, 46
culture-centered communication 35–36, 41, 47, 152, 534

development 627
development communication 10, 11–12
development journalism 238–241
development support communication 625–639
diabetes 256
dialogue 70–72, 75, 79, 179–180, 289–291
diarrheal diseases 82
diffusion of innovations 13, 17, 72
digital access 253
digital agenda 263
disabilities 135
deconstruction 47
Dominican Republic 106
donors 53, 56, 61

ecological model of communication for medical encounters 147
ecological model of human development 145
ecological model for health promotion 146
ecology 145
effectiveness 99
effects 106–107
efficacy 99, 282–284
  social side 282
Egypt 73, 83–85, 106, 125, 130, 374, 422
  building environment 385
  community health package 391–492
  community health program 390
  family planning 379
  fertility rate 375
  interpersonal communication and counseling 385
  maternal and child health 378
  national media campaign 385
e-health 165–166, 251–259
  impact 254
  and Maternal and Newborn m-health Initiative 268
  and mobile communication 259–262

empowerment 178, 235, 638
enabling environment 385, 437
England 104
entertainment-education 23–25, 121, 217,
        276, 387, 444, 446, 523, 586
    and identification 531
    second generation 444, 463
environmental health 133–134
ethnographic action research 611
ethnographic go-along 357–360, 369–370
European Commission (EC) 263
evaluation 98–117
    definition of Impact 98
    measuring processes 227
    of soap opera for Latinos 531–533
    of social change 293–295
    study designs 107–108
experimental design 111
experts
    criticism 490, 520
Extended Parallel Process Model
        (EPPM) 274

family communication and health 158
family planning 11, 17, 101–102, 114,
        375, 379, 395
    and entertainment-education 124–126
family relations 499–500
fear appeals 274–285, 412
    message design 283–384
female genital cutting 355
Femina HIP 616
formative research 80, 332, 338, 525
framing 197, 201
    effects 200–202
Freire, Paulo 179, 447, 635

Galway Consensus Report 565
Gates Foundation 1
gender 186, 453
Gender-Equitable Men (GEM) scale 475
    examples of GEM scale items 476
gender norms 215, 470–486
    and cost analysis 484
    and operations research 477
    roles 459–460
Ghana 109, 110, 265
global health 643–650

global health communication 645, 650
    definition 645
globalization 617
    challenges 618
government of India 1
grassroots participation 635
grassroots social activism 187–189
group education intervention 473–474

Hazipur eHealth Center 165–166
health
    activism 48, 187
    Amazonian conception 495–496
    citizenship 617
    communicators 56
    competence 77, 376–377, 381
    disparities 647
    integration across issues 381
    literacy 256
    programs 56
    promotion 45, 565
Healthcom project 73
Health communication
    achievements 608–612
    and campaign effects 100
    challenges 612–613
    definitions 148, 179
    as a field 608
    funding 65
    indicators and measurements 56
    as industry 59
    and institutionalization 582–605
    and international aid 58
    for malaria 62
    names 64, 97
    and participatory approaches 349
    rethinking of 52–68
Health Communication Partnership
        (HCP) 73, 77, 375
Healthy People 2010 253
Healthy People 2020 263
hearing safety 136
heterophily 534
hierarchy of influences model 195–197
HIV/AIDS 17, 20, 37, 41–42, 48, 54,
        63, 76, 85, 102, 105, 107, 114, 116,
        161–162, 163–164, 199–200, 281–284,
        288–304, 320–323, 381, 426–441, 491

and entertainment-education 126–129, 223
and interpersonal communication 158–159
maternal to child transmission 430
media's role 427
social and structural factors 291
social dimensions 291
social drivers of 289
homophily 534
Honduras 73
Hora comunitaria, La (radio program) 533
Human Development Index (HDI) 102
human rights 38–39, 189–190

ideation 17, 73
identification 127
impact 97–117, 227, 389
definitions 98–99
at national level 399–401
of training 439
India 106, 130, 132, 150, 161–162, 183–190,
    199, 240, 469–486
indigenous knowledge communication
    systems 241–243
individualism in health communication 18,
    40, 72
individual competence 90
individual rationality 19–20
Indonesia 82, 123, 422
information technologies 68
institutionalization 583
    measures by subsystems 587
Integrated Management of Childhood Illness
    (IMCI) 150
integrated marketing communication 384–385
integrated model for health
    communication 412
interactive theory of gender socialization 472
interactivity 326
international advocacy 189–190
international aid organizations 56
    see also donors
interpellation 447–448
interpersonal communication 144–168,
    389, 586
    and culture 159
    ecological perspective 145
    GATHER approach 586–587
    theories 150–152

Jamaica 121, 122
journalism
    and enabling environment 437–438
    and unidirectional messaging 435
journalistic culture
    transformation of 438–441
journalists 426–441
    role in HIV response 431

Kenya 125, 128, 160, 331
Know Yourself adolescent reproductive health
    communication program 164
knowledge–behavior gap 19
Korea 427

Latinos 523–524
life mapping 361–365, 369–370
Lippman, Walter 432
local knowledge systems 489
logical frameworks 294
lung cancer 198

Mabrouk! Initiative 374–408
Madagascar 331–346
malaria 53, 54, 57, 60, 61
Malawi 240
male involvement 518
malnutrition 509
marketing perspective 379
masculine ideologies 476
mass media and cultural change 85
Mass Media and Health Practices (MMHP)
    project 73
maternal health 53, 324, 395
maternal mortality 183–190
measurement 79, 80–81
measuring process 227
media 194–210
    advocacy 545–546
    coverage 435
    effects 10, 15, 18, 195
    and mediatization 618
messaging 435
Mexico 63, 123, 124
M-health 259–262, 311–327
Minga Perú 491–494
Millennium Development Goals 2, 53, 183,
    261, 265, 268, 625

minority audiences 527
modernization 11
monitoring and evaluation 56, 80, 97–118,
    292–297
  challenges 65, 229
  innovative approaches 296
  validity 113
most significant change 301, 448
Mozambique 426
multiple level analysis 598

narrative approach 115, 151
neoliberalism and health 38
Nepal 73, 135
Netherlands 121, 136
network and social networks analysis 299
network mapping 361–365, 369–370
New World Information and Communication
    Order (NWICO) 620
news
  framing 200–203
  production 195
  routines 203–204
  sources 433–434
  values 204–206
Nicaragua 215–230
Nigeria 60–61, 125, 163, 419
non-communicable diseases 2
nonexperimental designs 108
Norway 104, 260

obesity 46, 54, 65, 202
Operation Lighthouse (OPL) 161–164
operations research 470
oral rehydration therapy 54, 59, 65, 66
  and entertainment-education 129–130
Ottawa Charter 617
outcome analysis 415
outcome expectations 531
outcome mapping 300, 611

Pakistan 150, 512–517
Pan American Health Organization
    (PAHO) 566
Paris Declaration on Aid Effectiveness 559, 604
participatory approach 489
participatory action research 236, 244–247,
    349, 417, 636

participatory communication 10, 318,
    488–504
participatory research 80
participatory sketching 352–357, 369–370
patient-centered communication 156–157
patient-provider communication 154–156
peer facilitators 493
peer-to-peer communication 185–187
PEN-3 model 46
perceived efficacy 275
persuasion 12, 71, 72
  critique 178
Peru 64, 82–83, 106, 124, 488–504, 567
Philippines 73, 106, 239, 260
physician–patient communication 151, 153–154
population communication services 73, 584
Population Council 473
polio 1, 60–61
  communication 60–62
popular theater 415
Population Services International (PSI) 330–346
positive deviance 508–520
  approach 508, 519
  behaviors related to maternal and newborn
      care 516
  communication practices 519
  inquiry 515
  and male involvement 518
  and newborn mortality 512
poverty 177, 627
power 20, 35, 177, 181, 235
power-knowledge 181
primary health care 236
Program for Appropriate Technology
    in Health (PATH) 473
Program H 472
Promundo 473
P-Process 376, 595
propensity score matching 110
promotoras (peer facilitators) 495
protest action 546–548
Puntos de Encuentro 24, 215

qualitative comparative analysis 299
quasi-experimental designs 108

radio 427, 437, 522–536
randomized control trials 111

reflexivity 44
reproductive choices 498
reproductive health 73, 498
  see also family planning
right to communicate 637
risk communication 408–423
  approaches and theories 411
  community-based 414
  definition 411
  hazard and outrage 411
  integrated campaigns 412, 419
  lessons learned 418
  outcome analysis 415
  role of interpersonal communication and
    dialogue 422–423
  successes and challenges 416–418
risk perception 280, 420
  analysis framework 280
risk society 615
Rockefeller Foundation 567
Rotary International 1
Rwanda 260, 265

Schramm, Wilbur 58
Save the Children 513
Saving Newborn Lives (SNL) Initiative 513
self-confidence 496
self-efficacy 421
Sesame Street 129
severe acute respiratory syndrome (SARS) 410
sexual health 319–320, 445, 540
sexual imaginaries 450
sexuality
  dialogue about 450–452
  perceptions 453–455
sexually transmitted infections 126
  reduction of 126–127
Sexto Sentido (television series) 217
smoking cessation 54, 103–104, 201, 383
soap operas for Latinos in the United
    States 522–536
social and behavior change
    communication 571
  and competency-based curriculum 574
social change 26, 216, 218, 288, 318, 629
  communication 290
  and complex causality 293
  and dialogue 289–302

and income generation 502–504
  indicators 301
  scope of evaluation 295–296
  see also communication, for social change
social ecological model 22, 74, 81, 87, 97,
    145–148
social identity 180
social imaginaries 448
social justice 628–629
social learning 530
social marketing 14–15, 330–346
  evaluation 109–110
social media 257–259
social mobilization 292, 540–554, 634
  and alliances 553–554
social movements 292, 634
social networks 22, 299
social norm(s) 63, 376
social psychology 14, 22, 72
social security 550–554
social support 160–161
social system change model 638
social system equilibrium model 638
solidarity 45
Sonamoni (film) 130
Soul City 24, 128, 137, 540, 569
South Africa 63, 76, 85–86, 103, 104,
    128, 136, 159, 246, 261, 313, 317,
    321, 539–554, 614
stigma 65, 427
storytelling 526
story formats 436–437
strategic alliances 182
strategic design 382
substance abuse 54
Sudan 352
systems action research 298
systems thinking 296–297
Swedish International Development
    Cooperation Agency (SIDA) 136
Switzerland 258

Takalani (television series) 129
Tanzania 73, 126–127, 136, 260
technology 59, 60, 68
telemedicine 161, 167
  see also e-health
television 217–218, 386–387

Thailand 245, 324
The Lancet 54, 609
theater for development 244
theories of change 294
theory 9–27, 70–71
    behavioral and information
        processing 19
    communication 377
    complexity 297
    ecological model 472
    extended parallel process model 275
    participatory development 489
    post-colonial feminist 489
    role of 376
    of rupture 614
tobacco 201
transformative communication 179
Tsha Tsha (television series) 85–86
tuberculosis 20, 53
Twitter 80

Uganda 103, 320
UNAIDS 208, 291
UNESCO 58, 234
UNICEF 229, 414, 553
United Kingdom 260
United Kingdom Department for
    International Development (DFID)
    446, 574
United Nations 1, 408
United Nations Development Program
    245, 492

United Nations Environment
    Program 241
United Nations Population Fund 445
United Nations Roundtable on
    Communication for Development 617
United States 13, 104, 105, 130–132, 160,
    206, 260, 262, 319, 357, 438
United States Agency for International
    Development (USAID) 73, 77, 82, 83,
    101, 375, 567
United States Centers for Disease Control and
    Prevention 258, 412, 574
United States Government 53

vaccines 56
Viet Nam 508–512
voice 178, 612, 613

water 53
Web 2.0 257
women's empowerment 392
women's rights 492
World Health Organisation (WHO) 236–237,
    258, 450, 471, 628
World Wide Web 252–253

young people 444–464
    and courting 457
    and dialogue 450
    and edutainment 446
    and gender 453
    and sexuality 444

Printed and bound by CPI Group (UK) Ltd, Croydon, CR0 4YY

27/10/2024

14580249-0004